Joachim W. Dudenhausen

Practical Obstetrics

Joachim W. Dudenhausen

Practical Obstetrics

Founded by W. Pschyrembel
Assisted by M. Obladen
Translated by S. E. Travis

DE GRUYTER

Author
Dr. Joachim W. Dudenhausen, FRCOG
Professor of Obstetrics and Gynecology
Weill Cornell Medical College
Deputy Chief Medical Officer
Sidra Medical and Research Center
Qatar Foundation, POBox 26999
Doha, State of Qatar

Professor and Chairman Emeritus
Department of Obstetrics
Charité University Medicine Berlin
Augustenburger Platz 1
13353 Berlin, Germany
e-mail: joachim.dudenhausen@charite.de

Prof. Dr. med. Michael Obladen
Charité University Medicine Berlin
Augustenburger Platz 1
13353 Berlin, Germany

Translated by
Susan E. Travis
Mittenwalder Strasse 10
10961 Berlin, Germany
e-mail: suetee@gmx.net

The title is the english translation of "Praktische Geburtshilfe", 21th edition by J. W. Dudenhausen, De Gruyter 2012.
The book has 501 figures and 38 tables.

ISBN 978-3-11-027593-3
e-ISBN (PDF) 978-3-11-027611-4
e-ISBN (EPUB) 978-3-11-038135-1

Library of Congress Cataloging-in-Publication Data
A CIP catalog record for this book has been applied for at the Library of Congress.

Bibliographic information published by the Deutsche Nationalbibliothek
The Deutsche Nationalbibliothek lists this publication in the Deutsche Nationalbibliografie; detailed bibliographic data are available on the Internet at http://dnb.dnb.de.

Typesetting: PTP-Berlin Protago-TEX-Production GmbH, Berlin
Printing and Binding: Hubert & Co. GmbH und Co. KG, Göttingen
Cover image: Comstock/Getty Images
♾ Printed on acid-free paper
Printed in Germany

MIX
Papier aus verantwortungsvollen Quellen
FSC® C016439

www.degruyter.com

I dedicate this English edition of *Practical Obstetrics* to all women and their children, with the hope of optimal care for all.

Joachim W. Dudenhausen

Preface

The objective of this book is to provide a source of aid for health care providers for mothers and their unborn or newborn child. With enthusiasm, I looked forward to the translation and adaptation of the 21st edition of the German textbook *Praktische Geburtshilfe* into English and its publication under the current title *Practical Obstetrics*. The manuscript reflects the current state of the obstetrical and neonatal art in the globalized world of medicine. We were keen to reach a balance between the science of medicine and practical patient care, principles of practice, policies, and regulation of most professional and academic organizations, guidelines, and recommendations.

I am very thankful to Sue Travis for the careful translation of the German manuscript into English. I am indebted for advice from Dr. Paul Ogburn, New York and Doha, and Dr. Alfredo Gei, Houston, and also from Lisa Austin, Chicago and Doha, in the adaptation to American policies and procedures.

I received numerous tips and much advice from many colleagues and midwives. Thanks to everyone of them. Professor Wolfgang Henrich, Director of the Department of Obstetrics, Charité, University Medicine Berlin, helped me by supplying ultrasonographic illustrations and Doppler flow patterns. Thanks to Dr. Ulrike Mergner, Department for Radiology, Charité, University Medicine Berlin, for the MRIs of pregnant women.

I would like to thank Simone Witzel and Britta Nagl from De Gruyter Berlin/Boston for their assistance in accomplishing this task.

I would like to acknowledge the great contribution and help of my wife Dr. Ria Dudenhausen.

Joachim W. Dudenhausen
Doha / State of Qatar
June 2014

Content

1 Physiology

Definitions

Ovulation. Release of the ovum from the ovary on day 14 of the menstrual cycle of a woman of child-bearing age. The oocyte is flushed out of the Graafian follicle with the follicular fluid and consists of egg plasma with core, nucleolus, and zona pellucida. It is surrounded by follicular epithelial cells (corona radiata) and enters the fallopian tube through the fimbrial end. The passage of the ovum through the fallopian tube into the uterus takes five days.

Copulation. Sexual intercourse, cohabitation, coitus; copulation is coitus performed for the purpose of reproduction. The ejaculate (approx. 4 ml), containing 200 million sperm, is deposited in the posterior fornix. From there the sperm swim through the cervical mucus and the uterus to the entrance of the fallopian tube.

Conception. Coitus resulting in fertilization; fusion of ovum and spermatozoa in the ampulla of the fallopian tube.

Extrauterine fertilization (such as in the abdomen, the ovary or a section of the fallopian tube) may occur in cases of abnormal transport of the ovum to the uterine cavity.

Fertile period. The oocytes remain fertile for six to eight hours. Sperm can live for up to two days. The fertile period of the menstrual cycle is four days.

There are **two fertile phases**: impregnation and conjugation

- *Impregnation* (Fig. 1.1). The sperm penetrates the ripe ovum, thus creating a fertilized cell (zygote). The egg cytoplasm shrinks as a result of the sperm penetration, creating the perivitelline space between the zona pellucida and the ooplasm.
- *Conjugation.* Fusion of the nuclei of sperm and ovum; fusion of the chromosomes of the pronuclei on day one-two. They line up on the equatorial plane without fusing. Fertilization is now complete.

Cleavage. The development of grooves on the surface of the fertilized ovum, visible sign of cell division on day two to three after conception. Continued cell division results in the creation of many daughter cells.

Morula (Latin for mulberry). A ball of daughter cells or blastomeres, reaching the 16-cell stage on day three to five.

Blastocyst. Conceptus, product of conception. On day five the intercellular spaces enlarge and cavitation occurs, resulting in the creation of the blastocyst cavity. The morula becomes the blastocyst, consisting of the **trophoblast**, the outer cell layer, which develops into the chorionic epithelium (the fetal epithelium part of the placenta), and the **embryoblast**, or inner cell mass. The embryoblast develops into the embryo, amnion, yolk sac, allantois, and the chorionic mesoderm (fetal connective tissue part of the placenta).

Nidation, implantation. The blastocyst embeds itself in the endometrial wall of the uterus (decidua), which has been prepared for the pregnancy, on day six or seven after lysis of the zona pellucida has occurred.

Microvilli emerge from the endometrial cells and transform into smooth epithelial cells of the uterus (pinopods). These cells increase in size through the absorption of fluids from the uterine cavity and the influence of progesterone. Estrogens stimulate the release of the adhesive molecule Mucin 1, which facilitates the implantation of the blastocyst. The invasion of the im-

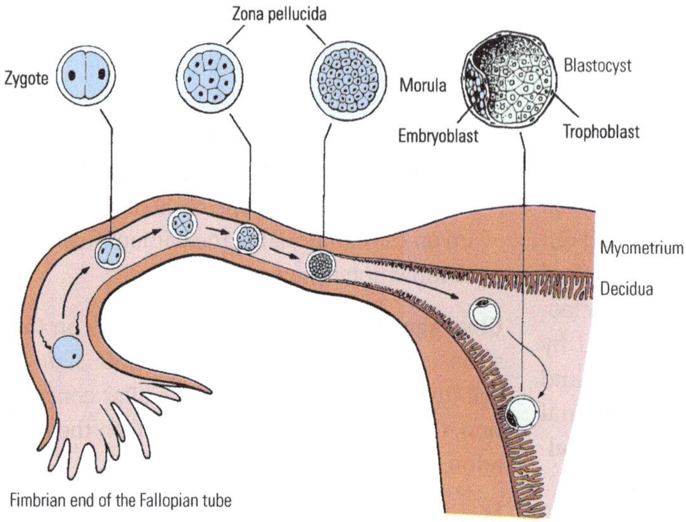

Fig. 1.1: Development of the fertilized ovum before implantation.

planted blastocyst is directed by interleukins, cytokines, and interferons. This leads to a production cascade of vascular endothelial growth factor (VEGF), nitric oxide, and prostacyclins.

Invading trophoblast. The cells of the implanted trophoblast surrounding the embryoblast erode the uterine epithelium with the help of enzymes, allowing it to embed in the endometrium, where rapid cell proliferation occurs. Some of the substances released in the process nourish the conceptus (histiotrophic phase). Numerous maternal blood vessels are eroded, and the first contact with maternal blood occurs. In this way the primitive maternal intervillous capillary system is constructed within the trophoblast. The histiotrophic phase is completed on days nine to twelve, and the hemotrophic phase begins.

Absorption trophoblast. Differentiation of the trophoblast; the intercellular boundaries fuse in the peripheral trophoblastic cells, forming the syncytium (syncytiotrophoblast), while the inner trophoblastic cells (those closest to the embryo) retain their cellular form (cytotrophoblast, Langhans cell layer). Finger-like projections grow from the cytotrophoblast into the syncytium, forming the primary chorionic villi.

Amniotic cavity. A gap forms in the originally solid embryoblast. The base of this gap is formed by the epiblast; the top by the amniotic layer of the embryoblast (hypoblast).

Formation of the germ layers (Fig. 1.2). The embryonic shield differentiates into the three germ layers: ectoderm, endoderm, and mesoderm.
- The ectodermal layer gives rise to the nervous system, skin, hair, nails, eyes, and ears.
- The mesodermal layer gives rise to bones, muscles, connective tissue, vessels, and the urogenital system.
- The endodermal layer gives rise to the gastrointestinal tract, liver, bile system, pancreas, thyroid, and lungs. The endoderm grows over the edge of the embryoblast into the inner cytotrophoblast until it surrounds a cavity: the yolk sac.

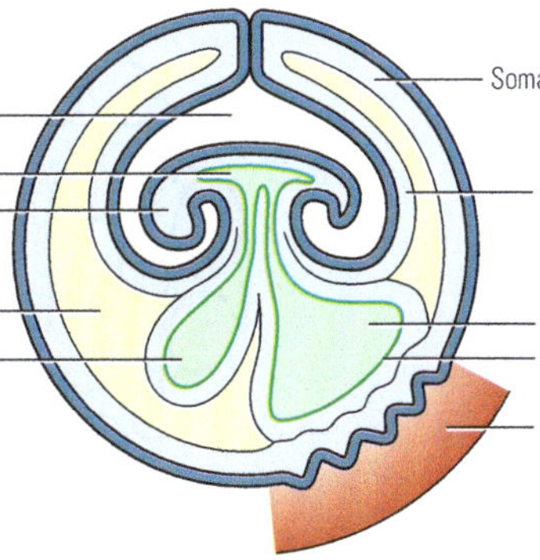

Fig. 1.2: Embryo three weeks after conception.

Extraembryonic mesoderm. Reticulum-like tissue which develops from the cells surrounding the embryoblast. In the 15-day-old embryo it covers the two close vesicles: the amniotic cavity and the yolk sac. It thickens to make up the chorion (somatic mesoderm) on the inner side of the trophoblast and on the outer side of the embryo the amnion, (sphlanchnic mesoderm).

Body stalk. Mesenchymal strand at the caudal end of the embryo, connecting chorion and amnion, later developing into the umbilical cord. The first blood vessels develop in the body stalk and in the mesoderm (blood islands and cells) on week three of embryonic development. The allantois follows, as part of the developing hindgut. During this rudimentary development, the blood vessels of the allantois penetrate the body stalk and later become the umbilical vessels.

Trophoblast invasion. Trophoblastic cells migrate into the decidua and the inner third of the myometrium to anchor the placenta and increase uteroplacental perfusion by remodeling the spiral arterioles. These trophoblastic cells are known as extravillous trophoblasts (in contrast to the villous trophoblast = placental villi). Extravillous trophoblasts take one of two paths:

- *Interstitial invasion.* Trophoblasts migrate from the villi into the decidua and myometrium, secreting an extra-cellular matrix which anchors the placenta in the decidua. They cause endothelial swelling in the spiral arterioles, edema, and a reduction of elasticity.
- *Endovascular invasion.* From week 10, trophoblasts are found in place of the intima and in the media of the spiral arterioles. This results in a pronounced vascular dilation, and thus an increase in the uteroplacental blood flow.

Development of the chorionic villi

Syncytial trabeculae border on blood-filled lacunae through which maternal blood flows in week 4. From these originate:

- Trabeculae. Radially arranged chorionic villi.
- Primary villi. Only epithelial cells. In week 4, cytotrophoblast cells grow into the inner trabeculae, which are overlaid with syncytial cells and have a cytotrophoblast core.

Mesenchymal cells have grown into the trophoblast and transformed primary into secondary villi.

- Secondary villi. Epithelial and connective tissue (= chorionic villi). They develop when extraembryonic mesoderm penetrates the cytotrophoblast. From outer to inner layers: syncytium, cytotrophoblast, basal membrane, chorionic mesoderm.

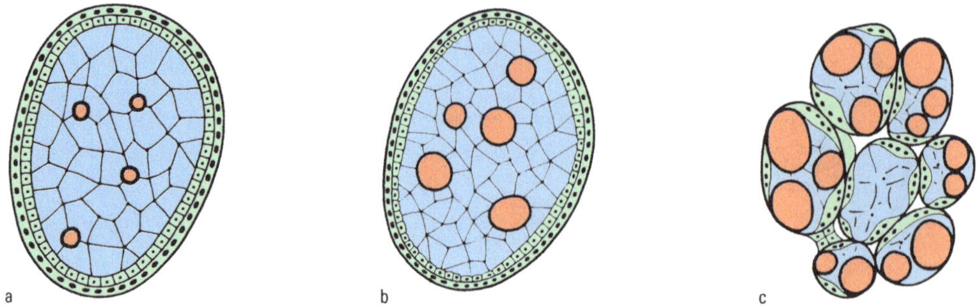

Fig. 1.3: Villous reduction and vascularization in pregnancy; (a) immature villus, week 16; (b) immature villus, week 24; (c) mesh of mature villi. Seven villi, interconnected by intervillous bridges, now occupy the same space. The widened capillaries (sinusoids) have displaced the villous stroma (after Becker).

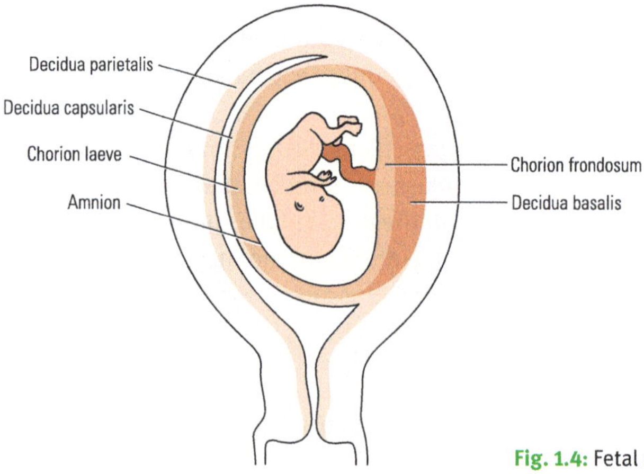

Fig. 1.4: Fetal and placental development 10 weeks after LMP.

- Tertiary villi. Contain blood vessels. Extra-embryonic blood vessels are present in the mesodermal nucleus from week 5. Once those vessels connect with the fetal circulatory system in week 6, substances are transported in the blood from placenta to the embryo, replacing diffusion, which was the main transport method until this time.

By week 14 of gestation the placenta has reached its definitive form. Continuing development takes the form of an increase in diameter and a decrease of the distance between the intervillous spaces.

Villi. The villi decrease in diameter throughout the pregnancy, from 140 μm in the first gestational week to 50 μm in the last weeks of pregnancy. The continuous decrease in villous volume goes hand-in-hand with the development of the villous vessels (Fig. 1.3). **The villi mature, adapting to the nutritional requirements of the fetus.** The distance covered by the substances being exchanged (diffusion between maternal and fetal blood = thickness of the syncytiocapillary membrane) grows smaller. The outer layer of the two-layered chorionic epithelium (syncytium and Langhans cell layer) contains plasma projections (microvilli) which increase the surface area of the syncytiocapillary membrane.

The inner surface area of the mature placenta amounts to 12–13 m².

Decidua graviditatis. After implantation has occurred, the functional portion of the endometrium (decidua) is divided into three sections (Fig. 1.4): decidua basalis, between conceptus and myometrium; decidua capsularis, which covers the embedded conceptus; and decidua parietalis, which lines the remainder of the cavity.

Chorion villosum, laeve. Whereas in weeks 1 to 8 the villi are evenly distributed on the chorion (→ chorion villosum), the villi on the decidua capsularis atrophy around week 8. This section becomes the chorion laeve.

Chorion frondosum. The villi in the decidua basalis hypertrophy to become the chorion frondosum. In weeks 12–14 the chorion laeve and decidua capsularis fuse with the decidua parietalis, so that the uterine cavity is no longer detectable.

By week 32 the placenta has reached its maximum thickness (20 mm). It continues to grow only in area, paralleling the growth of the uterus wall below it.

1.1 The mature placenta

1.1.1 Structure, function

The **mature placenta** is round or oval in shape, has a diameter of 20 cm, and weighs about 500 g.

Villous capillary system. The placenta consists of the chorion frondosum and the decidua basalis. Between them is a space filled with maternal blood, into which the villi are immersed (intervillous space), and a labyrinth-like capillary system (villous capillary system; Fig. 1.5). The chorion frondosum consists of the chorionic plate (a single layer of amnion epithelium, basal membrane, and chorionic connective tissue combined with chorionic epithelium) and the villi projecting from it.

Anchoring villi are the stem villi found in the chorionic plate which anchor in the decidua basalis or basal plate. Villi originate and branch from these stems, forming a spongy structure.

Umbilical cord. The umbilical vessels spread over the fetal side of the chorionic plate.
- Arteries cross veins.
- The umbilical cord contains three blood vessels: the umbilical vein and the two umbilical arteries.

The umbilical vein (vena umbilicalis) delivers oxygen-rich blood from the placenta to the fetus; deoxygenated blood is transported to the placenta via the umbilical arteries.
Approximately 100 ml of fetal blood volume can be found in the placenta at term.

The **decidua basalis** (basal plate) consists in
- Decidua compacta, the firm inner layer.
- Decidua spongiosa, the outer, softer layer.

Placental separation occurs in the decidua spongiosa. It is thus the decidua compacta and part

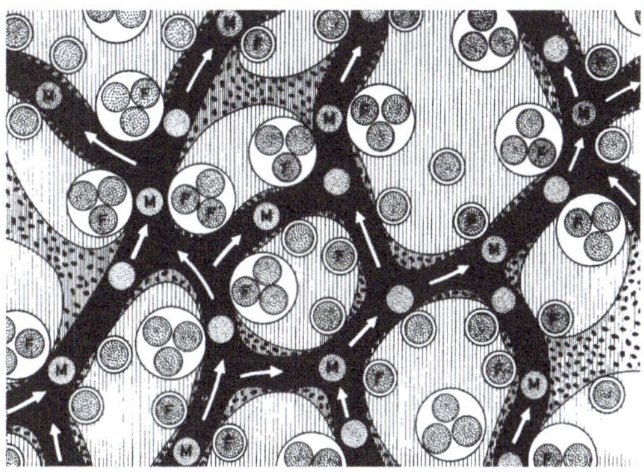

Fig. 1.5: Villi and the intervillous space of a mature placenta. Cross-sections of the villi, the blood-filled capillaries, and the maternal blood (M) circulating between the villi in the intervillous space. Microvillic brush borders in the syncytiocapillary membrane (after Lemtis).

of the decidua spongiosa which are expelled at birth from the placenta. The basal plate of the placenta is comprised of these two parts of the decidua.

Cotyledons. On average 19 separate sections (cotyledons) can be made out on the maternal side (i.e., the side facing the uterus in pregnancy) of a mature placenta.

The structuring of the placenta in cotyledons occurs due to projections of the deciduas compacta, which create placental septa. It is not possible to detect the cotyledons in situ. Maternal blood flows through the decidua via the uterine arteries and veins to and from the intervillous capillary system.

Spiral arterioles. These arterioles are very convoluted (hence the name), the veins have a funnel-like widening. According to Lemtis, seventy-two spiral arterioles supply the placenta. Maternal arterial blood flows out of the basal arterial openings towards the chorionic plate, where it flows over the villi and back to the basal plate:

Cotyledons are the main units of fetal and maternal blood flow in the placenta.
While the blood is in the intervillous space, oxygen and carbon dioxide are exchanged, and nutrients are transferred from the maternal blood in exchange for waste products from the fetal blood. Each cotyledon functions as a separate unit. Morphologically, however, they are not easily separated. Septa are not often present.

Function of the placenta

- Exchange of gas and nutrients between maternal and fetal blood.
- Endocrine organ-production of placental hormones (p. 7).
- Immunological barrier between conceptus and mother.

Placental exchanges

- Gases (oxygen, carbon dioxide).
- Nutrients (glucose, amino and fatty acids, vitamins, electrolytes).
- Medication (inhaled narcotics, lipophilic and hydrophilic substances of low molecular weight).
- Blood cells, macromolecules.

The exchange via the syncytiocapillary membrane occurs in one of two ways (Tab. 1.1): by passive diffusion following the concentration gradient, or via active transport requiring energy.

Tab. 1.1: Exchange of substances in the placenta.

Mechanism	Substance
Passive transport	
Simple diffusion	Oxygen, carbon dioxide, creatinine, medications
Simplified diffusion	Glucose
Diapedesis (through defects or pores of the syncytio-capillary membrane)	Erythrocytes, leukokytes
Active transport	
Enzymatic processes	Anorganic ions, amino acids, fatty acids, vitamins, hormones
Pinocytosis	Proteins, lipids, immunoglobulins

Example. Gases are exchanged via simple diffusion. An example of simplified transport is glucose. This method is faster than simple diffusion and involves structure- and stereospecific selection. It is assumed that transport molecules in the cells of the syncytiocapillary membrane play a role.

Fetal oxygen uptake is influenced by the difference in oxygen concentration between maternal and fetal blood and the circulation of blood in the intervillous space and the villi.

Example. Oxygen concentration in maternal blood is 80 mmHg, and in fetal blood in the villi 15 mmHg. Oxygen diffuses from maternal to fetal blood due to the concentration gradient.

Oxygen transport through the placental membrane follows the principle of simple diffusion, which does not require energy.
Oxygen concentration on both the maternal and fetal sides of the syncytiocapillary membrane depends on the blood flow. At term, blood circulates at a volume of 500 ml/min on the maternal side and 300 ml/min on the fetal side. There is no direct relationship between uterine and placental blood flow and oxygen absorption; however, if the circulating volume is reduced to 350 or 400 ml/min, oxygen absorption can be reduced.

Principle of multivillous flow. The oxygen content of the maternal blood decreases as it flows through the intervillous space, whereas that of the fetal blood in the villi increases.
- Higher oxygen-binding capacity of fetal blood (increased oxygen affinity) as a result of the different structure of fetal hemoglobin (HbF) compared to adult hemoglobin and the low diphospho-glycerate content of fetal erythrocytes. Oxygen affinity is also dependent on carbon dioxide content and blood pH level (Bohr effect: oxygen binding capacity is reduced when pH is low).
- Increased oxygen capacity of fetal blood due to relative polyglobulia (average fetal Hb at term 16 g% in contrast to the maternal 12 g%).

As the fetus develops, the diffusion process adapts to its growing oxygen requirements through increased blood volume, increased surface area of the capillaries, and thinning of the syncytiocapillary membrane. Increased fetal oxygen consumption results in reduced oxygen pressure in umbilical vein blood, increasing the concentration gradient and thus oxygen transport.

Exchange of carbon dioxide. Placental carbon dioxide exchange also occurs via simple diffusion. The diffusion rate is faster, because carbon dioxide is more soluble than oxygen.

Carbon dioxide (CO_2) is broken down into bicarbonate (HCO_3) and hydrogen (H) ions via hydration and dissociation; only a small amount is actually dissolved. More than 80 % is transported as bicarbonate (2/3 in plasma, 1/3 in erythrocytes). During pregnancy the maternal partial CO_2 pressure decreases from 40 to 32 mmHg due to hyperventilation. This respiratory alkalosis is balanced by a reduction of the CO_2 binding capacity so that the pH remains constant. The arterial pressure difference between maternal and fetal CO_2 amounts to 9 mm Hg.
Oxygenation of the blood reduces the CO_2 binding capacity (Haldane effect): increase in oxyhemoglobin facilitates CO_2 transport.

Fetomaternal CO_2 difference. The balance is not complete: the difference amounts to 3–5 mm Hg. The reasons for this are irregular placental diffusion and a delayed exchange of erythrocytes and plasma.

1.1.2 The placenta as an endocrine organ: hCG, hPL, progesterone, and estrogen

Placental hormones. The following hormones are synthesized in the placenta:
- *Protein hormones* (only produced in the placenta): human chorionic gonadotrophin (hCG), human placental lactogen (hPL), human chorionic thyrotrophin (hCT).
- *Steroid hormones*: estrogens and progestagens; synthesis in the placenta requires precursors of a steroid nature to be available from the fetus or mother.

Maternal-placental-fetal system. The placenta and fetus create a functional endocrine unit, also called the fetoplacental or fetoplacental endocrine unit. It is important to stress that it does not stand alone as an endocrine unit, however, but that a maternal endocrine influence also exists (maternal-placental-fetal unit).

Human chorionic gonadotrophin (hCG)

hCG was discovered in 1927 by Aschheim and Zondek at the Charité Hospital in Berlin. It is a gonadotropic (having an effect on the gonads) hormone with a protein structure and is produced in the syncytiotrophoblast.

The hCG molecule is made up of 2 peptide chains (alpha (α) and beta (β)). The β-chain is responsible for the hormone-specific activity.

hCG passes over to the mother from the trophoblasts (Fig. 1.6). Excretion via the kidneys (Fig. 1.7) begins a few days after implantation, peaking in the first trimester (50–80 days p.m.).

Detection of hCG is the basis of the immunological pregnancy test (see p. 60).

Function. hCG preserves the corpus luteum graviditatis, and thus the synthesis of estrogen and progesterone in the corpus luteum; the maternal pituitary gland is suppressed. As a result the ovary retains the decidua graviditatis until the trophoblast can produce enough progesterone itself.

Progesterone synthesis. The influence of hCG on placental steroid synthesis (progesterone synthesis) is in discussion, as is the stimulation of testosterone production in the testicles of the male fetus in weeks 10–12.

Human placental lactogen (hPL)

hPL, or human placental lactogen, is a lactogenic (milk-producing) hormone which was found by Ito and Higashi in 1961. It is a single-chain protein, chemically similar to human growth hormone (GH) and prolactin (PRL), produced in the syncytiotrophoblast.

hPL increase correlates with the number of functional syncytiotrophoblasts. The hPL level in maternal blood is an indicator for placental function.

Role. Not clearly understood. hPL is thought to mobilize glucose (antiinsulin effect) and free fatty acids in the mother and to regulate the placental transport of free fatty acids. Its mamo- and lactotropic properties do not appear to be important.

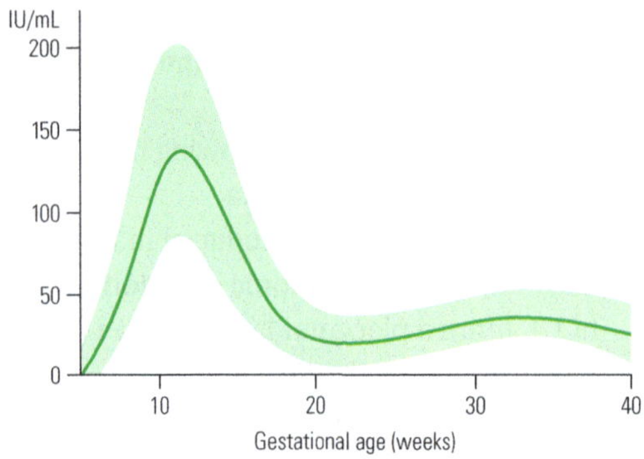

Fig. 1.6: Serum hCG levels in pregnancy; mean values and double standard variations (after Keller).

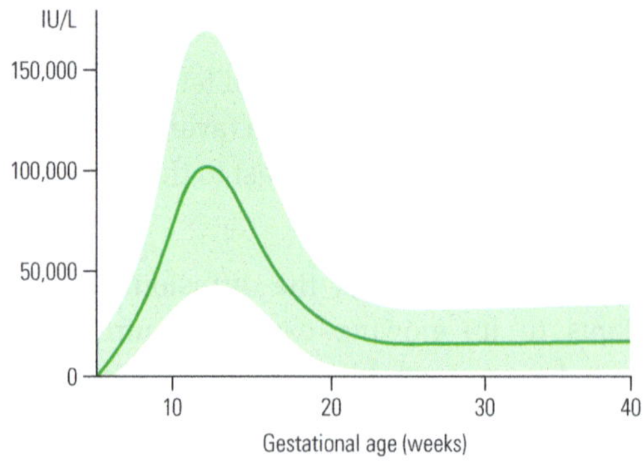

Fig. 1.7: Urine hCG in pregnancy; mean values and double standard variations (after Keller).

Progesterone

An increasing amount of **progesterone** is produced by the syncytiotrophoblast in pregnancy. It is produced by the adrenal glands of both fetus and mother and by the corpus luteum in the first weeks of pregnancy.

Towards the end of the pregnancy, 200–500 mg of placental progesterone are delivered to the maternal organism. Progesterone is produced in the placenta from cholesterol and pregnenolone, both of which are provided for the most part by the mother. The progesterone received by the fetus is mostly transformed to steroids: corticosterone, cortisol, androstenedione, and testosterone in male fetuses; some is reduced by the fetal liver to 20α- or 20β-dihydroprogesterone, which is returned to the placenta via the umbilical arteries.

Pregnanediol. 10–20 % of the placental progesterone (Fig. 1.8) returned to the maternal system is excreted in urine as pregnanediol (Fig. 1.9).

Note. As progesterone is produced by the placenta, pregnanediol excretion in maternal urine is an indicator of placental function.

Role. The assumed effect of pregnancy preservation is unproven. In experiments, Jung was able to demonstrate an inhibition of uterine contractions and a reduction of muscular tone, and of the frequency and amplitude of contractions.

Estrogens

Estrone (E1), estradiol (E2) and estriol (E3) are produced in the placenta, and the plasma concentration increases continually.

The **main form of synthesis** in the placenta is from maternal (10 %) and fetal (90 %) dehydroepiandrosterone sulfate (DHEA-S). After separation of the sulfate group, androstenedione and testosterone are transformed into estrone and estradiol.

As the placenta has no 16-hydroxylase activity, estriol cannot be produced from estrone and estradiol. These enzymes are found in the fetal liver and adrenal glands. Estrone and DHEAS produced in the placenta are then hydroxylated and converted to 16-OH-DHEAS or 16-OH-estrone, or provided as the hydroxylated precursors 16-OH-androstenedione and 16-OH-testosterone, which in turn can then be

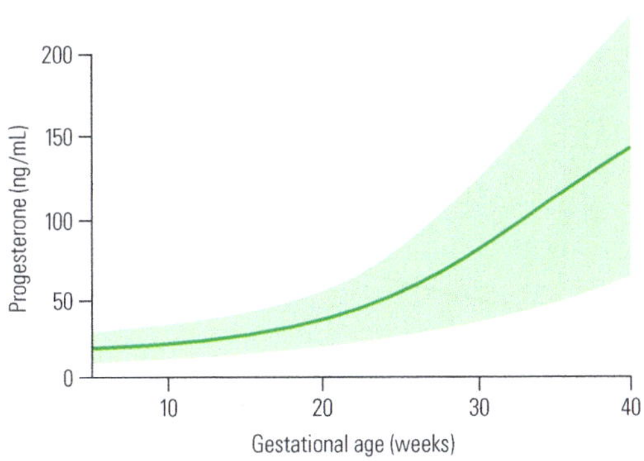

Fig. 1.8: Serum progesterone in pregnancy; mean values and confidence limit of 95 % (after Keller).

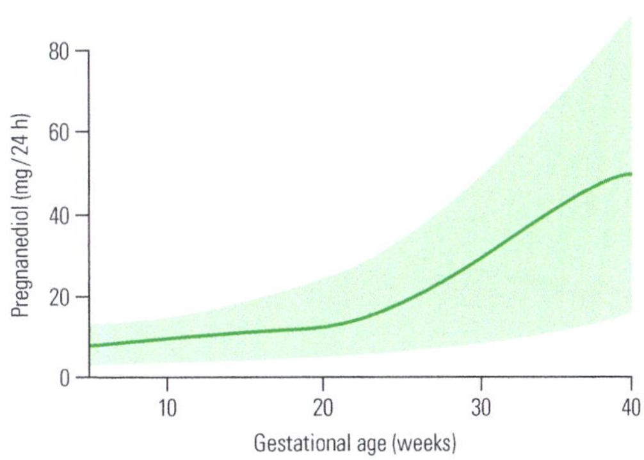

Fig. 1.9: Pregnanediol in urine in pregnancy; mean values and confidence limit of 95 % (after Keller).

transformed into estriol after separation of the sulphate group in the placenta.

The placental estrogens pass unconjugated into the maternal bloodstream. They are then conjugated to glucuronides, sulphates, and sulphoglucuronides – mainly in the maternal liver, but also in the bowel and kidneys. Only 10 % of the total estriol in maternal blood is free; the rest is made up of estriol glucuronide, estriol sulphate, and estriol sulphoglucuronide.

Excretion. Estrogens are excreted via the maternal kidneys; ten times as much estriol as estrone and estradiol. 80 % of the estriol originates from the fetus.

Practice tip. As the hydroxylation of estriol is performed by the fetus, the level of estriol in maternal serum (Fig. 1.11), or in maternal urine (Fig. 1.10) is an indicator of fetal wellbeing.

Physiological significance. Not completely understood. The main effect is to promote growth of the pregnant uterus by increasing contractile elements and energy-rich substances in the uterus.

An increase of intercellular calcium leads to increased membrane potential and nervous response in the muscle cells.

Administration of estrogen causes an increase in uterine contractions.

1.2 Amniotic fluid, liquor amnii

The **amniotic cavity** is enclosed by two membranes, the outer being the chorion, made up of trophoblasts, and the inner being the amnion, which originated from the embryoblast. Their function is the formation and absorption of amniotic fluid.

Amniotic fluid is initially a yellowish color, becoming opaque to transparent towards the end of the pregnancy. It contains suspended vernix, hair, and flakes of epidermis, particularly in late pregnancy.

Function

- Protection of the fetus/embryo from dehydration, mechanical trauma, temperature variations; space for growth and

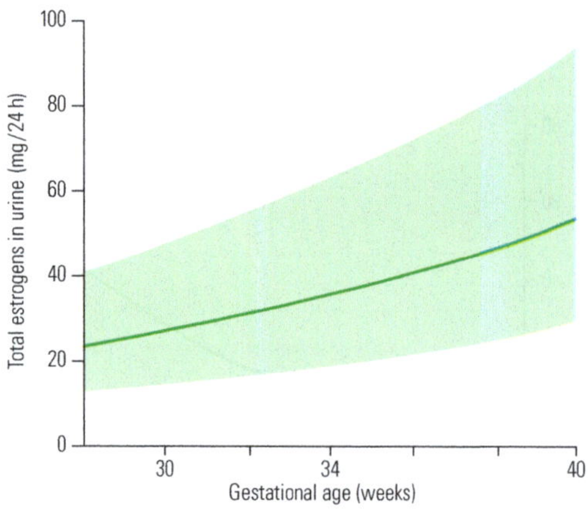

Fig. 1.10: Total estrogen excretion in pregnancy in 24 h urine; median and 95 % confidence interval (after Hull).

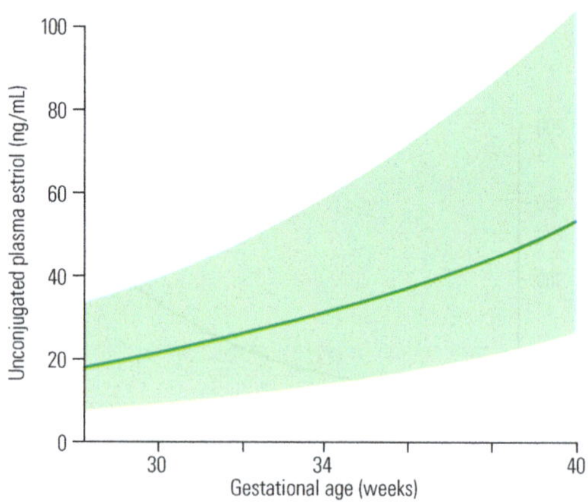

Fig. 1.11: Unconjugated plasma estriol in pregnancy; median and 95 % confidence interval (after Hull).

movement; cushioning the umbilical and chorionic vessels.
- Transport and exchange of nutrients and metabolic products.

Volume. 5–10 ml in week 9 (Fig. 1.12), increasing to 1,000 ml by week 36. After this point the amount decreases to about 800 ml by week 40.

Amniotic fluid exchange. Amniotic fluid is a dynamic substrate in constant exchange between mother and fetus.

Note. At term the complete amniotic fluid is exchanged every two hours.

Paraplacental substance exchange. Water and substrates are exchanged between amniotic fluid and maternal blood, and between amniotic fluid and the fetus. The amounts involved are less than those exchanged in the placenta:
- pH 7.0; acidotic compared to maternal blood. The blood gases oxygen and carbon dioxide only enter the amniotic fluid indirectly via the fetus.
- Urea passes directly from the amniotic fluid via the membranes into the maternal bloodstream; concentration increases from 23 mg% in early pregnancy to 33 mg% at term.

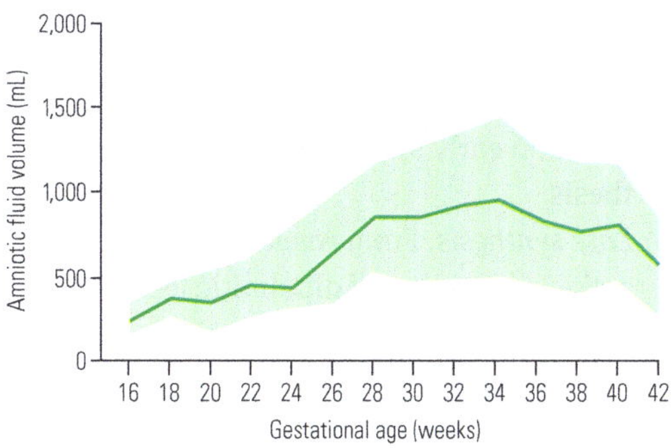

Fig. 1.12: Amniotic fluid in pregnancy (after Queenan, Thompson).

- Glucose level is lower than that of maternal blood at 22 mg%.
- Protein content at term 500 mg%.

Production. The epithelial cells of the amnion produce the amniotic fluid. The fetus contributes in the form of urine (up to 500 ml/day) and lung fluid (100 ml/day). Reabsorption occurs
- Directly via the membranes to the mother.
- Indirectly via the respiratory tract and digestive system after swallowing, and passing into the fetal bloodstream, umbilical cord and thus to the placenta.

Abnormal amniotic fluid volume. Production and absorption disorders lead to pathological amounts of amniotic fluid:
- Hydramnios: increase > 2,000ml.
- Oligohydramnios: decrease < 100ml.

1.3 Embryonic and fetal development

Normo-, teratogenesis. Normal development (normogenesis) passes through different stages in which development can proceed pathologically (teratogenesis).

Gametogenesis (ancient Greek gametes = husband, gamete = wife). Development of sex cell (gamete) in parental organisms.

Gametopathies are disorders in sex cells (ovum, spermatozoa) development: mutation, morphological and functional disorders.

Blastogenesis. Week 3–4 (ancient Greek blast = shoot, sprout); covers the period from fertilization up until implantation has been completed with development of the bilaminar embryonic disc.

Blastopathy. Blastogenesis disorder following the "all-or-none" principle: either the damage is reparable or the embryo dies (implantation disorder leads to loss of embryo; miscarriage = spontaneous abortion).

Organogenesis. Organ growth begins with the formation of the caudal and cranial protuberances on the embryonic shield. The period of organogenesis denotes the embryonic period (till the end of week 8 after conception).

Embryogenesis. Weeks 5–10 (ancient Greek embryon = unborn fruit of conception); begins with the trilaminar embryonic disc, includes organogenesis of the conceptus, which is now known as embryo.

Embryopathy. Developmental disorder in an embryo during the critical or sensitive periods of organogenesis. The damaging toxins do not threaten the survival of the embryo.

Fetogenesis. Week 11 (Latin: fetus) till birth. Longest period of the pregnancy, in which gestation and organ growth occur.

Fetopathy. Prenatal illness, intrauterine developmental disorder after organogenesis has been completed.

Intrauterine growth curve. Growth and differentiation of organ functions can be depicted in curves (Fig. 13.19, p. 452), which have been published for portions of the fetal period (e.g., Lubchenco curves).

Lungs

Anatomical lung maturation. The lungs begin to develop from a protrusion of the primitive gut (foregut) in the 26-day-old embryo. Beginning with the development of crude bronchial branches with a broad, loose mesenchymal sheath up to week 16 (pseudoglandular stage); followed by differentiation and division of the bronchioles (canalicular stage, weeks 16 to 24), lung growth is characterized by grape-like budding. Acini (Latin = berry) are the precursors of the mature alveoli. Transition to the alveolar or terminal sac stage takes place between weeks 25 and 27 and is characterized by tissue displacement, spreading of the pulmonary capillaries, and maturation of the type I and II pneumocytes, whose differentiation can begin as early as week 22. Type II pneumocytes contain globular insertions, which attain a lamellar structure on maturity.

Surfactant, biochemical maturation of the lungs. Maturation of type II pneumocytes with synthesis and release of surface-active substances: alveolar surfactant (antiatelectasis factor). This reduces surface tension on the layer between the air in the alveolus and the alveolar wall and allows the opening of the alveoli on beginning of extrauterine breathing.

Surfactant is a lipoprotein complex with lecithins in the lipid portion.
Type II pneumocytes are responsible for the biosynthesis of surfactant. The lamellar insertions serve as intracellular surfactant reservoirs; they empty their contents into the alveolus and build the surfactant layer. Surfactant is removed from the airways by ciliated epithelium and is continually replaced.

Lecithin biosynthesis in type II pneumocytes

- *Early synthesis.* In the immature fetus (week 22–35) palmitoyl-myristyl-phosphatidylcholine is mainly produced. Acidosis, hypoxia and hypocapnia have a greater inhibitory effect on early synthesis than on late synthesis.
- *Late synthesis.* From week 35 onwards, active production of dipalmitic lecithinis demonstrated by the steep increase of lecithins in amniotic fluid.

Glucocorticosteroids increase the enzyme activity of choline phosphotransferase in the fetal lung. The increase or stimulation of protein synthesis is thought to be transmitted via glucocorticosteroid receptors in fetal lung cells.

Practice tip. From week 26 the morphological prerequisite for exogenous lung maturation is fulfilled (Vogel).

Fetal respiratory movements were first observed by Ahlefeld in 1888. They are detectable with ultrasound and are useful to diagnose the condition of the fetus. These episodes occur in phases of varying lengths with a frequency of 60/min; up to 200/min has been occasionally observed. Temporal fluctuations, blood sugar levels, nicotine abuse, and medication all influence respiratory action.

Fetal circulatory system

Details are to be found in the appropriate textbooks. Here the focus is on those characteristics which are relevant from a clinical point of view (Fig. 13.7).

- Functionally, the foramen ovale lies between the inferior vena cava and the left atrium: blood from the lower half of the body and the placenta flows directly into the left side of the heart.
- Right-left shunt between the pulmonary artery and the aorta (ductus arteriosus). Most of the blood from the superior vena cava passes through the right atrium and pulmonary artery into the aorta.
- Circulation through the lungs is restricted.

Note. Blood pressure is higher in the pulmonary artery than in the aorta.

- Deoxygenated blood from the upper body (superior vena cava → right → pulmonary artery → ductus arteriosus) flows into the aorta after the coronary arteries and carotid artery. Arteriovenous blood is available for the lower part of the body.
- The coronary arteries and carotid arteries transport oxygen-rich blood in order to ensure a good supply of oxygen to the heart and brain.
- Most of the blood from the umbilical vein flows into the inferior v. cava via the ductus venosus.

1.4 The maternal organism

The maternal organism adapts to the increased demands which growth and nourishment of the child (before, during, and after birth) and the birth itself, place upon it. The physical and psychological adjustment processes are triggered by the hormones released by the fetoplacental unit.

The uterus

The most striking changes occur here.

Size and weight (from 60 to 1,000 g) increase due to growth and stretching.

- Characteristic of the first half of pregnancy: active growth with hypertrophy and hyperplasia of the muscle cells and an absolute increase in connective tissue. The proliferation of the muscle cells takes place primarily in the corpus uteri, as here the proportion of muscle cells is 30–40 % (5 % in the cervix).
- Characteristic of the second half of pregnancy: passive growth as a result of fetal growth.

Blood flow in the soft tissue is increased, and the uterus becomes softer in early pregnancy (see signs of pregnancy, p. 17).

Change in shape. In early pregnancy the uterus is pear-shaped; from week 12 it looks like a flattened ball, and from week 13 like an egg balanced on its pointed end. From week 13 the transitional zone between the corpus and the cervix is drawn up into the cavity. This zone develops into the lower uterine segment, which is 69 cm wide (craniocaudal view) at term.

Fluid household. The **fluid in the body** increases by 6–7 liters; the intravascular (35 %) and interstitial volumes increase; the intracellular fluid volume remains constant.

- Maximum blood volume is reached by 32–36 weeks.
- The increase in plasma volume is greater than that of the erythrocyte mass (→ polyglobulia), which results in blood thinning (→ pregnancy-related anemia).

Weight gain in pregnancy: 11 kg, half due to fetus, amniotic fluid, and placenta, the rest to uterus, breasts, fat storage, and fluid increase.

Cardiovascular function

The **cardiac output** (CO) peaks by 32 weeks: 6 l/min. Cause:

- Increase in stroke volume from 65 to 70 ml (→ increase in intravascular volume);
- Heart rate increase from 70 to 85 bpm.
- Decrease in peripheral resistance (minimum at week 32), followed by increase (see blood pressure).

The **mean arterial pressure** remains constant. The blood pressure amplitude is increased.

- Systolic blood pressure (BP) increases slightly or remains constant.
- Diastolic BP (which is a reflection of peripheral resistance) sinks in the first weeks of pregnancy. In the second half of pregnancy it increases by 10 mmHg over prepregnancy values.

Inferior vena cava syndrome (IVCS)

Supine hypotensive syndrome of pregnancy, venocaval compression of the inferior vena cava; shock symptoms (pallor, sweating, breathing difficulties, decrease in stroke volume) in pregnancy due to compression of the inferior vena cava by the uterus (particularly in a supine position). Venous blood flow to the heart and cardiac output are reduced, causing a reduction of blood flow to and in the uterus, which can lead to reduced fetal oxygen supply (causing a decrease in fetal heart rate) if it falls below the critical limit. 30–40 % of pregnant women suffer from mild forms of IVCS in a supine position during the third trimester. Therapy: lateral position.

Renal function

Renal blood flow increase of 30–50 %. Renal plasma flow (RPF) and glomerular filtration rate (GFR) increase equally due to the increase in intravascular and stroke volumes; peak in week 32, then slowly decrease to normal values by the end of the pregnancy.

Renal calices, renal pelvis, and ureters are dilated from week 10 on (right more so than left), due to the influence of progesterone, which predisposes to bacterial ascent and urinary tract infections.

Respiration

Respiratory minute volume (RMV) increases by 40 % by the end of pregnancy because respiratory and tidal volumes are increased; respiratory rate remains constant. Vital capacity, total lung capacity, and inspiratory reserve volume are reduced.

In early pregnancy hyperventilation causes a reduction of arterial carbon dioxide tension (P_aCO_2).

Dyspnea is experienced by one in two pregnant women on exertion, and at rest by 20 % of them. Progesterone is presumably responsible for hyperventilation, respiratory function changes, and dyspnea in pregnancy.

References

Boyd JD, Hamilton WJ: The 7human placenta. Heffers, Cambridge 1970

Kaufmann P, Castellucci M: Extravillous trophoblast in the human placenta. Troph Res 1997; 10:21–65

Zhu J-Y, Pang Z-J, Yu Y-H: Regulation of throphoblast invasion: The role of matrix metallo proteinases. Reviews Obstet Gynecol 2012; 5:e137-e143

2 Diagnosis of pregnancy

2.1 Early pregnancy

Clinical signs of pregnancy consist of probable (subjective) and positive signs.

Probable signs of pregnancy (changes to the reproductive organs):
- Amenorrhea.
- Enlargement and softening of the uterus.
- Enlargement of the breasts.
- Increased congestion (bluish-red flushing) of the vagina and introitus.
- Striae gravidarum: fresh (bluish-red) stretch marks, mainly on the abdomen, sides and outer thighs.
- Linea nigra: (black line) increased pigmentation results in a darkened vertical abdominal mid-line and darkening of the nipples.

Positive signs of pregnancy (occur only in the second half of the pregnancy)
- Fetal heartbeat is audible.
- Fetal movements are palpable, visible and audible.
- Fetal parts are palpable.

Vaginal examination

Practice tip. Request that women empty their bladder prior to the examination!

The vaginal examination consists of:

1. Observation of the introitus, labia and perineum
- Folds of the labia minora, examination of the introitus (in daylight!) for increased congestion.
- Inspection of the vulva: for the presence of ulcers, condyloma.
- Inspection of the perineum: high, low, scarred.

2. Speculum examination (cytology, colposcopy)
- Increased vaginal and cervical congestion.
- Early diagnosis of cervical carcinoma through observation, cytological (Papanicolaou) smear test and colposcopy of the cervix.
- Of 100 women with cervical carcinoma, 25 % are not yet 40 years old.
- Appearance of the external os: circular dimple-like appearance (nulligravida) or larger transverse slit (multigravida).

3. Bimanual examination

The uterine size is determined by palpation and compared with the information given on the LMP or gestational age.

Uterus size. Increase in size of the corpus uteri up to week 16
- No or minimal increase apparent at the end of week 4.
- Markedly larger, the size of a goose egg at the end of week 8.
- The size of a man's fist at the end of week 12.
- The size of a newborn's head at the end of week 16.

Differential diagnosis (in the case of discrepancies between findings and menstrual history)
- Smaller uterus, with bleeding: spontaneous abortion (threatened, inevitable, incomplete, complete) or ectopic pregnancy (p. 363).
- Smaller uterus, no bleeding: missed abortion (p. 357).
- Larger uterus: cystic or hydatidiform mole, hydramnios, twins.

Pregnancy test (see p. 60)
Sonographic diagnosis (see p. 44)

2.2 Diagnosis of late pregnancy

Signs of pregnancy. The diagnosis of late pregnancy is also made on the basis of the signs of pregnancy (see above).

Positive signs of pregnancy are found on **external examination**:

- Fetal heart sounds, palpation of fetal parts, observing and feeling fetal movements.
- Enlargement of the uterus.

Sonographic examination (see p. 44).

3 Prenatal care

3.1 Prenatal checkup

Normal pregnancy. Antenatal care is an important tool with which to reduce maternal and fetal morbidity and mortality. Antenatal checkups are to be performed every four weeks until week 32 and in the last 8 weeks every two weeks until the due date, a total of 12 consultations in normal pregnancy.

High-risk pregnancy. Pregnant women with one or several risk factors need more frequent apointments and comprehensive care.

Initial examination and consultation. Advantages of early (after missed period) consultations are information, advice, danger of infections (see p. 118), medication, and radiation, in particular for:

- Pregnant women working with infectous agents or nuclear medicine for example: physicians, microbiologists, nurses, technical assistants, nursing assistants, etc.
- Kindergarten or other teachers.
- Mothers of small and school children.
- All pregnant women must be advised to avoid contact with sick people, in particular those with colds or flu.

Risk factors signifying dangers for mother and child during pregnancy, labor, puerperium and the neonatal period are identified early.

- History
  - Name, age, obstetrical history (see p. 19).
  - Birth history (see p. 19).
  - History of current pregnancy: due date, course up till now.
  - Medical history (see p. 22).
  - Family history.
  - Social history.
  - Occupational history.
- Antenatal examination (see p. 22)
- Physical examination.
  - Blood pressure, weight, urine (see p. 32).
  - Blood group, rhesus factor.
  - Antibodies (see p. 33), hemoglobin.
  - Syphilis (see p. 132), German measles (see p. 119).
- Additional examination (see p. 35).

3.1.1 History

History-taking. Every examination begins with the history-taking which is broken down into 5 main points: **1.** name, age, obstetrical history; **2**, birth history; **3.** pregnancy; **4.** medical; **5.** social history

Name, age, obstetrical history

Definitions. Late age at first birth (or elderly primigravidae) are nulliparous women over 35 years of age. Young nulliparae are under 18.

Nulliparae, multiparae, and grand multiparae are differentiated as follows:

- First birth = primipara, para 1.
- Second to fifth birth = multipara, para 2, 3, etc.
- Six or more births = grand multipara.

During pregnancy women are referred to as being gravid:

- Nulligravida (e), primigravida(e), or multigravida(e).
- Primigravidae and nulliparae are women who are pregnant for the first time.
- A woman is parous once she is in labor.

Birth history

- Number and history of all previous pregnancies, miscarriages, births, puerperium.

- Ask about weak contractions, obstetrical operations, hemorrhaging, in particular post partum.
- Number of living children? Are they healthy? Were they premature?
- Birth weight? Malformations?

History of current pregnancy

Amenorrhea. The most important question is whether or not and when menstruation ceased.

Practice tip. If menstruation ceases in a healthy sexually mature woman with a regular cycle, it is to be assumed that she is pregnant until all other possibilities have been eliminated.

Menstruation ceases in pregnancy because the estrogens and progesterone produced in the corpus luteum and later in the placenta suppress ovulation and the progress of the menstrual cycle via the anterior pituitary gland.

DD. Common causes of spotting or brief vaginal bleeding episodes in the first half of pregnancy are threatened abortion (see p. 351); cervical polyp, bleeding cervical ectopy, or ectopic pregnancy (see p. 363); varicose bleeding from the vagina or clitoris, cervical cancer, vaginal injury.

Practice tip. In cases of bleeding, injury and ectopy are to be excluded by examination of the cervix and vagina using a sterile speculum.

Duration of pregnancy can be calculated according to the date of conception (→ post conceptionem), or the first day of the last menstrual period (LMP), post menstruationem (p.m.).

- Duration of pregnancy p.c.: day of conception to estimated date of delivery (EDD) 266 days = 38 weeks = 9 ½ lunar months (of 28 days).
- Duration of pregnancy from first day of LMP = approx. 280 days = 40 weeks = 10 lunar months.

Due date. Naegele's rule, date of conception, basal temperature, pregnancy test, fetal quickening

Three variations with which to determine estimated date of delivery:

1. From the first day of the LMP = Naegele's Rule (F.C. Naegele, 1778–1851, obstetrician in Heidelberg, Germany).
2. From the day of conception.
3. From the day of basal body temperature (BBT) increase.

A positive pregnancy test, fetal quickening and fundal height (see p. 23) are less important.

Naegele's rule. EDD is calculated by subtracting three months from day one of the LMP and adding one year and seven days:

LMP – 3 months + 7 days + 1 year = EDD.

Advantage: calculating 280 days backwards on a calendar is not necessary.
Example 1: 10.10.2013 – 3 months + 7 days + 1 year = 17.07.2014.
Example 2: If the menstrual cycle is longer or shorter than 28 days:
first day of LMP – 3 months + 7 days + 1 year ± x days (x being the number of days by which the cycle differs from the 28 day cycle).

Date of conception. Sometimes pregnant women are able to state the conception date, in which case the pregnancy duration (266 days after conception) is calculated: conception date – 3 months – 7 days + 1 year.

Example: 18.05.2013 – 3 months – 7 days + 1 year = 11.2.2014.

Practice tip. Less than 5 % of births follow Naegele's Rule. A deviation of eight to ten days earlier or later is to be expected. Statistically, two-thirds of babies are born within three weeks of the EDD (Fig. 3.1).

Basal body temperature (BBT) increase. Body temperature taken (orally or rectally) be-

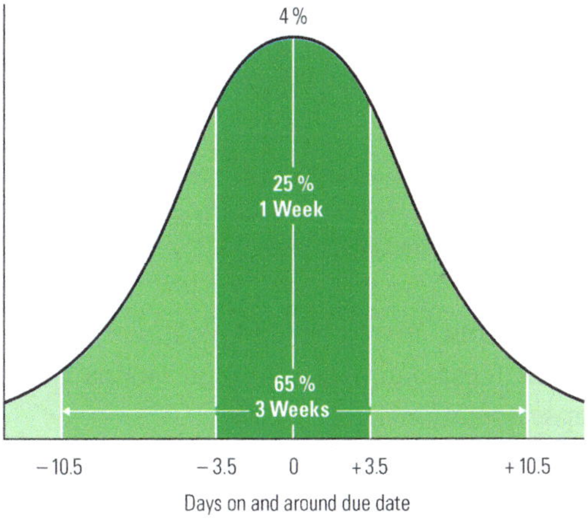

Fig. 3.1: Birth frequency on and around due date.

fore rising in the morning after at least six hours of rest. Fever alters the results.

The temperature curve of a sexually mature woman is 0.5 °C lower in the follicular (or proliferative) phase of the menstrual cycle (usually < 37 °C) than in the luteal (or secretory) phase (usually 37 °C). In a 28 day cycle the temperature increase (0.5 °C) occurs on day 14 or 15, the day after ovulation. It sinks again shortly before menstruation begins (Fig. 3.2).

The rise in temperature is due to the thermogenetic effect of progesterone on the temperature center in the midbrain.

In the case of pregnancy, the luteal phase continues, and the BBT remains the same (> 37 °C; Fig. 3.2b), often even increasing by 0.1–0.2 %. In order to calculate the EDD, the day on which the BBT rose is taken as the day of conception.

Positive pregnancy test. The immunological urine test (see p. 60) is usually positive 5–12 days after the menstrual period was due, i.e., five to six weeks after the last period. This date, once established at the initial visit, can be used to check the accuracy of other EDD calculations.

Date of quickening (Fig. 3.3) is usually by the end of week 20 for nulliparae, and the end of week 18, or even as early as week 16 or 17, for multiparae.

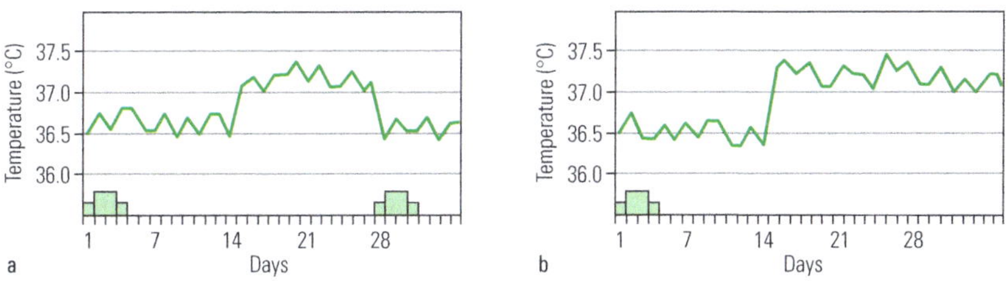

Fig. 3.2: Basal body temperature rise > 16 days indicates pregnancy (after Ufer).

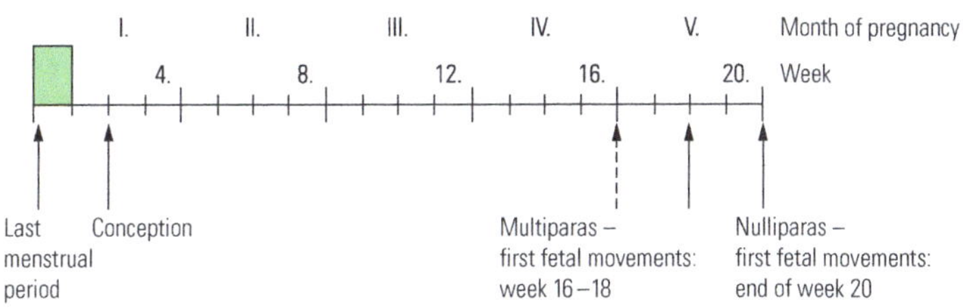

Fig. 3.3: First fetal movements (“quickening”) in nulli- and multiparae.

Ultrasound. Gestational age and EDD are usually clinically determined in the first half of pregnancy using sonography (see p. 44).

Practice tip. We recommend describing gestational age in completed weeks. A gestational age of 282 days would thus be 40+2 weeks.

Medical history

Preexistent illnesses are conditions which may predispose to the development of pregnancy-induced hypertension (PIH; pre-eclampsia, eclampsia – see p. 74) in the second half of pregnancy:

- Cardiovascular disorders, in particular essential hypertension; heart defects (see p. 84), thrombosis, embolism.
- Renal disorders: urinary tract infection, postinfectious glomerulonephritis, poststreptococcal glomerulonephritis.
- Liver disorders.
- Diabetes mellitus (see p. 87).

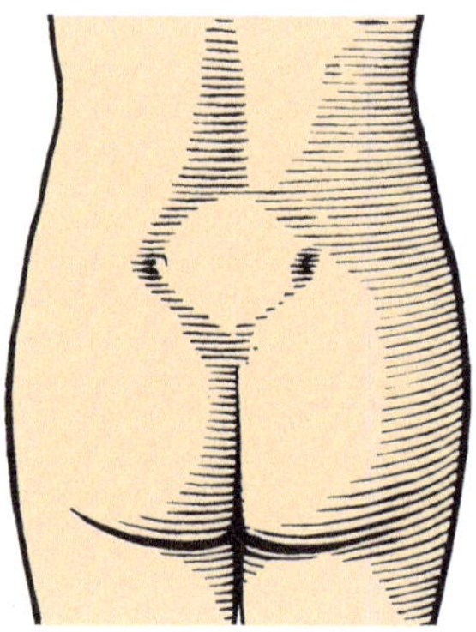

Fig. 3.4: Michaelis rhomboid – square standing on one tip.

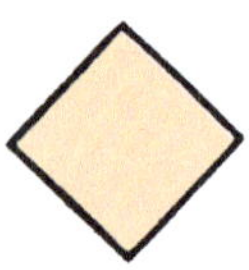

Fig. 3.5: Michaelis rhomboid, square shaped.

Pulmonary tuberculosis. (see p. 86)

Venereal diseases. Syphilis (see p. 132), gonorrhea, HIV.

Practice tip. All pregnant women should be tested for syphilis and offered an HIV test.

Operations. In particular operations on the uterus (Cesarean, fibroids), and vagina (prolapse operations).

Social history. Employment situation. Stress. Strain. Where applicable, maternity guidelines should be taken into account.

3.1.2 Obstetric examination

Pelvis, skin

Michaelis rhomboid (Fig. 3.4). Square (or rhombus) standing on one point above the os sacrum. Shape formed by four dimples.

- Upper point: dimple between the spinous processes of the lumbar vertebrae 3 and 4.
- Lower point: upper point of the anal cleft, formed by the edges of the gluteal muscles.
- Lateral points: posterior superior iliac spines (aka dimples of Venus), usually visible and palpable.

Normal pelvis (Fig. 3.4, 5). A pelvic anomaly is unlikely if the rhomboid is equilateral. A narrow or contracted pelvis is likely if this is not the case.

Contracted rachitic pelvis (Fig. 3.6). Kite-shaped rhomboid: flat, closer to triangular in form, in severe cases almost completely triangular with an obtuse upper angle.

Generally contracted pelvis (Fig. 3.7). Narrow rhomboid, with acute upper and lower angles, much higher than it is wide.

Long pelvis (see p. 303). The kite shape of the rhomboid (vertical deformation) can be due to:

- High position of the lateral points (elongation of the lower rhomboid half), common but not always the case in the long android pelvis.
- Low position of the upper point (flattening of the upper half of the rhomboid); see Fig. 3.8.

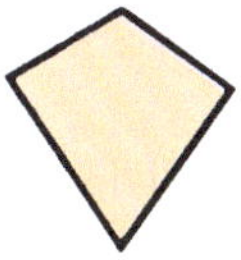

Fig. 3.6: Michaelis rhomboid of contracted rachitic pelvis = kite-shaped, almost triangular (-> obtuse upper angle).

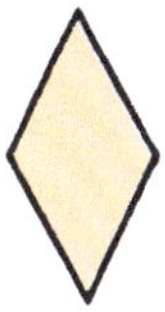

Fig. 3.7: Rhomboid of narrow (or contracted) pelvis = elongated shape, narrow, pointed at the top and bottom.

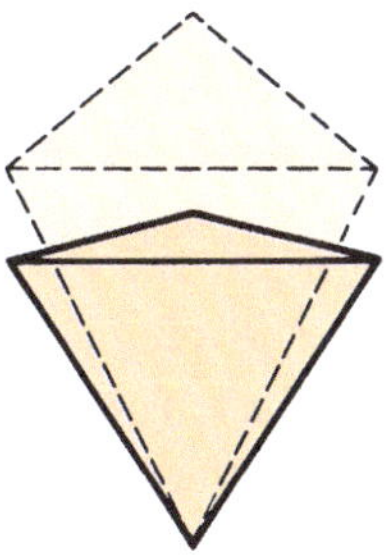

Fig. 3.8: Michaelis rhomboid of long pelvis (dashed) and of rachitic pelvis (outline; after Kirchhoff).

External examination: uterus, Leopold maneuvers

Note. The examination involves palpation, auscultation, measurement of abdominal girth, external pelvic exam.

Uterus

Fundal height (Fig. 3.9) at the end of
- Week 16 2–3 cm above the top of the pubis.
- Week 20 3–5 cm below the navel.
- Week 24 at navel height.
- Week 28 3–5 cm above the navel.
- Week 32 midway between navel and tip of xiphoid process.
- Week 36 level with the costal arch (highest fundal level).
- Week 40 2–3 cm below the costal arch, the same height as at the end of week 32.

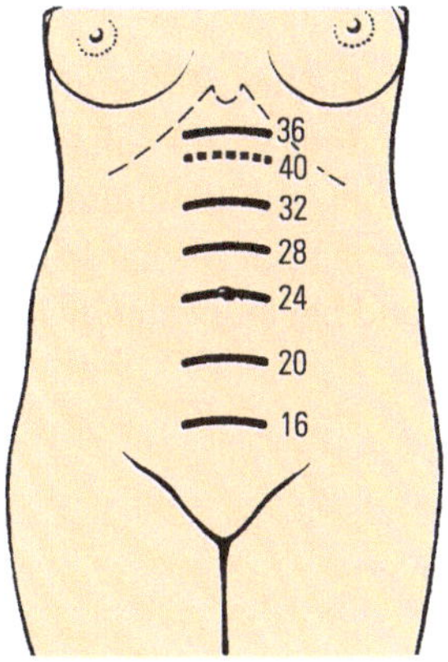

Fig. 3.9: Fundal height at end of corresponding week of pregnancy.

Decrease in fundal height (lightening) at the beginning of week 37 to the same height as at the end of week 32. Cause: descent of the fetus in nulliparae with a vertex presentation due to increased frequency of contractions (false labor) and engaging of the head in the pelvis. In parous women the baby's head does not descend so far, or engage, but remains above the pelvic inlet.
Lightening four weeks before the EDD is not so apparent in multi- and grand multiparae because the head does not engage, but remains above the pelvic inlet.

Irregularities in fundal height. If the fundal height is not appropriate to the gestational age, four questions are to be answered by sonographical examination:
- Has the gestational age been correctly calculated? Is the menstrual history correct?
- Have twins, hydramnios, macrosomia been ruled out?

- Malpresentation, deformity, intrauterine death?
- Intrauterine growth restriction (IUGR)?

Size. Fundal height (as explained above) and symphysis-fundus height measurement (Fig. 3.10, 3.11):

The distance from the upper edge of the pubic bone to the fundus is measured with a soft (not elastic) tape measure along the longitudinal axis of the baby. The woman lies on her back with an empty bladder and her legs extended.

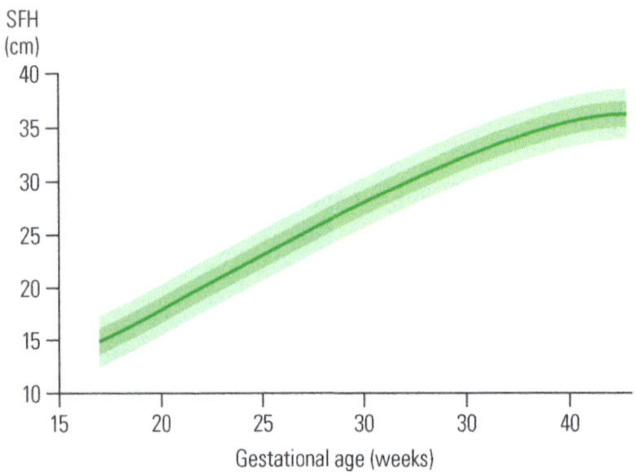

Fig. 3.10: Symphysis-fundus height (SFH) in pregnancy (mean value ± 2SD; after Westin).

According to Westin, the predictability for appropriate and small for gestational age (AGA and SGA) babies is around 75 % in each case. In addition to fundal height and fundal measurement, abdominal girth measurement also gives an indication of the size of the uterus.

Abdominal girth at navel height. 100–105 cm at term for a woman of normal height, normal amniotic fluid volume, and normal abdominal wall.

Charts are not provided, as great individual variations exist, and they would not be helpful in practice or the clinic.

Abdominal girth at term:
- Unusually large = large baby, twins, hydramnios.
- Unusually small = small baby (growth restriction, incorrect calculation of gestational age).

The Leopold maneuvers

Palpation of the abdomen. The pregnant woman lies stretched out on her back. For maneuvers one to three, the examiner sits next to her, facing her; for the fourth maneuver, the ex-

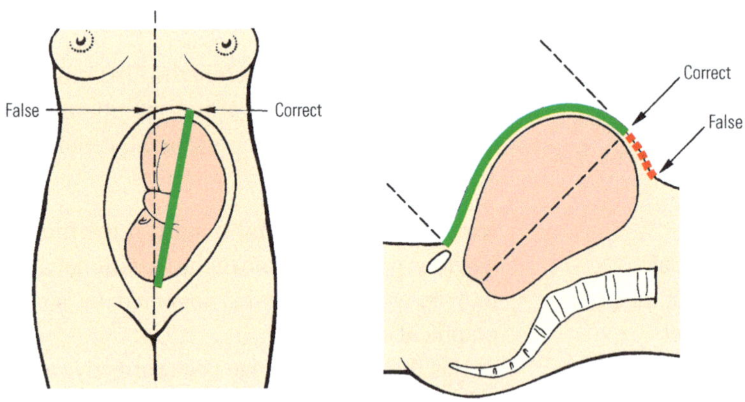

Fig. 3.11: Illustration of correct and incorrect techniques for measuring symphysis-fundus height, frontal and lateral view (after Westin).

aminer sits next to the supine pregnant woman facing her feet.

First maneuver (Fig. 3.12). The ulnar edges of both hands are pressed into the abdominal wall, so that they surround the fundus uteri and almost touch at the fingertips.

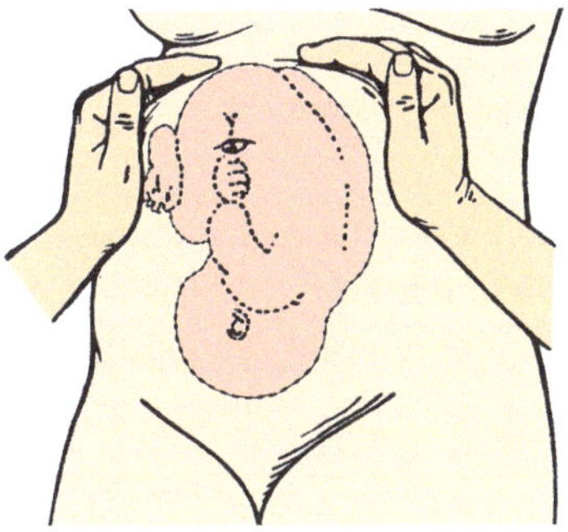

Fig. 3.12: First Leopold's maneuver.

This maneuver answers two questions:
- Where (how high) is the fundus uteri? → determination of pregnancy duration (fundal height/pregnancy; see p. 23).
- What fetal part is to be found at the uterine fundus?

99 % of the time one of the large fetal parts is felt:
- Breech (in 94 %): the smaller of the large parts, uneven, variable consistency, no ballottement, or
- Head (in 5 %): larger, even, round shape, firm, ballottement, or
- Part of the rump (in 1 %, transverse lie, see p. 264).

One differentiates between the large fetal parts (head, breech, back) and the small parts (legs, arms (→ arms are rarely felt)).

Second maneuver. Both hands slide, flattening and parallel to each other, from the fundus down either side of the abdomen (Fig. 3.13), to the level of the navel. In this way they come to lie on the sides of the uterus.

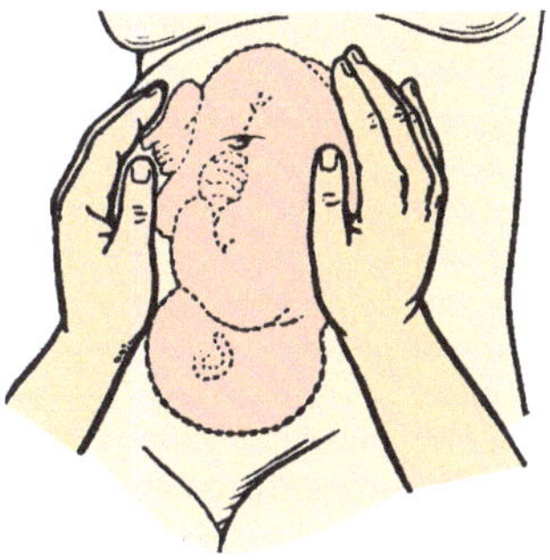

Fig. 3.13: Second Leopold's maneuver.

This maneuver clarifies where the back and the small parts are.

Procedure. Both hands are flat. Alternately, one hand palpates, with slightly bent fingers; the other remains immobile and exerts a gentle counter pressure.
- The back is long and even, almost cylindrical.
- The small parts, or limbs, are recognizably uneven, partly pointy and partly smooth bulges which can be moved or which move or slightly change position on palpation.
- The abdominal side is palpably sunken between breech and head.
- In transverse lie (see p. 264) large parts are felt on both sides: head and breech.

Third maneuver. Prerequisite: the presenting part is not fully engaged and is slightly mobile on palpation.
- The not-yet-engaged presenting part is grasped (gently, or the pregnant woman will tense her abdomen) between thumb and well-spread second and third fingers. In order to reach the presenting pole the fingers are pressed deeply into the suprapubic area (Fig. 3.14).

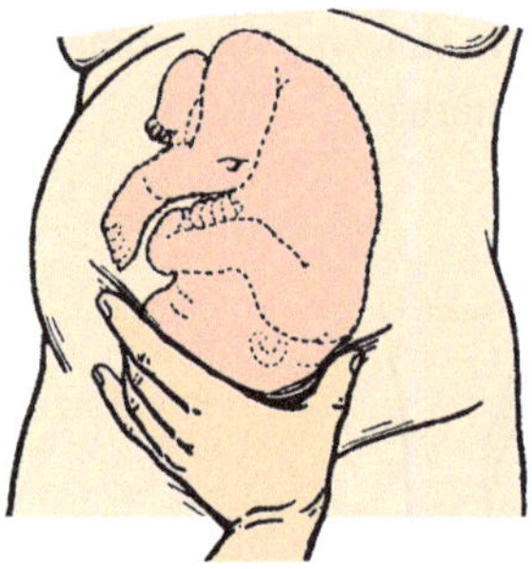

Fig. 3.14: Third Leopold's maneuver.

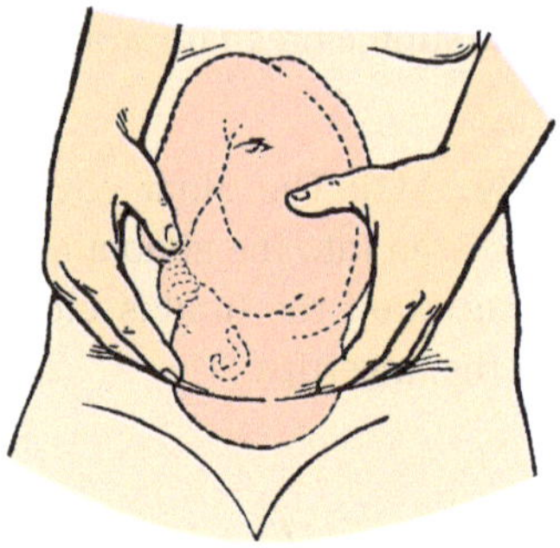

Fig. 3.15: Fourth Leopold's maneuver.

- Ballottement: once the presenting part is held, the examiner attempts to move it rapidly back and forth. The head "bounces" back and forth, the breech does not.

Fourth maneuver. Prerequisite: the presenting part is engaged.

- The examiner sits or stands on one side of the woman, facing her feet, places hands on abdomen (Fig. 3.15), and slides them along the lower uterus towards the pelvis, fingertips pointing towards each other.
- The penetration of the hands into the pelvic inlet takes place in two stages.
- Phase 1: gently, carefully, and under weak pressure, the hands are slowly pushed deeper into the pelvis from the original position. Resistance is felt as the pregnant woman tenses her muscles.
- Phase II: as soon as the muscles have relaxed, the hands are moved deeper and towards each other in several short, quick movements. In this way the examiner moves into the pelvis following the – engaged – presenting part and reaches it (depending on the station) in the depths of the pelvis (see p. 162).

Difference between the third and fourth maneuver. As long as the presenting part is mobile and not yet engaged, the third maneuver is used. If the presenting part is deeper, the fourth maneuver is used.

How much of the presenting part is above the pelvis, how much of it is engaged? The deeper the head is, the more relevant the fourth maneuver becomes.

Note. The fourth Leopold maneuver is the only external method of palpation with which the slow descent of the head into the pelvis can be followed.

Zangemeister maneuver (see p. 295)

Position of the fetus: lie, position, attitude, presentation

Four fundamental obstetric terms (Fig. 3.16)

Lie. Relationship of the longitudinal axis of the baby to the longitudinal axis of the mother: longitudinal, transverse or oblique lie.

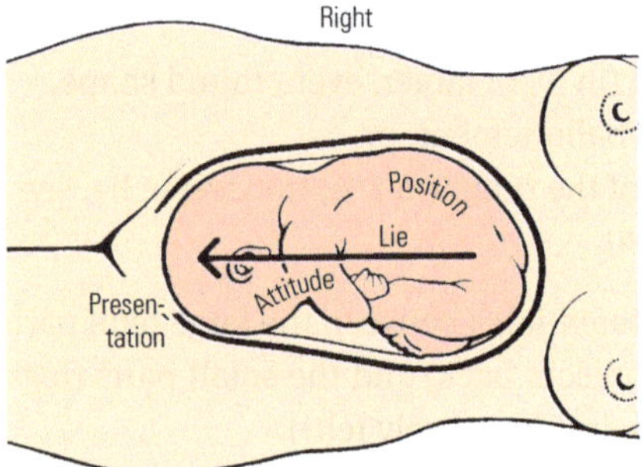

Fig. 3.16: Fundamental terms: lie, position, attitude, presentation.

Position. Relationship of the presenting part to the mother's right or left side and pelvis. Occiput left lateral, left anterior, left posterior, and so on.

Presentation. The relationship of the presenting part to the pelvic inlet. The presenting part is that which is encountered by the finger on vaginal examination (that which presents itself on internal examination). The presenting part is the lowermost part.

In a cephalic presentation (head first), the baby's back is on the mother's left side twice as often as on the right.
Cephalic presentations (head leading = longitudinal lies) are the most common, and are classified according to the position of the occiput (back of the head) as follows (Fig. 3.17, 3.18):
- Position: right (R) or left (L).
- Presenting part: vertex (O = occiput).
- Presentation: anterior (A), lateral (L) or posterior (P).
- Left occipito-transverse (or occipito-lateral): (LOT/LOL) Baby's back and occiput lateral, on the mother's left, baby is facing mother's right side.
- Left occipito-anterior. (LOA): Baby's back is on the left side of the mother, occiput frontal (= baby is facing mother's back).
- Left occipito-posterior (LOP): Baby's back is on the left side of the mother, occiput posterior (= baby is facing pubic symphysis).
- Right occipito-transverse (or occipito-lateral): (ROT/ROL) Baby's back and occiput lateral, on the mother's right side, baby is facing mother's left side.
- Right occipito-anterior. (ROA): Baby's back is on the mother's right side, occiput frontal (= baby is facing mother's back).
- Right occipito-posterior (ROP): Baby's back is on the right side of the mother, occiput posterior (= baby is facing pubic symphysis).

In breech presentations the sacrum (S) is the reference point rather than the occiput, and in cephalic malpresentations the chin (M = mentum).

Attitude. Relationship of the fetal parts to one another; how the baby "holds" itself. The relationship between head and trunk during passage of the birth canal is crucial.

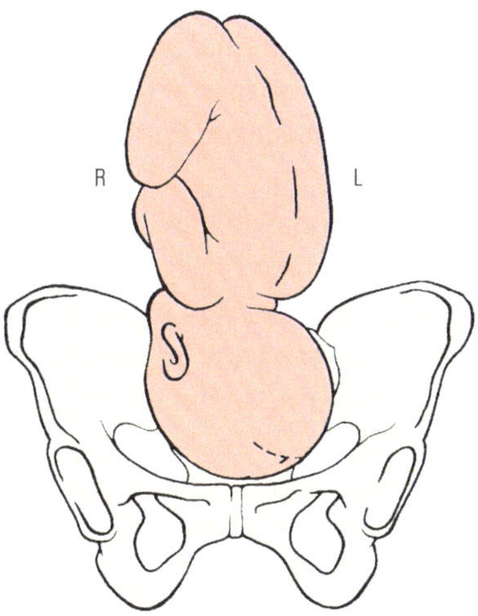

Fig. 3.17: Left occipitoanterior (LOA).

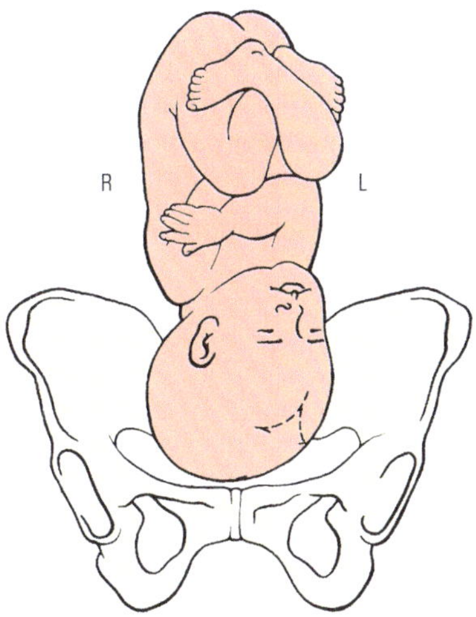

Fig. 3.18: Right occipitoposterior (ROP).

The normal or regular attitude is a deeply flexed head (chin on chest) passing into the pelvic inlet.
A malposition is any deviation from this attitude, extended or deflexed (extended attitudes; see p. 220).
Vertex/cephalic presentation. After adoption of the attitude (flexed or extended), the possible cephalic presentations are:
- Occiput (= normal vertex presentation) → posterior fontanelle, sinciput palpable → anterior fontanelle (bregma) palpable.
- Brow or face.
- Occiput, sinciput, and so on can be posterior, anterior, or lateral (position).

Breech presentations. The possible breech presentations are: frank breech (buttocks only), complete breech (buttocks and one or both feet), footling breech (one or both feet), or kneeling breech (one or both knees).

Transverse lie. The shoulder (arm) presents.

Statistics:
- Of 100 pregnant women 99 babies will be in longitudinal lie, one in transverse.
- Of 99 longitudinal lies, 94 will be in cephalic presentation at term, and 5 in breech.

Of the 94 cephalic presentations, 92 will be occipito-anterior in labor. In the remaining two of those 94 cases, another part of the head leads (sinciput, brow, face) or occipito-posterior; these cephalic presentations are known as malpresentations or malpositions (occipito-posterior).

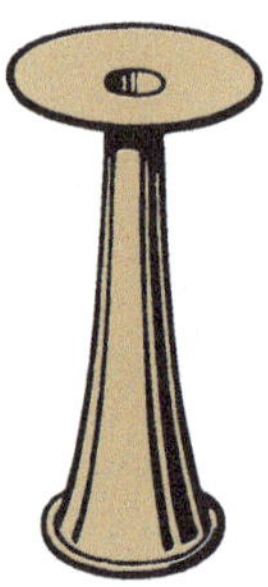

Fig. 3.19: Obstetric stethoscope (Pinard type).

Heart sounds, auscultation

Heart sounds

Six sound phenomena may be perceived on abdominal auscultation of the pregnant woman: three from the fetus, three from the mother.

From the fetus

- Fetal heart sounds. 110–150/min. The heart sounds are regular, strong double beats with the emphasis on the first sound. They are comparable to the “tick-tock” of the clock, but the rate of heart sounds is much faster. The double beat (the “tick-tock”) is counted as one beat.
- Instrument: obstetric stethoscope, Pinard type (Fig. 3.19).
- Cord sounds or funic souffle. 110–150/min. A blowing or scraping noise, synchronous with the fetal heart sounds. They originate from the foramen ovale or ductus botalli.
- Fetal movement. Scraping, rubbing or short abrupt sounds, particularly in the area of the feet (audible with the stethoscope), sometimes like quiet drumbeats.

From the mother

- Aortic pulse. 70/min (maternal heart rate). Loud tapping at the frequency of the maternal pulse; cannot be mistaken for the fetal heart sounds.
- Uterine soufflé. 70/min. Soft blowing sound in the dilated uterine blood vessels at the rate of the maternal pulse. Very easily and frequently heard, most clearly on the sides of the uterus. The uterine sound which is also to be heard in the case of large fibroid cysts (or myomas) is unimportant.
- Bowel sounds. Caused by movement of the bowels, particularly after meals; often very loud and polyphonous: rubbing, ringing, cooing, hissing.

Auscultation

Auscultation of fetal heart sounds has not become obsolete with ultrasound and cardiotocography; doctor and midwife must take the time to practice auscultation. The heart sounds are listened to attentively over a longer period and counted with a handheld watch, in particular in cases of fetal distress. Auscultation is performed shortly before and shortly after the contraction in order to detect fetal distress.

Practice tip. Always take the mother's pulse at the wrist while listening to the fetal heart sounds. This is the only sure way to differentiate the maternal from the fetal heart sounds.

Mother and child rarely have the same rate: elevation of maternal pulse (fever), decreased fetal rate (distress) or both.

When is the fetal heart audible for the first time? The well-trained beginner can hear the fetal heart from week 20. Experience and circumstances determine the time period: position of the fetal back, distance of the fetal heart from the abdominal wall, thickness of the abdominal wall, amount of liquor.

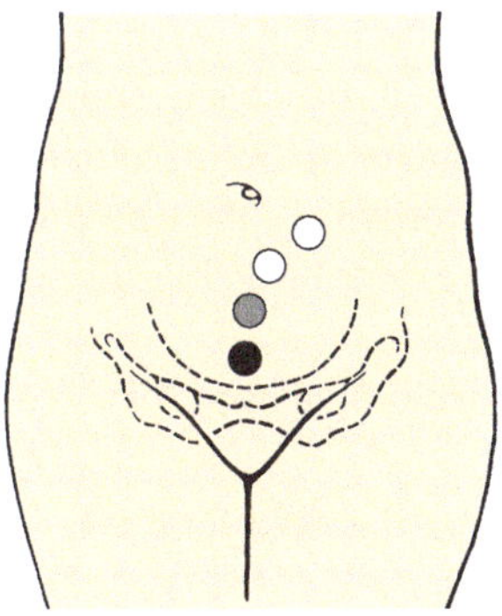

Fig. 3.20: Migration of fetal heart sounds in LOA. ○ = heart sounds in early labor ◍ = heart sounds at the beginning of second stage ● = heart sounds shortly before delivery.

Where are the heart sounds heard most clearly?

- Weeks 20–28: midline directly above the pubic symphysis or over the main abdominal protuberance.
- From week 28 focal point is the position of the fetal back. The fetal heart is best heard where its back lies against the wall of the uterus.
- Vertex lie, occipito-anterior: the heart is loudest where the fetal back lies against the uterus- LOA left, ROA on the right.
- As labor progresses, so do the heart sounds (Fig. 3.20).

External pelvic examination, pelvimetry

Four pelvic measurements are made (Fig 3.21, 22)
Inter-spinous diameter (distantia spinarum) 25–26 cm
Inter-crestal diameter (distantia cristarum) 28–29 cm
Distantia trochanterica 31–32 cm
External conjugate 20 cm

Measurement with the pelvimeter. The following measurements are to be taken:

Inter-spinous diameter (Fig. 3.21). Distance between the spinae iliacae anteriores superiores: 25–26 cm.

The points of the pelvimeter are taken and held on each of the spina and the measurement is read on the graduated bow.

Inter-crestal diameter (Fig. 3.21). The points of the pelvimeter are used to find the cristae iliacae (iliac crests), and these are followed until the points furthest from each other are found: 28–29 cm.

Distantia trochanterica (Fig. 3.21). Less important. Palpate to find the furthest apart points of the greater trochanters: 31–32 cm. In order to find them more easily, ask the woman to rotate her legs outwards.

External conjugate (Fig. 3.22). Best measured when the woman is upright or lying on her side. One point of the pelvimeter is placed on the dimple between the spinous processes of the lumbar vertebrae 3–4 (upper point of the Michaelis rhomboid), which is usually easily felt. The other point is placed in the middle of the upper edge of the pubic symphysis.

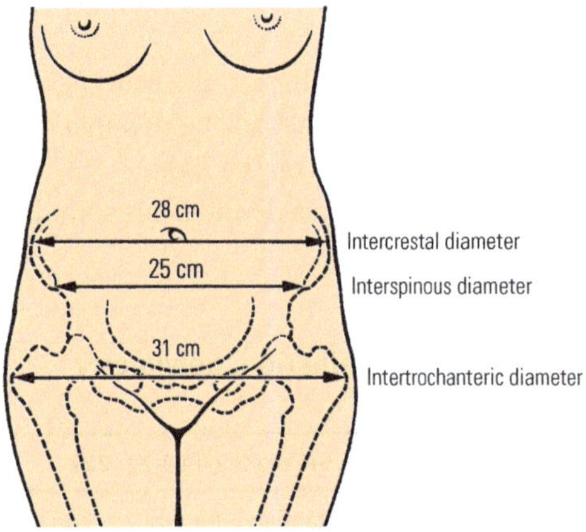

Fig. 3.21: Interspinous diameter, intercrestal diameter, intertrochanteric diameter.

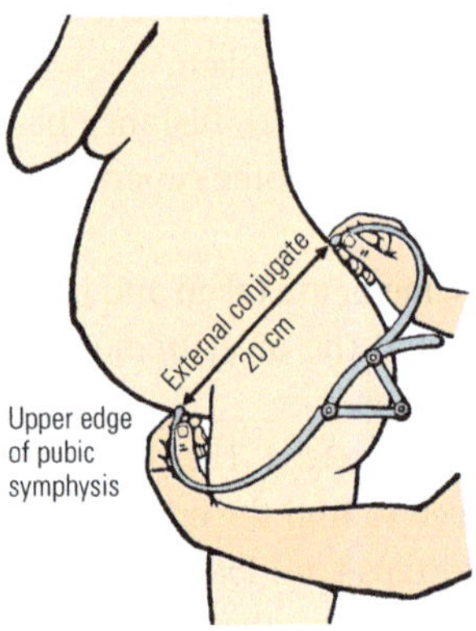

Fig. 3.22: External conjugate.

What use is external pelvimetry? The greater (or false) pelvis is measured in this way. However the internal bony frame of the birth canal which is of obstetric interest is the lesser (or true) pelvis (see p. 143). When a normal or small pelvis is referred to, it is the true pelvis which is meant, which cannot be measured externally (except by x-ray or NMR). Therefore it is important that midwives and obstetricians know about the anatomical relationships between the two.

Abnormal measurements of the false pelvis can indicate anomalies of the true pelvis.

Difference between interspinous and intercrestal diameters. The difference between the two main transverse measurements is more important than the actual measurements.

- A difference of three cm indicates that the false and most likely the true pelvis are of normal proportions.
- It must be assumed that the pelvis is contracted (the anteroposterior or conjugate diameter of the pelvic inlet is shortened; see p. 143) if the difference is 1–1.5 cm, if there is no difference, or if the intercrestal diameter is greater than the interspinous.

Reduced pelvic measurements. In the contracted pelvis (see p. 296), all external (and internal) measurements are smaller than the normal measurements; in this case the pelvis is a smaller version of the normal pelvis (Bumm).

It is possible to determine the important obstetric or true conjugate, anteroposterior diameter of the pelvic inlet, by subtracting 8–9 cm from the external conjugate. It has been shown, however, that this estimate is too inaccurate, so it is rarely used. Nevertheless, the true conjugate can to a certain extent be deduced from the external conjugate.

- > 20 cm means the true conjugate is of normal length.
- 20–19 cm normal length or slightly shortened.
- 18 cm shortened.

Practice tip. It must be clear that external pelvimetry can only give an approximate idea of pelvic shape and size.

Vaginal examination. Cervical status, pelvic exam

The internal examination fulfills two purposes: an indication of the risk of preterm labor and of progress in labor is gained from examination of the cervix, and the bony pelvis is examined. Antenatal care up until week 36 includes regular internal exams, in particular for early recognition of premature cervical ripening or cervical incompetence.

Cervical assessment score in pregnancy

Length of the cervical canal

3 cm (intact)	0 points
2 cm (partially effaced)	1 point
1 cm (considerably effaced)	2 points
0 cm (fully effaced)	3 points

Dilatation of the external os

Closed	0 points
Fingertip wide	1 point
Wide enough for insertion of a finger	2 points
≥ 2 cm open	3 points

Consistency

Rigid	0 points
Medium	1 point
Soft	3 points

Practice tip. Total score of > 3 risk of preterm labor! Use of transvaginal sonography advisable (see p. 101).

Labor progress score

Close to the due date or when a pregnancy needs to be brought to an end for medical reasons, the vaginal exam is performed to determine progress and also to deliver a prognosis on labor length and birth method.

Cervical effacement

≥ 2 cm (intact or partially effaced)	0 points
1 cm (considerably effaced)	1.5 points
0 cm (fully effaced)	3 points

Cervical consistency

Rigid	0 points
Medium	1.5 points
Soft	3 points

Cervical position

Posterior (sacral)	0 points
Mid-position	1.5 points
Anterior	2 points

Cervical dilatation

Closed	0 points
1 cm dilated	1 point
2 cm dilated	2 points
≥ 3 cm dilated	3 points

Fetal Station

2 cm above the ischial spines (–2)	0 points
1 cm above (–1) or zero station	1 point
2 cm below (+2)	2 points

Total score (labor progress points) > 7 means active labor and rapid cervical dilation is imminent.

Internal pelvic exam

First question: Does the middle finger, on examination with pointer and middle finger, reach the sacral promontory?

If the answer is no, the obstetric conjugate is not shortened (Fig. 3.23). The middle finger inserted into the vagina does not reach the sacral promontory of a regular sized pelvis. If the answer is yes, the obstetric conjugate is shortened, indicative of pelvic contraction.

Further questions

- Anterior sacral wall: Is it curved or flattened? Are any bony exostoses, tumors or projections to be detected on the anterior surface?
- Coccyx: Mobile? Protruding? At right angles to the sacrum? Immobile?
- Posterior wall of the pubis: Does the pubis appear particularly thick? Are any protuber-

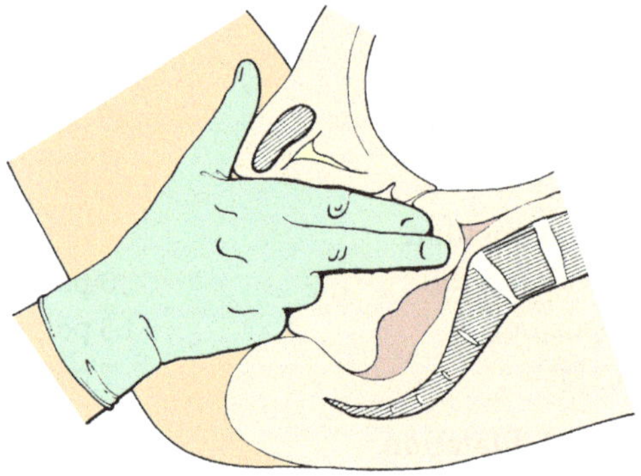

Fig. 3.23: Pelvic exam. If the middle finger does not reach the sacral promontory the pelvic inlet cannot be contracted.

ances to be felt such as internally projecting pubic crest? Exostoses are not rare here.
- Pelvic brim: Reachable? The lateral and posterior parts of the pelvic brim are not reachable in a normal pelvis. Equally rounded on both sides? Flatter on one side?
- Ischial spines: Easy or difficult to find, protruding, normal distance apart? If they are closer to each other than normal this indicates a transverse narrowing of the mid-pelvis, a so-called funnel pelvis (rare).
- Palpation of the soft tissue parts of the pelvis (pelvic floor, ligaments): Relaxed or unusually firm? Edema? Scarring?

3.1.3 General examination

Note. Obligatory examinations in addition to the obstetric exam:
- Blood pressure (meaning see p. 32): upper norm 135/85 mmHg.
- Mid-stream urine for protein (meaning see p. 33), sediment, bacteria (if applicable).
- Body weight (meaning see p. 33).
- Edema, varicosities. Weight gain during pregnancy 11–12 kg. 400–500 g/week in last trimester. Greater weight gain means edema and risk of PIH.

Initial serology
- Blood group, rhesus factor (meaning, see p. 113).
- Hemoglobin, rubella and irregular antibodies.
- Syphilis (meaning, see p. 132).
- HIV-test should be offered.

Obligatory check-ups at each antenatal visit
- Blood pressure.
- Mid-stream urine as at initial check-up.
- Weight check.
- Edema.
- Hemoglobin.

Blood pressure, urine, weight

The following check-ups assist in **PIH early recognition** (see p. 74).

Measurement of blood pressure. Result can be elevated (arterial hypertension) or low (arterial hypotension) blood pressure.

Arterial hypotension. Treatment decision should be made generously in the interests of the baby.
- Systolic < 100 mmHg, repeated measurements.
- Circulatory dysregulation. Dizziness, visual disturbance, fainting, profuse sweating, vegetative dysregulation on changing position, orthostatic syndrome.

Therapy. Support or compression stockings class 2 (20–30 mmHg).

Urinalysis

Methods. Examination for protein and sugar is vital.
- Dipstick. Qualitative and crude quantitative analysis. The dipstick is immersed in the urine and the color reaction interpreted.
- Laboratory analysis. The pregnant woman is given a urine glass into which she urinates.

- Proteinuria.
- Physiological proteinuria of pregnancy. Protein excretion is particularly frequent in the second half of pregnancy and "normal" at < 300mg/24h.
- Pathological proteinuria of pregnancy. ≥ 300mg/24h (increased capillary permeability, symptom of PIH; see p. 74).
- If protein is detected, a urine sediment test is required. Analysis for cells (epithelial, white, red) and casts (red blood cell or white blood cell casts).
- Midstream urine is spontaneous urination for bacteriological analysis. Procedure: cleansing of the genital area (orificium urethrae), then after discarding the first stream (flushing of the urethra), urine is collected in a sterile container.
  - More than 100,000 organisms/ml urine bacteriuria, urinary tract infection (UTI);
  - 10,000–100,000 organisms/ml urine requiring renewed check-up:
  - 1,000 organisms/ml urine caused by contamination with bacteria which colonize the urethra and genital area.
- Bacteriological analysis. In cases of preterm labor, UTI (frequent micturition, burning sensation on urination), elevated blood pressure, pathological urine sediment bacteriological analysis of mid-stream urine (urine culture, native urine) is the preferred method in order to be able to treat bacterial excretion (see pyelonephritis, p. 86).

Weight

Weight gain

- By week 20 → 5 kg have been gained.
- Weight gain in the last weeks of pregnancy 400 g/week.
- Total weight gain in pregnancy 11–12 kg.
- Desirable weight gain in relation to body-mass-index (BMI); see p. 66.

Weight distribution (11–12 kg)

- 3,300 g baby.
- 650 g placenta, 800 g amniotic fluid.
- 900 g uterine growth.
- 400 g breast growth.
- 1,250 g increase in blood volume, 2,000 g tissue fluids.
- 1,700 g fat depot.

Weight plunge. A few days before the birth the weight may drop by 0.5–1 kg.

Weight check

- In the first half of pregnancy weight is monitored in order to detect excessive weight loss (e.g., due to disrupted appetite, nausea, morning sickness) early.
- Regular monitoring in the second half of pregnancy, as PIH may be advisable in cases of marked weight gain.

Serology, blood group, antibodies

Determination of blood group and factors, antibodies, Obligatory blood tests are:

- Syphilis serology, see also p. 132,
- Rubella serology (p. 119),
- Blood grouping, rhesus typing (Rhesus blood group antigen D),
- Life-threatening hemorrhages necessitate fast transfusion, for which the blood group and factors must be known. In cases of rhesus incompatibility between mother and fetus, steps must be taken to keep the fetus alive (p. 113).
- Antibodies against the antigens D, C, c, E, e, Kell, Fy, S.

Irregular antibodies. Those antibodies which do not endanger the fetus (natural irregular antibodies) are listed in Table 3.1.

Dangerous antibodies cause a rapid destruction of fetal erythrocytes: hemolytic disease of the fetus and newborn, or erythroblastosis fetalis (Tab. 3.2).

Tab. 3.1: Natural irregular antibodies in pregnancy without therapeutic consequence (according to K. Fischer).

Lewis system	Anti-Lewis A Anti-Lewis B	
ABH system	Anti-A_1 in A_2 and A_2B Anti-H in A_1 and A_1B	
MN system	Anti M, Anti N	in negative indirect Coombs' test
P system	Anti P	

Tab. 3.2: Irregular IgG antibodies. Incidence in 2,000 babies with hemolytic disease of the newborn before introduction of the anti-D prophylaxis and without ABO erythroblastosis (according to K. Fischer).

Antibody	**Incidence (%)**
Anti-D including – Anti-D + C + E – Anti-D + K – Anti-D + S	98.04
Other antibodies	1.96
Anti-c	1.29
Anti-E	0.29
Anti-E +Fy(a)	0.05
Anti-C	0.05
Anti-K	0.19
Anti-Fy(a)	0.05
Anti-Jk(a)	0.05

Rules for antibody testing in maternal ABO, Rhesus system

- ABO System, blood group O. Hemolysin test only.
- Both parents Rhesus negative (no D-antigen!). Hemolytic disease unlikely (96 % caused by Rhesus factor).
- Test for irregular antibodies weeks 25–32 if none detected in initial test (anti-D prophylaxis in pregnancy, see p. 116).
- If antibodies detected in initial test. Check specificity and titer every four weeks.
- Titer is not a reliable factor in prognosis. If the woman has already been sensitized (from an earlier pregnancy or transfusion), antibodies will be produced in a subsequent pregnancy, even if the baby is Rh-negative, i.e., not in danger.

Practice tip. The only reliable methods to determine the condition of the fetus are ultrasound diagnosis and testing hemoglobin levels in fetal blood (cordocentesis).

Care in cases of hemolytic disease is discussed in detail on p. 113.

Note. Two questions must be asked after each prenatal check-up:
Is the pregnancy progressing normally? Which risk factors endanger the life of the mother, the fetus, or both?

Screening tests

Vaginal candidiasis. Some 35 % of women have vaginal yeast infections at term (mostly Candida albicans), which is then transmitted to around 80 % of newborns born vaginally. The resulting oral or ano-genital mycotic infection is unpleasant and will require treatment, but a mature newborn is not at risk; the danger for premature babies is greater.

Generalized screening is advisable, and if necessary treatment in week 34. If the diagnosis is confirmed by a yeast culture (e.g., Sabouraud-glucose-agar), intravaginal therapy with single-dose imidazole should be initiated.

Genital chlamydia. Around 1 % of pregnant women are infected with Chlamydia trachomatis of the urethra and cervix. This colonization may increase the risk of premature rupture of membranes (PROM) and preterm birth, but the literature is conflicting. The risk of newborns born vaginally becoming infected is significant: around 30 % develop conjunctivitis, 10 % develop an atypical pneumonia.

Prenatal screening for chlamydia is recommended. A swab of cervix and urethra and a tissue culture or enzyme immuno-assay. Treatment is with oral erythromycin (4 × 500 g for seven days), and the partner must also be treated.

Group B Streptococcus (GBS). Streptococci of the serological group B cause neonatal B streptococcal infection (see p. 468), a dramatic disease with high mortality and morbidity, and late complications; incidence of early-onset GBS in the US before the introduction of antibiotic prophylaxis 2 : 1,000.

Risk factors for early-onset neonatal GBS infection:
- Rectovaginal screening positive in pregnancy or at the beginning of labor.
- ≥ 18 hours between ROM and delivery.
- Temperature of ≥ 38 °C in labor.
- Preterm delivery < 37 weeks.

Around 10–30 % of pregnant women have asymptomatic GBS colonization of the anorectal and genital region, so the following recommendations apply:
Between weeks 34 and 36, a vaginal and anorectal swab is performed on all pregnant women, which is then sent for a bacteriological culture.
It is important to clarify which selective media the lab will use.
Rapid tests are unadvisable.
If the result is positive the woman receives a **peripartal prophylaxis** during labor (if vaginal birth is planned).
- **Penicillin G**, 5 million units IV initially, then 2.5 million units IV every four hours until delivery, or
- **Ampicillin**, 2 g IV initially, then 1 g IV every four hours until delivery.
- In case of penicillin allergy, Cefazolin, 2 g IV initially, then 1 g IV every eight hours until delivery.

If the GBS status of a woman in labor is unknown, but risk factors such as preterm delivery, ≥ 18 hours between ROM and delivery, temperature of ≥ 38 °C in labor are present, she should receive antibiotics prophylactically.
Symptomatic pregnant women < 37 weeks (preterm labor, ruptured membranes, at risk of preterm delivery) with a positive GBS test should receive antibiotics prophylactically in pregnancy and while in labor. Asymptomatic women with a positive GBS test should only receive prophylaxis in labor. Women who have already had a baby with GBS should be prophylactically treated in labor.

3.1.4 Examination of the woman at risk

High-risk pregnancy

Definition. Pregnancy in which mother or fetus are endangered due to one or more risk factors. 14 major risk factors are:
1. PIH. BP ≥ 140/90 mm Hg, proteinuria ≥ 0.5 g %; details see p. 74.
2. Prolonged pregnancy ≥ seven days; see p. 108.
3. Hemolytic disease of the fetus; see p. 113.
4. Diabetes mellitus (manifest, latent); see p. 87.
5. Preterm delivery, including cervical incompetence; see p. 99.
6. History of preterm delivery, miscarriage, stillbirth, cesarean section, difficult vaginal operative birth.
7. Age. Late age at first birth (over 35 years), or late multigravida (over 40 years), young primigravida (< 18 years).
8. Organ disease. Heart, circulatory system, lungs, liver kidneys, thyroid; see p. 84.
9. Anemia in pregnancy (Hb < 8 g%).
10. Malpresentation (transverse lie), breech, cephalopelvic disproportion (CPD), multiple birth, pelvic anomaly.

11. Weight. Obesity ≥ 15 kg overweight. Normal weight in kg = height above 100 cm minus 10 %. X = (height–100) – (height–100)/10.
12. Infectious diseases. Syphilis, tuberculosis, toxoplasmosis, AIDS, cytomegalovirus, herpes, listeriosis, viral diseases; see p. 118.
13. Discordance between uterus size and gestational age; see p. 108.
14. Hemorrhage; see p. 351.

Note. 30 % of pregnancies in central Europe are high risk.

Practice tip. High-risk pregnancy. Presence of a risk factor does not necessarily mean acute danger. It does, however, represent a potential danger requiring attentive care (intensive surveillance): frequency of visits, additional assessments (see below). The point of identifying risk factors and labeling high-risk pregnancies is not to scare the pregnant women. It is therefore doubtful that such labeling is useful.

Additional assessment. Investigative procedures which are performed in the care of high-risk pregnant women in order to obtain information about the fetus.

Note. All medical-technical or clinical-chemical procedures are only to be interpreted in connection with the clinical manifestation at the bedside.

Diagnostics

- The respiratory function of the placenta: cardiotocography, blood flow measurement.
- The nutritive function of the placenta: sonographic diagnosis, blood flow measurement.
- Fetal lung maturity.
- Genetic disorders (amniotic fluid).

Cardiotocography (CTG), electronic fetal monitoring (EFM)

Auscultation of fetal heart tones (see p. 28) has the following disadvantages: intermittent detection, heart rate variations associated with contractions will not be noticed in routine use, short-term heart rate variations will not be registered.

Definition. Cardiotocography is the continuous simultaneous recording (electronic fetal monitoring, EFM) of the fetal heart rate (FHR) and uterine contractions in late pregnancy (ante partum EFM) and during labor (intrapartum EFM), in order to monitor the fetus and recognize intrauterine hypoxia.

Pathophysiology of fetal heart rate regulation. The heart rate (HR) is influenced by biochemical, neural, and hemodynamic factors.
- *Biochemical factors.* Uterine contractions cause compression of the uterine arteries. This results in contraction-related reduction of oxygen for the fetus if the intervals between contractions are not long enough, and a decrease in FHR, typically following the contraction (late deceleration).
- *Neural factors.* Compression of the fetal head during the contraction causes stimulation of the vagus nerve, which leads to a simultaneous decrease in FHR (early deceleration).
- *Hemodynamic factors.* Interruption of the umbilical blood flow due to compression of the umbilical vein or arteries cause contraction-related HR decline which are variable in form and temporal in relationship to contractions (variable decelerations; venous backflow is controlled by baroreceptor reflex, according to Hammacher).

Cardiography. Heart rate detection involves PCG (heart tones), ECG (electric cardiac activity), and echocardiography (heart wall movements).

PCG (Phonocardiography). Registration of heart sounds from maternal abdomen with a special microphone.
- *Application.* Antepartum and in early labor, in particular as long as the membranes have not broken.
- *Disadvantages.* Difficult in obese women, active babies, anterior placenta, frequent repositioning of the microphone on change in maternal position, fetal movements.

ECG (electrocardiography). Transmission directly via an electrode on the fetus or indirectly via the maternal abdomen (abdominal electrocardiography).
- *Direct electrocardiography.* Application: intrapartum: flawless registration, regardless of position and movement (telemetry!); disadvantage: only once waters have broken (risk of infection).
- *Abdominal electrocardiography.* Ante partum and in early labor. Disadvantage: weak signal before week 36 (vernix layer).

Echocardiography (cardiac ultrasound). Registration of movement of, for example, the heart valves using Doppler Effect.
- *Application.* Ante- and intrapartum-minimal time expenditure.
- *Disadvantage.* Change of the reflection point causes alterations in the heart rate pattern (pseudofluctuation = jitter).

Beat-to-beat method (instantaneous heart beat registration). The interval between each heart beat (one heart cycle) is calculated.
Example. After electronic recognition (and filtering of disturbances), the frequency/minute is calculated from the interval between two R-peaks or from the beginning of the first heart sound. Thus the value is not calculated from a number of heart cycle interval measurements.

Tocography (recording of uterine contractions). Two methods are possible:
- Externally via a transducer on the maternal abdomen. Application: ante- and intrapartum, fetal movements are registered. Disadvantage: does not measure absolute intrauterine pressure.
- Internally, pressure variations in the amniotic cavity are registered via an open-ended fluid-filled catheter and transmitted to a pressure sensor; application intrapartum, in particular in cases of prior Cesarean section; measures absolute pressure. Disadvantages: only possible after rupture of

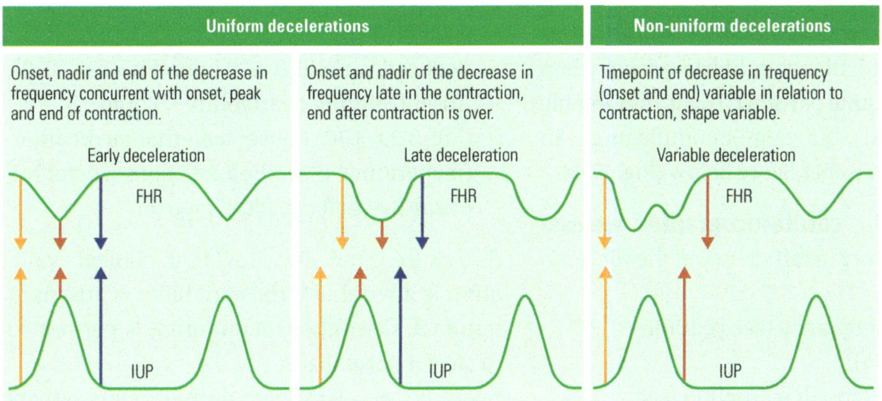

Fig. 3.24: Decelerations coincident with contractions (FHR = fetal heart rate, IUP = intra uterine pressure).

membranes, potential for bacterial ascent and chorioamnionitis.

There are **long-term**, **intermediate**, and **short-term** heart rate patterns.

Long-term HR patterns. Baseline frequency, extended rest period; in beats per minute (bpm):
- Normal cardiac rhythm: 110–150.
- Bradycardia: baseline deceleration ≥ 3 min:
  - mild bradycardia: 100–109;
  - (severe) bradycardia < 100.
- Tachycardia: Baseline acceleration ≥ 10 min:
  - Mild tachycardia: 151–160;
  - Moderate tachycardia: 161–180;
  - (Severe) tachycardia: > 180.

Intermediate HR patterns
- Increase of frequency (acceleration):
  - episodic, not associated with contractions;
  - periodic, associated with contractions.
- Decrease in frequency (deceleration) in association with contractions; see Fig. 3.24:
  - Uniform types: early deceleration, late deceleration;
  - Nonuniform: variable deceleration.

Short-term HR patterns. Variability (= oscillation; characterized by oscillation amplitude and frequency; see Fig. 3.25).

CTG scores. The cardiotocogram should be interpreted systematically and analytically. The beginner in particular should use a score when interpreting an ante partum CTG, as they enable not only analysis, but (semi)quantification. An example is the Fischer Score below (Fig. 3.26).

Indications for cardiotocographic assessment. Respiratory insufficiency of the placenta in cases of:
- Prolonged pregnancy (see p. 108).
- PIH (see p. 74).
- Intrauterine growth restriction (see p. 107).
- Heart sound alteration.
- Fetal hemolytic disease (see p. 113).

Only relevant for a fetus which will be viable on delivery.

CTG interpretation

Antepartal cardiotocography is almost always performed under stress-free conditions. In rare cases, stress can be used to simulate labor, which causes a reduction in uteroplacental circulation due to contractions; by observing the effect of this reduction on the FHR placenta function can be tested.

Nonstress-test (NST; Fig. 3.27). Test period 30 min.

Baseline
- Normal 110–150 bpm.
- Tachycardia > 150 bpm (Fig. 3.28); cause: fetal activity, fever, maternal medication (tocolysis!), hypoxia, fetal myocarditis.
- Bradycardia < 110; cause: maternal hypotension, supine hypotensive syndrome, prolonged contraction, vagotonus, fetal hypoxia, arrhythmia (in particular in cases of persistent bradycardia over a longer period).

Variability
- Moderate (normal) 10–25 bpm.
- Marked variability > 25 bpm; possibly an umbilical cord symptom.
- Reduced variability 5–9 bpm (Fig. 3.29, 3.30).
- Absent/minimal variability < 5 bpm (Fig. 3.29, 3.30) Cause: maternal medication (meperidine, atropine), rest phase, cerebral or cardiac defects, fetal hypoxia.

As a cause is not always evident, clinical evaluation is advisable if the variability is absent or minimal. Continuous monitoring is performed in case it normalizes.
Sporadic accelerations during fetal activity indicate fetal wellbeing (Evertson's Nonstress-

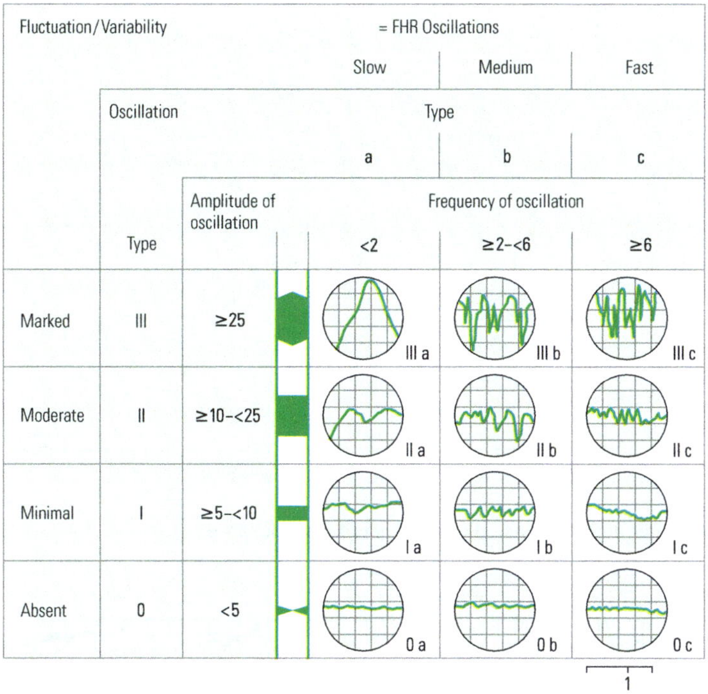

Fig. 3.25: Evaluation of variability using Hammacher's 12 oscillation types.

		0	1	2	Σ
Baseline FHR	Level (bpm)	<100 >170	100–110 150–170	110–150	
	Range (bpm)	<5	5–10 >30	10–30	
	Zero crossing/min	<2	2–6	>6	
FHR alterations	Accelerations	None	periodic	episodic	
	Decelerations	late, variable with non-reassuring characteristics	variable	none, sporadic dips	
	Score				
	Monitoring period 30 min Adding at least 10 min for baseline variability, in case of [green shading] non-reassuring trace				

Fig. 3.26: Score to evaluate fetal condition (after Fischer and colleagues, in the version altered acc. to FIGO guidelines). Five criteria are assigned 0–2 points each: 8–10 points normal, 5–7 points fetal wellbeing questionable, ≤ 4 fetal well-being endangered.

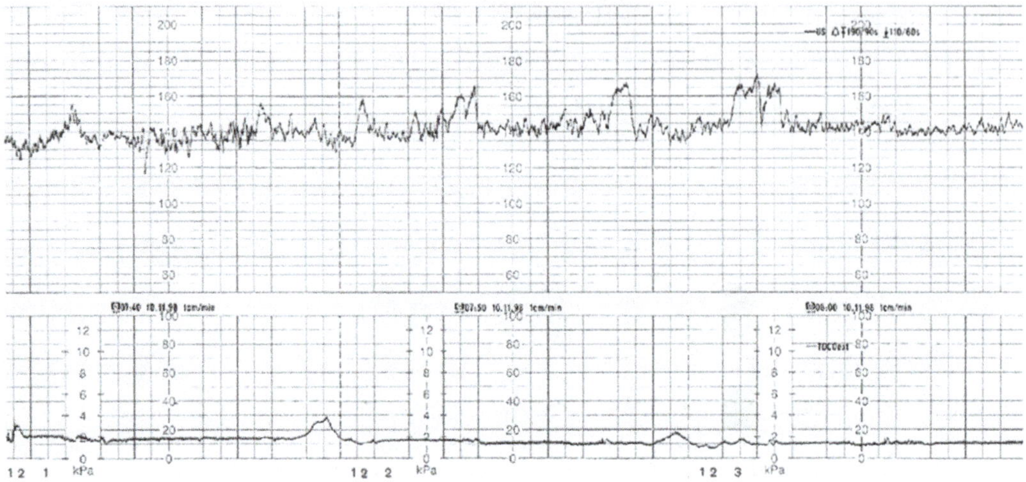

Fig. 3.27: Antenatal FHR tracing with sporadic accelerations. 31 year-old para 1 in week 37 + 6.

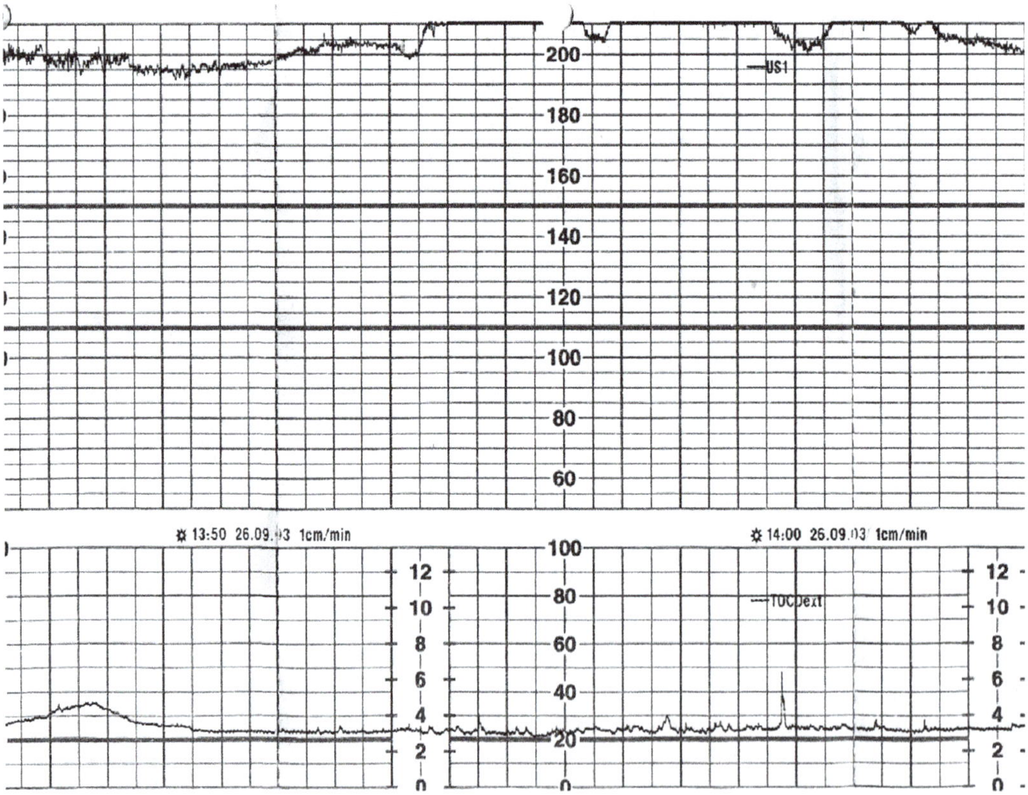

Fig. 3.28: FHR tracing showing tachycardia at 210 bpm. 43 year old para 8, week 37 + 4. Stable cardioversion after 7 days of digoxin therapy. Spontaneous delivery of a male, 3,310 g, 47cm, 36cm; Apgar 9/10/10, umbilical artery pH 7.32, umbilical vein pH 7.39; base excess −1.3 mmol/L.

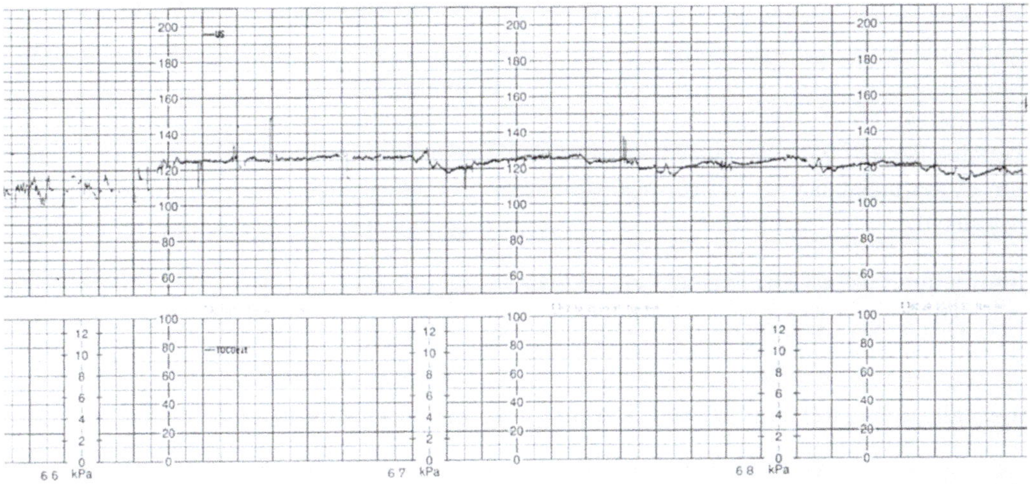

Fig. 3.29: Absent variability in admission trace of a 26 year-old para 3, week 26 + 1, with light vaginal bleeding and sonographically-detected retroplacental hematoma. Caesarean section: male, 37cm, Apgar 0, 0, 0; umbilical artery pH 6.7.

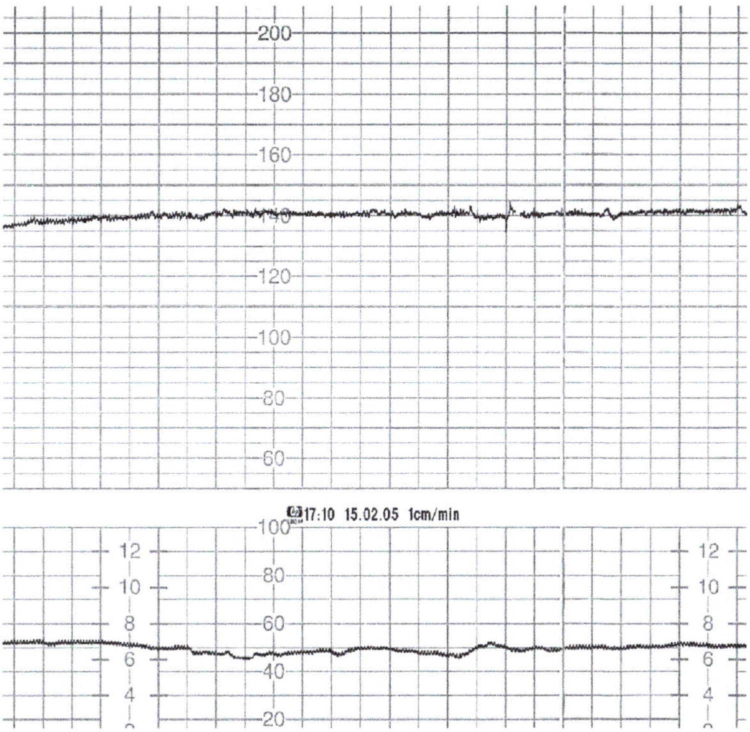

Fig. 3.30: Absent variability; 19 year old woman para 1, week 29 + 0, after sedation for an appendectomy (Midazolam 10mg/h, Fentanyl 1.5μg/h). Ultrasound: NGA fetus, arterial and venous Doppler normal, biophysical profile markedly reduced.

Test: 2 or more spontaneous accelerations of 15 bpm and lasting 15 s in 20 min).

Noninterpretable or pathological findings require continuous monitoring and sonography (Doppler, Fig. 3.31, 3.32); an immediate conclusion of the pregnancy will rarely need to be considered.

Contraction Stress CTG. Examination of the fetal heart frequency under medical induction. Indication: noninterpretable nonstress-CTG.

Medically induced stress CTG. Oxytocin challenge test. The mother receives IV oxytocin: 6 IU in 500 ml saline solution, 2 drops/min initially, increasing by 1 drop every 5 min until regular contractions are occurring, which should then continue for 30 min in order to be able to properly evaluate FHR. EFM is performed from the beginning. Result:

- Decelerations occurring in association with more than half of the contractions are pathological.
- Episodic decelerations require repeat CTG after 6 hours.

Clinical evaluation of the antepartal CTG. Normal CTG indicates fetal well-being. Repeated monitoring as follows:

- Every few hours in cases of IUGR, regular preterm contractions, PIH, after intrauterine procedures, external version.
- Every few days in prolonged pregnancy, diabetes.

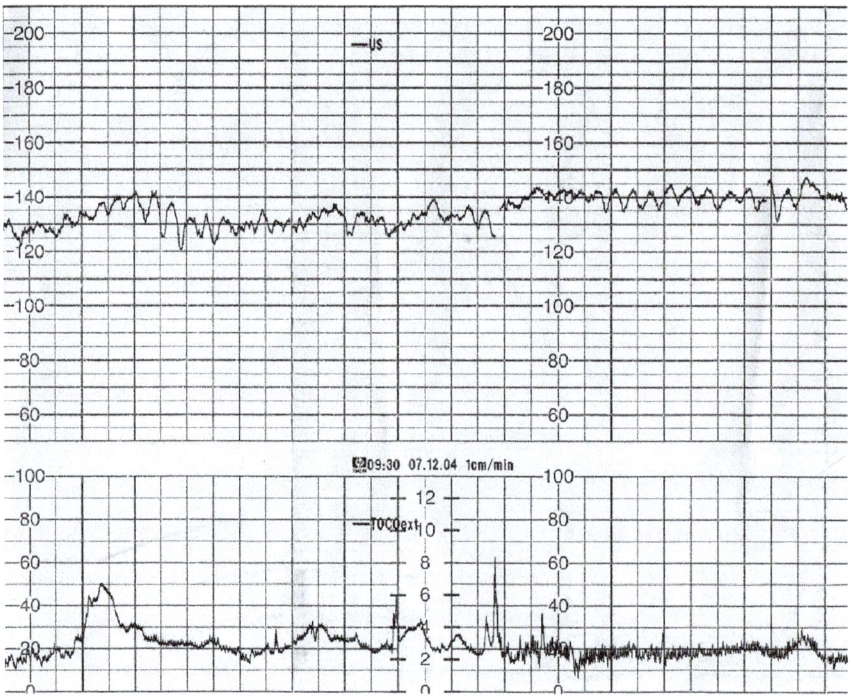

Fig. 3.31: FHR tracing on admission for decreased fetal movement; 26 year-old para 2 in week 32 + 1. Sonographic weight estimate 2,000 g, reduced movement profile, normal liquor volume, no abnormalities in umbilical Doppler, MCA with flow acceleration 114 cm/s. Cordocentesis: Fetal Hb 2.5 g/dl! Cesarean section. Delivery of a male, 2,140 g, 44 cm, 33 cm; Apgar 3/5/7; umbilical artery pH 7.33; Hb 2.7 g/dl; base excess –10.3 mmol/l; lactate 7.8 mmol/l; fetomaternal macrotransfusion.

If CTG findings are abnormal:
- Conservative measures: change of position in supine hypotensive syndrome, raising BP in arterial hypotension.
- Doppler sonography.
- If unsuccessful, conclusion of the pregnancy (danger of asphyxia) by induction or Cesarean section; gestational age, lung and cervical maturity must be considered.

Nonreassuring FHR. Doppler. Repeat monitoring in 1–2 hours necessary.

Amnioscopy

Amnioscopy. Inspection of the amniotic fluid in the forewaters (membranes still intact) with an amnioscope (Saling, 1961) inserted into the vagina and cervix (Fig. 3.33). Hypoxic risk to the fetus in late pregnancy and early labor may be recognized as long as the membranes are still intact. The calculated failure rate is 1 : 2,000.

Evaluation of the amniotic fluid: 1) color; 2) amount; 3) vernix content.
Amniotic fluid color:
1. Clear-milky is physiological.
2. Yellow indicates Rh-incompatibility (see p. 113).
3. Flesh-colored indicates stillborn fetus.
4. Green (pea-soup) liquor is an indication that meconium has been passed.

Cause of the passage of meconium (reduced intrauterine oxygen supply, most common risk to the fetus in late pregnancy) is the oxygen saving

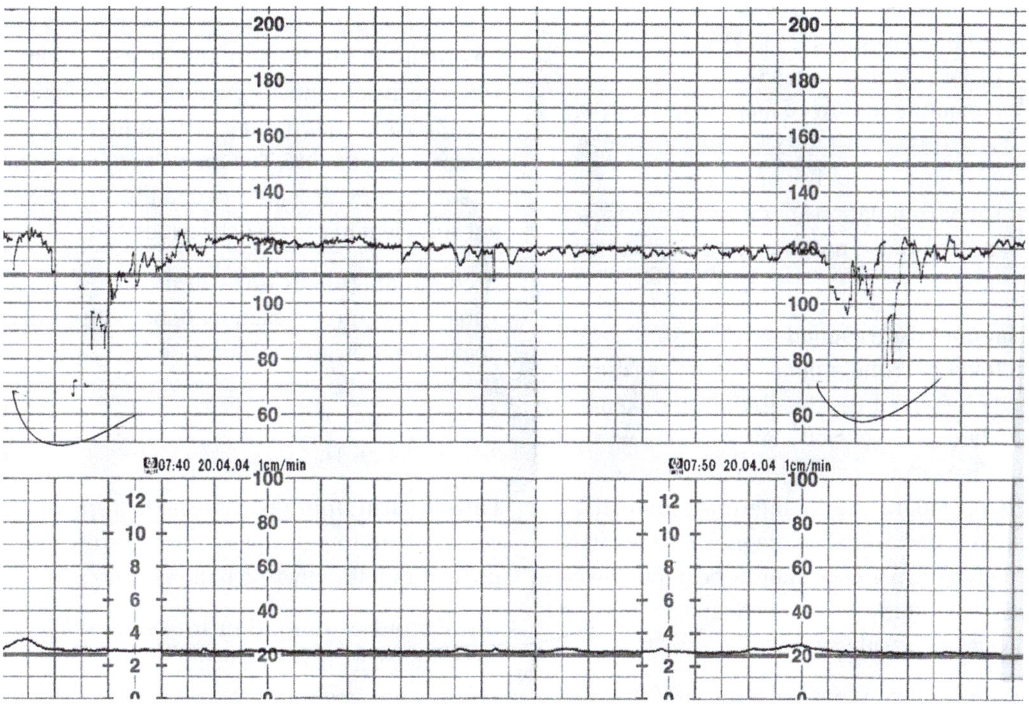

Fig. 3.32: Decelerations coincident with contractions; 19 year-old para 1 in week 24 + 4 with HELLP syndrome, fetal growth retardation, and end-diastolic zero flow in fetal Doppler. Caesarean section. Delivery of a baby girl, 595 g, 31 cm long, 23.5 cm head circumference; APGAR score 3/7/8, pH 7.25.

mechanism of the fetal circulatory system (see p. 284), which results in stimulation of the bowels.
Amount of amniotic fluid:

5. teduced or missing liquor in placental insufficiency, prolonged pregnancy.

Cause: imbalance between production and reabsorption of liquor.

6. Marked vernix content of liquor indicates a mature fetus.

Indication. Indicators of oxygen deficiency in the last 4 weeks of pregnancy (from 36 + 0) are PIH and prolonged pregnancy from the EDD on.

Frequency. Every second day.

Clinical evaluation. Pathological liquor necessitates fetal monitoring and intensive surveillance. Close to term and if the cervix is ripe, ending the pregnancy should be considered.

Complications. Low risk:
- Ruptured membranes in 1 %.
- Labor stimulation in 3 %.
- Premature rupture of membranes (PROM) 35 % (in contrast to 25 % of those women who have not had an amnioscopy).
- Labor stimulation at or post term 25 %, a desired effect, not strictly a complication.

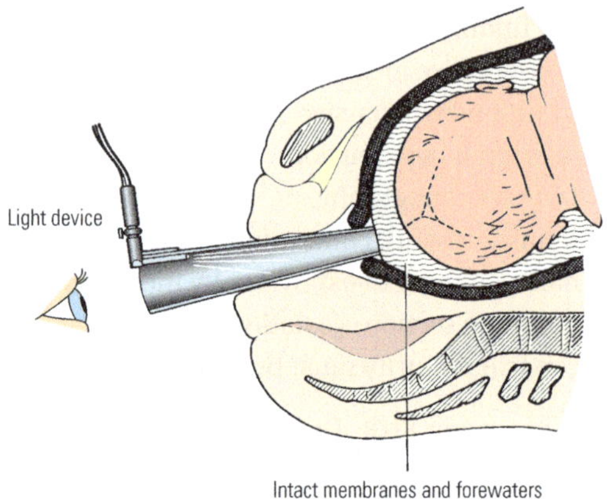

Fig. 3.33: Principle of amnioscopy.

Diagnostic ultrasound

Relevance. Sonographic imaging has dramatically increased the possibilities for examining the fetus. The obstetrician who has occupied him/herself intensively with the possibilities of the procedure and its interpretation can fully exploit the available diagnostic advantages. Practical experience should be supplemented with the study of detailed atlases and textbooks on the subject.

Ultrasound does not harm the fetus. Due to the biological effect on organic tissue, broad clinical experience shows that neither fetal damage nor a disruption of the pregnancy is to be feared. Thermic effects (hyperemia, necrosis, hemorrhage) due to tissue tearing caused by gas bubbles (cavitation) result from intensities in the therapeutic range (e.g., 15 watts/cm²) and above in the unmoving sound field. Alterations of all cell organs have been demonstrated ultrastructurally in in vitro and in vivo testing, whereby membranous structures such as mitochondria and endoplasmic reticulum were particularly susceptible. The intensity of diagnostic sonography (fractions of a milliwatt/cm²) is not sufficient to cause such lesions.

Prenatal diagnostic ultrasound

Three sonographic examinations with image documentation are recommended:

1. Weeks 9–12.
2. Weeks 19–22.
3. Weeks 29–32.

Pathological findings. Transfer to a specialist center should be arranged for high-risk pregnancies or if findings are pathological.

Ultrasound examination in weeks 9–12 focuses on six main questions:
- Intrauterine pregnancy?
- Is the embryo visible?
- Multiple pregnancy?
- Cardiac activity?

- Appropriate for gestational age (AGA) development?
- Fetal abnormalities?

Practice tip. Transvaginal (empty bladder) sonography is superior to transabdominal (full bladder). Abdominal sonographic findings in early pregnancy are to be cautiously interpreted.

Intrauterine pregnancy (= exclusion of ectopic pregnancy). Imaging of the intrauterine chorionic cavity 18 days p.c. or at the end of week 5 p.m. It is 4.5 mm large (Fig. 3.34).

Imaging of the embryo

- Proof of the yolk sac at the end of week 5 before the embryo is visible. A blighted ovum can be excluded.
- Embryo can be depicted by the end of week 6, and is 3 mm long. Crown-rump length (CRL) increases by 1–1.5 mm daily until week 13. By around week 10 it is 18 mm long and the chorionic cavity 31 mm.
- The amniotic cavity becomes visible at the end of week 7. It expands until week 10–12, when it meets up with the inner side of the chorion, thereby obliterating the chorionic cavity and the yolk sac lying within it.
- A chorionic cavity without clearly defined edges or which is no longer round, accompanied by bleeding into the trophoblast can be diagnosed as nonintact pregnancy (missed abortion, blighted ovum).

Differential diagnosis (DD) of abortion. Focus in early pregnancy is most commonly differential diagnostic of the abortion: intact pregnancy? Missed abortion? Incomplete abortion?

If the uterus is smaller on vaginal examination than it should be for gestational age the following questions arise:
- Missed abortion?
- Blighted ovum?

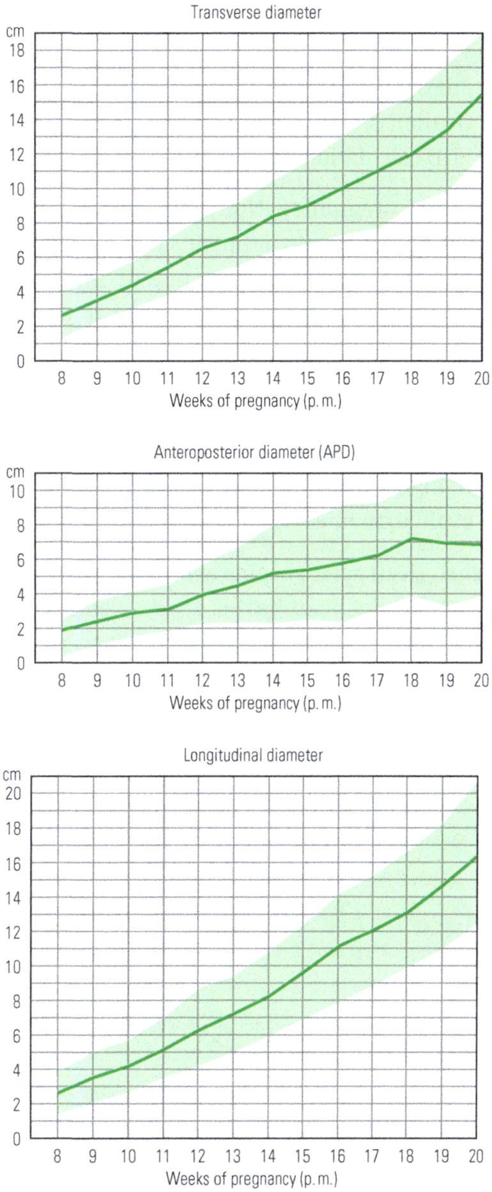

Fig. 3.34: Diameter of the amniotic cavity by week 20, mean and double standard deviation (after Reinold).

- Ectopic pregnancy?
- EDD calculation error?

If the uterus is smaller for gestational age than it should be on vaginal examination, the following questions arise:

- Hydatidiform mole?
- Multiple pregnancy?
- Fibromyoma in pregnancy?
- Ovarian cyst in pregnancy?
- EDD calculation error?

Multiple pregnancy. Not to be overlooked at first sonography appointment!
- Chorionic assessment (see p. 270). Dichorionic twins are at much lower risk than monochorionic.
- Only half of those twin pregnancies diagnosed in week 10 result in twins (see p. 270). Parents should be aware of this.
- In higher-order multiple pregnancies risk evaluation must be carried out.

Heart. Heart action begins at the end of week 5. By week 9 the heart beat is always detectable. This statement is invaluable in the diagnosis of miscarriage; hormonal diagnosis is unnecessary.

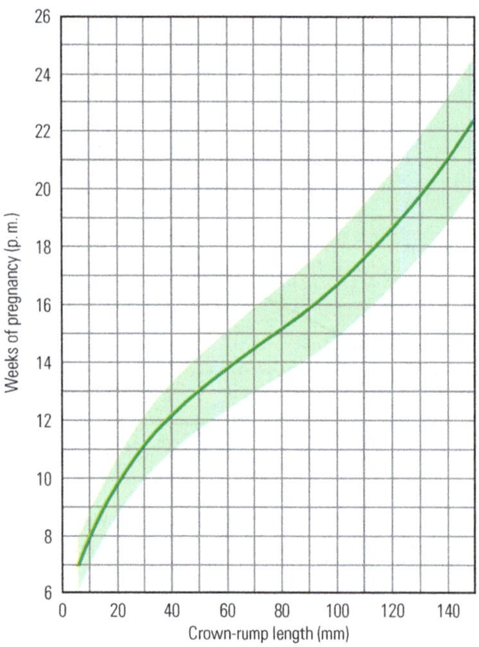

Fig. 3.35: Normal range curve. Estimate of gestational age from the sonographic crown-rump length, mean and double standard deviation (after Hansmann and colleagues).

AGA development. Measurement of crown-rump length (CRL) in week 9 and 12 (± 3 days) is the most reliable method of determining gestational age or due date (Figs. 3.35, 3.44). The EDD calculated according to menstrual data may need to be corrected.

Fetal abnormalities. Transvaginal sonography can detect anencephaly, Turner syndrome, and nuchal edema (trisomy 21).
- **Further diagnostics in early pregnancy. Nuchal translucency** is performed between weeks 11 and 14 with the fetus in sagittal section and the image zoomed (Fig. 3.37, 3.38). It allows an individual risk calculation with regard to chromosomal defects (in particular trisomy 21). An increased measurement is an indication of deformity. Nuchal translucency is not the same as nuchal edema. The nuchal translucency of every fetus is to be measured at this gestational age, and an increase of > 2 mm calls for further consideration, whereas nuchal edema is always an abnormal finding.

Ultrasound at week 19–22 and at week 29–32. Focuses on the following questions:
- AGA development? Developmental abnormalities?
- Localization and structure of the placenta?
- Amniotic fluid volume?
- Anatomical development, fetal structures?
- Body outline?
- Cardiac action?
- Movements?

Appropriate for gestational age (AGA) development. The following are assessed:
- Biparietal diameter (BPD)(Fig. 3.39).

Good imaging of the midline echo is required. This is created by sound reflected from the septum pellucidum, the falx cerebri, on the

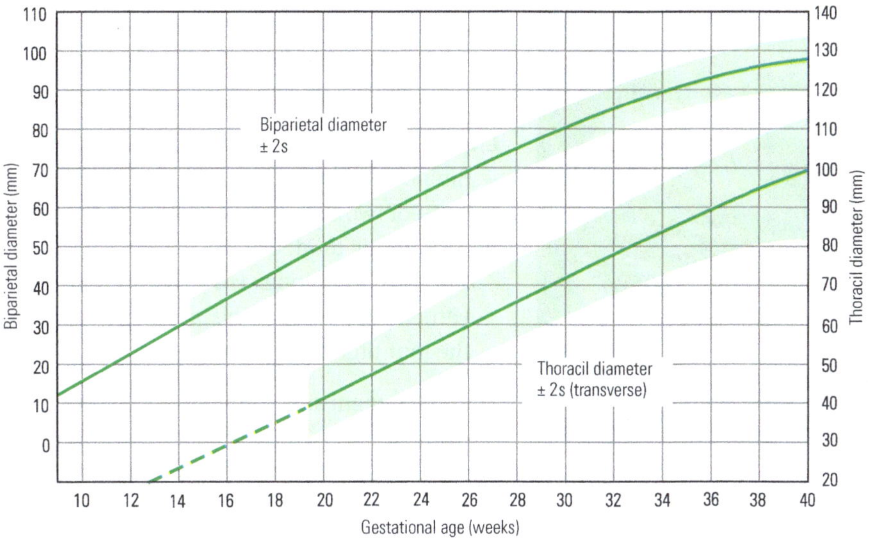

Fig. 3.36: Biparietal and transverse thoracic diameter in relation to gestational age, mean and double standard deviation (after Hansmann).

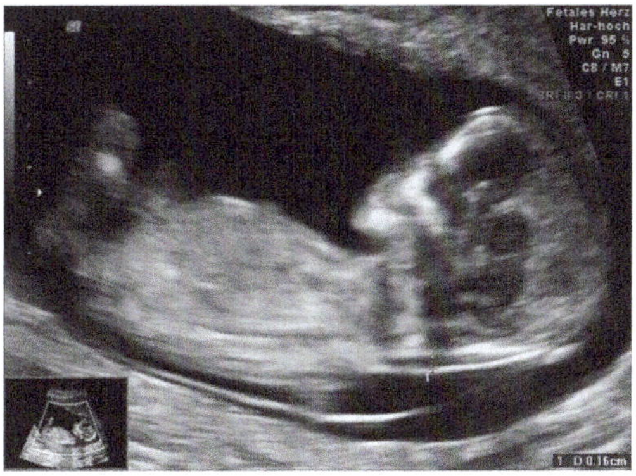

Fig. 3.37: Fetal nuchal translucency in week 13 + 2.

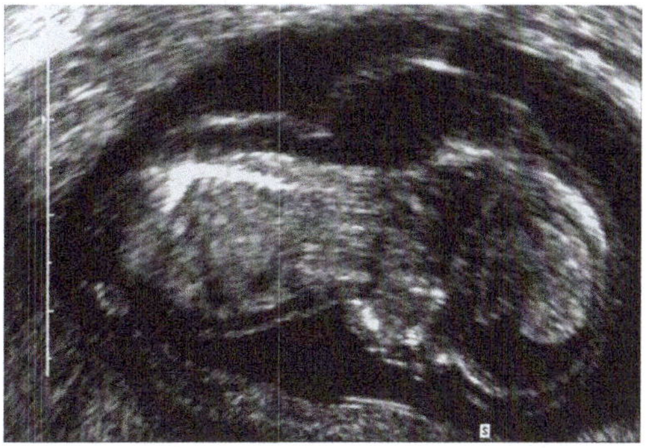

Fig. 3.38: Generalized edema with high nuchal translucency in Turner syndrome (week 12).

walls of the third ventricle, and on the cerebral aqueduct. It is reduced in breech presentation due to the elongated shape of the head. In such cases, the occipital frontal diameter or head circumference should be used instead and intrauterine growth assessed according to charts.

- Occipital frontal diameter (OFD) or head circumference.
- Transverse abdominal diameter (TAD), at the level of the portal sinus (Fig. 3.40). Abdominal circumference.
- Femur length. Each image should be documented (Fig. 3.36).

Placenta localization and structure. Placental development is followed from week 10 (chorion frondosum). Placental thickness and maturity are of limited diagnostic value.

Placental thickness (week 37, 35–40mm) is of use in monitoring nonimmune fetal hydrops, carbohydrate metabolism disorders, and fetal hemolytic disease.

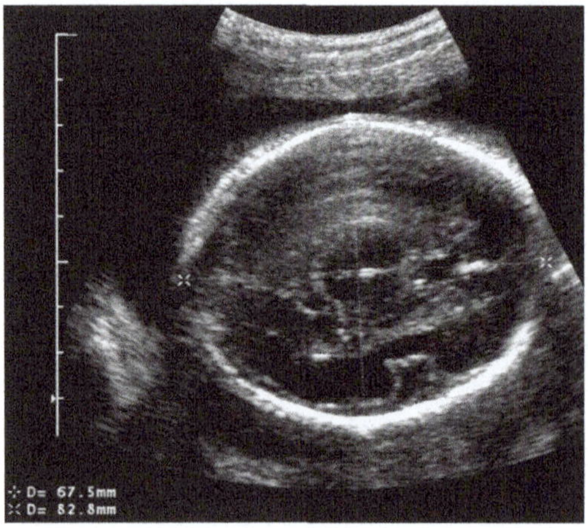

Fig. 3.39: Transverse view of the head, week 26. Biparietal diameter 67.5 mm, occipitofrontal diameter 82.8 mm.

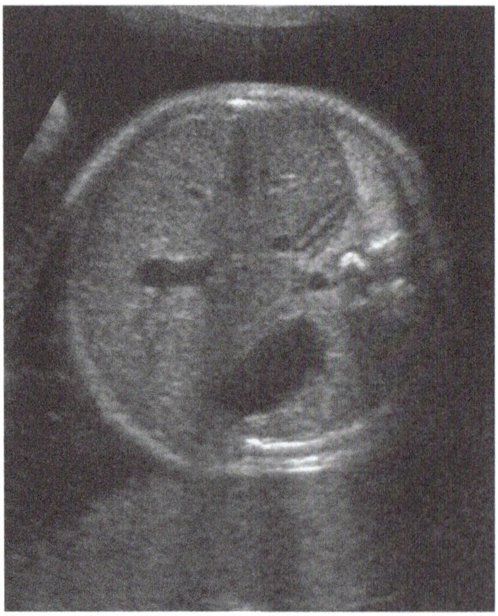

Fig. 3.40: Transverse view of the abdomen, week 30.

Degree of placental maturity. Placental maturity diagnostic is also of limited value (Monaghan and colleagues, 1987) despite the subtle grading (Grannum classification).

Localization of the placenta. Position of the placenta in relation to the cervix, measurement of the overlap; see p. 369.

Liquor volume. Semiquantitive evaluation.
- Single deepest pocket technique: measurement of two diameters of the largest pocket of amniotic fluid, or
- Amniotic fluid index (AFI): addition of the vertical diameters of the largest pockets in the four uterine quadrants.

The assessment may indicate too little liquor (oligohydramnios) or too much (hydramnios, or polyhydramnios).
- Oligohydramnios (Liquor volume < 100 ml) in renal dysplasia (Potter syndrome), obstruction of the ureter/s. This is particularly dangerous in weeks 20–25; Pulmonary hypoplasia, fetal deformities (DD: undetected PROM).
- Hydramnios (Fig. 3.41) is abnormally increased liquor volume (> 2,000 ml).

Liquor volume in hydramnios. 3–4 L are possible, but in exceptional cases volumes of 7–8 L have been described.

Etiology. Hydramnios is caused by excessive secretion from the epithelial cells of the amnion, or reduced liquor reabsorption. The cause cannot be determined in half of the cases.
- Reabsorption of liquor. The fetus drinks the amniotic fluid and absorbs it through the intestines, from where it enters the circulatory system.

Amniotic fluid at term	
Normal	500–1,000 ml
Copious	1,500–2,000 ml
Hydramnios or polyhydramnios	> 2,000 ml
Oligohydramnios	< 100 ml

Maternal etiology: frequently in connection with diabetes mellitus, syphilis and nephritis.

Fetal causes are usually malformations
- Esophageal atresia, intestinal atresia and oral teratoma hinder swallowing and intake of amniotic fluid.
- Congenital heart and kidney defects.

Placental causes: chorioangioma; hydramnios, chorioangioma, and PIH are often linked.

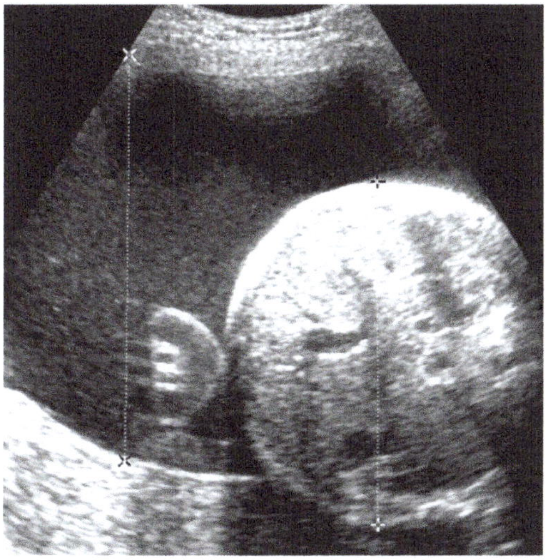

Fig. 3.41: Transverse view of the abdomen, week 33, polyhydramnios, 113.6 mm measured with the deepest-pocket method.

Incidence. Approximately 1 % of all births.

Clinical manifestation
- History (maternal diabetes mellitus).

There are two types: chronic hydramnios. In most cases hydramnios develops slowly, over weeks, and the increase in amniotic fluid causes no restrictions.
Acute hydramnios. Extreme increase in fluid volume within a few days (rare: never before 12 weeks, usually in weeks 16–24).
- Increase in abdominal girth (uterus enlargement), not corresponding to gestational age.
- Complaints due to compression: diffuse abdominal pain, in particular in the kidney or groin regions.
- Partial or complete ileus: stool and wind cannot be passed (acute abdomen).
- Oliguria, proteinuria.
- Pulmonary edema (cardiac decompensation), dyspnea, cyanosis, shock.
- Edema of the lower abdomen and legs.
- Anxiousness, agitation, insomnia.

Diagnosis. Ultrasonography is the leading diagnostic method.

DD. 1) Ovarian cyst. 2) Ascites. 3) Overfilled bladder. 4) Hydronephrosis. 5) Meteorism.

Delivery. Delivery is complicated in cases of extreme acute or chronic hydramnios. Labor usually begins before term. Characteristics are:
- Primary uterine inertia due to over distension of the uterus.
- Delayed cervical dilation because the uterus cannot relax after contractions.
- Presentation of the fetal part closest to the pelvic inlet on rupturing of the membranes.

Malpresentations or cord prolapse (cord is flushed out when the amniotic fluid pours out) frequently occur.
- Delivery is often rapid once the membranes have ruptured if the lie was a longitudinal one.
- Atonic hemorrhage is to be expected after delivery of the placenta.

Therapy. 1) No therapy for mild hydramnios. 2) Depending on the prognosis in cases of fetal malformation. 3) Treatment of the maternal cause (diabetes).
- Indomethacin (100 mg/day PO) is thought to be effective by reducing urine production, in particular before week 32. Its use is controversial due to the side effects (antepartum closure of the fetal ductus arteriosus).

- Amniocentesis. In acute cases of maternal dyspnea or discomfort due to displacement or other acute symptoms, amniocentesis is performed. This will bring relief in the short term, but relatively little in the long term.

Method. After sonographic localization of the placenta and fetus a thin needle, possibly a thin sterile tube, is inserted into the abdomen. Amniotic fluid (possibly several liters) is withdrawn; if necessary tocolytic medication can be given i.v.

Physical development. Normal development is assessed according to Table 3.3 and malformations of the most important organs are to be ruled out.

Body outline. Neural-tube defects are recognizable (1 : 1,000 births), of which anencephaly makes up approximately half.
- Spina bifida – in particular in the lower lumbal region – conspicuous because of ventricular enlargement. In order of severity: 1) Meningocele (contains no neural tissue). 2) Myelo-meningocele (contains spinal cord). 3) Spina bifida with myeloschisis (the spinal cord lies exposed on the surface).
- Intake of folic acid as a prophylaxis against neural-tube defects periconceptionally: 4 weeks before and 8 weeks after conception 0.4 mg/day. In cases of prior pregnancy with neural-tube defect 4 mg/day.
- Ventricular enlargement (ventriculomegaly) occurs due to disturbed cerebrospinal fluid (CSF) circulation as a result of incarceration of the brain stem and the cerebellum in the foramen magnum.
- External hydrocephalus. If the distance between the midline and the lateral wall of the lateral ventricle is greater than half of the maximum hemisphere width at week 24, an external hydrocephalus exists (enlargement of the subarachnoid space). Diagnosis is supported by presence of the lemon sign (lemon-shaped head form due to prominence of the forehead).

Practice tip. The diagnosis, prognosis, evaluation, and announcement of enlarged ventricles or an external hydrocephalus require thorough interdisciplinary antenatal consultation.

- Cleft lip and palate (see p. 463) usually (not always) become apparent on examination of the body outline (1 : 3,000 births).
- Defects of the abdominal wall are relatively easy to diagnose prenatally. Omphalocele (1 : 3,500 births): midline protrusion of intestines through the (enlarged) umbilical ring in the extra-embryonic coelomic cavity. A quarter of the cases are due to chromosomal aberration (→ chromosome testing advisable). Gastroschisis: lateral abdominal wall defect with no chromosomal disorder. Fetal bowel herniates into the amniotic cavity; as bowel paralysis is a risk, peristaltic movement must be monitored. Exchange of amniotic fluid may be advisable, possibly several times.

Cardiac action. Sonography of the fetal heart during this period often detects bradycardia and extrasystoles: supraventricular extrasystoles (SVES) due to tocolysis, nicotine, and caffeine use. Ventricular ES are usually indicators of heart defects: in 1 : 125 births very common!

Note. Fetal echocardiography should be performed at this point in time: four-chamber view and correct positioning of the great vessels.

Arrhythmia. Can be divided into two groups after hemodynamic and prognosis:
- Both supraventricular and ventricular arrhythmias can be harmless with spontaneous regression in the perinatal period.
- Some fetal arrhythmias require immediate attention, because cardiac function is inad-

Tab. 3.3: Normal findings in weeks 18–22 (according to Meinel 1995).

Body section	Finding
Head	
Biometry	AGA measurements
Shape	Normal ovoid
Internal structure	Midline echo, normal ventricle system, no cysts in the choroid plexus, no deformations of the cerebellum, cisterna cerebello-medullaris of normal width. No cysts or tumors (Figs. 3.42, 3.43)
Face	Distance between the orbits is one third of the orbital diameter (distance between the two outermost points)
Profile	Profile of forehead, nose, jaw, and lip contours normal (bearing ethnological differences in mind) (Fig. 3.45)
Thorax	
Lungs	Typical echogenicity. No foreign content (stomach, bowel). No pleural effusion. No cysts in lung tissue (Figs. 3.46, 3.47)
Heart	Four chamber view, correct localization of the great vessels (Figs. 3.48, 3.49)
Abdomen	Stomach of normal size and location. No double bladder. Liver – gall bladder. Spleen. Bowels. No bowel enlargement. No tumors or cysts. No ascites (Fig. 3.50–3.52)
Retroperitoneum	Adrenal glands. Kidneys of normal size, cyst-free. Bladder size and location normal. Renal pelvis not obstructed
Spine	Triangular vertebral ossification centers in horizontal view. Skin closed the length of the spine. Longitudinal sections: parallel ordering of the ossification zones (Figs. 3.53, 3.54, 3.55)
Skeleton	AGA ossification and biometry of the long tubular bones

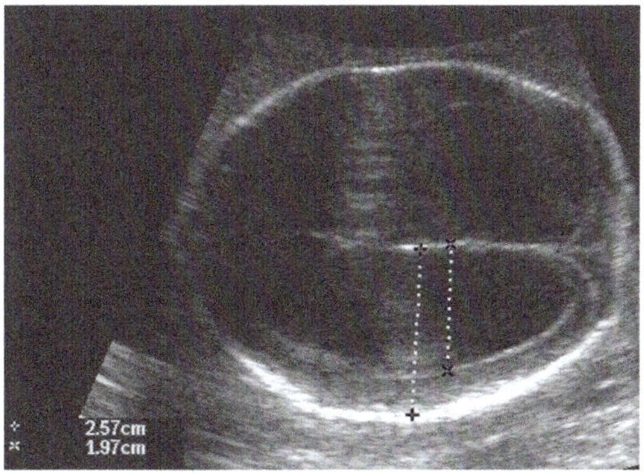

Fig. 3.42: Transverse view through the head, week 22, hydrocephalus internus; width of the hemispheres 2.57 cm, width of the lateral ventricle 1.97 cm, pathological ventricle-brain ratio (> 50 %).

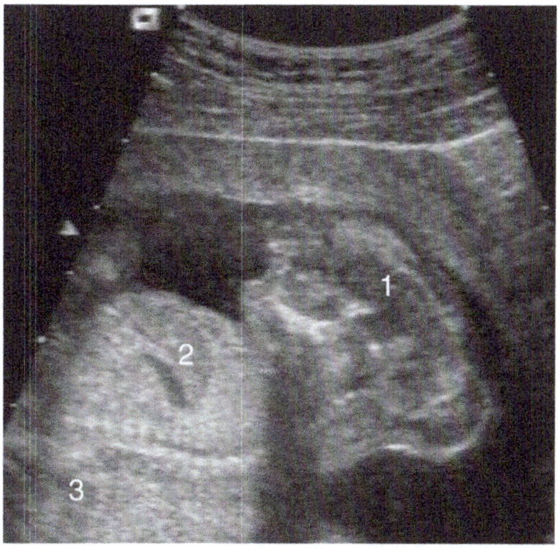

Fig. 3.43: Sagittal view through the fetus, week 19. Exencephaly; 1) cerebrum floating in amniotic fluid, ossification of the skull incomplete; 2) thorax; 3) abdomen.

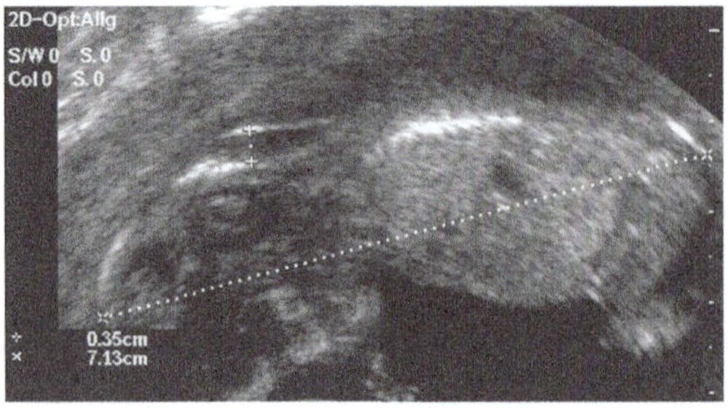

Fig. 3.44: Longitudinal view, week 13; crown-rump length 7.13 cm, nuchal edema 0.35 cm.

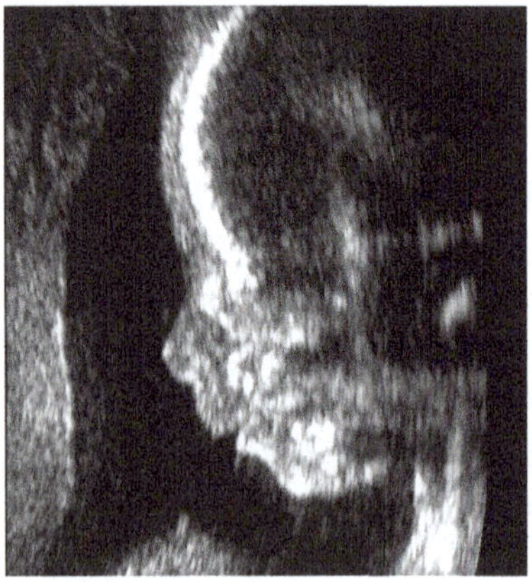

Fig. 3.45: Fetal profile, week 22.

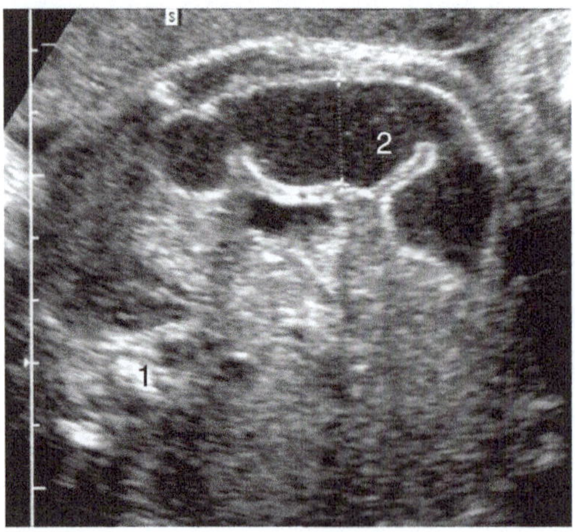

Fig. 3.46: Transverse view through the thorax, week 22, showing congenital cystic adenomatoid malformation (CCAM), cystic lung tissue (about 4 × 4 cm).

equate: supraventricular tachycardia, AV block, sinus tachycardia > 200 bpm, sinus bradycardia < 60 bpm, atrial fibrillation, and flutter.
- Signs of heart decompensation should be looked for sonographically: ascites, generalized edema.
- High lethality of 40 % and newborn morbidity of 60 % (Voigt and colleagues), therefore intrauterine therapy is advisable: maternal digoxin therapy or antiarrhythmic medication via umbilical vein.

Fetal activity. Fetal movements are recognizable from week 8. Detection of movement disorders, commonly linked with a syndrome. Analysis of fetal activity is particularly relevant in neuromuscular illnesses: myotonic dystrophy, Pena–Shokeir Syndrome, Arthrogryposis multiplex congenita. The fetal sleep-wake cycle must be taken into consideration when making an assessment.

Fetal movement patterns. Classification of movement patterns from week 8 (Prechtl and colleagues): slow and rapid movements follow a cycle (Fig. 3.57). Rest phases of 15–40 min (sleep phases) alternate with wakeful phases.

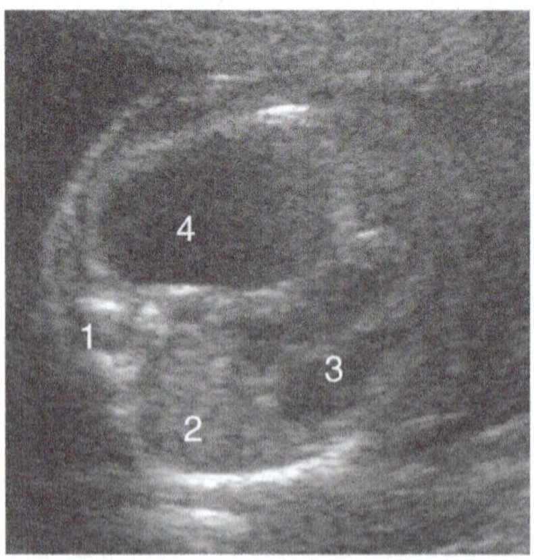

Fig. 3.47: Transverse view through the thorax, week 20, showing diaphragmatic hernia; 1) Spine; 2) lungs; 3) heart (right displacement); 4) stomach.

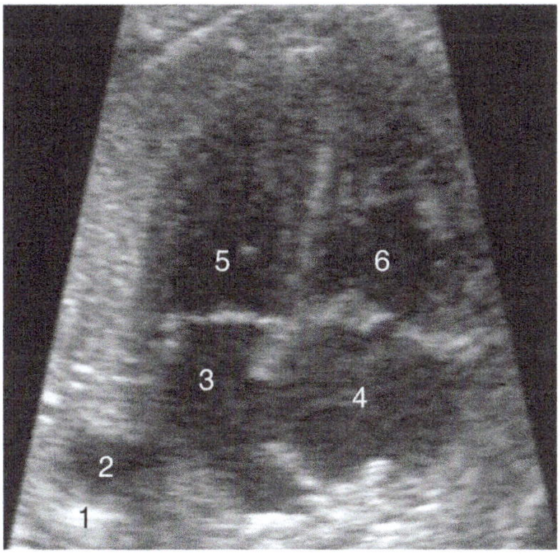

Fig. 3.48: Four-chamber view of the heart, week 28; 1) spine; 2) aorta; 3) left atrium; 4) right atrium; 5) left ventricle; 6) right ventricle.

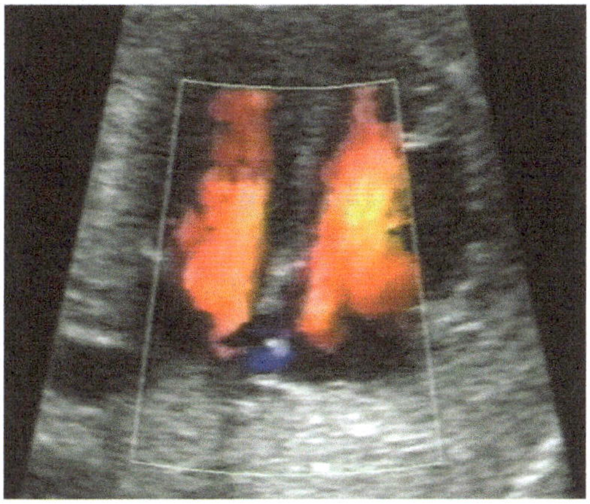

Fig. 3.49: Four-chamber view of the heart, week 28, color Doppler; the red area depicts the blood flow in the chamber-filling phase.

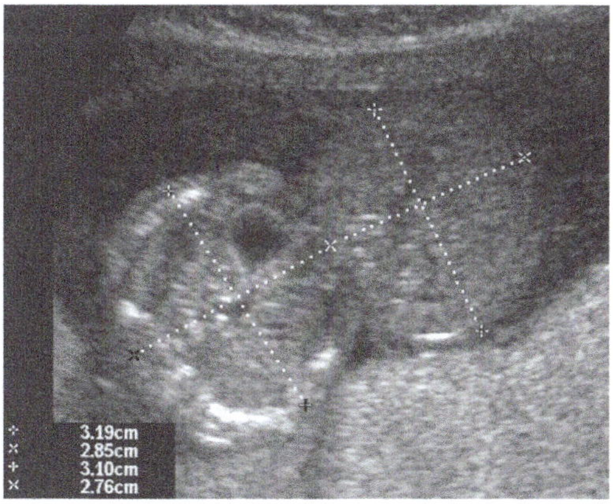

Fig. 3.50: Transverse abdominal view, week 19; omphalocele containing liver and small intestine. The hernia sac is the same circumference as the upper abdomen.

Doppler ultrasound

Definition. Method of diagnostic ultrasound used to determine blood flow velocity in the heart and blood vessels.

Biophysics. A piezoelectric crystal sends out ultrasound waves of constant frequency; if these waves meet a moving interface (such as an erythrocyte) the change in frequency (Doppler effect) will be reflected. The interference of incident and reflected wave is made audible as low frequency sound, or rather allows the calculation of the velocity and direction of the object.

The numerous variations in frequency are evaluated with the help of an analyzer, in which amount and distribution of the frequencies on a vessel cross-section are depicted. Blood flow in the arteries is pulsatile, the blood column moves from one section of a vessel to the next with each heart contraction (Fig. 3.58), influenced by blood viscosity, proportion of formed elements in the blood, elasticity of the vessel wall, and blood vessel diameter. Conclusions can be made about the influencing factors from the relationship between the heart phases (systole, diastole) and their respective flow spectrums.

Originally, continuous-wave Doppler was used, in which the piezoelectric crystal transmitter and receiver work continually and simultaneously. As a simultaneous B-mode ultrasound is not possible, pulsed-wave Doppler was developed, in which the same crystal functions

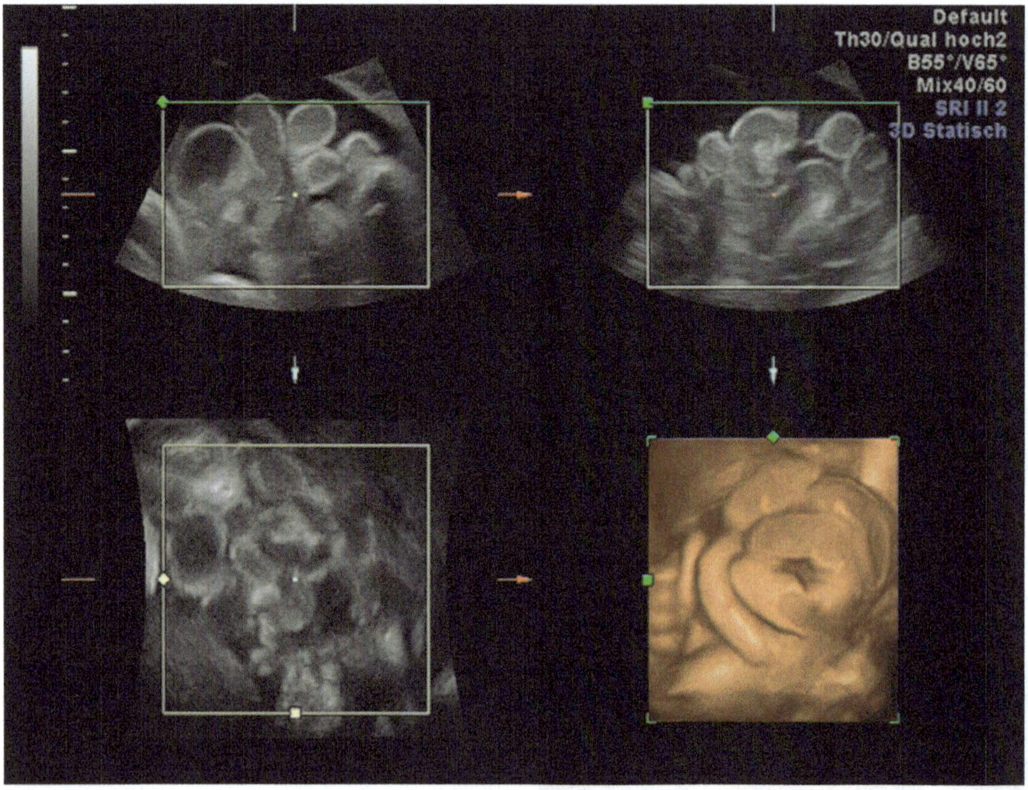

Fig. 3.51: Gastroschisis, week 35: dilated bowel loops in the amniotic cavity (no hernia sac). Multiplanar mode and 3-D sonography.

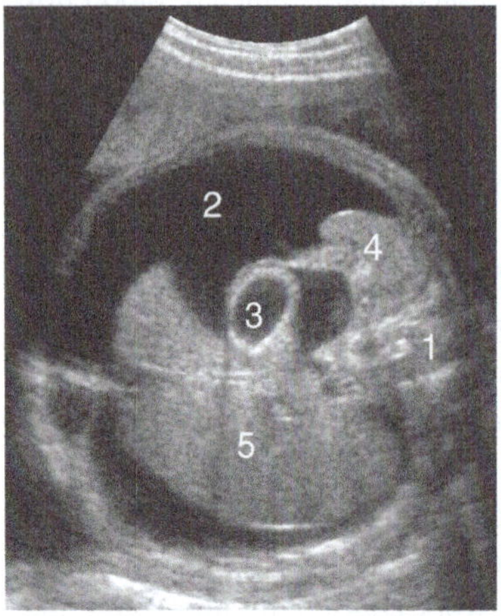

Fig. 3.52: Transverse view through the upper abdomen, week 30, with ascites. 1) Spine; 2) Ascites; 3) stomach; 4) spleen; 5) liver.

as transmitter and then receiver. B-mode ultrasound (duplex Doppler) is possible with this method. Flow direction is visualized with color coding (color-flow Doppler), simplifying the identification of certain blood vessels.

Measurement standards. Reproducible measurements require standards of technique such as measuring in maternal rest conditions in a semisupine position. Medication which may have an effect on blood flow (tocolytics, betablockers) must be taken into consideration in the interpretation. Likewise, measurements should be carried out during fetal rest phases and taking FHR into account.

Application. Additional to EFM and fetal anatomical assessment using ultrasound imaging. The fetal heart is examined, mostly with

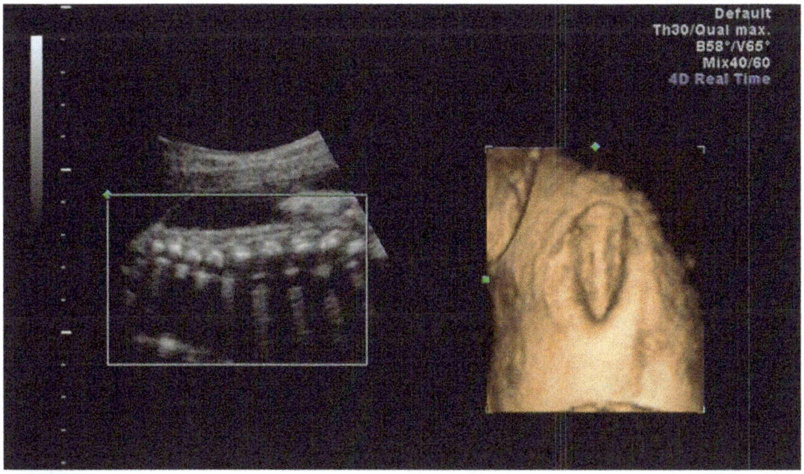

Fig. 3.53: Lumbosacral spina bifida, week 36; left, conventional B-Mode, sagittal view; right: surface-rendered 3-D image.

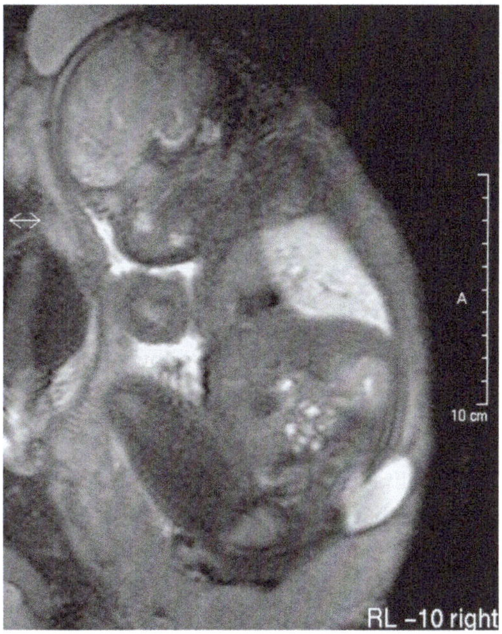

Fig. 3.54: Magnetic resonance image of spina bifida, week 32.

continuous-wave Doppler, as are the uteroplacental arteries, umbilical vessels, fetal aorta, middle cerebral artery (MCA), primarily with pulsed-wave Doppler.

The Doppler sonogram of a vessel depicts blood flow in relation to time. The spectrum corresponds with the velocity distribution of the erythrocytes in the blood vessel. It also provides information about blood flow characteristics, vessel width, blood flow velocity and disturbances.

Blood flow diagnostics

- Information about cardiac activity and resistance through acoustic and optical analysis of blood flow sounds.
- Two-dimensional (time vs. frequency) flow analysis. The Doppler spectrum describes a wave in constant change (= pulsatility) between peak systolic and end-diastolic minimum velocities. Indices which have been calculated from a number of uniform cycles (Fig. 3.58) are used to describe the blood flow spectrum, of which three are used internationally:
  - Systolic/diastolic (SD) ratio (A/B ratio, from Stuart and colleagues 1980).
  - Resistance index (RI) or Pourcelot ratio (PR).
  - Pulsatility index (PI) acc. to Gosling and colleagues 1975. The PI is considered the most accurate of the Doppler spectrum.

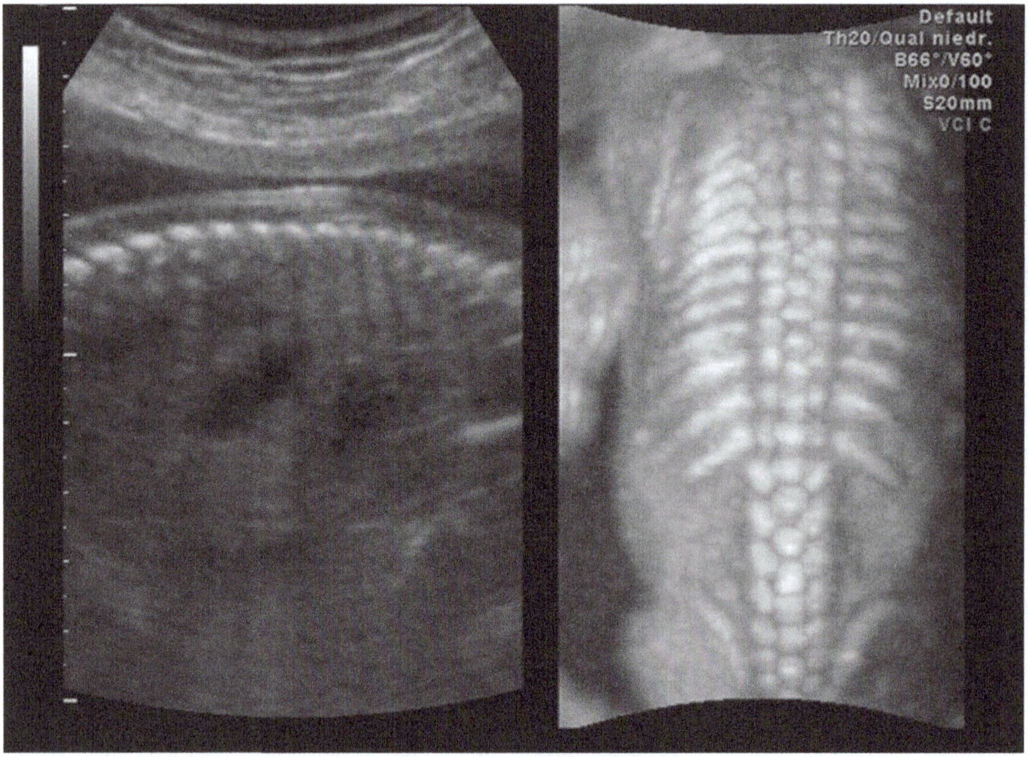

Fig. 3.55: Sonographic images of spine, and spine and ribs, week 21; left: conventional B-Mode; right: in 3-D skeleton mode.

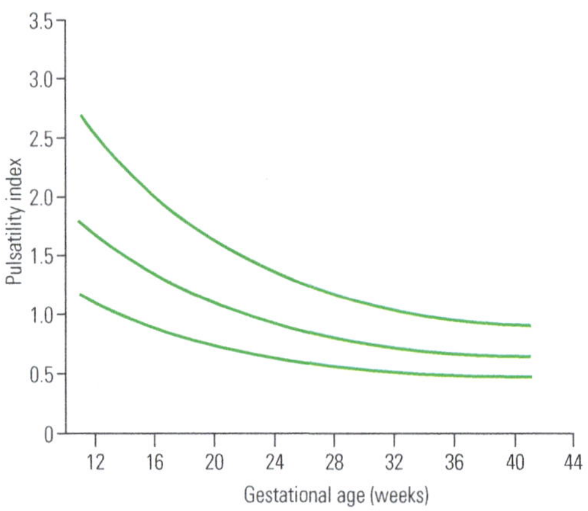

Fig. 3.56: Pulsatility Index (PI) of the uterine artery in relation to gestational age, 5th, 50th, and 95th percentile (after Gomez and colleagues 2008).

Uterine arteries. The uterine arteries best portray uteroplacental flow, allowing for gestational age and placenta location (Figs. 3.59, 3.60).

The qualitative analysis is introduced here, which is characterized by an increase in diastolic flow and the nondisappearance (after week 24) of the bilateral early diastolic notch. Persistence can be an indication of an incomplete trophoblast invasion. The notch is indicative of pulse-wave reflections which develop when the trophoblast invasion and the resulting dilation of the spiral arterioles fail to occur (Figs. 3.61, 3.62): PIH and IUGR are common in such cases. Furthermore, increased PI of the uterine artery (Fig. 3.56) can be an early warning sign for PIH, preeclampsia, and/or IUGR.

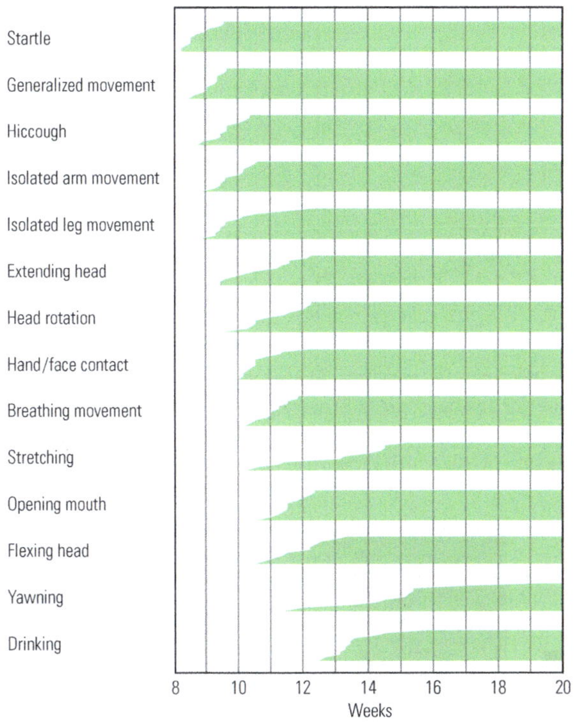

Fig. 3.57: Fetal movement patterns (after de Vries and colleagues). Startles are rapid synchronous movements, beginning in the extremities and spreading to neck and trunk; generalized movements are rough movements of the whole body, lasting from seconds to several minutes.

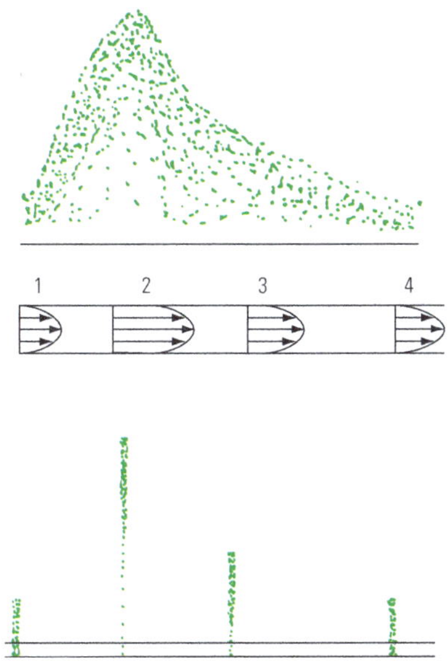

Fig. 3.58: Idealized flow profile in 2-D monitor image. 1) Laminar flow; 2) laminar flow, high peak velocity; 3) laminar flow, medium peak velocity; 4) laminar flow (after Vetter 1995).

Umbilical arteries. The blood flow is indicative of placental perfusion (Fig. 3.64). The diastolic flow increases over the length of the pregnancy. A reduction in blood flow to zero or reversed end-diastolic flow due to changes in placental vessels is pathological (Fig. 3.64).

Note. If the Doppler velocimetry of the umbilical arteries is pathological, intensive sonographic and cardiotocographic assessment is advisable.

Practice tip. If the blood flow pattern of the umbilical arteries is pathological, Doppler sonography of the middle cerebral artery (MCA) should be performed, because the fetal circulatory system reacts to disruptions in supply with oxygen-saving methods, i.e., increasing circulation in the brain when the peripheral circulation is reduced.

Fetal aorta. Blood flow reflects placental circulation (Fig. 3.66).

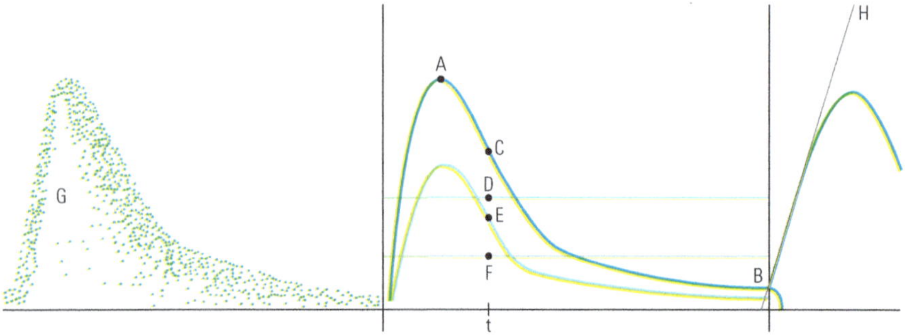

Fig. 3.59: Variables and indices for the analysis of flow spectrums (after Vetter). A) Peak velocity (PV); B) minimum PV; C) PV at an arbitrary timepoint t = PV (t); D) median PV of one heart cycle; E) average velocity at an arbitrary timepoint = space average velocity (t); F) median average velocity over one heart cycle = "median velocity"; G) spectral window; H) gradient. Indices: Resistance Index (RI): (A–B)/A; A/B ratio: A/B; pulsatility Index (PI): (A–B)/D.

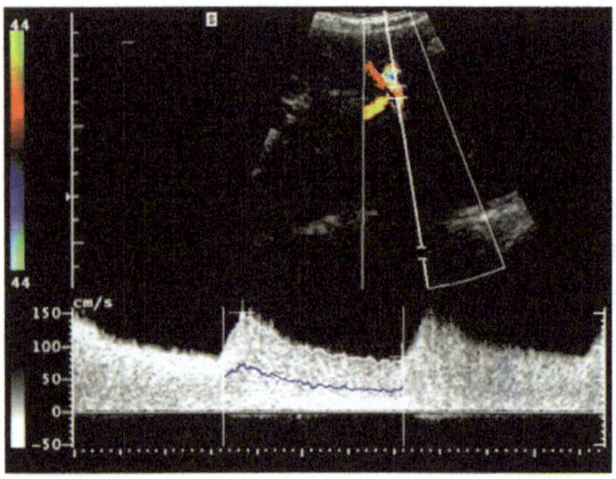

Fig. 3.60: Flow spectrum of the uterine artery in week 22.

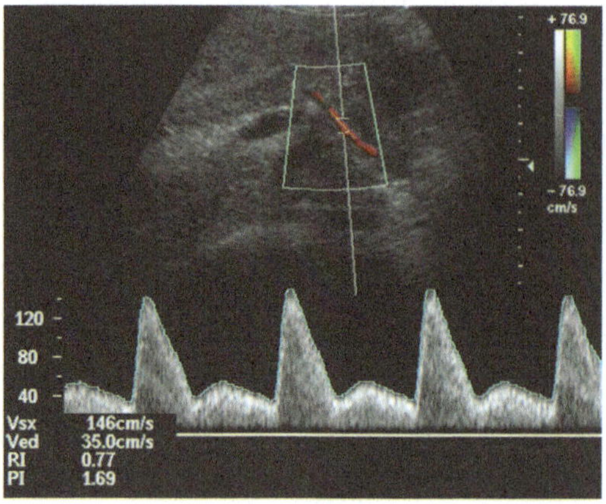

Fig. 3.61: Flow spectrum of the uterine artery in week 30 with postsystolic notch and reduced end-diastolic flow indicating increased resistance in uteroplacental circulation.

Middle cerebral artery (MCA). Blood flow in the MCA gives an indication of circulation in the brain (Figs. 3.66, 3.67, 3.68). It is constant up until week 36, after which it increases in the diastole. If increased diastolic flow occurs earlier, this is indicative of centralization of the fetal circulation in hypoxemia ("brain-sparing"). In such a case, blood flow will also be decreased in the umbilical arteries and the aorta.

Venous flow. Pathological patterns which may present are increased pulsatility in the precardiac veins (inferior vena cava, ductus venosus) and the occurrence of pulsations which are not breathing-related in the umbilical vein.

Indications (after week 20). Doppler velocimetry should be performed for the following risk groups:
- Small for gestational age (SGA).
- PIH/pre-eclampsia.
- Prior SGA or stillbirth.
- History of pre-eclampsia/eclampsia.
- Nonreassuring FHR.

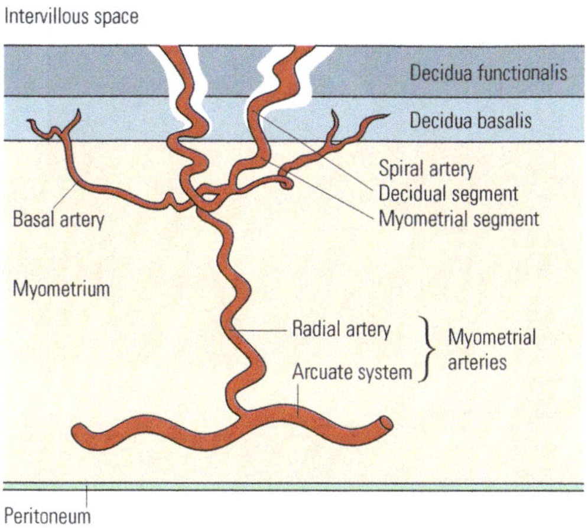

Fig. 3.62: Uterine blood vessels in pregnancy (Künzel and Wulf, 1993).

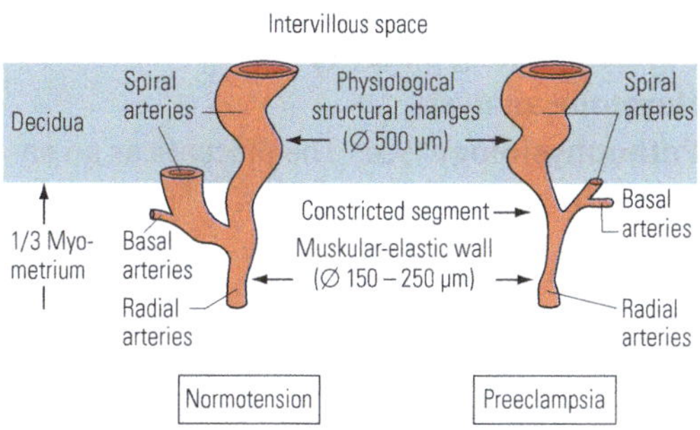

Fig. 3.63: Expansion of spiral arterioles due to trophoblast invasion in decidua and myometrium in normal pregnancy, and incomplete as the basis of pre-eclampsia (after Brosens 1973, from Künzel and Wulf 1993).

- Fetal malformation or disease.
- Multifetal pregnancy, particularly in cases of discordant growth.
- Cardiac defect or illness.

In addition it can be advisable in cases of:
- Diabetes mellitus.
- Autoimmune disease.
- Nephropathy.
- Preexistent hypertension.
- Coagulation disorders.

Assessment. If selectively is applied as indicated, Doppler sonography reduces perinatal mortality and morbidity. It is a valuable tool in best determining the date of delivery. The method has gained a firm footing in the diagnosis and surveillance of IUGR in particular. A disorder of this type due to placental disfunction is diagnosed by increased flow resistance in the umbilical arteries. If the disorder progresses, compensation occurs in the form of increased

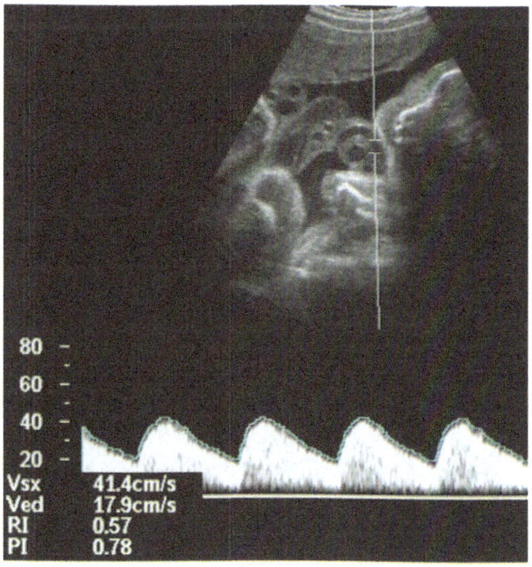

Fig. 3.64: Flow spectrum of the umbilical artery in week 30.

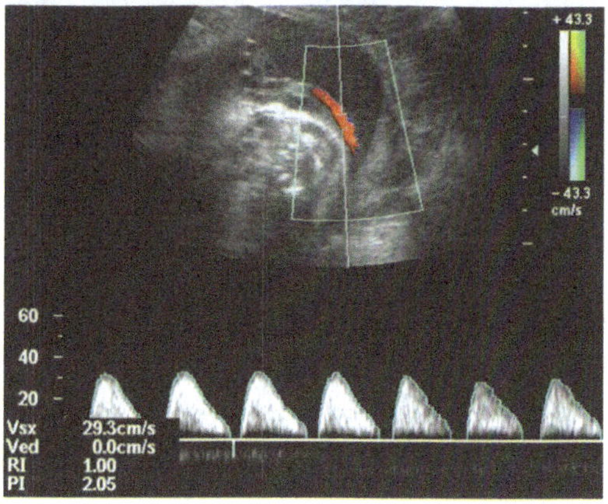

Fig. 3.65: Flow spectrum of the umbilical artery in week 30 showing diastolic zero flow.

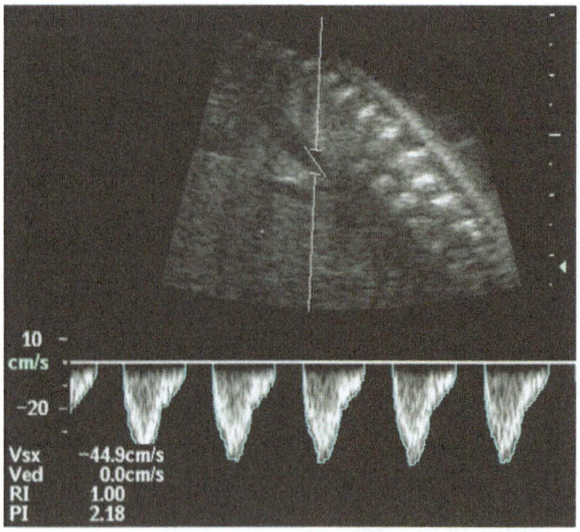

Fig. 3.66: Sagittal view through fetal aorta and spine, week 30, flow spectrum of the aorta showing diastolic zero flow.

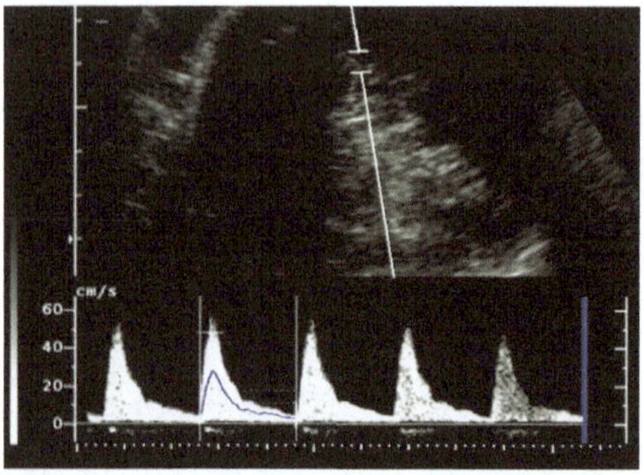

Fig. 3.67: Flow spectrum of the MCA in week 30.

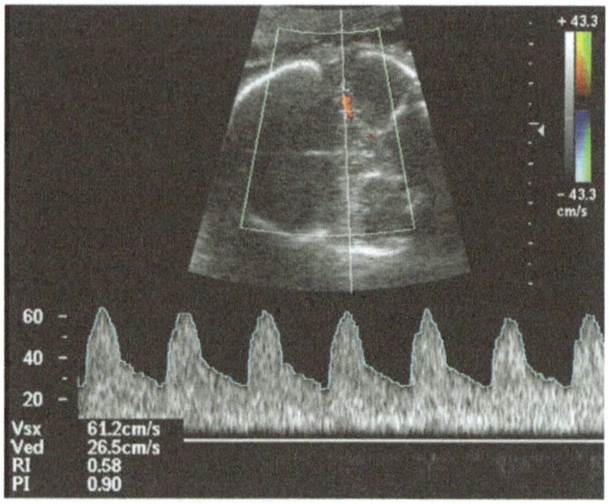

Fig. 3.68: Transverse view through fetal head in week 30; MCA flow spectrum right, increased diastolic flow signaling centralization of blood flow.

and intensified central blood flow (MCA!). The limits of this compensation make themselves known when the myocardial strain causes pathological venous blood flow patterns.

At present, Doppler sonography is not indicated for screening purposes. It is possible that mid-pregnancy Doppler ultrasound examination of the uterine arteries in the low-risk collective could be of use in predicting pathological pregnancies; a definitive and conclusive decision on this subject has not yet been reached.

Hormones, lung maturity

Hormone analysis

Pathophysiology (see "The placenta as an endocrine organ", p. 7).

hCG. Human chorionic gonadotropin is used to detect and monitor pregnancy. The synthesis of hCG by the trophoblasts is the basis of the immunological pregnancy tests in which the presence of hCG in blood or urine is detected.

Urine hCG test. HCG detection in urine (morning or 24 hour sample) via antigen-antibody reaction (between hCG and hCG antibodies). A positive result can be expected 5–12 days after the period was due. Reliability ≥ 95 %.

False positive results can occur in women with elevated gonadotropin levels, for example in menopause. In these women, elevated luteinizing hormone (LH) levels result in a cross-reaction of LH and hCG antibodies, causing the false positive result.
The pregnancy tests in use today (antibodies against the beta subunit of the hCG molecule, monoclonal antibodies) are more specific and sensitive and can detect pregnancy as early as the date the period is expected.

HCG detection in abnormal early pregnancy. hCG levels in threatened abortion, molar and ectopic pregnancies are to be interpreted as follows:

- Normal hCG levels and bleeding indicate a normal pregnancy.
- Reduced hCG levels and bleeding have a poor prognosis.

Ultrasonograph examination is more suited to detection of an intact pregnancy in cases of threatened abortion than hCG status.

- hCG levels are high in molar pregnancy (see p. 360).
- Low or no levels of hCG are indications of an extrauterine pregnancy (see p. 363).

Testing of fetal lung maturity. Lung maturity is assessed by means of the surfactant concentration, or rather the concentration of a part of surfactant (lecithin), in amniotic fluid, which is obtained via transabdominal amniocentesis. Lecithins are detectable from weeks 18–24 onwards. Concentration increases with pregnancy (Fig. 3.69).

In cases of lung immaturity (see “Embryonic and fetal development”, p. 11) the alveoli are in danger of collapsing after birth, leading to respiratory distress syndrome (RDS p. 447).

Measurement of the lecithin-sphingomyelin ratio (L/S ratio) according to Gluck, and modification of this method.

After extraction the phospholipids are separated out via thin-layer chromatography. An L/S ratio:

- ≥ 2 indicates less than 5 % probability of RDS.
- < 2 indicates a 25–90 % probability.

Enzymatic methods of lecithin measurement are more sensitive. The critical limit is thought to be around 5.0 mg lecithin/100 ml amniotic fluid.

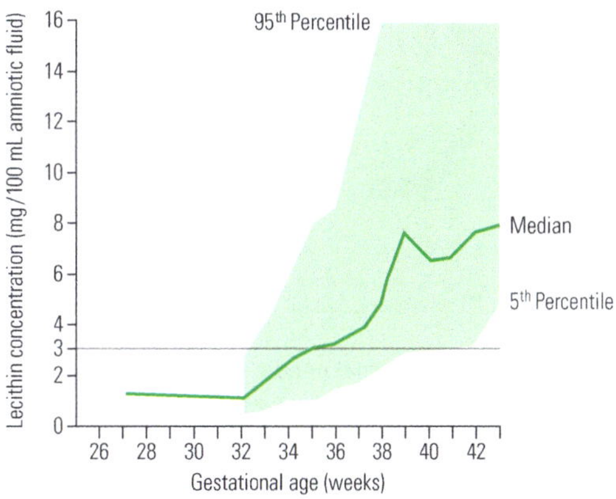

Fig. 3.69: Lecithin concentration (median, 5th percentile and 95th percentile) in amniotic fluid in relation to gestational age.

3.1.5 Prenatal diagnosis of genetic defects

Presumably > 30 % of all zygotes carry a chromosomal defect. The majority goes unnoticed or disintegrates before or on implantation. At least every third spontaneous abortion is due to chromosomal aberration (autosomal trisomies > 50 %, triploidies 17 %). Chromosomal defects are the cause of 5 % of stillbirths.

4–5 % of all live births exhibit genetic diseases, 2–3 % have recognizable, severe morphological disorders, and 0.6 % of all newborns have an altered set of chromosomes. 10 % of babies with severe congenital defects die in the first months of life.

Epidemiology. The most common disorders with chromosomal abnormalities are:

- Down syndrome: 1 : 1,000 live births.
- Fragile X syndrome: 1 : 1,000 live births.
- Klinefelter syndrome: 2 : 1,000 live births.
- Triple X syndrome: 1 : 1,000 live born girls.
- XYY syndrome: 1 : 1,000 live born boys.
- Turner syndrome: 1 : 2,500 live born girls.

The most common monogenic and polygenic disorders are hemophilia A, color blindness,

cleft lip, alveolus and palate, clubfoot, hip dysplasia, cardiac defects.
The most common morphogenetic disorder is fetal alcohol syndrome (FAS) →1–3 : 1,000 live births.

Genetic disorders. 4–5 % of newborns have a genetic disorder. Early recognition of these disorders is desirable in pregnancy.
- Diagnosis of chromosomal abnormalities.
- Diagnosis of congenital metabolic disorders.
- Determination of sex in inherited sex-chromosome abnormalities.
- Diagnosis of neural dysraphia.

Prenatal diagnosis is indicated
- Maternal age > 35 years (Tab. 3.5).
- Chromosomal translocation of one parent.
- Carriers of sex-chromosome abnormalities.
- Prior birth of child with chromosomal abnormality.
- Prior birth of child with neural dysraphia, or neural dysraphia in the family.
- Familial history of metabolic disorder.

Tab. 3.5: Maternal age and frequency of chromosomal defects (according to Knorr).

Maternal age in years	Rate of anomalies (%)
35–37	1.6
38–40	2.0
41–43	5.0
> 44	9.1

Note. The following methods are **suitable for prenatal diagnosis**: ultrasonography, amniocentesis and chorionic villus sampling (CVS), cordocentesis (Fig. 3.70) and biochemical tests.

Amniocentesis

Definition. Puncture of the amniotic sac under ultrasound guidance, usually transabdominally (through the maternal abdomen), and withdrawal of amniotic fluid from week 15 (liquor volume 180 ml).

Early amniocentesis is amniocentesis performed before week 14. Complications (spontaneous abortion) appear to be more likely the earlier amniocentesis is performed.

Technique. After disinfection of the puncture site, a single-use needle is inserted (with or without local anesthetic) under ultrasound guidance into the amniotic sac. 10 ml liquor is withdrawn for chromosomal analysis and the fetal cells it contains are cultured. Another 5 ml are withdrawn for biochemical tests. Rhesus negative women receive anti-D treatment.

Complications. Miscarriage 1 %; amniotic fluid leakage or light bleeding are common short-term complications; serious infections are rare.

An alternative method of prenatal diagnosis is chorionic villus sampling.

Chorionic villus sampling (CVS)

Definition. Biopsy of the chorion frondosum of the placenta (= chorionic villi biopsy, chorionic villus sampling, CVS) between weeks 11 and 13.

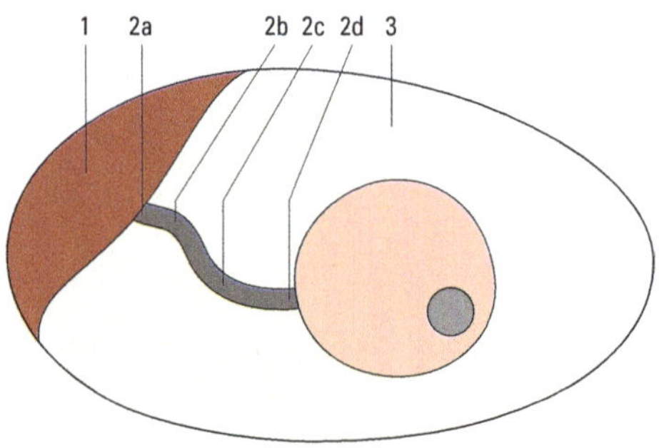

Fig. 3.70: Transabdominal needle insertion (under sonographic guidance) for prenatal diagnosis. 1) Chorionic villi sampling, placentesis; 2) cordocentesis, puncturing of the umbilical vein; 2a) transplacental insertion; 2b) puncturing at the placental cord attachment; 2c) puncturing of a free-moving umbilical cord; 2d) puncturing at the fetal cord attachment; 3) amniocentesis, amniotic fluid test (AFT).

Sonographic guidance is used to extract trophoblastic cells for cytogenetic, DNA, and biochemical analysis.

CVS is performed
- transabdominally with an 18–20 gauge spinal needle,
- transcervically with a flexible catheter (Portex or Angiomed catheters).

Advantages over amniocentesis
- Karyotyping of chorionic villi is faster, usually taking 1–2 days.
- Can be performed from week 11 + 0.
- Placenta biopsy. In cases of IUGR and sonographic evidence of dysmorphism, samples of chorionic villi can be taken in late pregnancy (= placenta biopsy); results are available sooner than from amniotic fluid.

Complications. The risks are no higher than for amniocentesis. The miscarriage rate after CVS is also 1 %.

The occasional diagnostic uncertainties in direct preparation and the possible association of deformities of the extremities, in particular if the CVS is performed before week 10 + 0, have restricted widespread use of CVS in recent years.

Biochemical tests

Alpha-fetoprotein (AFP). Definition. Single-chain glycoprotein which moves into the alpha-1 zone in serum electrophoresis. It is synthesized by the fetal liver and excreted by the kidneys into the amniotic fluid, from whence it enters maternal serum. Concentrations change with gestational age.

Screening method for neural-tube defects (NTD). In cases of open NTDs, AFP passes through cerebral spinal fluid to enter amniotic fluid and maternal serum; elevated levels in weeks 16–18 (Figs. 3.71, 3.72) are an indication of NTD (dysraphic syndrome): anencephalus, myelomeningocele.

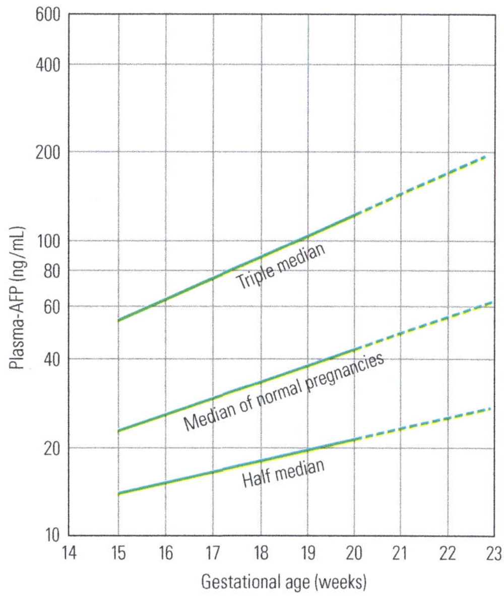

Fig. 3.71: Plasma concentration of AFP.

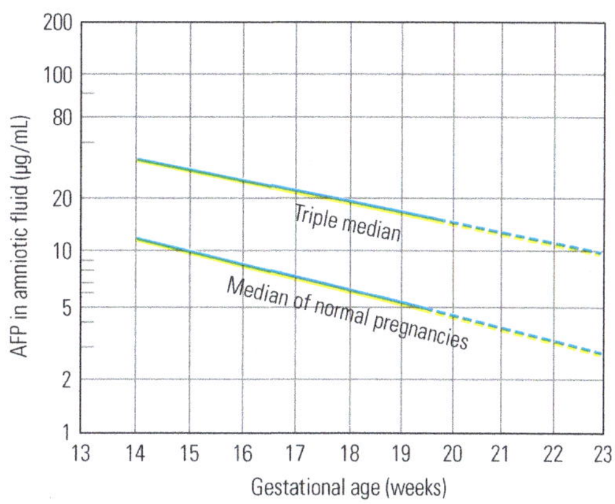

Fig. 3.72: Concentration of AFP in amniotic fluid.

Note. Elevated AFP levels require sonographic screening for fetal abnormalities to detect open NTD; nevertheless, 10 % of these defects are closed and cannot be detected by AFP screening.

Elevated serum AFP levels occur
- in EDD calculation errors,
- in multifetal pregnancies,

- if fetal death is imminent or has already occurred,
- in IUGR,
- in omphalocele, gastroschisis,
- in atresia of the fetal gastrointestinal tract,
- in fetal renal disease,
- in maternal liver disease.

Biochemical screening tests. In the 1980s statistical correlations were found between reduced AFP levels in maternal serum and trisomy 21. Wald and colleagues added hCG and unconjugated estriol in maternal serum as further markers for trisomy 21 (so-called *triple test*). This test has around a 60 % discovery rate, with a 5 % false-positive rate. Errors in method, inadequate standardization of laboratory technique and influencing factors such as gestational age, nicotine abuse, and the like have prevented a general introduction of this test.

In the first decades of prenatal diagnosis, age was the predominant indication for invasive diagnosis. This led to invasive methods not considered for women under 35, and thus trisomy 21 was not always prenatally diagnosed. The goal of screening all pregnant women without increasing the risk of miscarriage due to amniocentesis should be achievable with biochemical methods. Thus, the discovery that some biochemical serum markers could be useful in predicting trisomy 21 has been important, and attempts have been made to incorporate them in statistical risk calculations for trisomy 21.
Currently the serum parameters used consist of β-hCG, estriol, and PAPP-A (pregnancy-associated plasma protein A).

β-hCG. β chain of the placental protein hormone hCG. Serum levels are elevated in trisomy 21.

Estriol (E3). The steroid hormone is produced by the fetal adrenal glands with help from the liver and placenta. Serum levels are reduced in trisomy 21.

PAPP-A. A glycoprotein in maternal serum, levels of which steadily increase with increased gestational age, and whose physiological function is not yet known. Serum levels may be reduced in trisomy 21.

E3, β-hCG and PAPP-A are used today in the so-called *first-trimester screening* (weeks 11–14) for individual risk calculation. These parameters are also of predictive value for other chromosomal abnormalities (trisomy 21, trisomy 18, triploidy).
The detection rate of these markers is affected by many factors which influence serum concentration levels: multifetal pregnancy, maternal weight, parity, diabetes mellitus, nicotine abuse, ethnic group.

Tab. 3.6: Nutritional recommendations for pregnant women (> 16th week of pregnancy) from the German Nutrition Society – daily intake.

	Amount per day	Additional amount
Energy (kJ)	2,500	300
Protein (g)	58	10
Calcium (mg)	1,200	200
Iron (mg)	30	15
Iodine (μg)	230	30
Zinc (mg)	15	3
Vitamin A (mg RA)	1.1	0.3
Vitamin D (μg)	10	5
Vitamin E (mg)	14	2
Vitamin K (μg)	65	5
Vitamin B_1 (mg)	1.5	0.3
Vitamin B_2 (mg)	1.8	0.3
Niacin (mg)	17	2
Vitamin B_6 (mg)	2.6	1.0
Folic Acid (μg)	300	150
Vitamin B_{12} (μg)	3.5	0.5
Vitamin C (mg)	100	25

In the **combined first-trimester screening,** these biochemical methods are combined with measurement of nuchal translucency. Detection rates of > 90 % should be possible.
Prenatal diagnosis and the combined first-trimester screening must be preceded by **appropriate counseling**. The pregnant woman must be informed about the purpose, the potential problem, and the consequences, before screening is carried out. Although diagnosis should take place as early as possible in the pregnancy in order that possible consequences can be followed through early, adequate time must be allowed to impart all necessary information, provide counseling as required, and for making a decision. All impressions of routine are damaging.

3.2 Antenatal counseling

Comprehensive counseling. It is the doctor's job to inform the pregnant woman comprehensively about

- pregnancy, delivery, birth preparation methods, signs of impending delivery, methods of labor relief, monitoring in labor, birth place options,
- nutrition, iron supplements, other micronutrients,
- lifestyle, alcohol and nicotine use, travel,
- pregnancy complaints: heartburn, constipation, varicose veins.

Choice of birth place. Medical progress in obstetrics and family-oriented clinics have transformed hospital delivery into an option, and now have significantly lower risks for mother and baby while providing an emotionally-oriented environment. It is the job of the women's health care provider to provide adequate information about the possible advantages and risks of hospital and birth center or homebirths, so that an informed choice can be made.

Nutrition. Dietary habits only partially comply with the nutritional recommendations of the German Nutrition Society (Deutsche Gesellschaft für Ernährung, DGE; Tabs. 3.6. 3.7)

The 5th percentile of the intake section is lower than recommended for the nutrients listed, and for calcium, iron, and iodine even the median of the measured intake of young women is less than the DGE recommendations.
The intake of particular micronutrients (vitamins, zinc, and others) may be inadequate, especially in risk groups. How can this be assessed in individual cases?

Indirect nutritional indicators. Weight, weight gain. Biochemical indicators of nutritional deficiency are not reliable, analysis is cost intensive and not applicable to the entire population. For this reason, general indicators of nutritional status such as prepregnancy weight and weight gain, in addition to information about activity level and dietary habits, can be used as guides

Tab. 3.7: Nutritional recommendations of the German Nutricion Society for women from 19–24 years of age – daily intake.

	Energy (kJ)	Protein (g)	Calcium (mg)	Iron (mg)	Iodine (μg)	Folic acid (μg)
Median intake	2,108	68.5	690	12.2	100	114
90 percent range	(1,024–3,434)	(35–117)	(276–1414)	(6–23)	(33–284)	(49–344)
Recommendations (DGE) for women (19–24 years)	2,200	48	1,000	15	200	150
Pregnant women	2,500	58	1,200	30	230	400
Nursing women	2,850	63	1,300	20	260	225

for nutrient supply. Risk groups must be identified and counseled accordingly.

Risk factors for inadequate diet in pregnancy are
- teenager (younger than 15 years),
- one or more pregnancies in the last two years,
- previous history of IUGR, intrauterine death, premature birth,
- socioeconomically disadvantaged situation,
- alcohol, nicotine, drug consumption,
- dietary restrictions due to chronic systemic illness,
- prepregnancy weight < 85 % or > 120 % of standard weight.

Practice tip. Certain micronutrients (iron, iodine, magnesium) should be supplemented in all cases, whereas certain foods or methods of preparation should be avoided (e.g., raw fish, dishes containing liver).

Prepregnancy weight, weight gain

Weight deficiency. Low birth weight is a risk factor for perinatal mortality. Nutritional supplements in pregnancy are only able to promote weight gain to a certain extent.

In a US study, energy supplements led to higher birth weights in risk groups, not, however, in pregnant women with good nutritional status. The nutritional supplements reduced perinatal mortality by one quarter. Corresponding results from developing countries: birth weight increase of 200 g leads to a drop in underweight newborns of one-sixth, and perinatal mortality decreases by 37 %.
There is good data to support the hypothesis that intrauterine growth restriction is associated in the long-term with more frequent occurrence of coronary heart disease, arterial hypertension, and adult diabetes mellitus.

Obesity = risk factor. Excessive weight gain in pregnancy (as long as it is not due to edema) is a risk factor for high birth weight, complications in labor, diabetes, hypertension, and postpartum obesity.

Every normal birth adds 1 kg to age-standardized weight.
On the other hand, no diet should be recommended during pregnancy which might prevent adequate weight gain.
Recommendations based on empirical data for optimum weight gain (relative to pregnancy outcome) for each of three classes (low, middle, high) of pr-pregnancy body mass are listed in Tab. 3.8 below.

Tab. 3.8: Desirable weight gain in pregnancy.

Prepregnancy BMI (kg/m²)	Total weight gain (kg)
Low (< 19.8)	12.5–18
Middle (19.8–26.0)	11.5–16
High (> 26.0)	7.0–11.5

Postpartum weight. After delivery, the mother can aim for a weight loss of 2kg/month rather than the physiological 0.6–0.8, with no negative effect on lactation. In contrast, the lactation capacity of undernourished pregnant women cannot be improved with energy supplements.

Trace elements, vitamins, minerals

Iron. In developing countries, 65–70 % of pregnant women have diet-related deficiency anemias, which are responsible for 20 % of maternal mortality, in particular iron, B12, and folate deficiencies. Iron and folic acid supplementation raise hemoglobin concentration.

Iron deficiency in central Europe. As levels of iron and other indicators of iron supply were significantly higher in pregnant European women who had received iron supplements than in those who had not, it can be assumed that iron deficiency is also common in Europe.

Treatment. Maternal iron deficiency means fetal iron deficiency!

- Iron supplements are recommended from week 16 (10–30mg/day).

Iodine. Iodine deficiency exists worldwide: 1.5 billion people are affected. This is thought to be the single greatest cause of (avoidable) mental retardation (endemic cretinism), and is responsible for perinatal and infant mortality, neonatal hypothyroidism, and goiter.

Treatment. Central Europe is an iodine-deficient area. Iodized salt and a diet rich in fish are not sufficient to counteract the deficiency. One in four pregnant women have an iodine-deficiency goiter, and every second woman who has recently given birth an enlarged thyroid. Iodine tablets: 200 µg/day (recommendation of the German working group on iodine deficiency).

Folic acid. Deficiency is common and causes neural-tube defects (1 : 1,000 newborns): anencephaly, spina bifida, myelomeningocele, accompanied by early death or permanent handicap. The risk of recurrence in further children is 10 times as high. Distribution is highest where poverty and lack of education lead to poor nutrition and vitamin deficiency.

Interventional studies with multivitamin products and folic acid have shown that the risk of recurrence of NTD is significantly lower, and initial occurrence decreased.
The risk of development of orofacial clefts was also lower in a case control study of mothers who received a multivitamin product containing folic acid. The periconceptional intake of a multivitamin product was associated with low prevalence of cardiac defects in a case control study in the USA. 4 % of the German population has a low serum concentration of folic acid. A general enrichment of foods with folic acid seems hardly possible.

Prevention of cleft development with periconceptional folic acid supplementation: 4 weeks before and 8 weeks after conception 0.4 mg folic acid/day. In cases of prior pregnancy with NTD 4 mg folic acid/day.

Omega-3 fatty acids. These, and in particular docosahexaenoic acid (DHA), are essential building blocks of all cell membranes, including nerve cells in the brain and the retina. In late pregnancy and the first months of life, nerve tissue and photoreceptors store a particularly large amount of DHA. An adequate DHA supply for fetuses and newborns (200 mg/day) is important for the cognitive, visual, and physical development of children.

Calcium. The DGE recommendations for calcium intake in pregnancy (1,200 mg/day) are amongst the highest in comparison to other countries. In a normal diet the recommended intake could only be covered by the consumption of considerable amounts of dairy products. Adequate exposure to sunlight or sufficient vitamin D intake promote calcium absorption. In contrast, high phytate, oxalate, and cellulose intake, on a vegetable basis, for example by vegetarians, limit calcium absorption. Calcium depletion of the skeleton can be counteracted by calcium supplements.

Nonrecommended foods and stimulants

Risk groups. Dietary problems are often overlaid by low socioeconomic status, poor education, frequent infections, and chronic illness. Some stress factors suggest inadequate nourishment. These patients should be recognized and counseled by the doctor as early as possible.

Hypovitaminosis A is the most common vitamin deficiency worldwide and leads to 0.5 million cases of blindness and low resistance to infections, which are often fatal, in particular for children. The deficiency is rare in central

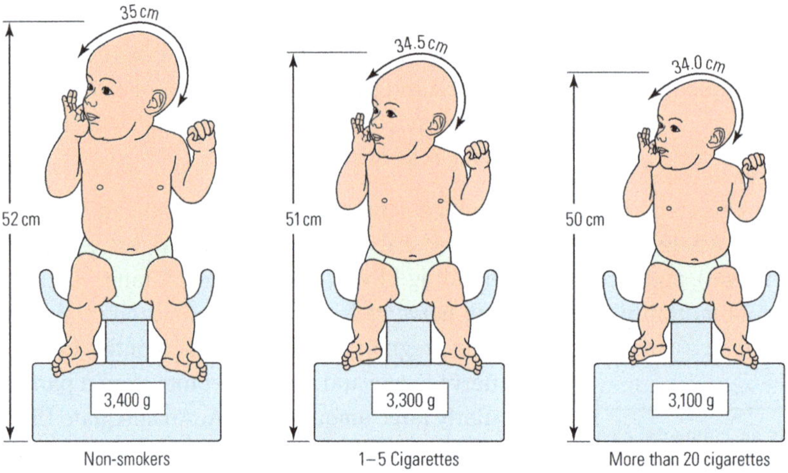

Fig. 3.73: Fetal growth restriction as a result of nicotine abuse in pregnancy.

Europe and does not occur with a carotene-rich diet with fruit and vegetables.

Practice tip. Vitamin A is a potential teratogen if taken in doses > 2400 µg/day (hypervitaminosis A). Multivitamin products for pregnancy contain up to 1,200 µg of vitamin A per dose, liver up to 13,200 µg/100 g. We recommend:
- No vitamin A supplements.
- Avoidance of dishes containing liver.

Stimulants. A link between consumption of stimulants such as alcohol and nicotine and perinatal mortality, morbidity, and premature birth rate, is difficult to establish, as consumption and environmental influences (social status, age) are difficult to separate.

Nicotine. The increase of intrauterine growth-restricted newborns with rising cigarette consumption in pregnancy (Fig. 3.73) has been established. Children of smoking mothers are 200 g lighter on average; there have been isolated reports of somatic and intellectual developmental retardation at the age of 1. The lag in height did not disappear by school age. Behavioral disorders and mental retardation were more common.

Alcohol. Dose-response relationship (exact data is not available!).

Daily alcohol consumption of > 17 g is considered dangerous. Beer contains 2–6, wine 7–17, liqueur 30–40, hard liquor 45, and rum 40–70 % alcohol.

Fetal alcohol syndrome (FAS). Children of chronic alcoholics are at risk for fetal alcohol syndrome (→ risk 30–50 %): low birth weight, microcephaly, physical and mental retardation, facial, and other malformations.

The rates of miscarriage and premature delivery are higher in cases of alcohol abuse. It is safest to avoid alcohol.

3.2.1 Lifestyle

Career, exercise, physical stress. Reliable data on the risks of sport and physical stress in pregnancy, for labor and baby, is rare.

In prospective studies standing for long periods, lifting and climbing were found to have no effect on fetal growth. On the other hand, studies conducted on risk groups with a history of obstetric complications in particular found an increased risk for another miscarriage after frequent lifting of > 9 kg or working longer than seven hours/day.

Effect on the pregnant woman. As pregnancy progresses, women feel less and less capable of physical labor. On the other hand, oxygen and energy consumption increase only minimally. Furthermore, training reduces the oxygen requirements, and maternal and fetal pH levels rise. Peak performances and stress should be avoided, both of which can bring on contractions.

Employment. Studies have shown working to have a positive effect. Certain professions or workplaces could be dangerous. The physician needs to know about the particular stresses and environmental conditions of the workplace.

A healthy pregnant woman cannot continue a stressful job.
Exercise which calls for steady exertion and the use of major muscle groups is recommended, for example swimming, cycling, cross-country skiing, and jogging.
Types of sport requiring abrupt spurts of action or ball games (abdominal trauma) are not advisable.

Swimming. The common fear of ascending infection is unfounded as water does not enter the vagina. Swimming is an ideal sport for pregnant women.

Effects on the fetus. Moderate exertion of the pregnant woman does not affect FHR; heavy exertion leads to light tachycardia. Extreme exertion is to be avoided.

The fetus adapts to the mother's physical condition, as demonstrated by FHR monitoring of a 10-week long swimming training. However, reports of severe fetal tachycardia on maximum maternal physical exertion also exist.

Travel
Air travel does not cause fetal oxygen deficiency. Nor does the alleged stress of flying negatively affect maternal blood circulation.
There is no argument against air travel for tourist purposes, in particular long distance flights.

Vaccinations. Destinations requiring vaccination with live viruses should be avoided.

Car travel. Pregnant women are not at greater risk of accidents, so car travel is not to be contraindicated as long as the three point restraint is properly positioned.

Staying in high-altitude areas. Pregnant women should not visit areas with an altitude over 2,000 m.

Sexual intercourse
Normal pregnancy. The majority of recommendations have no objection to sexual intercourse even in the last weeks of pregnancy.

Preterm labor symptoms. Orgasm can cause contractions. However, a link between frequency of coitus and premature delivery has not been established.

For safety's sake, however, if preterm labor threatens, or there is a history of it, sexual intercourse should be restricted.
The role of prostaglandins in stimulation of labor or preterm labor from semen deposited in the vagina is uncertain.

3.2.2 Common pregnancy complaints

Morning sickness, nausea, emesis gravidarum. Feeling nauseous and vomiting in the morning are typical complaints in early pregnancy. Thid begin at weeks 5–6, do not last longer than 3–4 months, and are more common in cases of multifetal gestation and molar pregnancy. A pregnant woman is not significantly restricted.

Causes are unclear; links between unwelcome and unplanned pregnancy as well as conflict in the mother-daughter relationship can only be revealed in longer conversations.
Treatment is usually not necessary and often unsuccessful. We recommend
- rest and avoidance of stress,
- avoidance of abrupt changes in position,
- Differentiation from hyperemesis with weight loss and disruption of the water-electrolyte household (in the clinic).

Heartburn is common. The cause is a hormone-related lowering of the resting tension of the cardia (entrance to the stomach, transitional zone between the two layers of esophagus into the three layers of the stomach musculature), with incomplete gastro-esophageal closure. Treatment:
- Avoidance of bending down and carrying heavy loads.
- Distribution of food intake over a number of smaller meals.
- Lying down, sleeping with elevated upper body (raising the head end of the bed).

Changes to skin and mucous membranes. Some typical changes in pregnancy: striae gravidarum, pigmentation of pregnancy, dilation and proliferation of blood vessels, and gum changes.

Stretch marks of pregnancy (striae gravidarum) affect 90 % of pregnant women in the last trimester. Fresh stretch marks are reddish-violet in color, easily distinguishable from old striae in multiparae, which are pale and wrinkled.

Striae gravidarum are the result of the hormone-related irreversible conformity changes of the collagen fiber network of the skin. Stretching does not play a major role.

Common location: lower abdomen, hips, breasts. Particularly affects obese women.
No prophylaxis or treatment exists.

Pigmentation in pregnancy. Local or generalized hyperpigmentation, due to stimulation of the melanocytes by increased levels of estrogen, progesterone, and MSH. Light pigmentation sometimes appears in early pregnancy.

Frequent locations: nipple, areola and area surrounding areola (secondary areola), vulva, anus; the linea alba becomes the linea nigra. Scars from operations or naevi become darker. Such pigmentation is more pronounced in brunettes than in blondes. Facial pigmentation (chloasma gravidarum): well-demarcated, irregularly shaped yellowish-brown patches on forehead, cheeks, chin. A symmetrical patch-shaped facial hyperpigmentation occurs in two-thirds of pregnant women in the second half of pregnancy. This is known as melasma gravidarum or "mask of pregnancy". Exposure to UV or sun rays increases pigmentation.
There is no treatment. In most cases spontaneous regression occurs in the weeks or months after delivery. However, 10 % of melasmas persist.

Dilation and proliferation of blood vessels. Under the influence of increased estrogen levels, 30 % of pregnant women develop palmar erythema and spider naevi (telangiectasias, spots with fine lines radiating out from them), which may persist to some extent after delivery.

Hemorrhoids. Hypervolemia, vasodilation, obstructed venous drainage, and pushing in the second stage of labor and in puerperium can all lead to the development of hemorrhoids, which can cause considerable discomfort.

Treatment:
- Local treatment with sitz baths, creams, suppositories.
- Ensuring that bowel movements are soft.

Varicosities. Primary varicosities. Result of a congenital blood vessel wall dysplasia, whose carriers often demonstrate other signs of mesenchymal weakness (hernia, hemorrhoids); secondary varicosites. Result of healed thrombosis.

Cause: hypervolemia and generalized vasodilation increase venous pressure in the legs. Promoted by blood flow obstructions (large uterus, constrictive clothing, working in a standing position).

Treatment. Medication is rarely successful. Elastic stockings (compression grade II) should be prescribed at an early stage.
- Daily elevation of the legs.
- Leg exercises and swimming.
- Low-dose heparin (3 × 5,000 IU Heparin S.C.) in extreme cases.
- Operative treatment several months after delivery, or sclerotherapy in weeks 28–32 (conflicting expert opinions!).

Muscle cramps. Cause unknown, mineral or pantothenic acid deficiency may be implicated.

Treatment: vitamin B, magnesium

Caries, gingivitis. The majority of pregnant women develop slightly swollen, hyperemic gums which bleed easily. The causes are hormonal influences and reduced pH of the saliva.

Treatment: visit to the dentist and regular teeth brushing.

Constipation. Common. Caused by elevated progesterone levels and relaxation of smooth muscles.

Treatment:
- High-fiber diet: large amounts of fruit, vegetables, dairy products, wholewheat bread, dried fruits, fruit juices, dried figs, or prunes which have been soaked in water overnight.
- Mild laxatives if necessary (→ increased peristaltic due to intraluminal volume increase).

References

American College of Obstetricians and Gynecologists: Anemia in pregnancy. Clinical Management Guidelines No 95, July 2008. Obstet Gynecol 2008; 112:201-7

American College of Obstetricians and Gynecologists: Prevention of early-onset group B streptococcal disease in newborns. Committee opinion No 485 April 2011. Obstet Gynecol 2011; 117:1019–27

Baschat AA, Gembruch U, Harmann CR: The sequence of changes in Doppler und biopysical parameters as severe fetal growth restriction. Ultrasouncl Obstet Gynecol 2001; 18:571–77

Brill-Edwards P, Ginsberg KS, Gent M, et al.: Safety of withholding heparın in pregnent women with a history of venous thromboembolism. Recurrence of clot in this pregnancy study group. N Engl J Med 2000; 343:1439

Blom HJ: Folic acid, methylation and neural tube closure in humans. Birth Defects Research (Part A) 2009; 85:285

Cancelo-Hidalgo MJ, Castelo-Branco C, Palacios S, et al.: Tolerability of different oral iron supplements: a systematic review. Curr Med Res&Opin 2013; 29:291–303

Chervenak FA, McCollough LB, Campbell S: Is third trimester abortion justified? Br J Obstet Gynaecol 1995; 102:434

Dizon-Townson D, Miller C, Sibai B, et al.: The relationship of the factor Leiden mutation and pregnancy outcomes for mother and fetus. Obstet Gynecol 2005; 106:517

Gomez O, Figueras F, Fernandenz S, et al: Reference rangers for uterine artery mean pulsatility indes at 11–41 weeks of gestation. Ultrasound Obstet Gynecol 2008; 32:128–32

Greer IA, Nelson-Piercy C: Low-molecular-weight heparins for thomboprophylaxis and treatment of venous thromboembolism in pregnancy: a systematic review of safety and efficacy. Blood 2005; 106:410

Haider BA, Olofin I, Wang M, et al.: Anemia, prenatal iron use, and risk of adverse pregnancy outcomes: systematic review and meta-analysis. BMJ 2013; 346:f3443doi:10.1136

James DK, Mahomed K, Stone P, et al: Evidence-based Obstetrics. 2nd ed. Saunders, London 2004
Kramer MS, Kakurna R: Energy and protein intrake in pregnancy. Cochrane Database Systematic Reviews 2003; 4:CD000032
Rey E, Kahn SR, David M, Shrier I: Thrombophilic disorders and fetal loss: a meta-analysis. Lancet 2003; 361:901
Royal College of Obstetricians and Gynaecologists: Amniocentesis and Chorionic Villus Sampling. Green-top Guideline No. 8. June 2010
Royal College of Obstetricians and Gynecologists: Late intrauterine fetal death and stillbirth. Green-top Guideline No. 55, October 2010
Royal College of Obstetricians and Gynecologists: Prevention of early-onset group B streptococcal disease in newborns. Green-top guideline No. 36, 2nd edition, July 2012
Royal College of Obstetricians and Gynecologists: The prevention of early-onset neonatal group B streptococcal disease. Green-top Guideline No. 36, August 2012
Royal College of Obstetricians and Gynecologists: Management of beta thalassaemia in pregnancy. Green-top Guidelne No. 66, March 2014
Van Dumme FM, de Craen AJ, Heijmans BT, et al.: Genderspecific association of the factor V Leiden mutation with fertility and fecundity in a historic cohort. The Leiden 85-plus study. Hum Reprod 2006; 21:967

4 Maternal disorders in pregnancy

4.1 Pregnancy-specific disorders

Disorders associated with pregnancy are: hyperemesis gravidarum, cholestasis, pregnancy-induced hypertension PIH, preeclampsia PE, eclampsia, HELLP syndrome.

4.1.1 Hyperemesis gravidarum

Definition. Severe vomiting of pregnancy. Escalation of nausea and vomiting (emesis gravidarum) in early pregnancy (begin week 5–6, ending week 12–16); gradual transition into severe vomiting of pregnancy.

Etiology. Unclear. The endocrine changes in the first trimester (placental hCG synthesis) are a possible cause. Psychological factors can modify or exacerbate.

Maternal ambivalence or fear associated with the pregnancy and/or may modify or exacerbate nausea and vomiting in pregnancy, contributing a psychosomatic component to the etiology of hyperemesis gravidarum.

Symptoms
- Vomiting is more severe and more frequent, up to 5–10 times a day, at any time, regardless of whether the stomach is empty or not.
- Severe thirst (fluid loss).
- Dehydration: flaccid and dry skin, dry tongue, skin folds persist for a long time after raising).
- Fetid breath (fetor ex ore).
- Rapid weight loss.
- Worsening general condition.
- Temperature increase.
- Jaundice (severe metabolic disorder of the liver).
- Central nervous system symptoms: drowsiness, delirium.

Laboratory findings
Urine. Elevated: protein, acetone, urobilinogen, porphyrin; casts in urine sediment.
Serum. In severe cases, bilirubin is increased by up to 2 mg %, a dangerous sign.

DD. Hepatitis (accompanied by nausea and vomiting), hyperthyroidism.

Treatment
- Hospital evaluation and treatment.
- Intravenous therapy (fluid, electrolyte, and glucose replacement) in severe cases, with the presence of acetone in urine, dehydration, electrolyte imbalance. To be continued until acetone is no longer found in the urine.
- Antiemetics, such as dimenhydrinate .
- The supplementation of ginger to combat morning sickness has been adopted from Asia (1 g/day).
- Psychological support and/or treatment for emotional disorders may be indicated.

Complications. Inadequate or wrong treatments can lead to irreparable organ damage, metabolic disorders, and loss of strength (temperature increase, delirium) followed by death.

4.1.2 Cholestasis

Definition. Disorder of the biliary tract or liver, with the main symptom of severe itching. Usually does not occur until the third trimester and disappears spontaneously after parturition.

Etiology and incidence. Hormonal influences on the biliary tract. Obstetric cholestasis occurs in 0.7 % of all pregnancies.

Diagnosis. Apart from the intense pruritus, results of liver function tests may be pathological, in particular the serum bile salts may be elevated. Normal liver function results and bile salt levels do not, however, rule out obstetric cholestasis. Viral hepatitis and obstructive jaundice must be considered as other possible diagnoses.

Prognosis. Contrary to earlier thinking, antepartum fetal mortality is not raised in obstetric cholestasis. Preterm delivery is, however, more common.

Treatment. First-line treatment with ursodeoxycholic acid (UCDA) or cholestyramine is recommended, although not evidence-based. Daily maternal supplementation with vitamin K is advisable in temporary liver function disorders, including clotting factors.

4.1.3 Pregnancy-induced hypertension (PIH), preeclampsia, eclampsia, HELLP syndrome

Definition. Group of pregnancy-specific disorders with hypertension as the cardinal symptom.

Incidence, relevance. 6–8 % of all pregnant women develop preeclampsia, 1 % develop HELLP syndrome, 0.1 % eclampsia. At 20 %, PIH is one of the commonest causes of maternal mortality. Eclampsia has a lethality rate of 1.8 %. The perinatal mortality rate of severe preeclampsia and eclampsia is as high as 20 %.

Pathophysiology (see Fig. 4.1). In recent decades, a large number of working hypotheses as to the causality and course of PIH and preeclampsia have been developed. Even today, however, a complete understanding and generally accepted pathophysiology of this group of disorders has not yet been achieved.

Central to today's explanations are impaired placental development, with defective trophoblast invasion into the spiral arteries and gradual reduction in placental perfusion. This leads to the release of substances in the maternal circulation which cause a generalized disfunction of endothelial cells. This produced generalized vasospasm with increased vascular permeability and can be associated with an intravascular activation of the coagulation cascade.

Genetic factors. According to a number of observations, a genetic predisposition seems likely:
- Primigravidae whose mothers and sisters suffered from preeclampsia have a two to five-fold increased risk of suffering from preeclampsia themselves.
- Partners of men who are the products of a pregnancy complicated by preeclampsia have an increased preeclampsia risk.
- Women impregnated by men whose earlier partner had preeclampsia are also at increased risk.

Both maternal and paternal influences on fetal genes probably contribute to inadequate trophoblast invasion and subsequent preeclampsia. While the evidence is not conclusive, some genes have been implicated in the pathogenesis of preeclampsia:
- T 235 variant of the angiotensinogen gene.
- The endothelial nitric oxide synthase (NOS) gene.
- Genes which cause thrombophilia.

Data ascribing etiological relevance to these findings is not convincing.

Immunological factors. The incidence of PIH in nulliparae is considerably higher than in parous women with the same partner, but it increases markedly with a partner change. The confrontation of the mother with paternal or fetal antigens appears to play a protective role. The finding that the duration of sexual intercourse, and thus exposure to the father's sperm, is inversely proportional to the risk of preeclampsia, must be similarly interpreted.

Endothelial disfunction. The substances produced as a result of placental ischemia cause generalized endothelial disfunction, as demonstrated by the following laboratory findings:
- Elevated fibronectin levels, increased Factor VIII and thrombomodulin.
- Reduction in vasodilatory and vasorelaxing substances.
- Decreased nitrous oxide (NO) and prostacyclin (vasodilatory effect).
- Increased production of endothelins and thromboxane (vasoconstrictive effect).
- Increased vascular response to angiotensin type II.

Since Gant's work in the early 1970s, it is recognized that women with preeclampsia demonstrate a vascular sensitivity to angiotensin type II, and a disrupted balance between vasodilation (prostacyclin) and vasoconstriction (thromboxane).

Impaired trophoblast invasion. In normal pregnancy the spiral arteries of the uterus are remodeled from small arterioles to large capacity vessels during the endovascular invasion and infiltration of the trophoblasts, providing the increased placental perfusion capable of meeting the increasing oxygen requirements of the fetus. The trophoblast invasion in women who later develop preeclampsia does not occur in this way (see Fig. 3.63). The physiological remodeling of the spiral arteries takes place at the end of the first trimester, and around weeks 18–20.

Vascular mediators. It has not been definitively determined whether these substances are cause or consequence of the placental ischemia. Two factors play a large role in the changes to maternal arteries: **VEGF** (vascular endothelial growth factor) and **PGF** (placental growth factor). These factors are expressed in the maternal

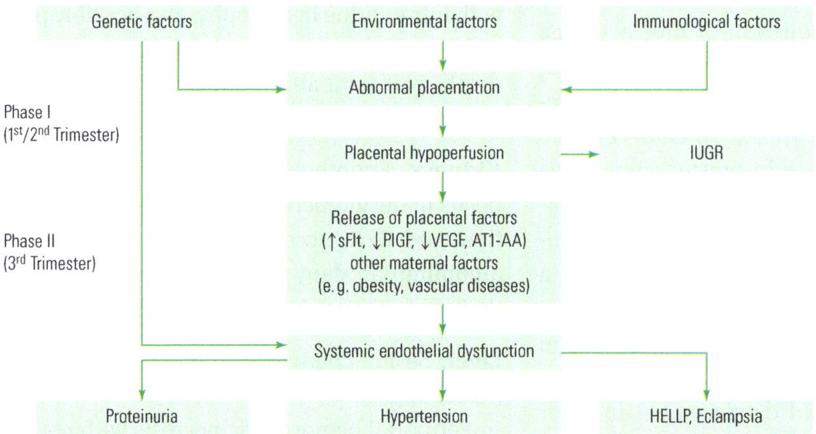

Fig. 4.1: The "two-stage theory" of preeclampsia: maternal factors such as genetic predisposition and environmental and immunological components cause abnormal placentation. The resulting placental hypoperfusion leads to ischemia and/or hypoxemia and triggers changes in expression of placental factors such as sFlT, PIGF, or Angiotensin I receptor autoantibodies. The release of those factors locally produced in the placenta into the maternal circulation results in systemic involvement of the maternal organism. The resulting vascular/endothelial disfunction leads to development of the maternal syndrome of preeclampsia, with hypertension, proteinuria; and potential deterioration to the complications of HELLP and eclampsia (modified, after Lamm and colleagues, 2005).

bloodstream by the growing trophoblasts. The soluble form of the VEGF receptor (= sFLT-1) binds VEGF and PlGF and is highly regulated in preeclampsia, with the result that free VEGF and free PlGF are significantly reduced in preeclampsia. It is not known what causes the increase in sFLT-1. It is remarkable that these changes can be detected in serum long before the clinical appearance of preeclampsia symptoms. A significant increase in sFLT-1 concentration has been described five weeks before the appearance of clinical symptoms. Substances which bind or inactivate sFLT-1 may be one hope for the early treatment of preeclampsia in future.

The angiotensin type-II hypersensitivity in preeclampsia, despite the fact that levels of angiotensin II remain constant, is due to the production of agonistic AT1 receptor autoantibodies (**AT1–AA**). They are also detectable before clinical manifestation of preeclampsia. AT1–AA generates reactive oxygen species (ROS) in trophoblastic cells, which are considered essential to the endothelial damage.

Prostaglandins. Production of prostacyclins, which have the physiological effects of potent vasodilation and inhibition of platelet aggregation, is decreased in endothelial cell disfunction. This decrease in prostacyclins plays a role in hypertension, because peripheral vasodilation does not occur. In contrast, thromboxane A_2, which is produced in the placenta and causes vasoconstriction and platelet aggregation, is seven times higher in PIH than in normotensive pregnant women. PIH is characterized by a marked displacement in favor of thromboxane A_2, and thus a predominating vasoconstriction.

RAAS (renin-angiotensin-aldosterone-system). A resistance to angiotensin type II is demonstrable in pregnancy, particularly after week 20. This resistance is missing in pregnant women with PIH.

NO (nitrous oxide) and **endothelin 1** (EDN-1). NO is a vasodilator and platelet aggregation inhibitor, while endothelin 1 acts as a peripheral vasoconstrictor. The endothelial disfunction causes increased expression of NO and EDN-1, whereby EDN-1 inactivates NO and contributes to vasoconstriction.

Central phenomena are:
- Generalized vasoconstriction, endothelial lesions with increased peripheral vascular resistance, microcirculation disorders.
- Activation of intravascular coagulation by fibrin deposits and platelet aggregation.
- Hypoperfusion of the terminal vascular bed and tissue hypoxia in organs.

Placenta. The reduced uteroplacental perfusion has morphological consequences:
- Increased fibrin deposits, proliferative endarteritis in the spiral arteries.
- Decidual hematoma, macro- and microinfarcts with fibrin precipitation.

The result is chronic placental insufficiency with intrauterine hypotrophy, and possibly placental oxidative stress with hypoxia and fetal death; placental abruption is more commonly observed.

Kidneys. Endothelial damage and fibrin deposits in the glomeruli reduce the renal plasma flow and GFR, accompanied by oliguria and albuminuria. Many glomeruli are returned to their normal state four weeks after parturition.

Liver. Severe changes in 10 % of women with preeclampsia:
- Periportal hemorrhagic necrosis with reduced blood flow in the sinusoids, subcapsular hematomas.
- Pain in the right upper abdomen or epigastric complaints are indicators of unfavorable developments.
- Periportal and focal parenchymal necroses cause elevated aminotransferase levels.

The changes cause thrombocytopenia and hemolysis, through mechanical-oxidative damage to erythrocytes (**HELLP syndrome**). The acronym for this group of symptoms (hemolysis, elevated liver enzymes, low platelet count), which 10 % of women with preeclampsia show, was coined by Weinstein in 1982. It is feared because of the maternal mortality rate of 4 %, and perinatal mortality rate of up to 23 %.

Classification, modeled on the National Institutes of Health (NIH) and the International Society of Hypertension in Pregnancy:

1. *Gestational hypertension (PIH):* elevated arterial blood pressure (systolic ≥ 140 mmHg, diastolic ≥ 90 mmHg) in the second half of pregnancy; without proteinuria.
2. *Gestational proteinuria:* protein excretion ≥ 300 mg/24hr in the second half of pregnancy.
3. *Preeclampsia:* gestational hypertension and gestational proteinuria.
4. *Eclampsia:* subjective symptoms and cramps in addition to the symptoms of preeclampsia.
5. *Chronic hypertension:* elevated arterial blood pressure (systolic ≥ 140 mmHg, diastolic ≥ 90 mmHg) before week 20 or preexistent hypertension, without proteinuria.
6. *Chronic renal disorder:* proteinuria before week 20 or preexisting.
7. *Chronic renal disorder with superimposed preeclampsia:* hypertension and proteinuria before week 20 or preexisting.

Symptoms of PIH

Hypertension. Blood pressure > 135/ 85 mmHg is pathological.

The diastolic measurement is the indicator for preeclampsia and is therefore of particular importance.

Standardized measurement of blood pressure (BP) seated, after a 10 min rest, on the arm.

Practice tip. Day-and-night BP regulation rhythm and white coat hypertension must be taken into account in the interpretation of the results.

Noninvasive 24-hour BP monitoring has advantages: registration of a 24 h BP profile. BP which does not sink at night is a symptom for PIH.

Systolic blood pressure. Alongside the international classification, which focuses on the diastolic measurement, the systolic measurement (> 135mmHg) and the relative BP increase systolic > 25 mm Hg and diastolic > 15 mm Hg are also relevant for diagnosis and therapy. In particular, the prepregnancy levels must be taken into consideration.

Both the level of sodium in the body and plasma volume are reduced in PIH. Hypovolemia intensifies the hypoperfusion of the fetal-placental unit and the reduced renal plasma flow.

Proteinuria. The increased permeability of the capillaries in pregnancy also affects the capillaries of the glomeruli. Protein is excreted in higher concentrations into the primary urine. Those albumins with the lowest molecular weight are primarily to be found; they can pass through capillary walls more easily than the higher molecular globulins.

- Total protein of < 0.3 g/l in 24 h urine is physiological.
- Total protein of > 0.3 g/l in 24 h urine is pathological.

Edema in late pregnancy was previously considered to be a symptom of renal insufficiency with increased tubular retention of sodium. The retained fluid is stored in the extracellular space and causes swelling of calves and thighs, feet, face, fingers, vulva, and the lower abdomen.

Edema usually develops slowly. Once several liters of fluid have been stored in the tissues it can be seen and felt.

Practice tip. Edema is only recognized early if regular antenatal check-ups are performed.
Diagnosis: weight gain: 500 g/week is the upper limit in the last trimester; test for pitting by applying pressure to the skin above the ankle, on the front edge of the tibia.

Note. According to epidemiological studies, edema is not a risk factor with regard to perinatal mortality on its own. It is not of predictive value for PIH or perinatal complications.

Friedmann examined 40,000 pregnant women and found a perinatal mortality of 2.8 %. 31 % had pretibial edema. The perinatal mortality of babies of women with edema was at 2.3 % not higher than that of the total group. The perinatal mortality of babies of women with proteinuria was, at 4.4 %, however, higher. At 11.5 %, the mortality of babies of women who had (diastolic) hypertension in week 24 was markedly higher.
In contrast, rapid weight gain (≥ 2 kg/week) is a warning sign for PIH (Rath 1999).

Upper abdomen. Pain in the epigastrium or right upper quadrant can be early cardinal symptoms of HELLP syndrome and call for laboratory tests: platelets, aminotransferase, haptoglobin.

Upper abdomen complaints such as nausea, vomiting, and epigastric pain can also be warning signs for eclampsia.
In addition:

Central nervous system symptoms
- Severe headaches, general restlessness, drowsiness.
- Hyperreflexia: intensified, widespread reflexes.
- Visual symptoms (flickering, double vision, hypertensive retinopathy), blindness.

Eclamptic seizure (convulsion caused by cerebral vasospasm). The eclamptic seizure develops from previous symptoms, and rarely occurs without pre-eclamptic signs; it is life-threatening for mother and fetus!

Symptoms:
- General restlessness; facial twitching, trembling of hands, arms, feet; mydriasis.
- Tonic seizure: hands balled into fists, jaw clamped shut (caution: tongue-biting!), apnea, cyanotic facial coloring, with abrupt transition into
- Clonic seizure, convulsions of all parts of the body. The convulsing woman throws arms and legs about, cramps in the neck muscles force the head backwards, cramps of the back muscles tense the spine like a bow. The patient foams at the mouth (increased saliva secretion).
- The cramp ceases after one minute with a deep snoring breath, and the patient usually remains unconscious for some time afterwards.
- Reflexes are absent during a seizure, and blood pressure is slightly increased.

Practice tip. Mortality increases with each seizure, and it is the obstetrician's task to prevent further seizures.

Asymptomatic eclampsia (eclampsia sine eclampsia), hepatic coma. Eclampsia can occur without seizure if hepatic insufficiency dominates (eclampsia sine eclampsia). The result is liver failure coma, with deep comatose breathing, jaundice, hyperbilirubinemia, and bilirubinuria.

The prognosis is particularly poor.
Differential diagnosis of eclampsia: 1) epilepsy, 2) tetany; 3) uremia; 5) meningitis; 5) diabetic coma.

Degrees of severity of PIH

1. Mild hypertension:
   a) Diastolic BP 90–110 mm Hg.
   b) Systolic BP 140–160 mm Hg.
   c) Proteinuria 0.5–5 g/ l/24 h.

2. Severe hypertension:
   a) Diastolic BP > 110 mm Hg.
   b) Systsolic BP > 160 mm Hg.
   c) Proteinuria > 5 g/ l/24 h.
   d) Oliguria < 400 ml/24 h.
   e) Hyperreflexia.
   f) Upper abdomen discomfort.
   g) Pulmonary edema, cyanosis.

3. Imminent eclampsia:
   a) Headache.
   b) Visual disturbances.

4. Eclampsia (most severe hypertensive disorder):
   a) Tonic-clonic convulsions.
   b) Apnea, coma.

Early diagnosis of PIH

Note. Measures for early diagnosis are: antenatal care, clinical (BP, weight) and laboratory (urine) findings in addition to the identification of risk groups.

Predisposition. Risk groups are:
- Young primigravidae, late age at first birth.
- Pregnant women with a family history of PIH or eclampsia (familial predisposition).
- Pregnant women with renal disorders.
- Multifetal pregnancies.
- Pregnant women with diabetes, lupus, antiphospholipid syndrome.
- Pregnant women with essential hypertension.
- Pregnant women with hydatididiform mole.
- Pregnant women with fetal hydrops.

Risk of recurrence of preeclampsia/eclampsia/HELLP syndrome. Pregnant women who previously suffered from preeclampsia/eclampsia have a risk of recurrence of
- 15 %;
- in the case of a known severe preeclampsia midpregnancy, the risk of recurrence is 40 %:
- the risk of recurrence of HELLP syndrome is 13 %.

Diagnosis and prevention in predisposition

Laboratory tests
- Hemoglobin (Hb), hematocrit (Ht).
- Platelet count every 14 days (thrombocytopenia < 150,000/μL is a warning sign).

Initial prospective studies on predicting preeclampsia in symptom-free women have demonstrated good prediction rates. The detection of PlGF and sFlt-1 in maternal blood is possible with *Triage PlGF*, from Alere Int. Sarl, Switzerland and Roche *Elecsys sFlt-1/PlGF*, from Roche Diagnostics.

Doppler ultrasound. An early diagnosis scan is recommended between weeks 20 and 24.

Sonography of the uterine artery is useful in assessing the relationship between PIH and uterine artery resistance. Pregnant women with late-onset preeclampsia have a nonreassuring Doppler scan at around 20 weeks. Further studies have shown that 60 % of high-risk women with a pathological Doppler flow in weeks 21–24 developed preeclampsia or IUGR, while in those with normal Doppler results only 8 % did.
Women with no known risk factors who had a pathological Doppler flow had a 6 % risk, andthose with normal results 5 %.

Prevention

Acetylsalicylic acid (ASA) inhibits the vasoconstriction caused by thromboxane and the isoenzyme COX-1, and through it the synthesis by mature platelets of Thromboxane-A_2, which restricts their ability to aggregate.

- Dosage: low dose oral ASA of 50–100 mg/day (Wallenburg).
- Prophylactically from week 12.

Randomized studies have shown conflicting results. Some studies (in particular the CLASP study), demonstrated that treating pregnant women with a history of preeclampsia before week 34 and high risk of recurrence, antiphospholipid syndrome, family history with low-dose ASA reduced the rate of preeclampsia and IUGR. An early start (before week 16) of ASA therapy, especially in the risk group with a pathological Doppler profile, is recommended for successful prevention.

Treatment of PIH

Principles. Early, rigorous treatment. In mild cases the risks of antihypertensive medication must be taken into account. In severe cases the mother's condition must be stabilized and a termination of the pregnancy considered.

General measures
- Fluids- no restrictions (allow to drink as desired).
- Protein-rich diet.
- Minimization of physical exertion, bed rest.

Low-sodium diet. ≤ 3 g NaCl/day. The low-salt diet usually recommended by internists for the treatment of hypertension is disallowed for obstetrical patients.

Antihypertensive medication only when BP is > 170/110 mm Hg.

Antihypertensive drugs are not recommended for mild hypertension (diastolic BP < 110 mm Hg) because of the possibility of uterine hypoperfusion. In addition, whether the drugs reduce the frequency of preeclampsia and improve fetal outcome is a point of contention.

Methyldopa educes total peripheral resistance.
- Dosage. 0.5–1 g/day, initial 0.5 g/day.
- Note: because of fetal side-effects (meconium ileus, lethargy) it should be combined with dihydralazine if doses of ≥ 2 g/day are required.

Calcium channel blockers (CCB, or calcium antagonists) cause peripheral vasodilation and have an anticonvulsive effect.
- Dosage: one 5 mg capsule, bitten open, repeated if necessary.
- after 20 min.
- Note: adequate information on fetal side-effects is not available, particularly regarding long-term usage.

Alpha-1 blocker. Urapidil reduces peripheral vascular resistance, without affecting HMV.

- Dosage. Intravenous, initially 6 mg/h, maximum 24 mg/h.
- Note: less likely to cause headache and tachycardia than dihydralazine.

Dihydralazine, effective, long-lasting BP reduction as a result of direct dilation of the peripheral blood vessels (improvement of renal circulation!), probably also due to its influence on central nervous centers. It can be given orally, IV or IM.
- Dosage: 1) orally 2–3 × 1 tablet/day up to 25 mg; 2) infusion: 50 mg Dihydralazine in 500 ml basic solution. Infusion rate initially 20 ml/h, dose according to BP; 3) single intravenous dose inject 1.25 to max 2.5 mg, slowly, whilst monitoring BP.

Practice tip. Continuous BP monitoring must be performed during injection. Slow BP reduction should be aimed for, not more than 20 % in an hour, e.g., from 200/120 mmHg down to 160/95 mmHg at most, and not lower than 140/95 mm Hg. A too rapid decrease can lead to maternal hypotension with reduced circulation to brain, kidneys, placenta, and constitute a threat to the fetus (acidosis).

- Combination. Caution should be applied when combining with tocolytics because of the combined vasodilatory effect.

- Side effects. Headache, palpitations, tachycardia, dizziness, nausea, vomiting, paresthesia of the extremities.

Diazoxide. Strongest antihypertensive substance, increases HMV by increasing pulse frequency, widening of the BP amplitude, and reduction of the peripheral vascular resistance.

- Dosage. (in a hypertensive crisis, diastolic BP > 150 mm Hg) 150 mg within 15 s (monitoring BP every 2 min!); repeat bolus injection after 15 min if necessary.

Beta blockers
- Dosage. Metaprolol 200 mg/day.
- Side effects. Significant fetal side effects are not known. Newborns tend to develop bradycardia if the mother has been treated with beta blockers.
- Note: end of treatment 1–2 days before birth because of tendency of newborns to be bradycardic, is usually not possible due to the necessity of treatment for hypertension. A reduced reactivity to hypoxia in growth-retarded fetuses has been reported, and avoidance of these medications is recommended. There is dispute on whether contractions are increased.

Practice tip. Treatment of PIH with beta blockers is not yet routine, because not enough large clinical studies have been performed.

Anticonvulsive therapy. Central to treatment of PIH is magnesium, which alongside its marked sedative effect, also causes a mild BP reduction.

Diuretics are not popular, because they cause placental hypoperfusion. Epidemiological studies have shown that attempts to reduce edema in pregnancy in nonhypertensive women are made at the risk of growth-restricted fetuses. Remaining indication: 1) only rarely in mild preeclampsia; 2) in cases of severe edema weak diuretics (Chlortalidone 3 times/week, 25–50 mg); 3) strong diuretics (furosemide) only in cases of severe PIH with threatened eclampsia and complications (pulmonary edema, renal failure).

Mild PIH
Outpatient treatment if diagnosed a number of weeks or months before EDD. Weekly monitoring of BP, weight, and urine for proteinuria. Hospital admission if additional risk factors are present (IUGR, multifetal gestation) or no response to treatment within 14 days.

General measures
- Bed rest, at least temporarily, as it
  - increases placental and renal perfusion and GFR;
  - prevents orthostatic edema.
- Protein intake: 100 g protein/day, more in cases of proteinuria. Dairy products, fish, meat, and eggs. Insufficient protein intake is detrimental for the fetus.
- Restricted fat intake.

Fluid and salt intake reduction diets are obsolete (see pathophysiology).

Severe PIH, imminent eclampsia
Prevention of convulsions via sedation of the central nervous system, BP reduction, diuresis, in particular in cases of oliguria or anuria.
- Infusion therapy (via cannula or venous catheter)

Practice tip. A central venous catheter (CVC) is the method of choice in cases of severe PIH, the treatment of which extends over a number of days. Advantage: continuous monitoring of central venous pressure (CVP).

CVP (central venous pressure 3–6, on average 4.5 H_2O). Used as a guide for infusion therapy.

- Low CVP is an indicator for hypovolemia (low blood volume).
- High CVP indicates hypervolemia (fluid overload) or right-sided heart failure.

Anticonvulsive therapy central sedation
Magnesium is the medication of choice. *Mechanism of action.* Peripherally: calcium antagonist at the interface between nerve end and motor end plate with reduction of muscle tone of both smooth and striated muscle tissue; centrally: sedation of perceptive, motoric and vegetative central nervous system function, overdose causes somnolence and respiratory failure. Magnesium has a strong spasmolytic effect, improves cerebral circulation and oxygenation.
It has a variable effect on blood pressure in PIH. It may have no effect, or a periodic one.
Dosage. Magnesium ascorbate/sulfate. 1) IM 0.5–1 g/day (5–10 ml of the 10 % magnesium-ascorbate solution); 2) slowly, IV in severe cases; in cases of imminent eclampsia: 2–4 g (10–20 %); 3) continuous IV drip appears the best method, as with an eclamptic seizure.

Practice tip. Magnesium is contraindicated if oliguria is present, as when not excreted (likewise in case of overdose) toxic reactions (somnolence, respiratory failure) may occur.

Blood pressure reduction, intravenous antihypertensive therapy (see p. 80)

Increased diuresis

Consequences of hypovolemia are:
Hemoconcentration. Increased hemoglobin (Hb) and hematocrit (Hct) levels (> 40–50 %; normal pregnancy 33–35 %).
Therapy. Hemodilution with low molecular weight dextran, hydroxyethyl starch or human albumin. Dosage according to Hct levels (ideal < 35 %)
Decrease of urinary output with threatened acute renal failure: oliguria, anuria, shock.
Therapy. Infusion therapy based on urinary output and CVP, to avoid the risks of life-threatening hyperhydration. Dialysis if infusion therapy is not effective in increasing diuresis.

Practice tip. Urinary output should not be less than 30 ml/h, CVP should not exceed 6–8 cm H_2O

Fetal monitoring in pregnancy
- Electronic (cardiotocography) (see p. 36).
- Ultrasonography (see p. 44).
- Doppler sonography (see p. 53).
- Diagnosis of lung maturity (see p. 60).

Fetal monitoring in labor
- Cardiotocography (see p. 168).
- Fetal blood sampling (see p. 177).

Eclampsia, eclamptic seizure
Interruption of the seizure and **prevention** of further seizures (most important measure) via:
- *Magnesium*
  - Magnesium ascorbate. Loading dosage 2–4 g (10–20 ml of the 20 % solution) IV, followed by maintenance dose of 1 g Magnesium ascorbate/h via continuous infusion.
  - Magnesium sulfate (acc. to Zuspan and colleagues). Loading dose 4–6 g (40–60 ml 10 % solution) followed by maintenance dose of 1 g Magnesium ascorbate/h via continuous infusion.
  - Dosage tip: dose based on serum Mg levels (3–4 mmol/l), clinically according to excitability of the patellar reflex (must be present!). Mg dose must be reduced if reflexes are missing. Respiratory rate should also be monitored: > 14/min!
  - Overdose tip: calcium gluconate is the antidote, injection of 10 ml of a 10 % solution if required.

- *Muscle relaxation*
  - Anesthetist should be involved if a seizure occurs: intubation, long-term ventilation under continuing antihypertensive therapy, diuretic treatment, and correction of metabolic acidosis.
- *Ceasarean section*
  - As early as possible after seizure in the interests of the fetus.
- *Additional measures*
  - Fluid intake and output must be monitored (oliguria: urinary output < 16 ml/h, anuria urinary output < 4 ml/h).
  - Indwelling urinary catheter is unavoidable! Disadvantages must be accepted.

Oxygenation. After sedation, adequate oxygen supply must be ensured: clear airways, artificial ventilation. Apnea occurs during the seizure, with the danger of suffocation; in coma respiratory failure, secretion of mucus with
- hypoxia or anoxia, coma;
- respiratory and metabolic acidosis;
- rise in BP.

Further dangers are
- cerebral hemorrhage, cardiac failure;
- regurgitation and aspiration of stomach contents.

Muscle relaxation and endotracheal intubation with artificial ventilation are imperative in serial convulsions (one convulsion after another causing extreme respiratory distress).

Blood pressure reduction (see p. 80).

Increasing diuresis (see p. 84).

General measures and laboratory analyses
- Rest in quiet, dim room, avoidance of noise.
- Automated BP monitoring.
- Airway tube or rubber wedge should be on hand to prevent tongue-biting.
- Examination of the ocular fundus.
- Daily fluid balance (intake and output).
- Daily monitoring of serum electrolyte, creatinine and urea levels.

Obstetric management in late pregnancy
Mild preeclampsia is treated conservatively for as long as possible (hospital admission; termination of pregnancy if indicated by maternal or fetal condition).
Fetal maturity is a requirement for active management.
Decisive factors in cases of severe PIH, imminent eclampsia or eclampsia are: threat to the mother, gestational age, or fetal weight, according to ultrasonography.

Note. A fetal weight of < 500 g (week 24) means the chance of survival is poor due to immaturity; therefore conservative management is advisable if the maternal condition allows it.
After brief conservative treatment (convulsive state resolved, BP reduced, metabolic status normalized), delivery is accomplished, usually via cesarean section.

Intensive surveillance is required in **labor** with preeclamptic symptoms; fetal blood sampling (see p. 177) may be required; electronic heart rate monitoring (see p. 167). Management of labor is initially conservative.
If fetal acidosis occurs, delivery by cesarean section, forceps, or vacuum extraction, depending on progress and stage of labor.
HELLP syndrome (see p. 77). Leading symptoms are: 1) epigastric discomfort in 80–90 %; 2) hypertension is missing in 20 %, proteinuria in 15 %. Required for diagnosis are: 3) thrombocytopenia; 4) elevated transaminase levels (SGOT, SGPT); 5) haptoglobin < 10 mg/dl.

Complications:
- Placental abruption, renal failure, pulmonary edema.
- Cerebral edema.
- Disseminated intravascular coagulation (DIC).
- Rupture of the liver.

HELLP syndrome doesn't result in an increase in fetal morbidity, however neonatal morbidity and mortality are higher as a result of treatment, which may necessitate preterm delivery.
Treatment. Rapid delivery, in order to avoid maternal complications.
Expectant management is suggested by some. The danger is that the mother may become ill due to complications. We advise against prolonging the pregnancy because of this risk.

4.1.4 Dermatoses of pregnancy

Definition. Typical skin disorders of pregnancy, including PUPPP (pruritic urticarial papules and plaques of pregnancy), herpes gestationis and pruritus gravidarum.

PUPPP. Occurs most commonly in primigravidae (and in particular in multiple pregnancies), in the third trimester. Extremely pruritic, polymorphic raised rash (also known as polymorphic eruption of pregnancy, or PEP), often with blisters, in particular on the lower abdomen. No apparent risk for mother and fetus. Risk of recurrence is low. Incidence: 1:160 pregnancies.

Treatment. Local anti-pruritic therapy, topical corticosteroids and antihistamines.

Herpes gestationis. HLA-associated autoimmune disorder of the second and third trimesters. Development of extremely pruritic erythematous papules and urticarial plaques followed by blistering in the periumbilical area. The rate of preterm delivery may be increased. Risk of recurrence is high.

Treatment. Topical corticosteroids and anti-histamines. Systemic corticosteroids if required.

Pruritis gravidarum. Result of intrahepatic cholestasis of pregnancy. Marked pruritus, mostly in the third trimester, followed a few weeks later by jaundice in half the cases. Hyperbilirubinemia is detectable, often a slight transaminase elevation also. Data on risks to the fetus is conflicting. Fetal surveillance by means of cardiotocography and Doppler velocimetry is indicated. The risk of recurrence is high.

Treatment. Topical corticosteroids and antihistamines, cholestyramine, ursodeoxycholic acid, and supplementation with vitamin K in cases of long-lasting cholestasis.

4.2 Disorders not specific to pregnancy

Not all disorders which may affect pregnant women can be mentioned here. We mention only those which, if they occur in pregnancy, require specialized diagnostic or therapeutic measures.
Some infectious diseases are covered elsewhere because of the high risk to the fetus: rubella (see p. 119), cytomegalovirus (see p. 121), viral hepatitis (see p. 125), listeria (see p. 129), gonorrhea (see p. 134), and toxoplasmosis (see p. 129).

4.2.1 Cardiac disease

Even pregnant women with healthy hearts complain not infrequently of palpitations, heart rhythm disorders, accidental heart murmurs, and dyspnea.
These are vegetative-nervous disorders as a result of the normal changes in pregnancy, in which the raised position of the diaphragm and the heart displacement in late pregnancy play a role. With the assistance of a specialist, these changes must be differentiated from organic cardiac.

Cardiac defects

Incidence. 1–2 %.
- Congenital heart disorders are the most common cardiac disorders in pregnancy, accounting for 75 %.
- 15 % are caused by acquired valve disorders.
- Cardiomyopathies, arrhythmias, and coronary heart disease are less common.

The following heart disorders are seen prenatally in particular in cooperation with cardiac specialists (incidence rates according to Gohlke-Bärwolf and Eichstädt 2004): mitral insufficiency (29 %) and stenosis (7 %), aortic stenosis (20 %) and insufficiency (4 %), atrial septum defect (21 %). Interdisciplinary care of these pregnant women with the cardiologist or a specialized center is strongly advised.
The assessment of pregnant women with heart disease is the job of the cardiologist.

New York Heart Association (NYHA) classification according to severity. Deciding factors for the prognosis are fitness and discomfort before and at the beginning of the pregnancy.

Class 1: no discomfort, no limitation in physical activity before pregnancy.
Class 2: light to moderate limitation in physical activity before pregnancy.
Class 3: marked limitation in activity before pregnancy. Cardiac decompensation occurs on mild exertion
Class 4: severe limitation before pregnancy even at rest (cardiac insufficiency at rest).

Mortality. The mortality of mothers in classes 1 and 2 is no higher than that of healthy mothers; that of class 3 is 5 %, of class 4 is 20–40 %.

The perinatal mortality of babies is higher, particularly in those of classes 3 and 4 (10 %).

Pregnancy. The following **contraindications** (based on guidelines of the German Cardiac Society) are important when considering continuation and management of pregnancy, or in preconceptional counseling:
- Severe pulmonary hypertension.
- Marked right- or left-ventricular disfunction.
- Woman with NYHA class 3–4.
- Severe left cardiac obstruction.
- Severe mitral stenosis.
- Cyanotic heart disease.

The question as to the risk of recurrence of congenital heart defects in the unborn baby is often posed. At 4 %, this risk is significantly higher than 0.7 % if neither parent has a congenital heart defect.

Management of labor. Admission 2–3 weeks before due date, in close cooperation with the internist: vaginal delivery is considered to be less strenuous for the heart and circulatory system than delivery by cesarean section, which is performed if there is an obstetric indication.
- First stage: epidural block, uterotonics should be avoided.
- Second stage: do not allow pushing; vacuum or forceps extraction.
- Third stage: hemorrhaging must be avoided.
- Puerperium: careful observation is required, as the risk of cardiac insufficiency (life-threatening pulmonary edema) exists in the first few days.
- Antibiotics should be given at the slightest increase in temperature, due to the risk of an endocarditis flare-up.

Endocarditis

Endocarditis is a rare occurrence in pregnancy (approx. 6 of 100,000 pregnant women).
Incidence is higher, however, in women with preexisting heart disease.

Treatment. Effective against the causative organism, commonly penicillin G, amoxicillin, erythromycin, mezlocillin.

Prophylaxis. The indications are not generally recognized and mandatory. Definite indications for antibiotic prophylaxis in pregnancy are valve replacement (mechanical or biological prostheses) or valve reconstruction, previous endocarditis, congenital heart defect, and heart transplant.

Cardiomyopathies

Incidence. Approximately one in 5,000 to 15,000 births.

Because of their rarity, the differing classifications and diagnostic criteria and the high risk of these disorders, recognition, and appropriate care are particularly important.
Peripartum cardiomyopathy with restricted ejection fraction and left ventricular dilation occurs in late pregnancy and in the first months after delivery.

Etiology. Unknown. An autoimmunological cause is in discussion.

Treatment. As a causal treatment is unknown, symptomatic treatment of cardiac insufficiency is advisable. Successful bromocriptine studies suggest a new therapeutic strategy.

4.2.2 Pulmonary tuberculosis

Note. Tuberculosis (TB) is not an indication for pregnancy termination! Combination therapy with isoniazid, rifampicin, and ethambutol. Aminoglycosides are contraindicated due to ototoxicity; protionamide should be avoided due to lack of data.

Latent TB. Neonatal infection is impossible if sputum does not contain the bacteria (Mycobacterium tuberculosis). Breast feeding is not contraindicated.

Active TB (bacteria present in sputum). The woman must be isolated during labor and puerperium. The newborn is to be isolated from the mother until she is no longer infectious (sputum culture negative).

The newborn of a mother with active tuberculosis is treated prophylactically with isoniazid. If the tuberculin test is negative after 3 months, the treatment can be discontinued. If tuberculin test conversion occurs, treatment should be continued (as chemoprevention) for another 3 months (once an x-ray has excluded a diagnosis of tuberculosis), for a total of 6 months.

4.2.3 Pyelonephritis in pregnancy

Definition. Ascending urinary tract infection, promoted by reduced tone and dilation of the urinary tract, usually in late pregnancy.

Incidence. 5 %, of which 30 % occur in the first trimester, 70 % later.

Etiology. Most commonly caused by E. coli bacteria. Further organisms are Enterococci, Proteus, and Klebsiella.

The infection ascends or descends (hematogenically via the liver or lymphogenic migration from the large intestine).
One in ten of all chronic cases of pyelonephritis occur in pregnancy. A relapse often occurs, whereby the initial infection occurred earlier, possibly in childhood. Kidney or urinary tract anomalies predispose to infections.
10 % of all pregnant women have asymptomatic bacteriuria, a precursor of pyelonephritis.

Predisposing factors for infection are

- reduced muscle tone of the renal pelvis and ureters (due to progesterone) → dilatation of the urinary tract;
- reduced muscle tone of the digestive tract → constipation of pregnancy;

– the enlarged uterus compresses the right ureter.

Location. In two thirds of cases, pyelonephritis occurs on the right.
Cause. Mild dextrorotation of the uterus; right kidney, renal pelvis, and ureter are connected to the large intestine via a larger number of lymphatic vessels than on the left. The left ureter may be somewhat protected by the sigmoid colon.

Clinical manifestation. Acute pyelonephritis. If a pregnant women suddenly develops a high fever (often with shivering) and complains of pain in the kidney region (usually on the right), the suspected diagnosis is clear. Detection of bacteria in the urine confirms this diagnosis.

Practice tip. Flank pain in pregnancy is to be taken seriously, as it has diagnostic consequences: 1) repeated urine culture and examination of urine for protein, sugar, sediment; 2) differential blood count.

Differential diagnosis. Cholecystitis, appendicitis, pancreatitis, pneumonia, ileus.

Complications. Preterm labor is common, even in afebrile cases, super-imposed preeclampsia (p. 74) in 50 %. A late consequence is chronic pyelonephritis with cirrhosis of the kidney in 30 % of cases. Fetal complication. Damage due to superimposed preeclampsia: placental insufficiency, hypoxemia, premature birth as a result of preterm labor brought on by fever.

Practice tip. Renal function must be bacteriologically monitored for two weeks after completion of treatment of acute and moderate pyelonephritis.

Treatment
- Hospital admission. Antibiotic therapy after antibiogram.
- If clinically necessary (high fever) empirical treatment with ampicillin or cephalosporins.
- Two urine cultures done three to four days apart must be negative before it can be considered healed.
- Prevention of relapse (tendency of recurrence during pregnancy and further pregnancies). Pregnant women with a history of nephritis (after angina, scarlet fever among others) must be thoroughly examined and possibly treated.

Note. Asymptomatic bacteriuria must be treated after antibiogram (identification of the responsible organism, sensitivity testing).

4.2.4 Diabetes mellitus

Definition. Pre-existing disorder of carbohydrate metabolism.

Incidence. 1–2 % of all pregnancies.

Etiology. Hereditary metabolic disorder with absolute (type 1 diabetes) or relative insulin deficiency (type 2 diabetes).

Diabetes mellitus is assumed to be a multifactorial genetic disorder involving autoimmune processes (e.g., autoantibodies against the insulin-producing β-cells of the islets of Langerhans of the pancreas). A viral infection can also cause or play a role in manifestation of the disorder, in particular in juvenile diabetes. The disposition alone does not lead to manifestation of the disease. There must be coinciding factors which support manifestation, such as obesity, stressful situations, and/or pregnancy.

Preconceptional counseling. An absolute contraindication for a diabetic woman to become pregnant is if she has had a myocardial infarction. Relative contraindications are advanced nephropathy, severe retinopathy, and marked occlusive disease of the pelvic arteries.

Hereditary risk. The risk of developing diabetes before the age of 30 is 1 % if one parent is diabetic. If both are diabetic the risk is 3 %.

Maternal mortality has dropped markedly. In the preinsulin era, every second pregnant diabetic died in a coma: the mortality rate was 50 %! Today pregnancy is still risky for a diabetic if she is not intensively cared for. **Child mortality** used to be 10–20 %, while today it is 1–2 %. Diabetes is dangerous for the fetus in the perinatal period, in particular if metabolic regulation is poor. The increased **neonatal morbidity** is due to the 20 % rate of premature delivery of diabetic mothers, the higher rate of defects, and diabetic fetopathy (see p. 452) with organ immaturity, hypoglycemia, polycythemia, and hyperbilirubinemia.
In the preinsulin era, diabetic women were usually infertile. Since insulin therapy, the incidence of sterility in diabetic women has dropped from 95 % to 2 %. Therefore we are confronted with diabetic women much more frequently in prenatal care.

Pathophysiology. Impaired carbohydrate conversion is the central problem, such as inadequate glucose conversion, in particular in muscle cells (limitation of glucose transfer via cell membrane), and increased synthesis of glucose from proteins and lipolysis, leading to an increase in serum fatty acids. Together these inhibit the conversion of acetyl-CoA for ketone body production.

The pregnancy is accompanied by a worsening of the metabolic situation:
- Decreased carbohydrate tolerance.
- Increased insulin requirement.
- Metabolism is generally less stable: tendency towards acidosis and coma, occasionally paradoxical hypoglycemia, hypoglycemic shock.

Fluctuations in the course of pregnancy
- *Early pregnancy.* The metabolism of the majority of women is unstable or worsens. In approximately one quarter it remains unchanged.
- *Midpregnancy.* Metabolism is therapeutically stabilized. Tolerance improvement for 2–3 months.
- *Third trimester.* Due to the continuing development of the fetus, metabolism is once again under greater strain, resulting in impaired tolerance and a tendency to develop acidosis, precoma, coma, from week 28 on.

Reduced insulin effectiveness. Three factors in particular cause a reduction in the effectiveness of insulin as pregnancy progresses:
- Placental hormones (estriol, progesterone, hPL) are insulin antagonists.
- Increasing maternal serum cortisol levels (insulin antagonism).
- Placental enzymes increase insulin breakdown.

Peripheral insulin resistance and increased insulin breakdown cause increased insulin release from the β-cells of the islets of Langerhans of the pancreas; this occurs only inadequately in gestational diabetes. The result is a relative insulin deficiency.

WHO and ADA classification. The classification of diabetes by the WHO and the American Diabetes Association describes 4 types:

I. *Type 1 diabetes mellitus.* Beta cell destruction with absolute insulin deficiency: 1) immunological; 2) idiopathic.
II. *Type 2 diabetes mellitus.* Insulin resistance with relative insulin deficiency or secretion deficit with insulin resistance.
III. *Other types of diabetes with known causes.* Genetic defects of the beta cells or effects of insulin, disorders of the exocrine pan-

creas, endocrinopathy, medicine-induced, infection, rare immunological forms and other syndromes associated with diabetes.

IV. *Gestational diabetes.* Disorder of carbohydrate metabolism, which begins in pregnancy.

White classification. The prognosis of the course of pregnancy and the maternal and fetal risks can be assessed using the White classification (Grazer modification):

- White A: limited glucose tolerance (mean blood-glucose concentration < 100 mg/dl) and/or amniotic fluid insulin < 7 μU/ml.
- White A/B. limited glucose tolerance (mean blood-glucose concentration 100–130 mg/dl) and amniotic fluid insulin < 7 μU/ml.
- White B0: mean blood-glucose concentration > 130 mg/dl or fasting blood-glucose concentration > 110 mg/dl, or oral antidiabetics prepregnancy.
- White B: Age at onset > 20 and/or duration of less than 10 years.
- White C: Age at onset and/or duration 10–19 years.
- White D: Age at onset < 10 or duration of > 20 years vascular calcification, hypertension, or benign retinopathy.
- White E: Calcified pelvic vessels.
- White F: Nephropathy.
- White R: Proliferative retinopathy.

Complications. The main pregnancy and obstetric complications are macrosomia, diabetic fetopathy (see p. 452), hydramnios with premature rupture of membranes, preterm delivery, umbilical cord prolapse, uterine inertia, errors of fetal position, shoulder dystocia, postpartem hemorrhage; hyperemesis, PIH, preeclampsia; urinary tract infections as a result of lowered defense against infections (five times as frequently as pregnant women with a healthy metabolism).

Treatment. Intensive and comprehensive monitoring of pregnancy in addition to metabolic adjustment are the basis of interdisciplinary (obstetric and diabetological) care in pregnancy.

Monitoring during pregnancy. As early as possible (in cases of overt diabetes, pre-conceptionally), as worsening of the metabolic condition in early pregnancy may cause malformations or fetal death.

The ocular fundi and the kidneys should be examined prior to conception or in early pregnancy.
Hospital admission is unavoidable if normoglycemic metabolism cannot be achieved with outpatient insulin treatment. Other short stays are often necessary in order to monitor and correct insulin regulation.
The fetus is very sensitive to acidosis and hyperglycemia. Metabolic decompensation can lead to intrauterine death.

Note. Metabolic check-ups include laboratory parameters, diet, and insulin treatment.

Laboratory parameters are blood glucose and glycosilated hemoglobin.
Blood glucose. Aim is normoglycemic capillary plasma glucose fasting below 90 mg/dl, 1 h postprandial < 140 mg/dl, 2 h postprandial 120 mg/dl.
Glycosilated hemoglobin (HbA1c). A small amount of the glucose absorbed by erythrocytes binds with the amino group of the beta globin chain, which correlates to the blood glucose level: the higher the blood glucose, the higher the HbA1c! Measurement of HbA1c is a method of controlling the long-term success of metabolic regulation over 3 months.
Normal value. Amount of glycosilated hemoglobin in total Hb is 4.8–6.0 % (HPLC method).

The differing validity of HbA1c measurement methods must be taken into account when interpreting results. Monthly HbA1c measurement.
Diet, exercise. Attention must be paid to regular physical activity during and after regulation.
Diet. 30 kcal/kg body weight are to be aimed for (ideal body weight = height (cm) – 100), whereby protein should make up 15 % and carbohydrates 50 % of the caloric intake.

Practice tip. Diabetics should also have a weight gain in pregnancy of 11–12 kg.

Insulin therapy. Intensive insulin therapy is the method of choice: 4 or 5 injections per day are required. Normal insulin is often given as a preprandial bolus, or slow-release insulin as a basal. However, individual treatment plans and individually selected forms of insulin are also possible.

Insulin pump. If near-normal blood-glucose levels cannot be attained with the conventional, intensive insulin therapy, an insulin pump may be used.

Regulation of the carbohydrate metabolism is controlled by the diabetic herself, under physician supervision. A semiquantitative reflectometer or test strips are used for blood sugar home testing.

24-hour blood sugar profile. A number of measurements must be taken to calculate a 24-hour profile: morning fasting, 90 min after breakfast, before and 90 min after lunch, before the evening meal, and before going to bed.

Instruction in selfmonitoring is an important task for the physician in antenatal care.

Note. Oral antidiabetic agents are obsolete in pregnancy.

Further checks. From an obstetric point of view, a pregnant diabetic is high risk, and as such requires frequent and intensive monitoring. Alongside specialized diabetes care the following are necessary:

- Sonographic examination to determine due date and to monitor fetal growth, in particular in the second half of pregnancy at 4-weekly intervals.
- EFM twice a week from week 28, every 2 days from week 36.
- Doppler velocimetry of maternal and fetal blood vessels to monitor the fetus.

Goal of care. Spontaneous labor close to due date (if carbohydrate metabolism is well-regulated and pregnancy has been unremarkable). Diabetes is not an indication for cesarean section; a significant delay in delivery should be avoided.

Long-term diabetic complications. It is unclear today whether pregnancy promotes the progression of long-term diabetic complications (diabetic retinopathy, diabetic glomerulosclerosis, gangrene as a result of the generalized diabetic microangiopathy; arteriosclerosis, diabetic neuropathy, arthropathy, bladder disorders), and to what extent an existing nephropathy is negatively affected.

Gestational diabetes mellitus (GDM)

Definition. Pathological carbohydrate tolerance or diabetic metabolism which manifests in pregnancy for the first time, or continues after delivery as diabetes mellitus type 1 or 2.

Incidence. 3–4 % of all pregnancies.

Diagnosis. An oral glucose tolerance test (OGTT) is recommended for all pregnant women between weeks 24 and 28 as a screening test for diabetes. GDM often goes undetected, which increases the risk of complications in pregnancy or delivery (see below).

An OGTT should be performed in early pregnancy in pregnant women with the following risk factors:

Anamnestic risk factors
- Family history of diabetes (in a first degree relative).
- Previous macrosomic child.
- Previous stillbirth of unclear etiology.
- Repeated premature delivery.
- Two miscarriages.

Presenting risk factors
- Glucosuria once in first half of pregnancy and again in the second half.
- Obesity (BMI > 27 kg/m^2, or prepregnancy weight > height–100 + 10 %).
- Extreme weight gain.
- PIH.
- Recurrent UTI.
- Suspected macrosomia, in particular if abdominal circumference > 90th percentile.
- Placental thickness > 6 cm.
- Fetal hydrops.
- Hydramnios.

OGTT procedure. The oral glucose challenge tests are performed after a carbohydrate-rich diet (150 g carbohydrates three days in a row). A single oral challenge after a 12 h fast has proven most effective. 75 g glucose in 300 ml liquid (tea or water) is to be drunk within five minutes. Plasma glucose is measured beforehand and then 90 and 120 min after the challenge. Threshold values:

Fasting blood glucose 90 mg/dl.

After 1 hour 180 mg/dl.

After 2 hours 155 mg/dl.

Evaluation. Two pathological results (above threshold values) are a definite diagnosis of gestational diabetes, one pathological result indicates impaired glucose tolerance and a repeat test in four weeks is advisable.

As an alternative. a two-stage diagnosis can be performed.
1. Oral glucose screening test with 50 g glucose and, if required.
2. Oral glucose challenge test (as described above).

The oral 50 g glucose screening test can be performed at any time of day, regardless of food intake. 50 g glucose is dissolved in 200 ml water and drunk within 3–5 min. Capillary blood glucose measurement one hour after drinking. Evaluation: > 140 mg/dl is indicative of GDM and must be followed up with an OGTT using 75 g glucose for confirmation.
Obstetric complications and **antenatal care** of pregnant women with GDM are the same as those for pregnant women with overt diabetes. The same basic treatment components are valid for women with GDM: exercise, diet, and insulin therapy.
Insulin therapy is indicated if the median blood glucose level in one day is above 100 mg % after 1–2 weeks of dietary therapy.

Practice tip. GDM rarely persists after delivery. On the other hand, a significantly higher number of women who had GDM develop overt diabetes later than women who did not.

4.2.5 Thrombophilia

Tendency to develop thrombosis (hypercoagulability) as a result of inherited or acquired deficiencies of the coagulation system.
Physiological changes to hemostasis parameters occur in pregnancy, resulting in an increase in factors VII, VIII, XII, and a decrease of the factors XI and XIII. Antithrombin decreases by 10–20 %, protein C increases by up to 50 %, protein S drops by up to 50 %, the platelets drop continually. Due to these pregnancy-related changes there is a four-fold risk of leg vein thrombosis in pregnancy, and a fourteen-

fold risk in the puerperium. Women at greater risk of thrombophilia in pregnancy and postpartum should be screened for thrombophilia in pregnancy. Medical history should be taken to check for previous thrombotic event/s before diagnostic laboratory methods are implemented (p. 420).

Coagulation analysis in this risk group for activated protein C resistance, usually factor V mutation, prothrombin polymorphism, protein C deficiency, protein S deficiency, antithrombin deficiency, elevated factor VIII levels, antiphospholipid syndrome.

Treatment. Heparinization is only indicated in the puerperium in heterozygous Factor V Leiden with no prior thromboembolism. In homozygous Factor V Leiden, protein C and protein S deficiencies heparinization is indicated in pregnancy and the puerperium (p. 420).

4.2.6 Thyroid disorders

Thyroid function increases in pregnancy, with an increase in hormone production and an accompanying hypertrophy (physiological increase of normal thyroid volume from approx. 18 ml by 10–15 %).

Thyroid hormone metabolism is characterized by a physiological hyperthyroxinemia. The increased production of thyroxine (T4) is a result of high estrogen levels, or rather the increase in the protein thyroid-binding globulin (TBG). TBG is synthesized in the liver and its breakdown is decreased. The increase in TBG results in the binding of more tri-iodothyronine (T3) and T4, which in turn means that hormone production must be increased in order to ensure constant levels of free hormones.

20 % of women experience a short-term placental hyperstimulation due to hCG, particularly during the serum hCG peak between weeks 8 and 14. This results in thyrotropin (thyroid-stimulating hormone, or TSH) suppression, despite adequate levels of free T3 and T4, causing subclinical hyperthyroidism. 1–2 % of women develop overt hyperthyroidism.

Hyperthyroidism. Women with hyperthyroidism have increased rates of miscarriage, premature birth, perinatal mortality and fetal malformations. They are at risk of triggering thyrotoxicosis in labor.

Treatment. The dose of the thyrostatic drug should be as low as possible, bearing in mind the fact that small amounts cross the placenta. The treatment goal is to establish thyroid hormone concentration in the upper norm levels, which will need to be monitored every 2–4 weeks.

- Initial dose 10–20 mg methimazole/day.
- Maintenance dose 2.5–5 mg/day.

Iodine supplementation is contraindicated; therapeutic radioiodine is absolutely contraindicated in pregnancy. In rare cases a thyroidectomy is necessary, usually between weeks 15 and 25.

Hypothyroidism. Women with hypothyroidism often do not become pregnant, or pregnancy is complicated by threatened miscarriage or preterm birth. Due to increased thyroid hormone requirements in many pregnant women, the daily thyroxine dose usually needs to be raised. The required dose is determined by the TSH level. The aim is normalization of the TSH level.

Euthyroid goiter. The most common cause for a visible, palpable, or sonographically measurable thyroid enlargement is iodine deficiency, increased due to pregnancy in iodine deficient regions.

Practice tip. Iodized salt is not an adequate prophylaxis against iodine deficiency in iodine deficiency regions. Daily supplementation with 200 μg of iodine is necessary.

4.2.7 Acute abdomen

Appendicitis, cholelithiasis (gallstones), choledocholithiasis (gallstones in the common bile duct), ileus, and ulcerative diseases in pregnancy can cause complaints and complications necessitating emergency surgery. The illness itself, the ensuing complications, the surgical procedure, and the anesthetics all pose risks for mother and fetus. At the same time, delayed diagnosis and treatment also frequently pose risks. The risks to the fetus depend on gestational age, fetal lung maturity, and oxygen supply. If surgery is required, deferment until the third trimester, antenatal enhancement of fetal lung maturation, and monitoring of the oxygen supply are advisable from an obstetric perspective.

Illnesses necessitating emergency surgery, and the risk to the pregnancy
Gastrointestinal symptoms frequently occur in pregnancy as a result of the physiological adaptation of the organs of the maternal digestive tract. In addition, preexistent gastrointestinal disorders can be exacerbated in pregnancy, and disorders related to or promoted by pregnancy can develop.

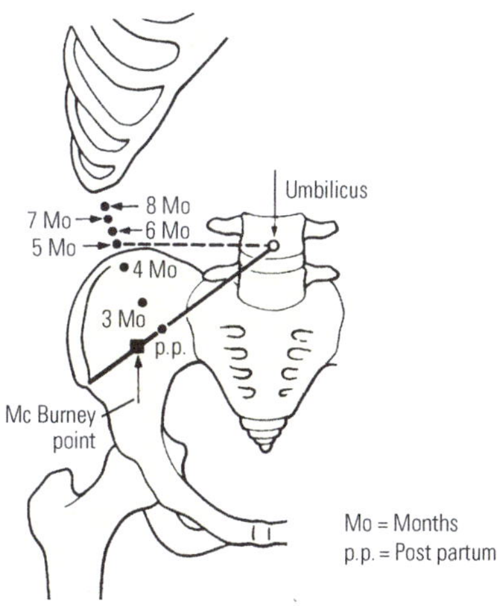

Fig. 4.2: Displacement of the appendix during pregnancy and in early puerperium.

Acute appendicitis. The incidence is calculated at 1 : 2,000 pregnancies. Delayed diagnosis is common due to the physiological changes causing atypical localization of the appendix (Fig. 4.2), the attribution of related complaints to obstetric complications, and the reluctance to operate on a pregnant woman. These factors in turn increase the risk of rupture, peritonitis, and septicemia, and also for miscarriage, preterm delivery, and stillbirth. Maternal mortality after rupture of an inflamed appendix is estimated at 17 %, and fetal mortality at 43 %. According to Swedish data a fetal mortality rate of 15–20 % has been observed. The causes of fetal and maternal mortality can be explained by delayed diagnosis and surgery.

With regards to the method of operation – laparascopic appendectomy vs. conventional appendectomy – the preferred method is laparoscopic for the following reasons:

1. Laparoscopic surgery makes it easier to find the appendix, which is not in its usual position due to the pregnancy.
2. Avoidance of strain and possible rupture of the scar of a conventional appendectomy over the course of pregnancy.

Ileus. Ileus is a common cause of abdominal complaints in pregnancy, usually as a result of adhesions from previous intraabdominal operations. In addition, volvulus, internal hernias, and Crohn's disease complications may be implicated. A maternal mortality rate of 10–20 %, and a fetal rate of 30–50 % have been reported.

Acute cholecystitis and cholelithiasis. The physiological reduction in motility of the gallbladder in pregnancy and the widening of the biliary tract increase the risk of gallbladder disorders. 3.5 % of pregnant women have an asymptomatic cholecystolithiasis, which is usually the cause of cholecystitis in pregnancy. 30 % of pregnant women present with sludge on the gallbladder and biliary tract. Diagnosis of disorders of the biliary tract and the gall bladder is unproblematic with abdominal sonography and nuclear magnetic resonance, which have replaced x-ray diagnosis. Gallstones are easily found sonographically, as they are echogenic and move when the patient moves. Diagnosis of biliary tract obstruction is possible with magnetic resonance cholangiopancreatography (MRCP) without exposing the fetus to radiation.

The diagnosis of cholecystolithiasis in an asymptomatic pregnant woman is not an indication for cholecystectomy. Pregnant women should, however, be operated on without delay if symptoms worsen under nonoperative treatment, if pancreatitis persists or worsens, or if obstructive jaundice develops. The golden standard method in pregnancy is also laparoscopy, using adapted pressure carbon dioxide insufflation. Pregnant women suffering from recurrent cholecystitis episodes should not be operated on before the early third trimester, in order to avoid the risk of an extremely premature preterm delivery. Acute gallstone-induced obstructive jaundice and secondary pancreatitis poses a particular problem. The incidence in pregnancy is calculated to be between 1 : 1,000 and 1 : 12,000. Immediate action is imperative. Whether ERCP (endoscopic retrograde cholangiopancreatography) with the option of stone extraction is appropriate must be decided individually, however the urgency of treatment must not be overlooked.

From an obstetric point of view HELLP syndrome must be considered as a differential diagnosis in cases of complaints in the upper right quadrant, as this syndrome poses high risks for mother and fetus.

Risks for mother and fetus are low in cholecystitis and cholecystolithiasis, whereas cholecystectomy in the second trimester has an intrauterine mortality rate of 5 %. There is an increased risk of preterm delivery after laparotomy, which rises markedly after rupture and peritonitis. Pancreatitis has a maternal mortality rate of 14 % and an intrauterine mortality rate of 20 %.

Bleeding and/or ruptured ulcer. The incidence of ulcerative diseases is estimated at 1 : 10,000 pregnant women. As ulcerative disorders frequently improve during pregnancy, complications are uncommon. On the rare instance of complications, a delayed diagnosis (usually via endoscopy) is a common criticism. Case reports are to be found in literature, but reliable statistics on maternal and fetal morbidity and mortality are not.

Emergency surgery in pregnancy can likewise be necessary if liver hemorrhage or rupture (also a complication of HELLP syndrome) occur, or aortic dissection in Marfan syndrome.

Risk of emergency surgery for the pregnancy. According to Swedish data, 1 in 500 women undergo laparotomies during pregnancy. The most common diagnoses resulting in surgery are appendicitis and gallstones.

Increased risk of miscarriage is described if laparotomy is performed in early pregnancy. As a result of the enlarged uterus, positioning of the abdominal organs and the danger of initiating a premature delivery are the main concerns in the third trimester. Nevertheless, the risks to mother and fetus posed by the problems described above are far greater than those of the operations themselves.

Operation timepoint and perinatal treatment

It is generally advisable to have an interdisciplinary consultation with the surgeon before every nonobstetric operation. Transfer to a perinatal center is recommended if the condition of

the mother allows it. Sonographic examination including fetal biometry, cervical length, biophysical profile, Doppler, and EFM should be performed both pre- and post-operatively.
From an obstetric point of view the risks to the fetus must be considered before an operation for a maternal indication is performed. The following factors must be taken into consideration: gestational age, survival probability, lung maturity, danger of hypoxia. If possible, the surgical procedure should be postponed to a later time in the pregnancy. Tocolytics should be given if operations are performed before 34 weeks.
In particular between weeks 24–34, if the disease/disorder allows it and the operation can be postponed for 48 hours, prenatal acceleration of fetal lung maturity with betamethasone (12 mg IM twice 24 hours apart) should be implemented. This procedure significantly reduces the risks of respiratory distress syndrome and intraventricular hemorrhage, typical complications of a preterm delivery.
Frequently, the surgical procedure must be accompanied by antibiotic therapy. Penicillin, cephalosporin, and erythromycin are suitable from an obstetric point of view. Paracetamol and opiates can be used pre- and post-operatively for analgesic therapy. If morphine is given in the last hours before delivery, neonatal care should be provided in case of respiratory difficulties of the newborn.

Risk to the pregnancy due to anesthetic and positioning

The anesthetic used depends on the operation and the requests of the pregnant woman and and of the surgeon. Both intubation anesthesia and regional anesthesia are possible in pregnancy. The risk of anesthesia in pregnancy is very low. From an obstetrical point of view, it is essential to avoid arterial hypotension and hypoxemia. The diastolic blood pressure should be kept above 70 mmHg, as maternal cardiovascular insufficiency and hypoxia endanger the fetus. Pulse oximetry enables noninvasive monitoring of the mother.
If the fetus is viable (from around the end of week 24), its oxygen supply should be monitored via cardiotocography (EFM). However, the effect of narcosis on fetal movement is also recognizable. Sedatives and narcotics crossing the placental barrier cause reduced fluctuations and oscillations in the fetal heart rate pattern.
It is important that the pregnant patient be placed in a left lateral tilt in the operating theatre before and during the procedure (tilt the operating table to the left by 15°). This reduces the risk of aortocaval compression (supine hypotensive syndrome). The left lateral position causes a direct improvement of the maternal cardiovascular situation and thus the fetal oxygen supply.

4.2.8 Adnexal tumors

Symptomatic or palpable tumors are discovered in 1 in 500 pregnant women. Ovarian tumors are found in routine sonographic examination in one in every hundred pregnancies.

Practice tip. Most ovarian masses are functional cysts.

In addition to these, which usually degenerate spontaneously, teratomas, mucinous and serous cystadenomas, and thecomas are found. The incidence of malignant ovarial tumors is 1 : 27,000.

Treatment. If symptoms are not acute (torsion, rupture) and sonographic examination does not suggest malignancy, an operative procedure should be postponed until midpregnancy. Spontaneously degenerating cysts will usually no longer be detectable, and the risk of the operation triggering abortion is lower. No prospective randomized study results are available; thus, the operation method (laparascopic or vertical laparotomy) is controversial.

4.2.9 Cervical cytology

1–3 % of all pregnant women have abnormal cervical epithelium: dysplasia (precancerous stages of the cervix). The incidence of cervical abnormalities appears to be on the increase.

Practice tip. Pregnancy-related cellular changes can be misinterpreted; in addition, spontaneous regression of atypical cervical epithelium, in particular low-grade dysplasias, is often observed after parturition. Evaluation of cervical cytology results requires specialized knowledge and skill (Tab. 4.1).

Tab. 4.1: Management of atypical cytological results in pregnancy (according to M.I. Schneider).

Low- to high-grade squamous epithelial lesions (LSIL–HSIL; CIN I–CIN III) in pregnancy	Cytological and colposcopical examination; if the results clearly indicate that the lesions are only pre-cancerous, then repeat examinations every 2–3 months until 6–8 weeks postpartum	If further children are desired, endocervical curettage should be performed 6–9 weeks postpartum; if the lesions are endo- or ectocervically located → conization, colposcopy of all women if no further children are desired → hysterectomy, cesarean hysterectomy only if delivery by cesarean section is medically indicated; better to perform hysterectomy 6 weeks postpartum
High-grade squamous epithelial lesions (HSIL; CIN III) or invasive cancer in pregnancy	Immediate clarification usually advisable if colposcopy and clinic suggest invasive cancer	Endocervical curettage or conization and endocervical curettage → if invasion not confirmed histologically, wait until delivery: hysterectomy 6–8 weeks postpartum in cases of micro-invasive cancer: conization, in some cases cesarean hysterectomy
High-grade squamous epithelial lesions (HSIL; CIN III) or invasive cancer in pregnancy	If clinic and colposcopy indicate invasive cancer	Colposcopy-directed biopsy and endocervical curettage: in cases of macroinvasive cancer in first half of pregnancy: Wertheim operation, in cases of small macroinvasive cancer in second half of pregnancy: → accelerated lung maturity → Wertheim operation, week 35

References

American College of Obstetricians and Gynecologists: Diagnosis and management of preeclampsia and eclampsia. ACOG practice bulletin No 33. Obstet Gynecol 2002; 99:159–167

Bujold E, Roberge S, Lacasse Y, er al.: Prevention of preeclampsia and intrauterine growth restriction with aspirin started in early pregnancy. A meta-analysis. Obstet Gynecol 2010; 11:402–14

CLASP: A randomised trial of low-dose aspirin fort the prevention and treatment of pre-eclampsia among 9364 pregnant women. Lancet 1994; 343:619–29

Davidson KM: Intrahepatic cholestasis of pregnancy. Semin Perinatol 1998; 22:104

Glasgow RE, Visser BC, Harris HW, et al.: Changing management of gallstone disease during pregnancy. Surg Endosc 1998; 12:241

Lapaire O, Shennan A, Srepan H: The preeclampsia biomarkers soluble fms-like tyrosine kinase-1 and placenital growth factor: current knowledge, clinical implications and future application. Eur J Obstet Gynecol Repro Biol 2010; 151:122–29

Mazze RI, Kallen B: Appendectomy during pregnancy: A Swedish registry study of 778 cases. Obstet Gynecol 1991; 77:835

McCrae KR: Thtombocytopenia in pregnancy: differential diagnosis, pathogenesis, and management. Blood Reviews 2003; 17:7
Plagemanrı A, Harder T, Kohlhoff R, et al.: Glucose tolerance and insulin secretion in children of mothers with pregestational IDDM or gestational diabetes. Diabetologia 1997; 40:1094
Sharp HT: Gastrointestinal surgical conditions during pregnancy. Clin Obstet Gynecol 1994; 37:306
Simmons DC, Tarnesky PR, Rivera-Alsina ME, et al.: Endoscopic retrograde cholangiopancreatography in pregnancy without the use of radiation. Amer J Obstet Gynecol 2004; 190:1467
Verlohren S, Galindo A, Schlembach D, et al.: An autornated method for the determination of the sFlt-1/ PIGF ratio in the assessment of preeclampsia. Am J Obstet Gynecol 2010; 201:161
Than NG, Romero R, Hillermann R, et al.: Prediction of preeclampsia – a workshop report. Placenta 2008; 29:S83-5

5 Problems in the second half of pregnancy

5.1 Preterm birth (PTB)

Definition. Birth before 37 completed weeks (based on length of pregnancy from last menstrual period). Earlier, preterm birth was referred to a birth weight of less than 2,500 g.

Birth is defined as delivery of a stillborn infant with a birth weight greater than 500 g, or of a living infant regardless of birth weight or gestational age.

Incidence. 9.2 % in Germany (2010); 1 % with a birth weight below 1,250 g; preterm birth rate in the US 11.5 % (2012).

Etiology. Multifactorial; causes are usually unclear in individual cases. A number of risk factors are usually involved (Tab. 5.1): poor socioeconomic status, history, complications in pregnancy.

Pathophysiology. Just as unclear as the onset of spontaneous labor at term.

1. *Chorion/decidua cells.* It has been proven that chorionic and neighboring decidual cells are involved in the genesis of preterm delivery. Ascending infection and vascular alterations involving impaired placental circulation are considered important triggers, supported by maternal stress, placental hypoxemia, decidual hemorrhage. The production of corticotropin-releasing hormone (CRH) and the cellular prostaglandin production in chorion/decidua are stimulated in vitro by bacterial endotoxins and the inflammatory cytokines Interleukin 1 (IL-1) and tumor necrosis factor (TNF). The production of IL-6 by choriodecidual cell cultures is stimulated by IL-1 and TNF. In addition, IL-6 stimulates decidual prostaglandin production. Inflammatory mediators can thus induce uterine contractions.
2. *Choriodecidual abruption, rupture of membranes.* Preterm delivery is associated with progressive tearing of the extracellular matrix (ECM) of the cervix, which leads to dilatation and tearing of the choriodecidual-ECM interface, choriodecidual abruption, and rupture of membranes. Cultured cervical and decidual cells exposed to IL-1 release collagenases which break down ECM. The amount of IL-8, a granulocyte chemotactic and activator, is elevated in amniotic fluid at preterm birth. Activated granulocytes release collagenases, which are capable of breaking down certain substances: collagen I–III (components of cervical ECM), elastase (which breaks down elastin), collagen IV, proteoglycans, and fibronectin (components of choriodecidual ECM).

Prevention. A reasonable level of health-awareness and lifestyle changes serve to reduce the long-term PTB rate.

Risk assessment in prenatal care is based on clinical experience or performed with the help of risk classifications. It is important to inform pregnant women and the general public about the dangers of preterm delivery and the risk factors which could indicate a preterm birth. The need for more frequent prenatal checkups, early discontinuation of work, and, if necessary, early admission to the hospital must be understood by the patient.
The sociomedical environment of women at risk for preterm delivery requires particular attention.

Practice tip. The effects of prophylactic tocolysis and prophylactic cerclage have not been validated.
Focus is on preventing ascension of infection from the vagina into the endocervical canal or membranes.

Tab. 5.1: Preterm birth (PTB) risk factors.

Socioeconomic risk	History	Pregnancy complication
Low socioeconomic status	Prior PTB	Ascending infection
Maternal age < 18 or > 35	Prior stillbirth	Impaired placentation and disturbed placental development
Multiparous	More than 2 miscarriages	Uterine pathologies
Single	(spontaneous or induced)	Fetal causes such as malformations and multiples
Smoker		

Vaginal pH. The pH of the vaginal introitus in an uncomplicated pregnancy is 4.4 (Riedewald and colleagues 1990). The high acidity of the vaginal milieu is a natural form of protection against infection. Lactic acid bacteria (lactobacilli or Döderlein bacteria), which multiply in pregnancy, are responsible for this acidity. Disrupted vaginal flora and colonization of the vagina with atypical bacteria are frequently associated with an increase in vaginal pH.

Regular vaginal pH self-testing is a useful marker for risk of premature delivery (Saling). Therapeutic lactobacillus products reduce high vaginal acidity.

Bacterial vaginosis. Two indicators are:

- Excessive leucorrhea (vaginal discharge): milky, thin liquid, fishy smell, pH > 4.5, clue cells visible microscopically in vaginal secretion.
- Pathological bacteria: reduction of lactobacilli in favor of Gardnerella vaginalis and Bacteroides spp.

Wet preparation (or wet mount). A direct preparation of the vaginal secretions (phase contrast microscopy) is of differential diagnostic value: Trichomoniasis, mycosis, or bacterial vaginosis are recognized, and the extent of the bacterial colonization estimated.

Cervical swab. In cases of pathological colonization, a cervical swab may be performed for bacteriological diagnosis after the native preparation.

Bacterial vaginosis increases the rate of ascending infections, resulting in preterm labor, premature cervical ripening, premature rupture of membranes, and preterm birth. To reduce the danger of preterm birth it is advisable to treat women in the high-risk collective (pregnant women with a history of PTB) with a 7-day systematic antibiotic therapy (Metronidazole oral 2 × 500 mg/day or Clindamycin oral 2 × 300 mg/day after the first trimester), and women in the low-risk collective (those with no history of PTB) with an intra-vaginal Clindamycin therapy with vaginal cream (Clindamycin 2 % vaginal cream 5 g for 7 days).

Clinical manifestation, diagnosis. History: Risk factor assessment according to Tab. 5.1; symptoms: premature labor (presence of contractions), premature cervical ripening (cervical examination).

Uterine contractions

- Contractions felt. The simplest method is for the pregnant woman to note uterine contractions (contraction calendar).

Up to 10 contractions in 24 hours are normal.

- External monitoring of contractions (external tocometric monitoring). Electromechanical pressure converters which register contractions are fastened around the most prominent point of the gravid abdomen with a belt:

Frequency of contractions. Normal: 3 per hour up to week 30, then 5 per hour (acc. to Zahn).

Two types/forms of contractions (Fig. 7.19). Alvarez contractions are weak, uncoordinated local uterus contractions before week 20, Braxton-Hicks contractions are stronger, rarer uterine contractions from week 20.
The frequency and strength of uterine contractions necessary to cause cervical ripening varies individually.

Preterm cervical ripening. Of relevance are:
- Cervix length.
- Cervical consistency.
- Cervical dilatation.

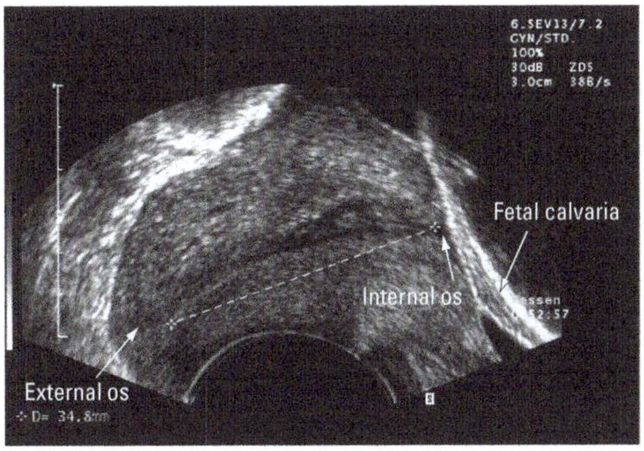

Fig. 5.1: Transvaginal sonography for cervical measurement, cervix length 35 mm.

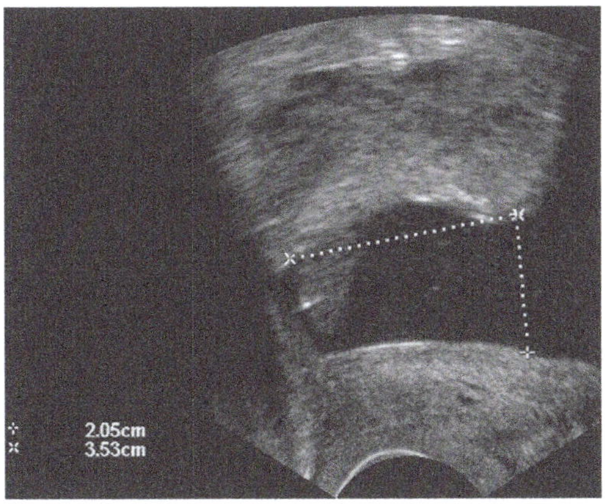

Fig. 5.2: Transvaginal sonography (TVS) with amniotic sac prolapse and cervical dilatation.

An increased readiness for labor is indicated by effacement and softening of the cervix, in addition to dilatation of the cervical canal. The cervix is viewed with the help of a speculum or palpated with the finger.
- **Transvaginal sonography (TVS).** In order to monitor women at risk of PTB, or to make a prognosis in women experiencing preterm labor, cervical measurement via transvaginal ultrasound is more reliable and easier to reproduce than digital assessment of the cervix (Figs. 5.1, 5.2). Cervix length is measured from the internal to the external os, ideally between weeks 22 and 24: a cervix length ≤ 15 mm is to be found in < 2 % of all pregnant women, however 90 % of all women who will have a preterm birth before week 28 are in this group.

The following classification has proven practical:
- ≤ 15 mm very high PTB risk, also in the next few days.
- 16–24 mm increased risk of PTB.
- ≥ 25 mm singleton: low PTB risk.
- ≥ 30 mm multifetal pregnancy: low PTB risk.

Repeated measurements are advisable, in particular of pregnant women with preterm labor. Incompetent cervix is cervical dilatation without preterm labor, a disturbance of the cervical closure mechanism (rare!) Cervical ripening due to uterine contractions before week 37/0 (premature cervical ripening) is commonly, and incorrectly, equated with cervical incompetence.

Fibronectin release as PTB marker. Choriodecidual separation releases ECM proteins, which are then detectable in the cervical or vaginal area. One particular fibronectin has been found which features a specific oncofetal domain (FFN). This means that fibronectin released into cervicovaginal secretions can be an indicator of threatened PTB.

Studies show that the presence of FFN in cervical/vaginal fluid predicts PTB with a sensitivity and specificity of 80 %. User-friendly tests are available, for example Rapid fFN 10Q System (Hologic Inc USA; Hologic GmbH Germany). The combination of TVS and the detection of FFN in cervical fluid appears to have the best predictive value for threatened PTB.

Threatened PTB. Approximately one third of all premature babies are born too early because of maternal or fetal risks (e.g., pregnancy termination due to PIH, HELLP Syndrome, placenta previa hemorrhage, IUGR), one third are born prematurely as a result of membrane rupture, and in one third of cases PTB occurs spontaneously.

Note. Fetal well-being, as determined by ultrasonography and EFM, is a prerequisite for treatment to prolong pregnancy. The prolongation of pregnancy in threatened PTB (contractions, premature cervical ripening) of a viable fetus is contraindicated if the fetus is at risk because of placental insufficiency and hypoxia. Treatment includes 1) rest, 2), tocolysis, 3) antibiotics, 4) progesterone, and 5) cerclage.

Rest. Mandatory rest can be increased in the following stages: certificate confirming inability to work, support in the household and rest at home; in higher risk cases, or where compliance with rest recommendation is uncertain, hospital admission with moderate bed rest (physical and medicated anti-thrombosis prophylaxis is advisable in long-term cases). Strict bed rest is not recommended.

Although physical rest has proven to make sense clinically, it should be stressed that there is evidence-based data for the practice of bed rest as therapy in threatened.

Tocolysis. The aim of tocolysis is the prolongation of pregnancy for at least 48 hours. In this time fetal lung maturity enhancement (see p. 104) is implemented and the pregnant woman can be transferred to a perinatal center if necessary. In certain cases tocolysis may be indicated over a longer period of time (for example symptomatic placenta previa). It must, however, be emphasized that despite frequent, impressive clinical experience, evidence-based data on the effectiveness of long-term tocolysis is not available.

Indications
- Gestational age 24 + 0 to 34 + 0 weeks.
- Spontaneous premature labor = painful, palpable contractions lasting longer than 30 seconds and > 3 every 30 min.
- Shortening of the functional cervix length, TVS.
- and/or cervical dilatation.

Contraindications
- Intrauterine infection.
- Intrauterine death.
- Nonviable fetus due to malformations.
- Fetal indication for termination of pregnancy.

Medication in use today
1. Beta$_2$ sympathomimetics.
2. Oxytocin receptor antagonists.
3. Calcium channel blockers.
4. Magnesium sulfate.
5. Prostaglandin inhibitors.
6. Nitric oxide donors.

Of these substances only the beta$_2$ sympathomimetics and the oxytocin receptor antagonists are permitted for use as tocolytic agents in Germany, and in the USA only the beta$_2$ sympathomimetics. Use of the other substances is off-label, and the pregnant woman must be informed and give her consent.

Beta$_2$ sympathomimetics. Bind with the beta$_2$ receptors in the cell-membrane of the myometrium and bring about an increase in intracellular cAMP, which causes relaxation of the myometrial cells by inhibiting the phosphorylation of myosin light chain kinase (MYLK). The efficiency of $beta_2$ sympathomimetics as tocolytics for 48 hours has been **proven.**

Practice tip. Oral administration of $beta_2$ sympathomimetics is ineffective.

Dosage. Continuous infusion via intravenous pump 1–4 µg/min fenoterol; bolus infusion (with less side effects) begin with 3–5 µg/min; reduce once effective.
Despite the reported $beta_2$ selectivity, sympathomimetics also bind with $beta_1$ and $beta_3$ receptors giving rise to side effects (palpitations, tremor and pulmonary edema: 1 : 400 cases!).

Practice tip. Due to maternal side effects, fluid intake must be limited, and if certain predisposing factors such as multifetal gestation or maternal cardiac disease exist, an alternative tocolytic should be considered.

Oxytocin receptor antagonists. Bind competitively to oxytocin receptors, thus suppressing oxytocin-induced contractions. Data is available verifying the efficacy of atosiban in prolonging pregnancy by 7 days. Though the clinical effects of atosiban and $beta_2$ sympathomimetics are considered equivalent, atosiban is associated with with far less maternal side effects. Severe maternal side effects are unknown.

Dosage. Continuous infusion via intravenous pump: 6.75 mg for 1 minute, 18 mg/h for 3 h, 6 mg/h for 15–48 hours.

Calcium channel blockers (CCB). Inhibit the entry of calcium into the cell and promote its exit. The reduction of the intracellular calcium level leads to inhibition of myosin light chain kinase (MYLK) and thus relaxation of the uterine myocyte. Studies on nifedipine have shown that it is as or more effective as a tocolytic than $beta_2$ sympathomimetics. The function of peripheral vasodilation explains the maternal side effects (arterial hypotension). They are generally minor, in particular in normotensive women.

Dosage. Oral! There is no generally recognized dosage as yet. Suggested doses are: 10 mg nifedipine every 20 min., up to 40 mg, then 20 mg every 4–8 h or 3 times 30 mg/day.

Practice tip. Calcium channel blockers must not be taken with magnesium sulfate! Severe fetal bradycardia and fatal complications have been observed with this combination.

Magnesium sulfate. Acts as intracellular calcium channel blocker, thus inhibiting phosphorylation of MYLK and bringing about relaxation of the myometrial cells. Randomized controlled studies have shown no efficacy as a tocolytic agent, but an increased fetal mortality at an adequate maintenance dose.

Dosage. Continuous infusion via intravenous pump, 4–6 g in 30 min, then 1–2 g/h.

Prostaglandin inhibitors. Inhibit COX enzymes, which take part in prostaglandin synthesis, which in turn participate in the stimulation of myometrial cells. Only indomethacin has been tried and shown to be effective, similarly to $beta_2$ sympathomimetics. Although no maternal side effects have been described, severe fetal side effects have been publicized. If given for more than 48 hours, fetal anuria; after week 32, if used for more than 48 hours, premature closure of the ductus arteriosus (DA, or ductus Botalli) can be expected in 20–50 % of cases.

Dosage. Rectal 100 mg, then 25 mg every 4–6 h.

Nitric oxide donors. Nitric oxide stimulates guanylate cyclase which results in an increase in intracellular cGMP, which in turn intensifies calcium outflow and thus relaxation of the uterine myocyte. A number of studies have shown a similar effect to that of $beta_2$ sympathomimetics, while others were unable to confirm it. Ultimately, there is not yet enough data. Known maternal side effects are headaches caused by the widening of the cerebral arteries, which lead to discontinuation of therapy in about 25 %.

Dosage. Transdermal! No dosage guidelines have been accepted yet. Suggested dosage levels till now: 10 mg/day to 100 mg/day.

Antibacterial therapy. There is a correlation between ascending (intrauterine) infection and PTB. Clinical trials have demonstrated pregnancy prolongation under antibiotic therapy in cases of threatened PTB; this was not confirmed in other extended trials (Egarter and colleagues 1996).

A general antibacterial therapy in cases of threatened PTB (with intact membranes!) is currently not indicated.

Progesterone. The prophylactic administration of progesterone to pregnant women at high risk of PTB reduces the PTB rate. A multicenter randomized double-blind placebo-controlled study demonstrated – at least for singleton pregnancies with a sonographically confirmed shortened cervix – a significant reduction of the PTB rate after daily vaginal application of progesterone gel (Coomarasamy and colleagues 2006). There is no international consensus on dosage, application method, and time frame; the current recommendation appears to be 100 mg progesterone intravaginal daily.

Operative cervical closure, cerclage (MacDonald cerclage). Indication. Closure of the cervix in cases of (genuine) cervical incompetence.

Further indications (prophylactic cerclage, emergency cerclage, cerclage because of premature cervical ripening) are controversial. It was not possible to statistically demonstrate the effectiveness of cerclage in reducing the PTB rate.

Pessary insertion. A minimal invasive alternative to cerclage is the insertion of a pessary. Different models are available, such as the Arabin pessary. Insertion is possible prophylactically or therapeutically in cases of cervical shortening. A conclusive statement is not possible due to insufficient studies.

Prenatal enhancement of lung maturation. Disturbed adaptation of the fetal lung (respiratory distress syndrome) is a danger of PTB (see lung maturity, pp. 12, 60). The mother is given corticosteroids, which increase the fetal intraalveolar synthesis of surfactant.

Procedure in cases of threatened or actual preterm labor (gestational age of 24 + 0 to 34 + 0 weeks):
- Postponement of birth with tocolytic agents by a minimum of 24 to 48 hours (if justifiable).
- 12 mg betamethasone IM twice 24 h apart.
- No repetition.

Management of preterm birth

Birth method. The sensitivity of the immature fetal brain and avoidance of hypoxia are important considerations for deciding the method of delivery in preterm birth.

Indications for cesarean delivery:
- Breech presentation or transverse lie.
- Premature placental abruption.
- Intrapartum hypoxia.
- Prolonged labor, PROM, amnionitis.

Factors speaking for a vaginal delivery:
- Vertex presentation.
- Rapid progression of preterm labor.
- Imminent delivery.
- Fetal wellbeing.

Birth trauma. Epidural block is recommended in order to relax the birth canal: reduction of fetal skull trauma.

Membrane preservation. The recommendation of maintaining the membranes intact is secondary to fetal monitoring!

Generous episiotomy and speculum-assisted delivery (insertion of a broad speculum in order to stretch the perineum) reduce birth trauma!

5.2 Premature rupture of membranes; chorioamnionitis

Premature rupture of membranes (PROM)

Definition. Rupture of membranes and loss of amniotic fluid before labor contractions begin.

Incidence. 10–20 % of all births.

Causes

- Premature cervical ripening.
- Hydramnios.
- Multifetal gestation.
- Chorioamnionitis of the lower part of the fetal membranes.
- Iatrogenic (amniocentesis, cerclage).

Diagnosis

- Assessment of the pH value of vaginal fluid with litmus paper: if the red paper turns blue, this indicates loss of amniotic fluid.
- Detection of fetal cells with Nile blue staining
- Detection of insulin-like growth factor binding protein-1 (IGFBP-1) in fluid found in the posterior fornix
- IGFBP-1 is not normally found in vaginal fluid; in amniotic fluid its concentration is 100–1,000 times higher than in maternal serum. It is detectable in vaginal fluid in cases of PROM, which is the basis of the Actim PROM test: during a sterile speculum examination a sample of vaginal fluid is taken with a polyester swab and extracted with a puffer solution. With immune chromatography, in which monoclonal antibodies against IGFBP-1 are used, the presence of IGFBP-1 can be detected on a test strip. Test **limitations**. If PROM occurred some time ago, amniotic fluid may cease to flow. If blood is also present in the fluid a false positive result may occur.
- Detection of placental alpha-microglobulin-1 (PAMG-1) in cervicovaginal fluid.

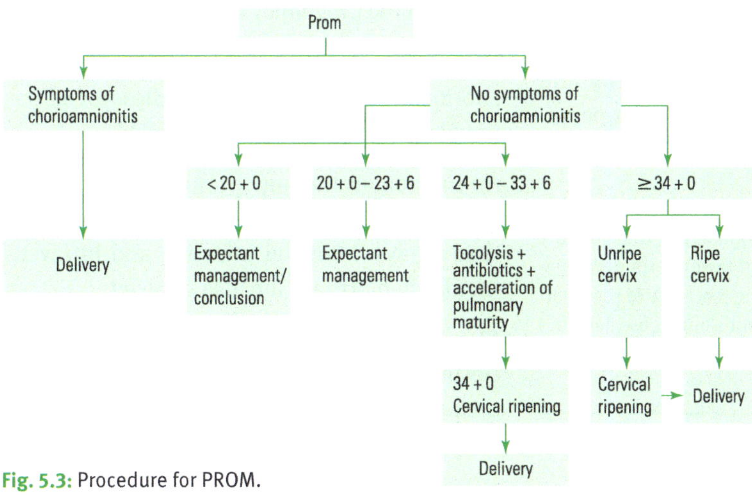

Fig. 5.3: Procedure for PROM.

- The concentration of PAMG-1 is approximately 1,000 to 10,000 times higher in amniotic fluid than in cervical secretion if the fetal membranes are intact. A bedside immunoassay test (**Amnisure ROM Test**) makes detection simple.
- Cervical swab for microbiological diagnostics!
- Avoid digital examination of the cervix and TVS for measurement of cervix length!

Classification. PROM close to due date or with mature fetus, or PROM before 33 completed weeks and immature fetus (Fig. 5.3).

Membrane rupture ≥33 completed weeks (34+0). Unproblematic prognosis, spontaneous delivery usually within hours, low risk of infection.

Complication. Chorioamnionitis. The danger of ascending infection increases with the latency period between membrane rupture and birth (chorioamnionitis).
- Wait for 12 hours for contractions or cervical ripening to begin spontaneously (if cervix unfavorable).
- Oxytocin infusion or local administration of prostaglandin to induce delivery or cervical ripening.
- Antibiotics between weeks 34 and 37.

Membrane rupture from completion of weeks 23 to 33. The risks of prematurity and infection must be weighed up against one another.

Practice tip. The younger the pregnancy is, the more the management should be inclined towards its prolongation; the older the pregnancy, the more active the treatment should be! Chorioamnionitis must be detected early in cases of PROM, in particular in early pregnancy with an immature fetus.

- Monitoring of temperature and CRP every 6–24 hours, EFM twice daily, regular ultrasonography.
- Expectant management, administration of tocolytic agents, and acceleration of pulmonary maturation.
- 2–4 % of fetuses have an infection within 24 hours of PROM, and 20 % after 48 hours Antibiotics should be given prophylactically; this often occurs too late because women are admitted too late after PROM. Bacterial invasion occurs within hours of PROM. Suggested antimicrobial therapy for 7 days:
- Cefotiam: 2 × 1 g/day.
- Amoxicillin/clavulanic acid: 3 × 1–2 g/day.
- Erythromycin (4 × 500 mg/day) if chlamydia has been detected in the cervical canal.
- **Once 33 weeks have been completed, proceed as described above.**

PROM from 19 to 23 completed weeks
Expectant management, regular monitoring of temperature and CRP; antimicrobial therapy (controversial), no tocolytic agents, and no acceleration of fetal lung maturity (but possibly to be considered after completion of 23 weeks).

PROM < week 20. Expectant management is possible. Poor prognosis for the fetus due to pulmonary hypoplasia, among other things. Termination of the pregnancy must be discussed.

Expectant management is contraindicated if chorioamnionitis occurs, regardless of gestational age. Pregnancy must be ended.

Antimicrobial therapy prolongs the latency period (ROM to beginning of labor) by more than 7 days. Neonatal infection and intraventricular hemorrhage are also reduced.

Chorioamnionitis
Definition. Threat to mother and child by an unspecific infection of the amniotic cavity with

the common substrate of amnionitis and chorioamnionitis; uncommon if membranes are intact.

Pathogens. Gram-negative rods, in particular E. coli; in addition Streptococcus (or Enterococcus) faecalis, β-hemolytic streptococci, Staphylococci.

Clinical manifestations

- Maternal temperature increase ≥ 38°C.
- Leukocytosis ≥ 15,000/μL.
- CRP increase.
- Fetal tachycardia.

Diagnosis. Daily monitoring of

- Temperature.
- Blood count, differential blood count.
- Fetal heart rate.

Treatment

Note. Termination of the pregnancy! The danger to the fetus is considerable: the perinatal mortality rate doubles with amnionitis and chorioamnionitis, neonatal infection (possibly with fetal tachycardia, puerperal fever, postnatal respiratory adaptation difficulties, septicemia).

5.3 Intrauterine growth restriction (IUGR)

A **growth-restricted or small for gestational age (SGA) baby** is defined in relation to the gestational age: a small for gestational age newborn is a newborn below the 10th percentile of the standard weight curve (see Fig. 13.19). Definition criteria are: birth weight, gestational age, length, or other body measurements.

Low birth weight (LBW) newborns (birth weight < 2,500 g) are babies born too early or too light.

Clinically, a differentiation is made between symmetrically and asymmetrically growth-restricted newborns.

- *Symmetrically grown- restricted babies.* All body measurements are equally growth-restricted. It is assumed that the growth restriction began around mid-pregnancy.
- *Asymmetrically grown- restricted babies.* Length is appropriate for gestational age, whereas weight is low. This growth restriction occurs in the last weeks of the pregnancy.

Etiology. Approximately 85 % of SGA babies are genetically small, which means that they have grown according to their genetic potential. Approximately 15 % have underlying external or internal factors which restricted their growth:

- Placental insufficiency (see below).
- Ionizing radiation, long-term corticosteroid administration, alcohol abuse, smoking, heroin.
- Viral or bacterial infection (rubella, cytomegalovirus, herpes zoster).
- Chromosomal abnormalities (Turner syndrome, trisomy).
- Deformities (osteogenesis imperfecta, duodenal atresia).
- Maternal illness (PIH, essential hypertension, severe anemia).
- Maternal malnutrition.

Note. The major cause of placental insufficiency is anatomically or functionally reduced placental function:

1. Acute placental insufficiency occurs within minutes or hours (typical: placental abruption).
2. Subacute placental insufficiency occurs over days (typical: prolonged or post-term pregnancy).
3. Chronic placental insufficiency occurs over weeks and months (typical: IUGR).

Diagnosis

- *History.* Identification of risk factors: PIH, renal disease, multifetal gestation, smoking in pregnancy, women who have previously given birth to an SGA baby.
- Reduced growth of uterine fundus (flat fudal height curve; see p. 23).
- Reduced amniotic fluid volume (diagnosis, see p. 48).
- Sonographic assessment (in particular biparietal diameter and first abdominal or thoracic measurement; see p. 46)
- Doppler sonography (see p. 53).

Complications. Intrauterine hypoxia (typical complication during labor). IUGR is often linked with respiratory insufficiency, leading to a higher incidence of operative delivery. Babies are at risk of hypoglycemia and hypothermia after birth.

Treatment

- Bed rest is the most important measure (promotion of uterine circulation).
- Removal of external factors such as smoking and drug use, treatment of underlying illnesses such as hypertension, anemia. Low-dose aspirin treatment of pregnant women with a history of preeclampsia and IUGR may be appropriate for prevention of preeclampsia; significant changes to IUGR risk have not been found.
- Intensive fetal monitoring and waiting for spontaneous onset of labor at the latest until EDD, or
- Ending the pregnancy in cases of growth standstill or respiratory placental insufficiency before spontaneous onset of labor, if necessary after antenatal lung maturation, induction (see p. 282).

Prognosis

Late infant morbidity appears to be low, as infancy is usually characterized by a catch-up in growth. Nevertheless a difference in weight between former SGA children and those who were appropriate for gestational age (AGA) is common. On their sixth year, 30 % of former SGA children are undersized. Intellectual development is often impaired. 50 % are classified as abnormal.

IUGR, similar to maternal diabetes mellitus and perinatal overeating, has permanent consequences, in that it creates a predisposition to obesity, insulin resistance, disturbed glucose tolerance, increased risk for DM type 2, cardiovascular disease (**adult metabolic syndrome**). In this concept of pathophysiological development (**fetal/perinatal programming**), the cause of the process of defective programming is seen as mal-programming of neuroendocrine control systems (Plagemann): Programming describes a process, by which, during a critical developmental phase (prenatal/neonatal), external factors such as diet, hormones etc. have a permanent effect on the future functioning of organs and organ systems, resulting in chronic disorders.

5.4 Postterm pregnancy

Definition. Continuation of pregnancy after the EDD, which has been determined according to history and sonography before week 20. Prolonged pregnancy continues more than 7–10 days after the EDD.

Most prolonged pregnancies are due to errors in calculation, mistakes, or deliberate falsification of dates. Genuine postterm pregnancies are rare.

Precise EDD calculation (± 4 days) is possible via sonographic measurement of **crown-rump length** between weeks 8 and 11, and between weeks 19 and 22 EDD calculation ± 8 days is still possible.

Sonographic results from later in the pregnancy should not be used for determining the gestational age or EDD.

Causes. The main cause is impaired excitability of uterine musculature.

Complications. Children are endangered in genuine postterm pregnancy. Perinatal mortality increases because placenta function decreases.

Mistakes. Those with experience know that postterm pregnancy cannot definitely be established. For this reason, pregnant women not yet at term are often induced (see below). This results in dystocia: rigid soft parts, inadequate contractions, difficulties in stage 3, which in turn lead to an increase in infant morbidity and mortality rates.

Treatment

- Intensive monitoring (Fig. 5.4), EFM every 2 days for early recognition of placental insufficiency, and weekly for measurement of AF volume.
- Cervical ripening 12–14 days after EDD with prostaglandins applied locally. Clinicians today prefer – in particular in cases of unripe or unfavorable cervix–local (intravaginal or intracervical) or oral application of prostaglandins for induction and cervical ripening.
- Induction – in particular if the cervix is ripe: rupturing of the membranes, continuous oxytocin infusion (p. 282).

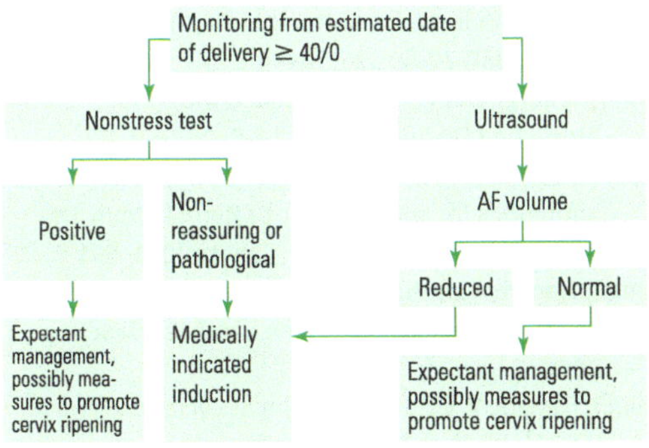

Fig. 5.4: Procedure for postterm pregnancy. EFM; see p. 168. Amniotic fluid (AF) volume is determined sonographically: the vertical diameter of the largest AF pocket is measured (normal 2–8cm), in postterm pregnancy often < 2cm.

5.5 Stillbirth

Definition. Fetal death in the second half of pregnancy.

Incidence. 0.4 % of all pregnant women.

Causes. Placental abruption, diabetes mellitus, umbilical cord prolapse, hemolytic disease of the fetus, deformity, infections, hypoxemia (placental insufficiency) in PIH (p. 74), and postterm pregnancy (p. 108).

Maceration. The fetus which dies and remains in utero undergoes maceration and autolysis due to enzymes on the body surface and bile acids in the excreted meconium. Maceration occurs aseptically and has nothing to do with bacterial decomposition. Differentiation:

- *First degree maceration.* The skin is greyish white and the umbilical cord has a greenish tinge.
- *Second degree maceration.* The skin lifts in blisters and peels away in strips (within 1–3 days after death).
- *Third degree maceration.* As a result of hemolysis, the fetus is a dirty greyish-brown. The joints have lost their firmness, are loose and floppy. The cranium is unevenly sunken due to separation of the bony joints. The skin is flaccid, the fetus is shrunken in general, its weight reduced (complete development of third degree maceration takes 3–4 weeks).

Diagnosis
- Subjective. Fetal movements are no longer felt.
- Objective. Fetal HR missing, no palpable fetal movements or sonographic lack of heart activity, fetal movements, breathing movements.
- Signs of maceration. Flesh-colored amniotic fluid (ooze of blood pigments),
- Loose cranial bones on vaginal examination.

It is not possible to determine the time of death by the degree of maceration, as it occurs at variable rates.

Complications. If intrauterine death occurred more than 3–4 weeks previously, release of tissue factor from the fetoplacental unit can cause disseminated intravascular coagulation (DIC, hemorrhage due to disturbed coagulation).

As stillbirth is often recognized early due to antenatal care, disturbed coagulation is rare (Reister and colleagues 1996).

Treatment. Generally (90 %), the dead fetus is born spontaneously within 14 days of death. Induction procedure in the clinic depends on the ripeness of the cervix:
Unripe cervix: Prostaglandin E2 (PGE2) intracervical gel (Minprostin®) every 6 hours until adequate ripening or begin of active labor occurs.
Ripe cervix: continuous infusion of Sulprostone (Nalador®) or IV oxytocin and artificial rupture of membranes (AROM; amniotomy).
Children who die in labor should be born spontaneously. The fetal cranium can be perforated on crowning, also in cases of breech delivery before manual assistance for delivery of the head.
Vacuum or forceps extraction is a possibility in extreme cases of uterine hypotonia.

For prophylaxis of hemorrhage due to fibrinogen deficiency, management, see p. 377.

References

American College of Obstetricians and Gynecologists: Management of preterm labour. Clinical Management Guidelines for Obstetricain-Gynecologists No. 127, July 2012

American College of Obstetricians and Gynecologists: Oral health care during pregnancy and through the lifespan. Committee opinion No 569, August 2013. Obstet Gynecol 2013; 122:417–22

Coomrasamy A, Thangaratinam S, Gee H, Khan KS: Progesterone for the prevention of preterm birth: A critical evaluation of evidence. Eur J Obstet Gynecol Reproduc Biol 2006; 129:111

Duley L, Henderson-Smart D, Knight M, et al.: Antiplatelet drugs for prevention of pre-eclampsia and consequences: systematic review. Br Med J 2001; 222:329

Fuchs IB, Henrich W, Osthues K, Dudenhausen JW: Sonographic cervical length in singleton pregnancies with intact membranes presenting with threatened preterm labor. Ultrasound Obstet Gynecol 2004; 24:554

Goldenberg RL, Cliver SP, Bronstein J, et al.: Bed rest in pregnancy. Obstet Gynecol 1994; 84:131

Growther CA, Hiller JE, Doyle LW, Haslam RR: Effect of magnesium sulphate given for neuroprotection before preterm birth. JAMA 2003; 2090:2669

Honest H, Bachmann LM, Gupta JK, et al.: Accuracy of cervicovaginal fetal fibronectin test in predicting risk of spontaneous preterm birth: systematic review. BMJ 2002; 325:301–4

Iams JD, Berghella V: Care for women with prior preterm birth. Am J Obstet Gynecol 2010; 203:89–100

Kenyon SL, Taylor DJ, Tarnow-Mordi W: Broad spectrum antibiotics for spontaneous preterm labour: The ORACLE II randomised trial. Lancer 2001; 591

King J, Flenady V: Antibiotics for preterm labour with intact membranes. Cochrane Database Syst Rev 2000; 2

King J, Flenady V, Cole S, Thornton S: Cyclo-oxygenase (COX) inhibitors for treating preterm labour. Cochrane Database Syst Rev 2005; 2:CD 001992

Lamont RF, Khan KS, Beattie B, et al.: The quality of nifedipine studies used to access tocolytic efficacy – a symptomatic review. J Perinat Med 2005; 33:287

Lee SE, Park JS, Norwitz BR, et al.: Measurement of placerital alpha-microglobulin-1 in cervicovaginal discharge to diagnose rupture of membranes. Obstet Gynecol 2007; 109:634

Maher MA, Abdelaziz A, Ellaithy M, Bazeed MF: Prevention of preterm birth: A randomzed trial of vaginal compared with intramuscular progesterone. Obste&Gynecol Survey 2013;68:411–3

Manuck TA, Eller AG, Esplín MS, et al.: Outcomes of expectantly managed preterm premature rupture of membranes occuring before 24 weeks of gestation. Obstet Gynecol 2009; 114:29–37

McKinlay CJD, Crowther CA, Middleton P, Harding JE: Repeat antenatal glucocorticoids for women at risk of preterm birth: a Cochrane systematic review. Amer J Obstet Gynecol 2012; 206:187–194

Meis PJ, Aleman A: Progesteron treatment to prevent preterm birth. Drugs 2004; 64:2463

Mittendorf R, Dambrosia J, Pryde PG, et al.: Association between use of antenatal magnesium sulfate in preteirm labor and adverse health outcome in children. Am J Obstet Gyecol 2002; 186:1111

Plagemann A: Fetal programming and functional teratogeriesis: an epigenetic mechariism and prevention of perinatally acquired lasting health risks. J Perinat Med 2004; 32:297

Royal College of Obstetricians and Gynecologists: Antenatal Corticosteroids to reduce neonatal morbidity and mortality. Green-top Guideline No. 7, October 2010

Royal College of Obstctricians and Gynaecologists: Cervical Cerclage. Green-top Guideline No. 60. May 2011

Royal College of Obstetricians and Gynecologists: Magnesium sulphate to prevent cerebral palsy following preterm birth. Scientific Advisory Committee, Opinion Paper 29, August 2011

Royal College of Obstetricians and Gynecologists: The investigation and management of the small-for-gestational-age fetus. Green-top Guideline No. 31, February 2013

Royal College of Obstetricians and Gynecologists: Preterm labour, antibiotics, and cerebral palsy. Scientific Impact Paper No. 33, February 2013

Royal College of Obstetricians and Gynecologists: The investigation and management of the small-for-gestational-age fetus. Green-top Guideline No.31, January 2014

Sanchez-Ramos L, Kaunitz A, Delke I: Progestational agents to prevent preterm birth: a metaanalysis of randomized controlled trials. Obstet Gynecol 2005; 105:273

Smith V, Devane D, Beglay CM, et al.: A systematic review and quality assessment of systematic reviews of fetal fibronectin and transvaginal length for predicting preterm birth. Eur J Obstet Gynecol Reprod Biol 2007; 133:134

Simhan HN, Caritis SN: Prevention of preterm delivery. N Engl J Med 2007; 357:477

The GRIT Study Group: When do obstetricians recommend delivery for a high-risk preterm growth-retarded fetus? Growth restriction intervention trial. Eur J Obstet Gynecol Reprocl Biol 1996; 67:121

Tsalsaris U, Papatsonis D, Goffinet F, et al.: Tocolysis with nifedipine or beta adrenergic agonists: a meta-analysis. Obstet Gynecol 2001; 97:840

Waters TP, Mercer BM: The management of preterm premature rupture of the membraries near the limit of fetal viability. Am J Obstet Gynecol 2009; 21:230–40

6 Disorders of the fetus

6.1 Hemolytic disease

Definition. Immune hemolytic anemia of the fetus or newborn, with erythroblastosis (immature nucleated red blood cells), as a result of increased regeneration of red blood cells due to the transplacental transfer of maternal blood group antibodies against fetal blood groups (in particular D, also E, c, Cw, C, e). It is usually (> 85 %) caused by Rhesus incompatibility in pregnancy.

Incidence
Before introduction of the anti-D immunoglobulin:
- Incidence of Rhesus sensitization of D-negative mothers 40–50 in 1,000.
- Incidence of Rhesus D:
  - hemolytic disease: 4–5 in 1,000 live births.
  - mortality (prenatal): 0.8–1.0 in 1,000 live births.

After introduction of the anti-D immunoglobulin
- Incidence of Rhesus D:
  - hemolytic disease: 0.5–1.0 in 1,000 live births.
  - mortality: 0.05–0.1 in 1,000 live births.

Pathophysiology, pathogenesis. Maternal antibodies. Fetal blood group antigens (Rhesus, ABO) pass via transplacental diapedesis of erythrocytes into the maternal circulation during pregnancy, in particular during labor with feto-maternal bleeding, and induce antibody production (alloimmunization; Fig. 6.1). Maternal antibodies are produced if the mother does not possess the fetal blood factor and thus recognizes it as an antigen. Blood group incompatibility implies that the fetal blood group differs from the maternal one (autosomal inheritance from the father; see Tab. 6.1).

Common blood group combinations resulting in incompatibility are listed in Tab. 6.1; in reality, alloimmunization rarely occurs.

Note. An Rh-negative woman and Rh-positive man in 15 % of all partnerships. This means that they can expect an Rh-positive child. Only 5 % of these mothers will become alloimmunized, because D antibodies are rarely detected in Rh-negative women in the first pregnancy (no preimmunization). In 50 % of these partnerships the heterozygosity of the Rh-positive father and the corresponding production of a number of Rh-negative children is to be expected.

Further factors which influence maternal antibody production:
- Prior incompatible blood transfusions.
- Prior pregnancies (also miscarriage or ectopic pregnancy) with blood group-incompatible fetus promote antibody production.
- ABO-Rh antagonism results in isoantibody destruction of fetal erythrocytes (hemolysis before Rh-system alloimmunization of the mother).

Tab. 6.1. Common blood group incompatibilities in the Rhesus and ABO system (sensitization of the mother to differing fetal blood group antigens inherited from the father).

Blood groups	Father	Child	Mother
CDE/Rhesus blood groups	D C-D-E	D C-D-E	d cc-dd-ee
ABO blood groups	A B	A B	0 0
In rare blood groups – Kell system – Duffy system – MNSs system	 $Kell^+$ Fy^b S	 $Kell^+$ Fy^b S	 $Kell^-$ Fy^a s

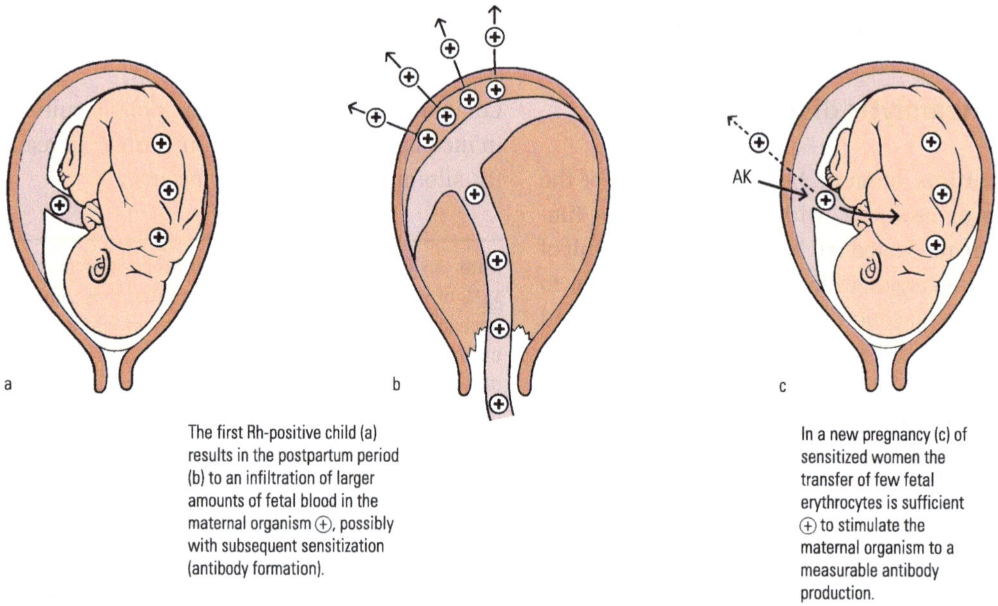

Fig. 6.1: D-isoimmunization (after Ballowitz). The first Rh-positive child (a) causes an inundation of large amounts of fetal blood into the maternal system (+) in stage 3 (b), which may cause sensitization (production of antibodies). In a subsequent pregnancy (c), the crossing over of a few fetal erythrocytes (+) can be enough to stimulate detectable production of antibodies in a sensitized woman.

Further irregular antibodies. Those incompatibilities not due to Rhesus incompatibility are unaffected by the anti-D-immunoglobulin: mother-child constellation: C-c, O-A,O-B, Fy^a-Fy^b, Fy^b-Fy^a, S-s, s-S. Comparatively, their incidence has increased.

Practice tip. Blood group incompatibility, in particular through Rhesus-D, followed by Rhesus-C, causes severe hemolysis, which begins in-utero.

- *Rhesus-incompatibility:* intra- and extrauterine damage to the child.
- *ABO-incompatibility:* only extrauterine damage to the child.

Clinical manifestations

Low-grade hemolytic disease (newborn anemia; 30 % of the Rhesus erythroblastoses) begins in utero with:

- *Anemia.* Maternal antibodies pass through the placenta to the fetus and destroy its erythrocytes, as indicated by the hemolytic anemia. This can be evaluated with Doppler sonography.
- *Hyperbilirubinemia.* A further indicator of the demise of erythrocytes is excess bilirubin (hyperbilirubinemia), which first manifests itself extrauterinely after birth. The infant reacts with rapid regeneration of erythrocytes, erythroblastemia, reticulocytosis, and enlargement of the extramedullary blood-building organs (enlargement of liver and spleen).

Medium-grade hemolytic disease (→Icterus gravis, 60 % of Rh-erythroblastoses) begins after birth.

- Alongside the reduction of fetal erythrocytes and hypoxia, the yellow coloring of the amniotic fluid is noted.

– Hypoxia (severe anemia, Doppler-sonography!) and hyperbilirubinemia can have serious consequences for the child.

Note. Erythrocyte destruction begins prenatally and damages the fetus. The dangerous increase in bilirubin only takes place after delivery.

Bilirubin. In the newborn, bilirubin not bound to glucuronic acid is not water-soluble, so it cannot be excreted in bile. Instead, it is deposited in the blood and connective tissue. Being liposoluble, it easily penetrates organs rich in fat (CNS), where it has a cytotoxic effect (inhibition of phosphorylation in the cells of the basal ganglia, which have the most active metabolism in the newborn brain): kernicterus and bilirubin encephalopathy are serious consequences.
– Oxygen deficiency increases the permeability of the nerve cell membrane.
– Hypoxia promotes bilirubin encephalopathy in icteric newborns.

High-grade hemolytic disease (hydrops fetalis; < 10 % of Rhesus erythroblastoses), begins in utero:
– Hydrops (fluid accumulation in preformed cavities and tissues). Hydrops of fetus and placenta occurs in cases of severe anemia (Hb < 8 g%), as a result of increased blood vessel permeability and inadequate protein synthesis (hypoproteinemia < 3 g%) in the liver. It has both fetal and maternal consequences (Tab. 6.2).
– Such babies are frequently stillborn or die shortly after birth.
– The most common form of hemolytic disease is immune-mediated hydrops fetalis (IHF).

Diagnosis

– *Sonography.* Among other things, prenatal detection of congenital hydrops.
– Prenatal sonographic detection of hydrops necessitates further differential diagnostic considerations (Tab. 6.2).
– *Doppler-sonography.* MCA peak systolic velocity measurement is a suitable, non-invasive method for estimating the danger to the fetus. Umbilical vein pulsations are more likely late signs of fetal compromise. The current method of choice for monitoring hemolytic disease of the fetus (HDF) is noninvasive Doppler-sonography, in preference to the invasive method of AF spectrophotometry.
– *Serodiagnosis.* Blood group incompatibility is detectable at the latest by week 16:
– – Fetal **blood typing** (ABO, Rh) and antibody screen (D, C, c, E, e, Kell, Fy and S) at the first prenatal visit and again in weeks 24–27.
– – **Cordocentesis** to determine fetal Hb.
– – It is possible to perform fetal D genotyping from maternal plasma via **DNA analysis**
– – **Amniotic fluid (AF) spectrophotometry** with maximum absorbance of 450 nm for evaluation of the degree of fetal anemia

Pathological pigment additives, for example products of fetal hemolysis, alter the normal AF curve, whereby indirect bilirubin demonstrates a characteristic peak (maximum absorbance) at 450 nm.

Practice tip. The color intensity of AF correlates with the degree to which the fetus is endangered in Rh (D) alloimmunization.

Tab. 6.2: Causes of fetal hydrops.

Maternal causes	Immune-mediated hemolytic disease Alpha-thalassemia Diabetes mellitus PIH
Placental	Chorionic vein thrombosis Umbilical vein thrombosis
Fetal causes	Anemia, e.g., feto-maternal or feto-fetal transfusion syndrome Cardiac, e.g., severe heart defect, fibroelastosis, supraventricular tachycardia Pulmonary, e.g., pulmonary hypoplasia Hypoproteinemia, e.g., nephrosis, renal vein thrombosis Infectious, e.g., cytomegalovirus, virus hepatitis, syphilis, toxoplasmosis Anomalies, e.g., chromosomal
Idiopathic hydrops	

Anti-D-immunoglobulin, Rhesus desensitization (mother Rh-negative, child Rh-positive). Anti-D-immunoglobulin is to be injected

- in an Rh-negative woman directly (at the latest 48–72 hours) after delivery of an Rh-positive baby;
- after every miscarriage, abortion, ectopic pregnancy, amniocentesis, chorionic villus sampling;
- if bleeding occurs in pregnancy.

The initial Rhesus alloimmunization occurs when fetal erythrocytes pass into the mother's bloodstream during birth of the first Rh-negative baby. The mother produces Rhesus antibodies postpartum. The second Rh-positive fetus induces a repeat alloimmunization ("booster") in pregnancy via transplacental erythrocyte transfer. The critical factor in alloimmunization of the Rh-negative woman is the initial antigen contact during delivery of an Rh-positive baby. The passive application of IgG anti-Rh(D) hinders the synthesis of anti-D. In addition, the passively introduced anti-D-immunoglobulins bind to the fetal erythrocytes and promote their rapid elimination from the maternal bloodstream before the body can begin to produce its own antibodies.

Practice tip. Prophylaxis only makes sense if the mother does not show antibodies (indirect Coombs' test), i.e., if simply the combination of an Rh-negative (d) mother and a Rh-positive (D) fetus exists:

1. 300 µg anti-D-immunoglobulin IV or IM within 48 (at the latest 72 hours) postpartum.
2. If the pregnancy did not last longer than 12 weeks, the dose is reduced to 100 µg.

The maternal immune system is protected from 20–30 ml fetal Rh-positive blood with the standard dose of 300 µg. Studies using the Kleihauer-Betke test have established feto-maternal transfusion in 75 % of all pregnancies (3 % in the first trimester, 45 % in the third) and 64 % during delivery (Bowmann 1988). The amount transfused was below the detection limit (0.05 ml fetal blood) in 80 %, > 20 ml in 1 %.

In order to detect a maternal-fetal macrotransfusion and an inadequate anti-D dose, it is advisable to count fetal erythrocytes in the mother's blood 3 days after anti-D application. Should such a case (≥ 1 ‰) occur, a calculable dose of anti-D should be readministered: 300 µg anti-D IM per estimated 20 ml of transfused fetal blood.

Example. Results of the Hb-F cell count: 8‰. Maternal blood volume 5,000 ml. This means

that around 40 ml fetal blood has entered the maternal bloodstream, and therefore 600 µg anti-D should be injected IM.
If anti-D-immunoglobulin is given during a continuing pregnancy (after amniocentesis, chorionic villus sampling, possible miscarriage), a standard anti-D dose every 12 weeks is recommended in order to avoid an increase of the following injections (Schneider).

General prenatal isoimmunization prophylaxis
All Rh-negative women (showing no antibodies) are given a 300 µg IM injection. Antibodies are to be checked beforehand!

Practice tip. The incidence of hemolytic disease has been reduced due to systematic anti Rh (D) prophylaxis and its course is milder.

Treatment. Intrauterine transfusion. The donor blood cells are injected (under ultrasound guidance) into the umbilical vein (cordocentesis).

The procedure was introduced by Liley (1963) in order to avoid a premature delivery (immaturity!): injection of serologically compatible (usually O D negative) concentrated erythrocytes into the abdominal cavity of the fetus.

Practice tip. Obstetrical procedure during and after delivery of a baby in whose mother antibodies have been detected:

- Cut umbilical cord immediately, to prevent transferal of the reserve blood which contains erythrocytes loaded with antibodies.
- Leave the remaing cord long (3–4 cm) in case an exchange transfusion (best performed via catheterization of the umbilical vein) should be necessary.
- Immediate testing of umbilical vein blood (if this has not already occurred during labor):
  - Direct Coombs' test (detects antibodies bound to fetal erythrocytes).
  - Detailed blood typing (blood group, Rh factor).
  - Detection of free maternal antibodies in the newborn's serum and determination of their nature (using the indirect Coombs' test and an enzyme test).
  - Red and white blood count with erythroblasts (nonreassuring > 10 erythroblasts: 100 leukocytes, hemoglobin level (nonreassuring: Hb < 16 g% = 10 mmol/l), reticulocytes (nonreassuring > 50 ‰).
- Immediate treatment is unnecessary. Frequent monitoring of clinical, serological and hematological status gives the indication for phototherapy or exchange transfusion:
  - Pale?
  - Spleen or liver enlargement? Worsening of hepatosplenomegaly?
  - Jaundice? Worsening of jaundice or increased bilirubin levels?
  - Drop in Hb level < 14 g% = 9 mmol/l.
  - Increase in erythroblasts.
- Immediate treatment if: direct Coombs' test is positive, Hb < 10 g% (7 mmol/l), hydrops:
  - Intubation, mechanical ventilation (O_2!).
  - Withdrawal of 50–100 ml of blood and transfusion of prepared (before delivery!) erythrocyte concentrate of the universal donor group O-negative (10–20 ml per Kg body weight slowly IV). The addition of oxygen carriers can be a lifesaving measure to reduce the period of hypoxia.
  - Prepare and perform exchange transfusion.

Postnatal exchange transfusion. The exchange transfusion is obligatory in newborns presenting with clinical HDN, regardless of maternal antigen specificity. This is, however, relevant for the selection of donor blood. Maternal antibodies damaged fetal erythrocytes and bilirubin are removed. Fresh, functioning blood cells are transferred.

- Donor blood in cases of Rh-incompatibility is the relevant ABO blood type, Rh-negative.
- Donor blood in cases of ABO-incompatibility:
  - Type-A_2 blood, if the baby is blood type A, or
  - Type O blood, which must be low in α-lysine in babies with blood type A, or low in β-lysine in babies with blood type B,
  - Type O erythrocytes in plasma (complicated).
- Hyperbilirubinemia progress chart. The serum bilirubin level is a critical indicator for exchange transfusion. The higher it is, the greater the danger of bilirubin encephalopathy (= kernicterus). Progress charts are employed; one by Polacek is commonly used.

Phototherapy p. 456.

Prognosis. Irregular antibodies are not relevant for the prognosis of an infant, regardless of the titer! Crucial for the prognosis are studies of fetal blood (acquired by cordocentesis performed under ultrasound guidance).

6.2 Fetal alloimmune thrombocytopenia

Definition. Fetal thrombocytopenia as a result of the transfer of platelet-specific maternal antibodies into the fetal bloodstream.

Incidence. Around 1 in 3,000 to 1 in 5,000 births.

Pathophysiology. The transplacental passage of maternal IgG antibodies against a fetal platelet-specific antigen inherited from the father accelerates platelet breakdown and thrombocytopenia (< 30,000 μl), in particular in the second half of pregnancy. Maternal alloimmunization can occur in the first pregnancy.

Clinical manifestation. Intracranial hemorrhage (ICH) is at the forefront of hemorrhage symptoms such as petechiae, hematomas, and others. The risk is greater (20 %) if the platelet count is below 30,000 μl, in particular during the perinatal period.

Diagnosis. Possible by detection of maternal antibodies against platelet surface antigens. The first fetal blood sampling for platelet count and antibody tests takes place at around weeks 20–22.

Treatment. As the therapeutic value of noninvasive measures has not been demonstrated, the invasive procedure of platelet transfusion is the method of choice. It is initiated at the diagnostic cordocentesis (and possibly at weekly intervals thereafter) in weeks 20–22. A preterm delivery (at around 35 weeks) may reduce the risks. If the fetal platelet count is below 10,000 μl, a cesarean delivery is considered to be less traumatic. None of the therapeutic suggestions have been clinically proven.

6.3 Prenatal infections

Infection is the transmission, adherence and penetration of microorganisms (viruses, bacteria, fungi protozoas) into a macroorganism (pre-, peri-, and postnatally), followed by reproduction in the host; they are the prerequisite for an infectious disease. Viruses, bacteria (e.g., spirochetes), and protozoa can infect the fetus prenatally via the mother. Bacterial infections are formost during the perinatal period.

Paths of infection are (in order of decreasing frequency):

- Ascending, after ROM; more rarely if membranes are intact.

– Hematogenous via the placenta in cases of maternal viremia, bacteremia or parasitemia.
– Descending, via the Fallopian tubes.

Infection timepoint. The timing of the infection determines whether it manifests pre- or postnatally. Prenatal infections can develop into blasto-, embryo-, or fetopathies.

Blasto-, embryopathy. Developmental disorder of the embryo during the embryonic period (organogenesis; blastopathy during the first 2 weeks after conception).

Note. Blasto- (weeks 3–4) and embryopathies (weeks 5–14) are phase-specific (timing of infection is critical) and not cause-specific (pathogen) and encompass the following spectrum: 1) miscarriage and stillbirth; 2) preterm baby with birth defect; 3) term baby with birth defect; 4) clinically healthy preterm baby; 5) clinically healthy term baby. The type of defect (affected organ) makes it possible to determine retrospectively when the prenatal damage (e.g., rubella infection) occurred.

Fetopathies. Defined prenatal illnesses with specific causality in the fetal period (weeks 15 till birth) after organogenesis has been completed (embryonic period).

The fetus develops the ability to defend itself, which can lead to morphological (inflammation) and functional (developmental disorder) changes.

Practice tip. Late-onset prenatal infections are clinically relevant. They can manifest during later childhood. Late-onset symptoms of prenatal infections can cause challenging diagnostic problems:
Growth and developmental disorders such as dwarfism, psychomotor retardation, hearing defects ranging from hearing impairment to deafness, type 1 diabetes and possibly other regulating disorders, recurrent diarrhea, respiratory illnesses, hepatoma, malignant tumors.

TORCH complex (acronym, stands for): toxoplasmosa gondii, other infectious microorganisms, rubella-, cytomegalo-, herpes-simplex viruses.

T =	Toxoplasmosis	Protozoa
O =	Other (syphilis, listeria, TB)	Bacteria
R =	Rubella	Virus
C =	Cytomegalovirus	Virus
H =	Herpes-simplex	Virus
H =	Hepatitis	Virus
HIV =	AIDS	Virus

6.3.1 Prenatal rubella infection, congenital rubella syndrome

Definition. Prenatal differentiation disorder caused by the rubella virus in the first trimester (= congenital rubella syndrome, CRS, Gregg syndrome). The severity of the classical triad of symptoms (deafness, congenital heart disease, cataracts) varies.

Gregg syndrome. In 1941, the Australian ophthalmologist Gregg first described a syndrome which he could trace back to a rubella infection in pregnancy. In the USA in 1964 a very extensive rubella epidemic broke out with several million infected, of which more than 10,000 prenatal infections were observed and studied.

Incidence. During the great rubella epidemic of 1964 in the US, the rate of congenital malformations was expected to be 4‰ and in nonepidemic periods 1‰. The CRS rate is currently 1 : 100,000.

Etiology. Infection with viremia (only occurs in the initial infection) of a pregnant woman who has never been infected with the rubella virus (togavirus family) or immunized against it. The presence of the virus in the blood (= viremia) is necessary for prenatal infection to occur.

Practice tip. Classic rubella embryopathy is caused by prenatal infection before week 16; rarely up until week 20.

Pathogenesis. Persisting inflammation of the placenta with necrosis of the epithelium of the chorionic villi and blood vessels, intravascular clotting, hemorrhage. Hematogenous spread with necrosis in the fetal heart.

The classical rubella embryopathy presents a relatively consistent prenatal malformation syndrome which could also be relevant for other virus embryopathies (virus embryopathy model; influenza, mumps, varicella-zoster virus).

Incidence of malformations. The timing of the infection determines the rate of infection (Enders):

Time of infection	Incidence of infection (%)
Before 3 completed weeks	~ 50
Weeks 5–8	~ 25
Weeks 9–12	~ 15
Weeks 13–16	~ 10
From 16 completed weeks	< 3.5

Clinical manifestations

Practice tip. The earlier the infection, the more serious the damage. The typical rubella embryopathy occurs before week 14, with disruptive morphological disorders. After week 14 hypotrophy, hemolytic anemia, thrombocytopenic purpura, hepatosplenomegaly, interstitial pneumonia. The organs most commonly organ affected are ears, eyes. and heart.

Classical symptoms:
- Ear (sensorineural deafness, often partial).
- Eye (cataract, microphthalmia).
- Cardiopathy.
- Prenatal dystrophy (LBW, underdeveloped neonates).
- Disturbed psychomotor development (commonly microcephaly).
- Milk teeth defects (hypoplasia, aplasia).

Extended rubella syndrome, acute congenital rubella:
- Prenatal dystrophy (LBW neonates).
- Hepatosplenomegaly with or without jaundice.
- Maculopapular ("Blueberry muffin") rash.
- Thrombocytopenia.
- Bone disorders (e.g., calcification disorders in the long bones).
- Myocardial injury (congenital aortic stenosis is possible).
- Glaucoma.
- Renal changes (e.g., renal artery stenosis).

The clinical picture of CRS conforms with a severe generalized viral infection.

Prevention. Previous infection or immunization provide life-long immunity.

There are conflicting opinions as to whether immunization of newborns provides life-long immunity during puberty.
- Active immunization with childhood vaccination programs in combination with mumps and measles vaccines is advisable, as are repeat immunizations for all girls from 6–12 years of age (before puberty). Antibody titers are measured before planned pregnancies. Women with rubella serum negativity are immunized. Rubella antibodies (hemagglutination inhibitions titer (HAI) > 1 : 16) indicate immune protection for mother and embryo.
- Pregnant women who have had contact with people infected with rubella are tested for immunity (detection of rubella antibodies).
- If rubella antibodies (IgG and IgM) are not detected or the HAI titer is < 1 : 32, the following procedure applies: 10 ml anti-ru-

bella hyper-immunoglobulin IM (exposure shouldn't have occurred more than 7 days previously) or Repeat test in 10 days:
  - Titer increase (> 2 dilutions) or rubella IgM detected mean recent infection
  - If the titer remains low, infection has not occurred. As a result, chorionic villus sampling should be performed after week 9, or amniocentesis using the PCR method.
  - Unclear result. Fetal blood sampling via cordocentesis in week 20 is recommended. Fetal blood is tested for rubella IgM antibodies. If IgM antibodies are detected, infection has occurred. The potential damage can be calculated by analysis of the timing of the infection.

Practice tip. If viremia is already present (rash!) immunoglobulins are pointless.

- If a high titer (e.g., 1 : 512) is detected at a prenatal check-up, recent infection is possible. Repeat test in 7–10 days to observe changes in titer levels.
- Pregnant women should only give care to children with rubella if they are immune to the disease.

6.3.2 Cytomegalovirus (CMV)

Cytomegalovirus, pre- and postnatal viral infection.

Incidence. Commonest prenatal infection!

A generalized cytomegaly of newborns was first described in 1904. Infection with CMV is widespread; 1 % of all newborns are infected in utero. Infection occurs more often than is diagnosed.

Etiology, pathogenesis. The cause is infection with cytomegalovirus (CMV), an RNA-virus. CMV infections are often not apparent, regardless of when the infection occurred; the cells of the infected organism host the virus. The latent infection can manifest in immune-compromised patients (malignant tumors or systemic disorders, immune-suppressive therapy, organ transplants).

Infection in pregnancy places the fetus at risk of infection; it is possible for the mother to experience recurrent infection, but the risk for the fetus in such cases is lower.

Clinical manifestations. Broad range of symptoms! Most infected children (90 %) are healthy on delivery. Later, mental retardation and hearing defects can occur.

Prenatal infection. 10 % of infected neonates are symptomatic.
- Microcephaly, meningoencephalitis, intracranial calcifications.
- Hepatosplenomegaly, anemia.
- Prenatal dystrophy, thrombocytopenic purpura.
- Interstitial pneumonia, myocarditis.

Postnatal infection. Also seldom symptomatic:
- Similar to infectious mononucleosis (with characteristic serological changes), in some cases organ manifestations can be the main symptoms: hepatitis, pneumonia, myocarditis, gastroenteritis

Diagnosis. Detection of the virus is crucial.
- Detection of the virus in urine, saliva, cervical secretion; in biopsies of liver, kidney, lung, brain.
- Antibody detection is of epidemiological interest; a titer increase in a recent infection is rarely detectable.
- If maternal serology and sonographic evidence (ascites, hydramnios, hypotrophy, hepatosplenomegaly) are inconclusive, invasive methods of prenatal diagnosis are used: PCR of chorionic villi or AF, from week 22 fetal blood.

- Cytology (cytomegalic cells containing the virus with "owl's eye" form) and histology (cells containing the virus in infected organs) are significantly inferior to virus culture.

DD.
1. *Numerous neonatal diseases.* Clinical manifestation of pre- and postnatal CMV infection shows few typical characteristics and is similar to other illnesses of the newborn period, in particular in cases of organ manifestation in postnatal infection. This explains the difficulty of clinical diagnosis.
2. *Infectious mononucleosis.* Postnatal infection causes symptoms which are also typical for other illnesses, often bringing glandular fever (Pfeiffer's disease) to mind because of the typical serological findings.

Treatment. Symptomatic therapy (treatment of the cause is not possible!). Transfusions, human gamma globulin, corticosteroids. Passive immunization with CMV hyperimmuneglobulin in cases of primary infection in pregnancy appears to be effective (Nigro and colleagues). Fetal antenatal therapy with transabdominal IV CMV hyperimmune globulin has been suggested (Bald).

Prognosis. Poor!
- Symptomatic infection: 20 % lethality.
- Late sequelae. Restricted vision, hearing impairment, development of cerebral seizures, sensory-motor and mental retardation, tooth defects.
- Asymptomatic infection. Less than 1 % lethality. 5–15 % develop late sequelae!

Prevention. Serological screening of mothers at risk (e.g., nurses). Seropositive mother: minimal risk of giving birth to a sick baby. Seronegative mother: hygienic measures to be followed. Care must be taken with the urine and saliva of infected persons. A CMV vaccination is not available.

6.3.3 Varicella-zoster-virus (VZV)

Definition. Highly contagious viral disease which manifests itself as chicken pox on initial infection and can reactivate at a later date as herpes zoster or shingles. Risk of embryo- or fetopathy if the mother is infected with the herpes zoster virus and shows with viremia in the first half of pregnancy (congenital varicella syndrome).

Incidence. Chicken pox during pregnancy is rare, due to the high number (95 %) of women of child-bearing age who are VZV seropositive. Congenital varicella syndrome affects 20 % of infected newborns.

Etiology, pathogenesis. The pathogen is the varicella-zoster-virus (alpha virus of the herpes family). Transmission is via contact or airborne, initially the nose and throat are affected; viremia, virus reproduction in the skin. Shingles is endogenous reinfection. Congenital varicella syndrome is a serious illness, as maternal antibodies cannot be produced and transferred to the baby in perinatal infection (a few days prior to or after delivery).

Clinical manifestations

Note. Congenital varicella syndrome: perinatal infection 4 days before and 2 days after delivery is a life-threatening illness.

- *CNS.* Microcephaly, cortical atrophy, cerebellar hypoplasia, development of hydrocephaly, calcifications.
- *Eyes.* Atrophy of the optic nerve, microphthalmia, chorioretinitis, anisocoria, cataracts.

- *Peripheral nerves.* Sensory-motor retardation, hypoplasia of the extremities, anal and vesical sphincter disorders, scarring.

In cases of infection in late pregnancy (30–5 days prior to delivery), the course of the infection is milder as a result of maternal IgG antibody transmission: 25 % of newborns develop blister-like skin lesions; rarely pneumonia.

Diagnosis. Maternal history of prenatal chicken pox infection. IgM antibody detection in newborn directly after delivery.

Treatment. Isolation of mother and baby!

Procedure if a pregnant woman has had contact with an individual infected with VZV:
- Determine VZV immunity status.
- If immunity exists (VZV antibody positive), no further action.
- If immunity does not exist, IM application of 0.2 ml/kg Varicella-zoster immune globulin within 72–96 hours after exposure.

Procedure if infection occurs in pregnancy:
- Before 20 completed weeks: risk of congenital varicella syndrome 1.5 %. No varicella-zoster immune globulin, parents should be counseled.
- 30–5 days before delivery: newborn should be given varicella-zoster immune globulin.
- Perinatal infection, 4 days before and 2 days after delivery: mother should be given varicella-zoster immune globulin (0.2 ml/kg) and the neonate also, after birth (2.0 ml).

Prognosis. The mortality rate is 30 % without varicella-zoster immune globulin treatment; permanent neurological damage is common. Maternal shingles during pregnancy, labor, or puerperium is not dangerous.

6.3.4 Herpes simplex virus (HSV)

Definition. Primary infection (herpes labialis or genitalis) with the herpes simplex virus (HSV) or reactivation of the virus, which persists in the ganglia.

Incidence. The most widespread viruses; as evidenced by high seropositivity: HSV-1 antibodies are found in 85 % of young adults and over 90 % of older adults; HSV-2 in 20–40 % of adults.

Etiology. Pathogen is HSV, a DNA alphavirus of the family of herpes viruses. 2 types: 1) HSV-1 (herpes labialis; orofacial or oral herpes); 2) HSV-2 (herpes genitalis; genital herpes).

Distribution. Viruses in saliva, urine and stool; infection via micro lesions in skin and mucous membranes (urogenital tract, digestive tract, conjunctiva). HSV penetrates the nerve ends as a nucleocapsid and enters the corresponding ganglia via the axonal flow. Active, productive infection begins after 1–2 days. Symptoms do not appear until after day 6, and viral shedding lasts until day 10.

Pathogenesis. Transmission. Initial infection usually occurs in children under 5 via contact or airborne from herpes lesions and is commonly asymptomatic.

Only 1 % of infections (predominantly in children) are clinically apparent: gingivastomatitis, herpetic vulvovaginitis, herpetic keratitis. Genital herpes (HSV-2) and oral herpes (HSV-1) of the laboring mother or care provider pose a threat to the newborn. Severe forms are recognized: neonatal herpes sepsis, eczema herpeticum, herpes meningo-encephalitis. Prenatal HSV infection is linked to miscarriages and malformations.

Clinical manifestations
- Itchiness, tense sensation.
- Grouped blisters on a reddened area which develop a crusty scab on drying out.
- Even the smallest, most unapparent genital lesion in the mother poses a life-threatening danger to the fetus in labor. PROM promotes ascension of all infections including HSV-2.
- Scar-free healing after 8–10 days.
- Swollen and painful regional lymph nodes.
- Favored localizations: lips (herpes labialis), vulva (herpes genitalis).

Maternal diagnosis
- Clinical manifestation.
- Cytological (Papanicolaou smear). Results within hours.
- Virus serology is only diagnostically relevant in primary HSV-2 infection or an extremely serious case involving the lymph nodes. Only in such a case can an antibody increase be expected within 8–10 days.
- Results of virological tests from lesion content or tissue within 1–2 days.
- Electron microscope, immunofluorescence, ELISA.

Distinctive feature. An HSV-2 infection can be expected in 0.1–1 % of all pregnant women – reactivation of a latent infection due to the pregnancy, usually asymptomatic, rarely with groups of blisters on skin and mucous membranes of the genital area. The affected areas are often painful; the cervical region is not sensitive to pain. The infection is often noticed by chance at an prenatal checkup. Regular relapses (herpes simplex recidivans), often at the same location (herpes simplex recidivans in loco) as a result of irritation of infected neurons after febrile infection (herpes febrilis), exposure to sunlight, menstruation (herpes menstrualis), trauma (herpes traumaticus), digestive disorder, immunosuppression, hormonal and psychological factors.

Treatment. Symptomatic local therapy during HSV outbreak:
- Herpes labialis in the vesicular stage. Clioquinol (2 % Clioquinol in lotio alba aquosa) 3 × daily as drying, antiseptic treatment. Crust removal in the healing phase with, for example, Dexpanthenol.
- Herpes genitalis. Bathe twice daily with chamomile extract, followed by direct application of antiseptic dyes (e.g., 0.5 % gentian violet solution). Healing phase: povidone-iodine applied to the erosions.
- Local antiviral therapy: application up to 5x daily of tromantadine, idoxurine, or acyclovir; care should be taken to avoid development of contact allergies.

Prognosis
- Prenatal HSV infection causes miscarriage in 30 % of cases.
- Herpes genitalis after week 32 in pregnancy will result in neonatal HSV- infection in 10 % of cases.
- Herpes genitalis in pregnancy results in:
  - neonatal infection after vaginal delivery in 40 % of cases;
  - no neonatal infection after cesarean delivery (if performed ≤ 4 hours after membrane rupture).
- Neonatal HSV-infection clinically manifests in 50 % of cases resulting in:
  - death in 30 %;
  - severe neurological damage in 30 %.

Prophylaxis
- Avoidance of trigger factors (e.g., UV light), regular application of sun screen if necessary.
- Aim for nonactive herpes at the latest by EDD.
- Caesarean delivery (under 4 hours after membrane rupture), if seropositivity or active herpes genitalis persist until delivery to avoid neonatal infection.

Practice tip. Prevention of transmission of HSV-1 to a neonate requires isolation. Those with active herpes labialis (mother, nurse) must not be caregivers for neonates.

6.3.5 Virus hepatitis

Definition. Acute inflammation of the liver with hepatitis viruses A–G and disease duration <6 months. One of the most widespread infectious diseases worldwide.

Differential diagnosis. See Tab. 6.3.

Hepatitis A
- Pathogen: hepatitis A virus (HAV).
- Transmission: usually fecal-oral. Virus shedding 2–3 weeks after disease begins.
- Prenatal risk: probably only 3–4 weeks before and during labor, if at all.
- Protection: human gamma globulin.

Hepatitis B
- Pathogen: hepatitis B virus (HBV).
- Transmission: parenteral.
- Virus shedding: weeks to months after disease begins, in particular in HBe-antigen (HBeAg) carriers.
- Prenatal risk: second–third trimester via transplacental transmission, during delivery.
- Protection: hepatitis-B immune globulin (HBIG), hepatitis B vaccination.

Hepatitis C
- Pathogen: hepatitis C virus (HCV).
- Transmission: parenteral.
- Virus shedding: unknown.
- Prenatal risk: transplacental transmission.
- Protection: no prophylaxis.

Hepatitis D
- Pathogen: hepatitis D virus (HDV).
- Transmission: parenteral.
- Virus shedding: unknown.
- Prenatal risk: as for HBV and HCV.
- Protection: no prophylaxis.

Tab. 6.3: Differential diagnosis of liver disease in pregnancy.

Pregnancy-specific liver disease	Preeclampsia, HELLP syndrome (see p. 74) Acute fatty liver of pregnancy Cholestasis (see p. 73) Virus hepatitis A–G
Nonpregnancy-specific liver disease	Hepatitis with Epstein-Barr virus (EBV), cytomegalovirus, Herpes simplex virus, Coxsackie virus Autoimmune hepatitis (ANA, AMA, LKM and others) Wilson's disease Cholelithiasis

Hepatitis E
- Pathogen: hepatitis E virus (HEV).
- Transmission: mainly fecal-oral.
- Virus shedding: unknown.
- Prenatal risk: as yet undetected.

Hepatitis G
- Pathogen: hepatitis G virus (HGV).
- Transmission: probably parental.
- Virus shedding: unknown.
- Prenatal risk: as yet unknown.

Hepatitis B

Note. Hepatitis B is the most dangerous for the fetus because it is transmitted across the placenta and is the most common form of hepatitis in northern and central Europe.

Pathogenesis. The risk of infection for the newborn depends on the time of infection and maternal antibody production.
- Infection in the first 6 months of pregnancy, fetal infection 10 %.
- Infection in the last weeks of pregnancy and during labor, fetal/neonate infection 75–80 %.

Maternal anti-HBs and even more HBe cross the placenta and protect the fetus from hepatitis B infection or ensure a milder course of the disease.

Clinical manifestations. Usually asymptomatic! Development of chronic hepatitis is possible (see complications).

Diagnosis. Serodiagnosis (HBsAg) is recommended for all pregnant women after week 32.
- Liver enzymes (AST, PT, alkaline phosphatase), bilirubin.
- HBeAg.

Practice tip. Pregnant women with HBeAg are highly contagious with regards to the fetus!

Complications. Prolonged duration of disease progressing to cirrhosis: chronic persistent hepatitis (CPH), chronic active hepatitis (CAH). Specialist pediatric care (monitoring) is therefore strongly advisable in the first year of life.

Prevention of neonatal hepatitis
- Neonates of HBsAg seropositive mothers should be simultaneously treated with hepatitis B immune globulin and hepatitis B vaccination immediately (within 12 hours) after birth.
- Hepatitis B immune globulin (0.5 ml IM) directly after birth.
- Hepatitis B vaccination. Dosage 10 µl directly after birth, parallel to gamma globulin. Repeat administration in 4 weeks and 6 months, 10 µl each time.

6.3.6 Parvovirus B19

Definition. Erythema infectiosum, fifth disease; rare, not very contagious viral infection with typical skin rash (erythema).

Etiology, pathogenesis. Pathogen: parvovirus B19, parvovirus family (single-stranded DNA virus). Transmission is airborne or hand-to-mouth contact, or parenteral. After the viremic phase there is a temporary disruption in erythrocyte maturation (main target cell: erythropoietic stem cell). There is a marked tropism of erythroid precursor cells, which results in impairment of hematopoietic organs. Once synthesis of specific IgG and IgM antibodies has begun, these serological changes disappear. The infection is thus detectable in healthy people, but basically meaningless.

Epidemiology. 50 % contagion rate; incubation 6–14 days, contagiousness persists until rash appears; lifelong immunity is likely.

Clinical manifestations
- Butterfly-shaped facial rash (tense, itchy), also called “slapped cheek” syndrome. After 1–2 days, spread to the extensor sides of the extremities and buttocks, later flexor sides and trunk. The rash takes on a lace-like appearance, with a red edge and pale center.
- Pathognomonic is that the rash periodically pales and flares up again (duration 8 days)
- Swollen lymph glands, flu-like symptoms, polyarthralgia (in 10 % of children and 60 % of adults), stomach ache, acute gastroenteritis.
- Complications are more likely in the unborn child with low immunity.

Diagnosis
- Clinical manifestation (rash).
- Possibly thrombo-, neutro-, reticulocytopenia, anemia.
- Hb-level can drop markedly (3–4 g%).
- Serology (12 days after infection). IgM and IgG antibodies, (ELISA).
- Ultrasound diagnosis and Doppler sonography, if necessary AF and fetal blood sampling for virus – DNA.
- PCR assay.

Characteristics. 50 % of infections are asymptomatic (occult immunization). Patients with rash are no longer contagious.

Complications. Transplacental transfer to the fetus resulting in anemia, edema, nonimmune hydrops. Fetal symptoms develop 2–6 weeks after acute maternal infection. Risk of intrauterine death 1–2 %.

Treatment

- In prenatal infection with hydrops, cordocentesis, Hb level, and intrauterine transfusion.
- High-dose immune globulin can be indicated, especially if organs are affected.

Prevention. Pregnant women should avoid contact with infected persons, as far as possible.

6.3.7 AIDS, HIV seropositivity

Definition. Acquired immune deficiency syndrome; first described in 1981, viral infectious disease with lowered cellular immunity, recurrent infections with opportunistic pathogens, parasites, and potential for malignant tumors (Kaposi's sarcoma, malignant lymphoma).

Etiology. Pathogen is HIV-1 (human immunodeficiency virus) and, particularly in Africa, HIV-2; the virus is a retrovirus with marked polymorphism.

Transmission. The infection occurs primarily via sexual contact, or parenteral via blood contact (transfusions, injections). HIV has been detected in blood, seminal fluid, vaginal secretions, saliva, breast milk, and other body fluids such as ascites, joint fluids, cerebrospinal fluid, and lymphatic tissue.

Transmission via parenteral inoculation of body fluids, blood, and blood products containing the virus has been epidemiologically proven:

- Sexual intercourse.
- Injection/transfusion.
- Pre- or perinatal transmission.

The HIV virus is rapidly inactivated with standard disinfection methods.

Pathogenesis. HIV target cells are a subpopulation of T-lymphocytes, the T4 lymphocytes, $CD4^+$ helper cells, as well as cells of the monocyte macrophage or reticuloendothelial system (RES), mucosal Langerhans cells, dendritic lymphatic cells, and microglia. Macrophages are considered to be the HIV reservoir in the organism.

HIV causes reduced cellular immunity via cell destruction, autoimmune phenomena, and immune dysregulation. T4 lymphocytes are particularly affected.
The tropism of the virus explains the phase-like course of the infection (weeks, months up to many years). Serological changes such as those for infectious mononucleosis are detectable in a number of those infected with the virus directly after infection and then disappear. The subsequent latent phase can last up to 15 years!

Pre- and perinatal infection. Timing and path of maternal-fetal transmission have not been definitively clarified. It is certain that infection occurs in late pregnancy or during labor; contractions appear to increase virus transmission considerably. Preterm birth, chorioamnionitis, and membrane rupture present an increased risk of HIV infection.

In the 1980s, the risk of perinatal virus transmission was 30 % in developed countries. Since the introduction of preventative measures in pregnancy and for neonates it is lower <1 % now.

Diagnosis. HIV serology:

- HIV-antibodies (ELISA-test, suitable for screening).

- HIV-virus material (Western- or Immunoblot method).

Three laboratory categories are defined according to the number of $CD4^+$ cells: > 500/µl, 200–490/µl, and < 200/µl.

Viral load. The concentration of HIV-RNA is prognostically relevant for the course of the disease, treatment success and maternal-fetal transmission:
- < 10,000 genome copies/ml allows a more favorable prognosis.
- > 10,000 genome copies/ml, the risk of transmission increases proportionally to the viral load.

Prevention. Central to prevention of maternal-fetal virus transmission are:
- Antiretroviral therapy (ART) of pregnant HIV-1 positive women.
- Avoidance of contractions and cesarean delivery from a contraction-free uterus.
- Antiviral therapy of the neonate.
- Breastfeeding prohibition for HIV-1 positive mothers.

The majority of HIV-seropositive pregnant women belong to primary risk groups (e.g., drug addicts), some belong to secondary risk groups (partners of HIV-seropositive drug addicts or HIV-seropositive hemophiliacs), whereby some pregnant women are not aware of their HIV-seropositivity or HIV infection. In order to take preventative measures, **HIV antibody screening of all pregnant women is indicated.**

All pregnant women should be offered HIV-screening; blood taking and testing must only be performed with the woman's consent!

Obstetric care of pregnant HIV-positive women should take place in a center specializing in care of pregnant, laboring, and puerperal HIV-positive women and their babies and should involve:
- Monthly checks of
  - $CD4^+$ cell count;
  - Viral load;
  - Hb level.
- Wet mount microbiological culture in vaginal secretions.
- STD diagnosis: chlamydia, gonorrhea, trichomoniasis, syphilis.
- Screening for toxoplasmosis.
- Hepatitis serology.
- Cytological cervix swab, colposcopy and HPV high-risk-type-DNA test.
- Nuchal translucency between weeks 11 and 13.
- Malformation scan between weeks 20 and 22.

Invasive prenatal testing should be avoided! When making a decision regarding invasive diagnostic methods, viral load should be considered, and if necessary the procedure performed with concurrent antiretroviral prophylaxis.

Pregnant women not requiring treatment with ART, with no obstetrical risk factors and a viral load of < 10,000 copies/ml take zidovudine (ZDV) orally from week 32 (2 × 250 mg). A primary cesarean section is performed after completion of 36 weeks, with the aim of delivering the child in intact membranes. Directly before the operation, IV zidovudine is given (beginning 3 h before the operation, 2 mg/kg over 1 h, then 1 mg/kg). If the viral load directly before delivery is below the detectable level and there are no obstetrical contraindications, a vaginal delivery is possible without increased maternal-fetal risk of infection. Directly after delivery the neonate is given oral zidovudine (2 mg/kg every 6 h) for between 2 and 4 weeks. Pregnant women, with a viral load of > 10,000 copies/ml receive prenatal prophylaxis with a combination therapy (zidovudine + lamivudine + neviparine) from week 32.

Pregnant women with obstetrical risk factors receive an modified HIV-transmission prophylaxis: due to the risk of preterm delivery, prophylaxis should begin from week 29 in multifetal gestations. In cases of preterm labor and tocolytic therapy or ROM, an ART combination therapy should be initiated.

The ZDV prevention scheme is not suitable for pregnant women requiring ART; recommendations on adult HIV-treatment must be followed for the mother's treatment. Due to the relatively poor data available on the embryotoxicity of ART combination therapy, individual consultation with a specialized clinic is advisable.

It is important to note that the indication for this therapy is not only maternal. Mothers with a high viral load or low $CD4^+$ cell count have a higher rate of HIV transmission to the fetus hence the fetal indication for ART. The decision as to whether a maternally indicated therapy requirement can be interrupted in the first trimester because of embryotoxic side-effects must be made based on clinical, immunological and virological presentation of the mother.

6.3.8 Pregnancy and neonatal listeriosis

Definition. Listeriosis is a zoonosis (cattle, sheep, goats, pigs; poultry; rodents) and is transmitted from animals to humans.

Incidence. Serological testing of central Europeans indicates a high seroprevalence in the population (50–80 %). Incidence of the disease is affected by regional fluctuation, and the connection between listeriosis-infected pets and infected foods is controversial; on the whole it is rare.

Etiology. Pathogen is Listeria monocytogenes, a gram-positive rod bacteria.

Practice tip. Listeriosis is only of pathogenic relevance for pregnant women and newborns.

Clinical manifestations. Listeriosis in pregnancy: pain in the kidney region, urinary findings (as in pyelonephritis).

Neonatal listeriosis. The timepoint of the infection is critical:
- Early infection (early fetal, i.e., intrauterine during pregnancy) causes septicemia (granulomatosis infantiseptica): hypotonia, rejection of food, hepatosplenomegaly with hyperbilirubinemia (elevated levels of direct bilirubin), tendency to respiratory distress and fever. Changes in blood count and proteins are often not detected.
- Later infection (perinatal): pneumonia, meningitis.

Diagnosis. Leading diagnostic tool is detection of the pathogen in:
- Blood culture, maternal urine and lochia, ear canal of the baby, AF, meconium, secretions from nose and throat, cerebrospinal fluid, urine, granuloma.
- Repeated serological testing of the agglutinin titer of mother and child is only of use for diagnostic purposes. Listeriosis agglutinins do not cross the placenta to the fetus.

Treatment
- Ampicillin (for newborns 100–200 mg per kg body weight in 2 doses over 24 h). The sooner it is begun, the more effective it is.
- Gentamycin (4–5 mg/kg in 2 doses over 24 h) in serious, generalized disease in combination with ampicillin.

Prevention. Avoidance of contact with animals, unpasteurized milk, and raw meat (prevention of exposure).

6.3.9 Toxoplasmosis

Definition. Zoonosis (cattle, sheep, goats, pigs; poultry; rodents). Infection is asymptomatic, acute or chronic, and can occur pre- or postnatally.

Incidence, epidemiology. High, regionally varying, seroprevalence in adults of 50–80 %. Prevalence in Europe ranges from 30 % (England) to 50 % (Switzerland). The risk of infection with toxoplasmosis in pregnancy is 0.4–2.6 % in Europe.

Note. 1–3 neonates in 1,000 births have congenital toxoplasmosis in Europe, one of the commonest infectious fetal diseases (1–8 in 1,000 neonates).

Etiology, pathogenesis. The pathogen, Toxoplasma gondii, is transmitted from animals to humans. Very few toxoplasmosis infections become clinically manifest; most remain latent. Cats are host and source.

Toxoplasma gondii is an intracellular parasite that can be found as single organisms or groups of parasites, which can be found in parasitophorous vacuoles (pseudocysts) or in genuine cysts (encapsulated by a cyst-wall). It causes circumscribed local inflammations and necrosis with CNS affinity (cerebral form), in particular in the fetal period and in childhood.

Source of infection. Raw or undercooked meat (slaughtered animals, pets as intermediate hosts, cattle, sheep) with live toxoplasma cysts and oocysts from infected soil or unwashed vegetables; congenital, intrauterine infection of the fetus by the infected mother.

Transmission. Ingestion of cysts with raw or undercooked meat, oocyst infection with cat feces or prenatally (transplacentally) from the infected mother.

Prenatal toxoplasmosis (= congenital, nonnatal toxoplasmosis). Passage of toxoplasmas across the placenta occurs in 30 %; 90 % of transmissions take place at the end of pregnancy and 1 %, in the first weeks.
The severity of damage to the fetus is inverted: infections in the first trimester are serious, whereas those in the last trimester are mild and subclinical. The greatest danger for the child is when the mother undergoes the initial toxoplasmosis infection in pregnancy and develops parasitemia, which is a prerequisite for the prenatal form.
Previous maternal toxoplasmosis infections are not dangerous.

Clinical manifestation.

Prenatal toxoplasmosis. Triad of hydrocephalus, chorioretinitis and intracerebral calcification.

- Generalization (Dissemination ?) of the pathogen in liver, spleen, lymph nodes, lungs, and heart.
- CNS- and eye-invasion of the pathogen: with encephalitis, chorioretinitis, hydrocephalus, intracerebral calcifications, and further CNS damage, because the permanent forms (cysts) settle in the CNS and muscles (up to several thousand toxoplasmas).
- Generalized disease, active encephalitis to postencephalitic stage.
- Toxoplasma fetopathy (preterm or stillbirths).

Postnatal toxoplasmosis (incorrect name: “acquired toxoplasmosis”):
- Mostly asymptomatic in older children and adults (> 60 %).
- Milder course (30 %): fever, lymphadenitis.
- Serious symptoms (< 10 %) with encephalitis.
- No lasting damage.

Prevention, diagnosis, and treatment during pregnancy
1. Toxoplasmosis testing (toxoplasmosis-specific IgG and IgM antibodies, see below) of all women in early pregnancy (first trimester). Screening in pregnancy is advisable, usually only performed if acute

infection is suspected. Results of this test allow classification between

a) noninfected women without antibodies,
b) women with prior infection and continued presence of antibodies,
c) women with fresh toxoplasmosis infection.

Toxoplasmosis-specific antibody detection (Fig. 6.2) allows calculation of time of maternal infection and determines the fetal risk:

a) IgM antibodies are still detectable 1–2 years after the acute stage of the infection. Due to the long postinfection persistence of the IgM antibody titer, diagnosis of primary maternal infection is only possible if prior seronegativity is known.
b) IgA antibodies 6 months.
c) IgE antibodies 4 months.

Practice tip. A single titer diagnosis is insufficient, as IgM antibodies are detectable 2–3 years after infection. On the other hand, in AIDS patients, IgG titer is often low, and IgM titer is hardly ever detectable.

2. Seronegative women are at risk in pregnancy, and must avoid infection (primary prevention): Serology every 4–6 weeks (seroconversion permits exact dating of the infection).
3. Nutritional hygiene:
   a) Ingestion of well-cooked meat.
   b) Ingestion of well-cleaned and – cooked vegetables or salad.
   c) Regular disinfection of cat litter.
4. Women with IgG and IgM antibodies receive after a repeat test:
   a) Cordocentesis after week 22 and testing for IgM, IgA antibodies, platelets, further indicators of inflammation in fetal blood.

Practice tip. Diagnostic sensitivity in fetal blood is 60–70 %.

   b) AF removal via amniocentesis (after week 18, at the latest, however, 4 weeks after maternal infection): PCR positive, titer increase, antibody titer several times higher that of the mother's.

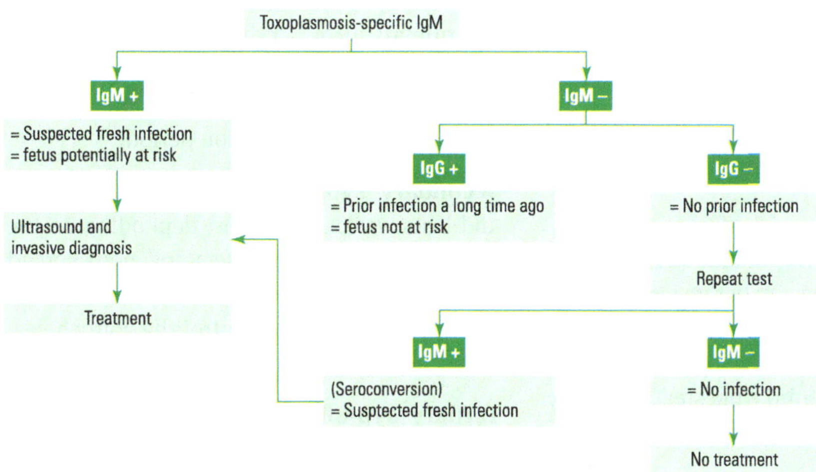

Fig. 6.2: Procedure if toxoplasmosis-specific IgM is detected.

c) A sensitivity of 90 % has been reached with the rDNA gene (Cazenave and colleagues, 1994).
d) Ultrasound diagnosis: if symmetrical ventricle enlargement or ventricular dilatations with cerebral calcifications are found (indication of an early infection!), the prognosis is extremely poor, and termination of the pregnancy appears indicated.

Treatment

- With seroconversion and fresh infection: spiramycin 2–3 g/24 h in 4 doses over 4 weeks, in particular in the first trimester.
- With fetal infection (from week 16) pyrimethamine (1 mg/kg in 24 h in 2 doses) + sulphadiazine (50–100 mg/kg in 24 h in 4 doses) combined over 3 weeks.
  - Repeat dose after at least 3 treatment-free weeks.
  - Supplemental folic acid (15 mg/day) and weekly blood count.

The results of prenatal treatment of toxoplasmosis infection in an unborn child are not encouraging. Thiebaut and colleagues found no significant reduction of clinical manifestations in 550 infected live births after prenatal therapy.

Prognosis. Severe brain disfunction with permanent defects (post-encephalitic damage); need for long-term care, depending on time of infection.

- Early infection. Low risk of transmission, usually resulting in spontaneous miscarriage if infection occurs before week 16. Embryopathies have not been observed. Severe consequences of fetopathy!
- Late infection (in third trimester). High risk of transmission, asymptomatic.

Prevention. No raw or undercooked meats; contact with cat feces is to be avoided; raw vegetables are to be washed thoroughly, and hands must be disinfected after garden work or other soil contact.

6.3.10 Syphilis

Definition. Lues, sexually transmitted disease caused by Treponema pallidum; congenital (Syphilis connata), or acquired (Syphilis acquisita).

Incidence. Two cases of registered disease in 100,000 inhabitants (2002). The real disease prevalence is calculated to be ten times this rate.

Epidemiology. Humans are the source of infection; transmission via sexual contact.

Pathogenesis. Pathogens penetrate microscopic lesions of skin or mucous membranes.

The early stages of syphilis consist of primary and secondary syphilis.

Primary syphilis. A lesion (chancre) develops after 5–21 (up to 90) days (incubation period) at the point of entry. The regional lymph nodes are involved. Primary lesion: rapidly disintegrating papular, coin-sized, indurated, painless primary ulcer (= primary syphilitic lesion). Most frequent location: Genitals, perioral. The activated immune system heals the primary lesion during the incubation period.

Secondary syphilis begins 3–6 weeks later and lasts weeks to months, depending on the systemic immunity. The hematogenous spread of the spirochetes causes a macular rash. If immunity is sufficient to control the spirochetes, it may be asymptomatic (latent syphilis).

Tertiary syphilis. After a latency period of 1–20 years in which the spirochetes survive in immunological niches (e.g., in CNS), about one third of untreated patients develop tertiary syphilis (gummatous syphilis, cardiovascular syphilis, neurosyphilis).

Congenital syphilis. Transplacental transmission from an infected or inadequately treated mother to the fetus. Fetal infection is possible at any time during pregnancy, most common however, after weeks 16–18.

Clinical manifestations

Acquired syphilis. Early syphilis. At the point of entry a rapidly disintegrating papule develops which becomes a coin-sized, indurated, painless ulcer: the primary syphilitic lesion.
Secondary syphilis. Nonpruritic, maculopapular rash, patchy, psoriasis-like rash on the soles of the feet and palms. Oozing, broad-based, proliferative, spirochete-rich perianal and perigenital papules; highly infectious condylomata lata and mucous membrane lesions; sore throat, hair loss, syphilitic leukoderma (in particular on the neck: Venus collar).

Congenital syphilis (Fig. 6.3). As in all prenatal infections, the clinical presentation depends upon the time of infection: the earlier, the more severe: early stillbirth in early syphilis of newborns and infants. Recurrent syphilis of the toddler, late syphilis of the schoolchild (lues connata tarda).

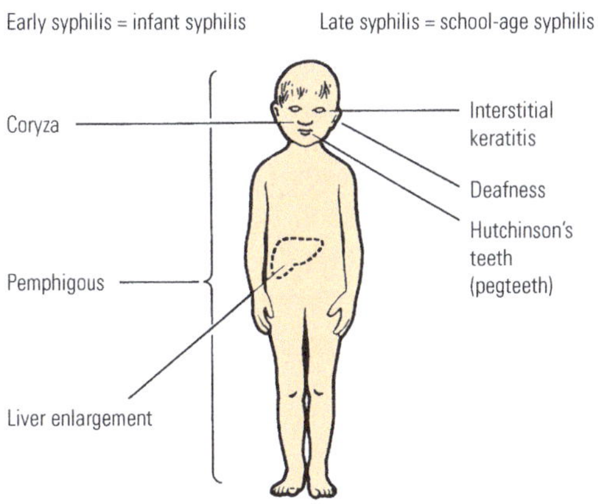

Fig. 6.3: The most common manifestations of congenital syphilis.

Early syphilis manifests in the neonatal period, more commonly in weeks 6–10.
The clinical manifestations are varied and can be classified into 4 grades of severity.

Asymptomatic. Most neonates have no clinical symptoms in the newborn period.

- Oligosymptomatic. Anemia, hepatosplenomegaly, skin changes (shiny skin) on palms and soles of feet.
- Marked (highly contagious) skin and mucosal condition with blisters (pemphigus syphiliticus).
- Visceral syphilis. Severe manifestation of internal organs: liver, skeleton, nose (coryza), CNS.

Main symptoms. Syphilitic rhinitis (coryza syphilitica; puss with bloody nasal discharge from affected nasal mucosa), pemphigus, hepatomegaly.

Late syphilis occurs in school age children, commonly between 6 and 14 years of age.

Note. Main symptoms are the Hutchinson triad: interstitial keratitis (IK; most common); deafness of the inner ear; Hutchinson's teeth (only on the two permanent, upper middle incisors → peg-shaped with crescent-like indentations).

Diagnosis. The diagnosis is to be made prenatally with history and serology: Treponema pallidum hemagglutination (TPHA) test on initial prenatal check-up.

Infection can also occur after the initial prenatal check-up.
- TPHA-test becomes reactive 3 weeks after infection. Principle: positive if macroscopically visible agglutination of the test

erythrocytes (treponemal) with the serum; sufficient for routine diagnosis
- FTA-Abs (fluorescent treponemal antibody absorption) test becomes reactive 2 weeks after infection. Principle: dead spirochetes are mixed with patient serum on a slide. If an antibody reaction occurs it is made microscopically visible by fluorescent antibodies.

Both tests have a high specificity and often remain reactive for life even after treatment. They detect not only venereal, but also non-venereal (Yaws, Bejel, Pinta) infections, so are only suitable for diagnosis of treponemal infections (care must be taken with pregnant women from endemic regions!) and not for evaluating treatment success.
- IgM FTA-Abs (immune globulin M fluorescent treponemal antibody absorption) test: provides information about the activity of the infection, about the need for treatment and assessment of therapy. Principle: detects treponema-specific IgM antibodies.
- If a primary lesion is suspected, direct microscopic detection of T. pallidum in the chancre, or smear test using dark-field microscopy and direct immune fluorescence possibly in addition to genome detection.

The serological results must be carefully evaluated:

TPHA	positive	Repeat test necessary
FTA-Abs	negative	
TPHA	negative	Most likely “old” healed syphilis (“serological scar”)
FTA-Abs	positive	
TPHA	positive	Possibly “old” healed syphilis (“serological scar”), Primary syphilis a possibility, therefore differential diagnosis using IgM-FTA-Abs test
FTA-Abs	positive	
TPHA	positive	Syphilis (all stages) requiring treatment
FTA-Abs	positive	
IgM-FTA-Abs	positive	

Treatment. Indication: history and clinical findings–laboratory detection of active syphilis and direct detection of spirochetes in darkfield examination.

Clemizole penicillin 1 million units IM daily over 14 days (if duration of infection < 1 year), over 21 days (if duration of infection > 1 year).

6.3.11 Gonorrhea

Definition. Infection caused by Neisseria gonorrhoeae affecting mucose and connective tissues of the genitals (purulent urethral and vaginal discharge) and extragenital regions (anorectal gonorrhea, pharyngeal gonorrhea, arthritis, endocarditis, meningitis, ophthalmoblenorrhea). In newborns, the eyes are primarily affected (gonococcal conjunctivitis, ophthalmia neonatorum).

Epidemiology. Most common sexually transmitted disease (STD). Peak age of infection in men 20–24 years, in women 15–19.

Infection. Perinatal: vertical transmission (newborns are usually infected during delivery if the mother has gonococcal cervicitis).

Etiology, pathogenesis. Pathogen: gonococci (Neisseria gonorrhoeae) have cell structures (pili, fimbriae, membrane proteins) with which they attach to nonciliated epithelial cells of mucose tissue; after phagocytosis, they manage to survive in the phagocytes.

Incubation period: 3 (2–7) days.
Purulent infection with copious exudate and polymorphonuclear leukocytes!

Contact infection of mucosal tissues of urethra, cervix, rectum, pharynx or conjunctiva, and in some cases the vagina with Neisseria gonorrhoeae.

Clinical manifestations

- Gonococcal conjunctivitis of the newborn. Purulent-bloody inflammation of the eye a few days after infection, with chemosis and swollen eyelids. Unlike other pathogens, ulceration of the cornea, necrolysis, and blindness can rapidly occur. In addition: bacteremia, scalp abscesses, vaginitis, arthritis, meningitis, endocarditis.
- Adults (with sexual contact). Primarily infection of the genital tract. Women frequently have vaginitis, inflammation of the internal genital organs (salpingitis, adnexitis, peritonitis). Youths/men: urethritis, epididymitis. In addition, depending on the point of entry, proctitis, pharyngitis, and conjunctivitis can occur. In systemic dissemination skin and joints are affected.

Diagnosis. Maternal history: discharge, dysuria, changing sexual partners in pregnancy.

- Swab and gram-staining (detection of intra- and extracellular gram-negative diplococci).
- Culture on chocolate agar in 5–10 % CO_2 atmosphere; culture immediately, as gonococci are sensitive to heat and dessication.

Characteristics. Ophthalmia neonatorum, or gonococcal conjunctivitis of the newborn, has become rare in developed countries due to regular prenatal checkups and Credé's prophylaxis method (see below).

Complications. Anorectal and pharyngeal gonorrhea with a small number of uncharacteristic symptoms: gonoblenorrhea, benign gonococcal septicemia, meningitis, arthritis (usually monoarthritis), endocarditis, skin lesions. In women, adhesion of the fallopian tubes causing sterility, Douglas abscess. In men, urethral stricture.

Treatment. Sexually transmitted disease requiring treatment.

- Uncomplicated. Single-dose treatment with ceftriaxone (250 mg IM), spectinomycin (2 g IM), or ciprofloxacin (500 mg orally).
- Pregnant women. Ceftriaxone (oral).
- Ophthalmia neonatorum. 7 day courses of either ceftriaxone (daily 25–50 mg/kg) or cefotaxime (twice daily 25 mg/kg).
- Gonococcal septicemia. 7 day courses of either ceftriaxone (1,000 mg/day IV) or spectinomycin (2 g twice daily), in addition to eye rinsing. Mother and her sexual partner must be treated.
- If pathogen persists, treat according to sensitivities.

Further action. Due to the worldwide increase in penicillinase-producing and tetracyclin-resistant neisserias, treatment with penicillin or tetracyclins should only be pursued if the infecting agent is sensitive to the antibiotic (antibiogram).

- No sexual intercourse until cure has been ascertained.
- Examination of and treatment (as required) of all sexual partners.
- Serology for syphilis (6 weeks after conclusion of treatment), and HIV infection (3 months after conclusion of treatment) is advisable due to possible concomitant infections.

Prevention. Credé's method. One drop of 1 % silver nitrate solution into the lower conjunctiva after delivery. We recommend continuation of this antiseptic preventative method, although its necessity is currently being argued.

Prognosis. Good cure rate dependent on early recognition and treatment. Poor if ophthalmia and corneal ulceration have already occurred.

6.3.12 Vaccination in pregnancy

Vaccinations are necessary! Pregnant women are more susceptible to infections than non-pregnant women, in particular to viral infections, which are promoted by the increased metabolism of the pregnant woman.

Vaccination specifics. Embryo and fetus, with their rapid tissue growth, offer an ideal breeding ground for viruses and other pathogens.. For this reason, vaccination with live vaccines (measles, mumps, rubella, yellow fever) is out of the question, particularly in the first trimester.

Practice tip. Vaccinations in pregnancy are to be limited to imperative indications (rabies) or unavoidable travel abroad (yellow fever, typhus; Tab. 6.4).

6.4 Malformations

A large number of congenital malformations (see also Chapter 13.9) can be detected prenatally with ultrasound. The diagnosis of fetal malformation as early as possible can have consequences such as invasive diagnosis, counseling of the parents as to the ramifications, prenatal consultations with neonatologists, pediatric cardiologists, pediatric surgeons, and other disciplines, choice of ideal birth location and method, planning of competent neonatal care, and discussion of the prognosis.

6.4.1 Hydrocephalus

Definition. Hydrocephalus ("water on the brain"), ventriculomegaly. 2 forms: external hydrocephalus (enlargement of the subarachnoid space: collection of fluid between the meninges; very rare) and internal hydrocephalus (enlargement of the ventricles).

Communicating hydrocephalus. External and internal hydrocephalus, continued connection between the ventricles and subarachnoid space.

Incidence. 0.5 % of all births (1 hydrocephalus in 2,000 births).

Tab. 6.4: Vaccinations in pregnancy.

Antiviral vaccines		Antibacterial vaccines	
Poliomyelitis (inactivated polio vaccine)	yes	Tetanus	yes (if possible, not in first trimester)
Rabies	not generally recommended	Diphtheria	not generally recommended
Yellow fever	not generally recommended	Typhus, paratyphus	not generally recommended
Measles	no	Cholera	no
Influenza	not generally recommended	Tuberculosis	no
Hepatitis A	not generally recommended, lack of clinical data	Meningococcus	yes, if at risk of infection in endemic areas
Hepatitis B	not generally recommended, lack of clinical data		
Western tick-borne encephalitis	not generally recommended		

Etiology. Aqueductal stenosis in 80 % of cases; neural-tube defects, intracerebral malformation, fetal brain hemorrhage, aneuploidy, intracranial tumor, infection (CMV, toxoplasmosis).

Pathogenesis. Result of disturbed CSF dynamics. Caused by: excessive CSF secretion due to inflammatory or toxic irritants, choroid plexus papilloma (CPP); disturbed resorption post-meningitis; obstruction of CSF flow: aqueductal stenosis or obstruction of the foramen of Monro (e.g malformation, tumor, inflammation).

Diagnosis. Based on palpation and ultrasound diagnosis.

Palpatory findings. Four characteristics (Fig. 6.4) on vaginal examination:
- Broad sutures and extremely wide fontanelles.
- Thin, yielding cranial bones.
- Rustling sensation on palpation of cranial bones .
- Abnormal mobility of the bone edges in the interval between contractions or (if the hydrocephalus is very large): sensation of an extremely full, fluctuating cyst.

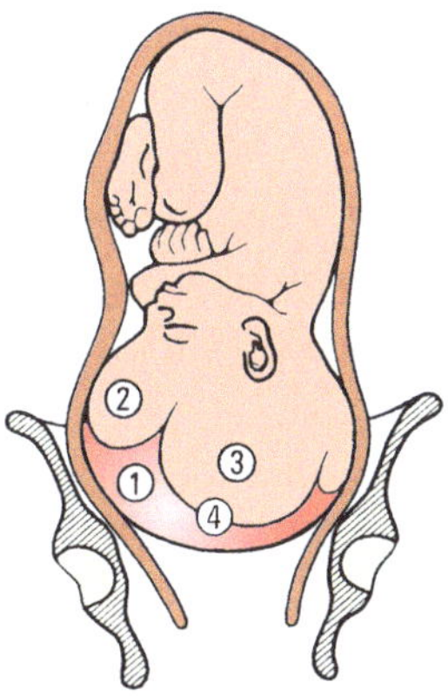

Fig. 6.4: Hydrocephalus: (1) widened sutures and fontanelles; (2) soft cranial bones; (3) rustling of the cranial bones; (4) mobile bone edges.

This sensation is particularly marked when the anterior fontanelle show in the cervix, although it is difficult to differentiate between anterior fontanelle and amniotic sac. If fetal death has occurred, the cranial bones are very thin and soft, and can be moved ("wobbled") back and forth.

Ultrasound diagnosis (see Fig. 3.42). Prenatal diagnosis is the goal through:
- Increase in BPD after week 20.
- Measurement of ventricle diameter, or ventricular/hemisphere ratio.
- In cases of ventricular enlargement, check for accompanying defects (e.g., spinal openings) and infections (see characteristics).

Characteristics. Hydrocephalus is also possible in microcephaly (normotensive), e.g., in connatal cytomegalovirus. The incidence of congenital hydrocephali not associated with spina bifida, is 0.5/1,000 live births; of these, 30 % have an aqueductal stenosis! 2 % of all hydrocephali (most with aqueductal stenosis) are inherited on the X-chromosome. Hydrocephalus also occurs in combination with spina bifida and Chiari malformations: displacement of parts of the cerebellum and medulla through the foramen magnum into the spinal canal, frequently with myelo-meningocele. In the Dandy–Walker syndrome (DWS), malformation of the cerebellar vermis causes cystic enlargement of the fourth ventricle with and without obstruction of the foramina of Lushka and Magendie; secondary hydrocephalus often results. Symptoms: increased intracranial pressure with bulging cranial sutures, possibly tetraplegia, and disorders of caudal cranial nerves.

Complications. Primarily caused by uterine overdistension: early ineffective labor; postpartum hemorrhage (PPH); uterine rupture.

Mechanism of labor

- Cephalic presentation (in about two thirds) – dangerous! The presenting hydrocephalus lies in the lower uterine segment in pregnancy and distends it. Uterine rupture threatens when contractions begin. As the head cannot budge in severe hydrocephalus, every contraction is futile when the hydrocephalus is presenting. In fact every contraction increases the stretching of the lower uterine segment and brings the laboring woman closer to a potential catastrophe.

Note. Hydrocephalus is extremely dangerous for the mother! Early diagnosis is particularly important in (hydro-)cephalic presentation because of the risk of uterine rupture in the first stage of labor.

- Breech presentation (one third). Delivery is uncomplicated until the shoulders have been delivered. The head remains stuck above the pelvic inlet and the distension of the lower uterine segment then begins in the last part of second stage. In contrast to cephalic presentation, the over-distension of the uterus does not begin until the trunk has been delivered, which means that the uterine content is much smaller.
- Transverse and oblique lie (rare).

A large or medium-sized hydrocephalus at term does not enter the pelvic inlet with strong contractions, or enters only partially. Characteristics are:

- Ineffective labor. Active labor does not develop over a number of days due to uterine overdistension.
- Painful contractions. If strong contractions do eventually begin, they are extremely painful.
- Distension of the lower uterine segment, no labor progress. At the same time, the abdomen is more or less sensitive to pressure above the symphysis. The lower uterine segment is extremely distended in both width and height over the hydrocephalus and labor does not progress, despite contractions. If cesarean section is not performed, rupture or septicemia will occur.
- Uterine rupture. The rupture occurs very suddenly, without the classical signs (silent rupture), also if the cervix is not fully dilated (in general: uterine rupture occurs only after complete cervical dilatation). Vertical and transverse tearing has been observed, which can be explained by the spherical swelling and distension of the lower uterine segment.
- The rupture may go unnoticed for some time because it occurred while the operator was unsuccessfully attempting manual delivery assistance.

Treatment

Mild hydrocephalus or sonographically detected **ventriculomegaly.** In these cases, the primary concern is not management of delivery, but rather the prognosis for the fetus.

- In late pregnancy delivery at term should be the goal in cases of:
  - moderate worsening of ventricular enlargement,
  - further malformations.
- Labor inducement should be considered if ventriculomegaly increases, so that vaginal delivery might be allowed and neurosurgical treatment expedited.

Practice tip. Antenatal cephalocentesis and drainage (shunt or screws) are not recommended because the results are disappointing.

Severe hydrocephalus. Severe and overt hydrocephalus mean that a vaginal birth is impossible because of cephalopelvic disproportion; despite contractions the head cannot enter the pelvic inlet. Result: extreme distension of the lower uterine segment, possible uterine rupture (relatively common) or septicemia (see labor progress).

Practice tip. Management is determined by the risk to the mother, prognosis for the newborn, and the parents' decision regarding the option of vaginal birth with removal of CSF during delivery if the prognosis is unfavorable.

Perforation of the skull (see p. 343) with the perforator (cervix should be at least 3 cm dilated).

With perforation the hindrance is removed, the mother is out of danger, and birth can proceed spontaneously.

Cranial perforation. If the cervix is not 3 cm dilated, the cranium is punctured with a long canula and CSF is withdrawn.

Transabdominal cephalocentesis for CSF removal is an exception.

Because the mother is typically exhausted from the long labor, when the cervix is fully dilated the fetus can be extracted: 1) by hand – it is simplest to extract the hydrocephalus which has collapsed to a limp sac with the hand by pulling on the bony parts; 2) with forceps – if the above is not possible, even with strong pressure from above, the head is grasped with forceps, Boer craniotomy forceps or a cranioclast; 3) in breech presentation the after-coming head is perforated through the interparietal bone or foramen magnum.

References

American College of Obstetricians and Gynecologists: Viral hepatitis in pregnancy. Educational bulletin 1998; 248

Centers for Disease Control: Rubella and congenital rubella syndrome – United States 1994–1997. MMWR 1997; 38:350

Demmler G: Congenital cytomegalovirus infection and disease. Adv Pediatr Infect Dis 1996; 11:135

Mari GC, Deter RL, Carpenter R, et al.: Noninvasive diagnosis by Doppler ultrasonography of fetal anemia due to maternal alloimmunization. N Engl J Med 2000; 342:9

Montoya JG, Liesenfeld O: Toxoplasmosis. Lancet 2004; 363:1965

Nigro G, Adler SP, La Torre R, Best AM, Congenital Cytornegalovirus Collaborating Group: Passive immunization duiing pregnancy for congenital cytomegalovirus infection. N Engı J Med 2005; 353:1350

Thiebaut R, et al.: Effecıiveness of prenatal treatment for congenital toxoplasmosis: a meta-analysis of individual patients' data. Lancer 2007; 369:115

WHO: Syphilis. Guidelines for the management of sexually transmitted infections. 2001; 38

7 Normal labor

7.1 Birth factors

Note. Birth is influenced by three main factors: fetus, birth route, and the force of labor (contractions).

7.1.1 Fetus

The **mature** (term) fetus is 48–52 cm long, weighs 3,000–3,500 g, and has large and small parts:
- large parts are head, back, buttocks;
- small parts are legs and arms (limbs, extremities).

Note. The head plays the most important role in the mechanism of labor; it is the largest and hardest part of the fetus and is the presenting part in 94 of 100 births (p. 25).

Head. The head fills the pelvis, apart for a small gap; the head/pelvis (cephalopelvic) proportions determine the course of labor.

Head diameter, planes, circumferences (Fig. 7.1, Tab. 7.1) are signs of maturity (see p. 199), and also criteria relevant to the mechanism of labor, in order to understand the birth process in normal and abnormal cephalic presentations.

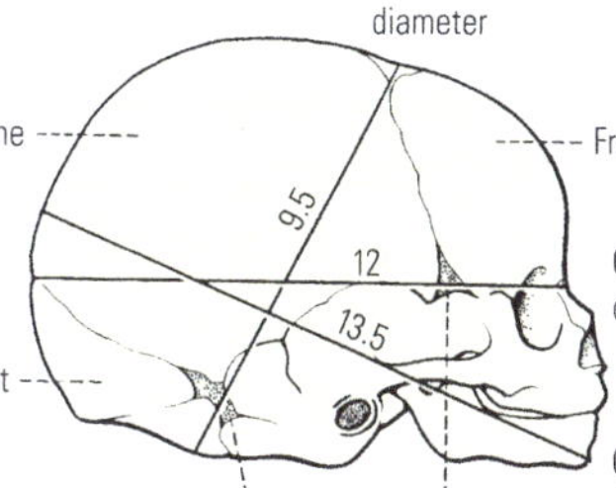

Fig. 7.1: Three longitudinal diameters of the skull (measured with the pelvimeter): 1) suboccipitobregmatic (→ 9.5 cm); 2) occipitofrontal (→ 12 cm); 3) occipitomental (→ 13.5 cm).

Cranial sutures are (Fig. 7.6):
- Sagittal suture, between the parietal bones.
- Lamboid suture, between parietal and occipital bones.
- Coronal suture, between frontal and parietal bones.
- Frontal suture, between frontal bones.

Fontanelles (Fig. 7.6). Two spaces between the bones of the fetal skull:
- Anterior fontanelle (greater, bregmatic or frontal fontanelle; Fig. 7.7). Diamond-shaped; juncture of 4 sutures: sagittal, frontal, and both branches of the coronal suture.

Tab. 7.1: Head, longitudinal diameters, planes, circumferences.

Diameter	Length	Plane	Circumference
Suboccipitobregmatic[1](see Fig. 7.1; from neck to the middle of the anterior fontanelle)	9.5 cm	Suboccipitobregmatical	32 cm (see Fig. 7.2)
Occipitofrontal (Fig. 7.1; from glabella to the furthermost point of the occipital bone)	12 cm	Occipitofrontal	34 cm (see Fig. 7.3)
Occipitomental (Fig. 7.1; from chin to the furthermost point of the occipital bone)	13.5	Occipitomental	35 cm (see Fig. 7.4)

[1]bregma = sinciput.

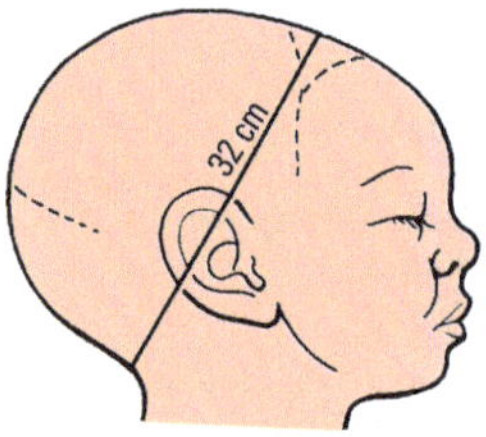

Fig. 7.2: Suboccipitobregmatic circumference (32 cm).

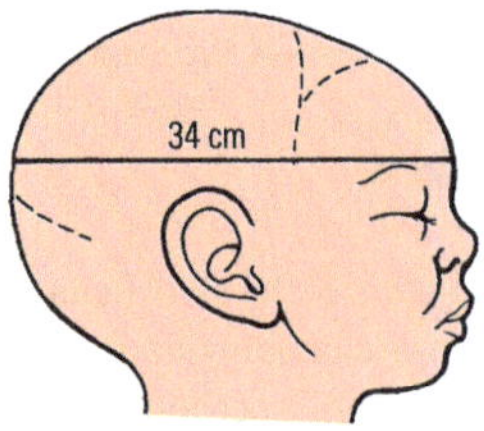

Fig. 7.3: Occipitofrontal circumference (34 cm).

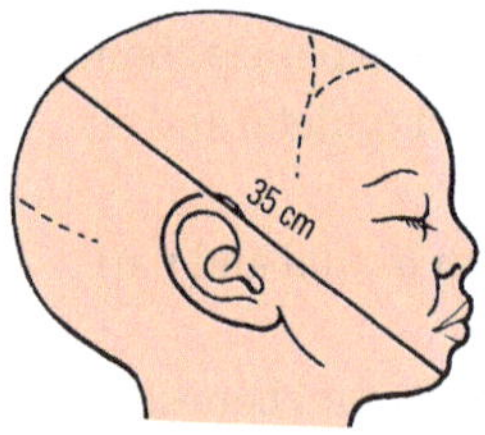

Fig. 7.4: Occipitomental circumference (35 cm).

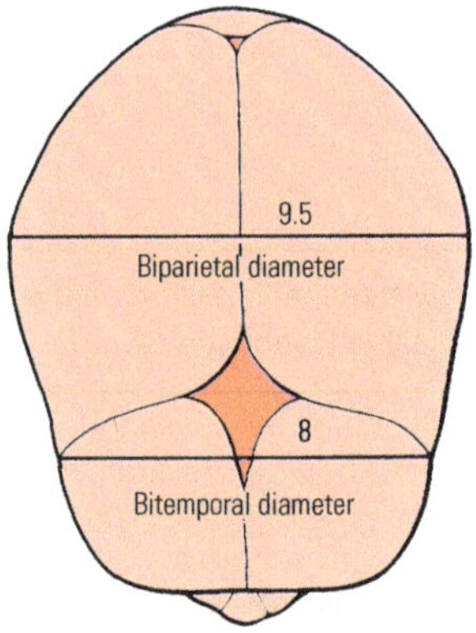

Fig. 7.5: Transverse diameters of the head: 1) biparietal diameter (9.5 cm); 2) bitemporal (8.0 cm).

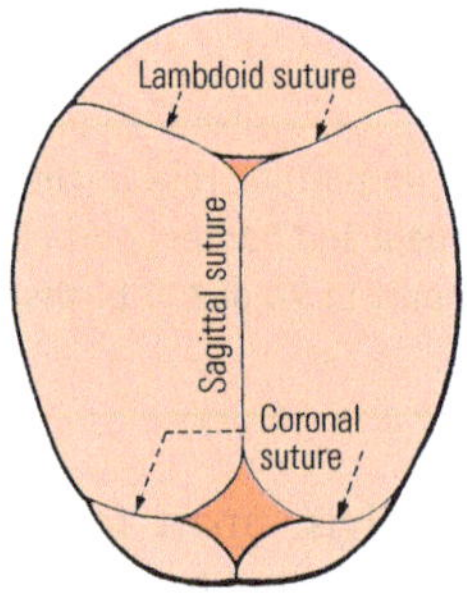

Fig. 7.6: Cranial sutures, posterior (lesser), anterior (greater) fontanelles.

- Posterior fontanelle (lesser or occipital fontanelle; Fig. 7.8). Three-pointed; juncture of 3 sutures: sagittal and both branches of the lamboid suture.

Finding. A fontanelle can be palpated when the cervix is slightly dilated.

Differential diagnosis:
- Anterior fontanelle (Fig. 7.7). This is the juncture of 4 sutures. This is not an infallible method for finding the fontanelle, or rather for differentiating it from the posterior fontanelle. We recommend the following method: follow the course of the sagittal suture (see Fig. 7.7) until a fontanelle is reached. If the fontanelle is crossed in the same direction (continuation of the sagittal suture) and another suture is reached, this can only be the frontal suture and the palpated fontanelle the anterior fontanelle.
- Posterior fontanelle (Fig. 7.8). If the continuation of the sagittal suture over the fontanelle does not lead to another suture, it is the posterior fontanelle.

Trunk measurements
- Shoulder width (bisacromial diameter): longest transverse diameter of the shoulders 12 cm.
- Shoulder circumference: 35 cm.

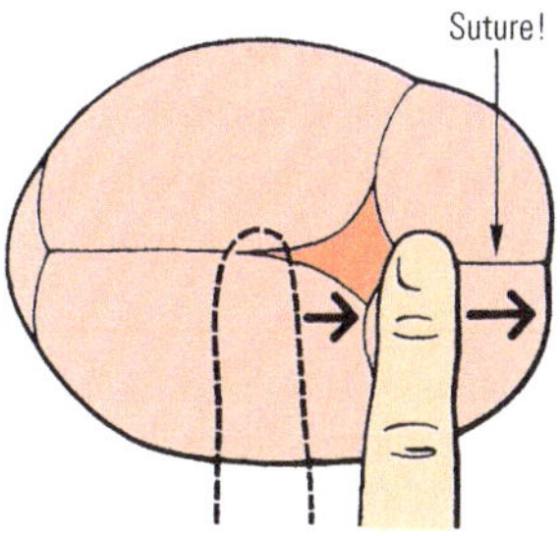

Fig. 7.7: Palpation of the anterior fontanelle. Following the sagittal suture and crossing over the fontanelle, another suture is reached, the frontal suture.

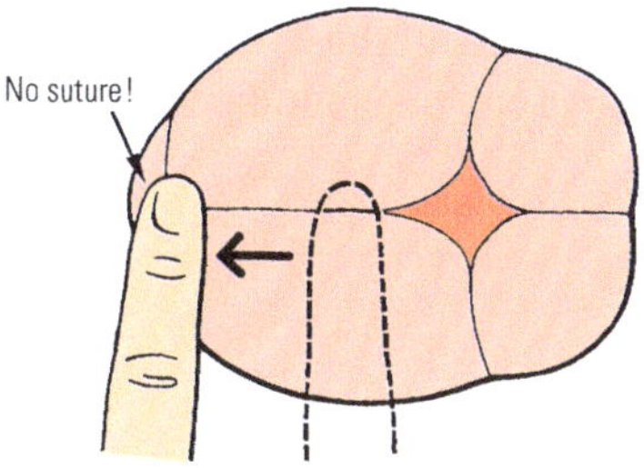

Fig. 7.8: Palpation of the posterior fontanelle. This can only be the posterior fontanelle, because when the sagittal suture is followed across the fontanelle, no further suture is palpable.

- Hip width: longest transverse diameter of the hips 10–11 cm.
- Hip circumference: 25 cm.

7.1.2 Birth route

Definition. The birth route is the birth canal, a bone-connective tissue canal: the bony canal is made up of the bony pelvis (bony walls of the true pelvis). The soft tissue canal is made up of the lower uterine segment, cervix, vagina, vulva, pelvic floor.

Bony canal

Definition. The bony walls of the true or lesser pelvis are the scaffolding or frame of the birth canal. The bony canal determines the shape,

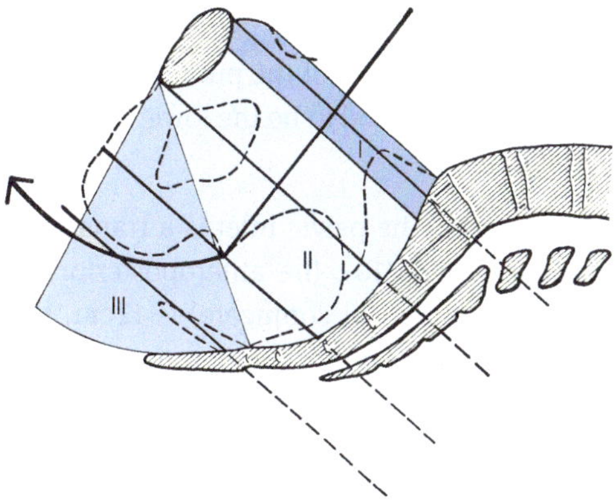

Fig. 7.9: Three planes of the pelvis: I) pelvic inlet, II) midpelvis, III) pelvic outlet.

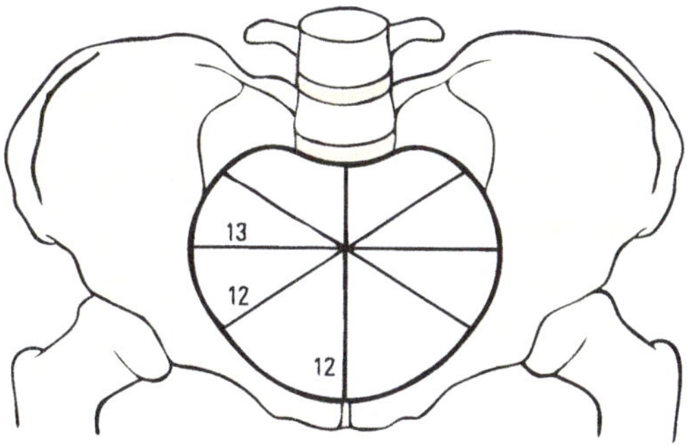

Fig. 7.10: Transverse oval pelvic inlet.

width, and direction of the birth route and reinforces the soft tissue canal.

Pelvic inlet (Fig. 7.9, 10). The obstetrically relevant structures in the uppermost part of the birth canal are:
- Sacral promontory.
- The innermost point of the pubic symphysis.
- Transverse, anteroposterior and oblique diameters of the pelvic inlet.

Boundaries. Two parallel planes bound the pelvic inlet:
- Upper pelvic inlet plane from the pubic tubercles to the sacral promontory.
- Lower pelvic inlet plane through the Linea terminalis (→ terminal plane; Fig. 7.9).

- The parallel plane which passes through the innermost point of the pubic symphysis is often understood to be the lower pelvic inlet plane.

Measurements. The pelvic inlet is a transverse oval shape (Fig. 7.10); the anteroposterior diameter (→ anatomical conjugate) is 12 cm, the transverse diameter (in the terminal plane) 13 cm. Both oblique diameters are 12 cm long.

Note. The longest diameter is the transverse diameter.

Directional terms in obstetrics (Fig. 7.11). Typical beginners' mistakes result from referring to the woman in a supine position (in examination or birthing position) instead of in an upright position: front is confused with up, back with down:
- front (ventral/anterior) → towards the pubic symphysis,
- back (caudal/posterior) → towards the tailbone or sacral promontory,
- up → cranial, towards the head,
- down → towards, the feet.

Obstetrical conjugate: 12 cm. The diameter of the pelvic inlet is an orientation guide. It is the line connecting the sacral promontory with the innermost point of the pubic symphysis (Fig. 7.13), the conjugata vera.

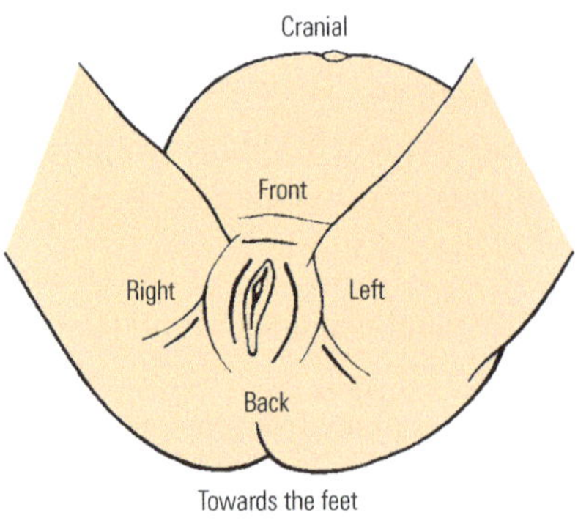

Fig. 7.11: Directional terms in obstetrics.

Left and right oblique diameters (Fig. 7.12). When looking at the pelvis from below, from the perspective gained on internal examination, two oblique diameters are determined.

Practice tip. Left oblique diameter (LOD) runs from left anterior to right posterior, the right oblique diameter (ROD) runs from right anterior to left posterior (Fig. 7.12).

Pelvic cavity = midpelvis (Fig. 7.13). Once the presenting part has passed through the pelvic inlet, it enters the pelvic cavity, which makes up the largest part of the space enclosed by the bony walls of the cavity of the true pelvis. It is the shape of a large cup or a round pot.

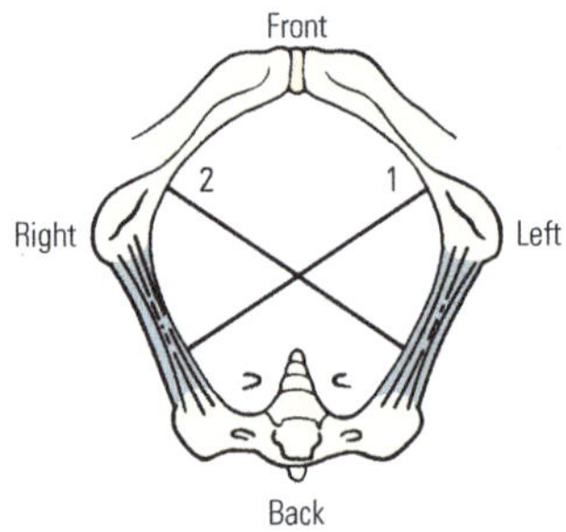

Fig. 7.12: Oblique pelvic diameters (as seen from below).

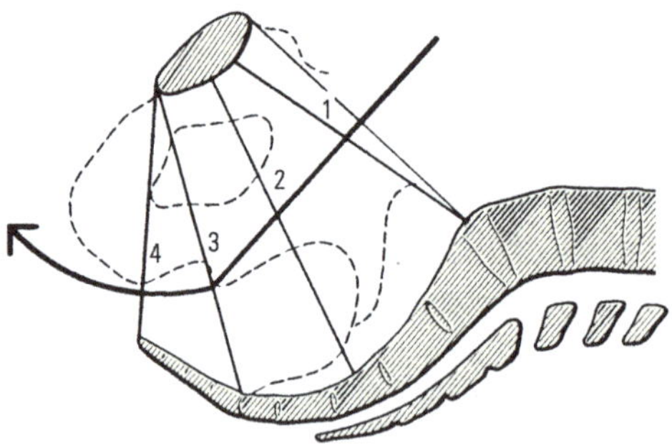

Fig. 7.13: Classical pelvic plane system (median sagittal section through the pelvis) with 4 anteroposterior diameters: 1) plane of pelvic inlet; 2) pelvic plane of greatest dimensions; 3) pelvic plane of least dimensions; 4) plane of pelvic outlet.

Division according to the classical plane system of pelvic planes: plane of the pelvic inlet (superior strait), pelvic plane of greatest dimensions, pelvic plane of least dimensions, plane of the pelvic outlet (inferior strait)

The pelvic plane of greatest dimensions is bounded

- anteriorly from the middle of the surface of the pubic symphysis,
- posteriorly through the middle of the third sacral vertebra (deepest point of the sacral cavity),
- laterally through the posterior surface of the acetabula (socket of the hip joint).

On this plane, the pelvic cavity is almost round, anteroposterior, and transverse diameters are both 13 cm.

The pelvic plane of least dimensions is bounded

- anteriorly from the lower edge of the pubic symphysis,
- posteriorly through the tip of the tailbone (articulus sacrococcygeus),
- laterally through the ischial spines.

Anteroposterior diameter 12 cm, transverse (interspinous) diameter 11.5 cm (distance between the ischial spines, spinae ischiadicae).

Pelvic outlet (Fig. 7.14). Oval shape, consisting of two semicircular planes, almost vertically on top of one another.

Tab. 7.2: Anteroposterior (AP) and transverse diameters of the bony birth canal.

Plane of the birth canal	Anteroposterior diameter	Transverse diameter
Pelvic inlet	**12 cm**	13 cm
Plane of greatest dimensions	13 cm	13 cm
Plane of least dimensions	12 cm	**11.5 cm**
Pelvic outlet	9.5 (to 11.5)	12 cm

The anterior semicircle is bounded by: the ischial tuberosities, the pubic arch and the middle of the pubis.

The posterior semicircle has the same base: the ischial tuberosities; laterally it is bordered by the sacrotuberous ligaments and posteriorly the tip of the tailbone.

The anteroposterior diameter (distance between tailbone tip and midline of the pubic symphysis) is 9.5 cm. As the tailbone can be bent backwards, this diameter can be lengthened by 2 cm. Transverse diameter (distance between the ischial tuberosities): 12 cm.

Practice tip. The following characterizations are widespread (Tab. 7.2): pelvic inlet (PI), midpelvis, (pelvic cavity), and pelvic outlet (PO).

The pelvic axis (Fig. 7.13) is the line connecting the midpoints of the classical planes (see above). This axis of the birth canal runs in a straight line through the pelvic inlet and midpelvis, then curves anteriorly towards the pubis (→ curve of the birth canal, or curve of Carus).

Soft tissue canal

Definition. Soft birth canal or soft tissue canal, made up of two interconnected cylinders: the long inner cylinder, and short outer cylinder.

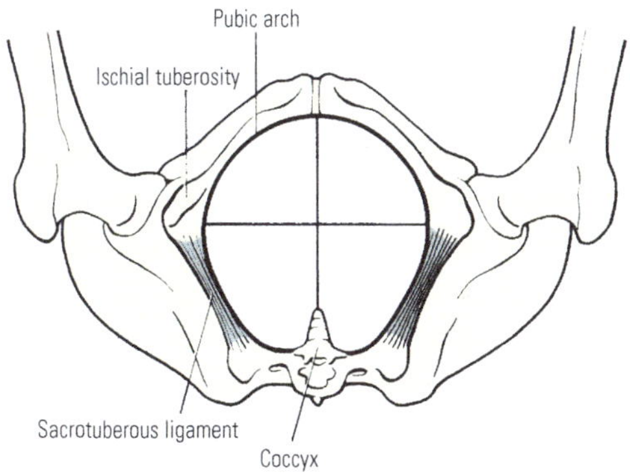

Fig. 7.14: Pelvic outlet showing both diameters.

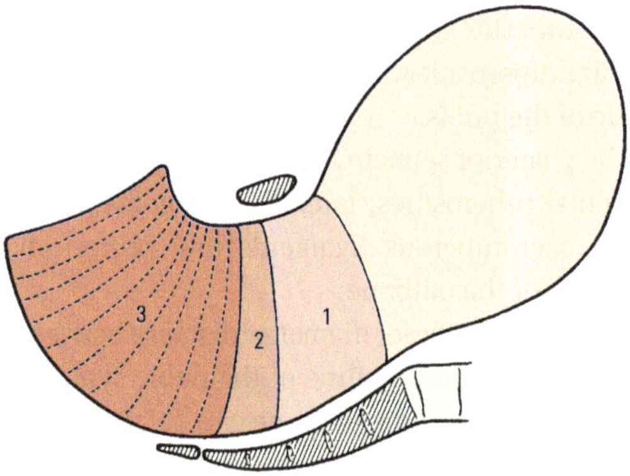

Fig. 7.15: Fully extended inner soft tissue canal at the end of second stage, internal view: 1) lower uterine segment; 2) cervical canal; 3) soft tissue canal extension (vagina and vulva).

The **inner cylinder** (Fig. 7.15) is made up of the lower uterine segment, cervix, vagina, and vulva. Fig. 7.15 shows it after cervical dilatation and extension of the vagina and vulva, as it occurs at the end of second stage.
The outer cylinder is made up of the pelvic floor.

Pelvic floor (Fig. 7.16). At rest (not during labor), flat, roof-tile-like interwoven muscle-fascia system 4 cm thick, which is stretched/extended in second stage to a 15 cm long cylinder.

The pelvic floor is the muscular closure of the pelvic outlet by (from inner to outer layer): pelvic diaphragm (M. levator ani and M. coccygeus), the urogenital diaphragm (M. transversus perinei profundus and superficialis, Lig. Transversum perinei), which – from caudal – lies in front of the gap between the muscles of the levator ani, which urethra, anal and genital canals pass through.

Details:
Pelvic diaphragm. Broad sheet of muscles, mainly composed of M. levator ani, and its two parts (Pars pubica and Pars iliaca).
Levator funnel. The levator ani muscle is arranged like a steep funnel-shaped sloping layer (→levator funnel), its role in rotation of the head is discussed on p. 157.
Hiatus urogenitalis. An opening towards the pelvic outlet is created by the two medial arms of the levator ani, a longitudinal soft tissue gap, the vulvo-vaginal opening, which is anteriorly hemmed in by the urogenital diaphragm, the second muscle layer of the pelvic floor.

Urogenital diaphragm. The transverse perineal muscle, embedded in the anterior part of the pubic arch, forms the base. It contains outlets for urethra (M. sphincter urethrae) and vagina.

The plate is supported by: M. sphincter urethrae, Lig. transversum perinei, and the Fascia

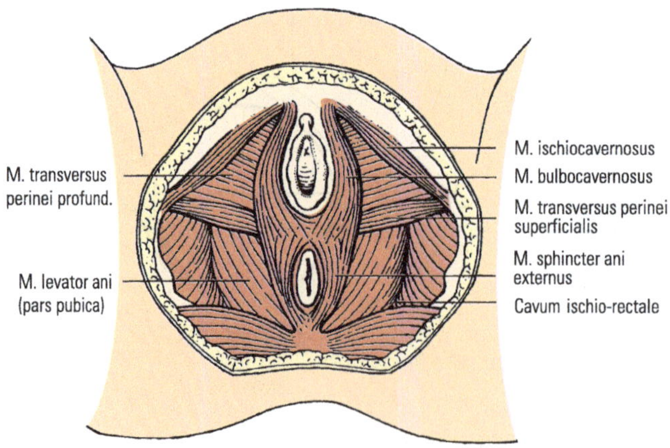

Fig. 7.16: Pelvic floor (not in labor). In labor the pelvic floor is extended to become the outer canal, see Fig. 7.17.

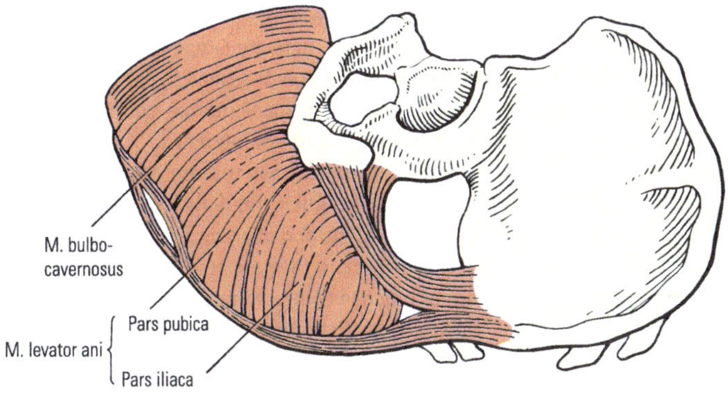

Fig. 7.17: Extended outer canal of the birth route, external view (after Sellheim).

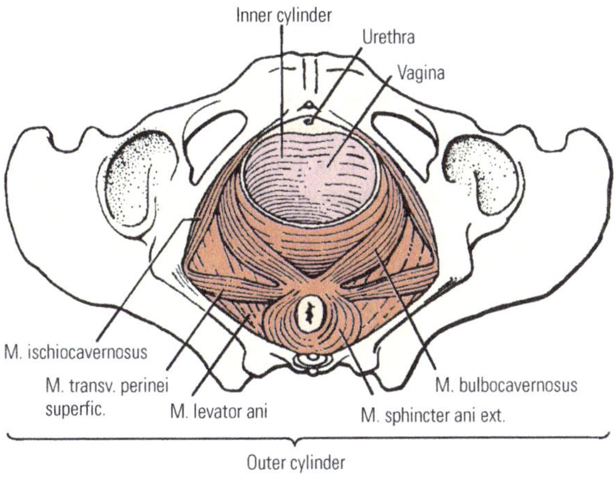

Fig. 7.18: End part of the extended soft tissue canal with both soft tissue canals telescoped over one another (after Jaschke).

diaphragmatis urogenitalis superior et inferior which covers it.

Outer layer (sphincter layer). Main components are two strong muscles: M. bulbocavernosus (sive bulbospongiosus: outlet opening of the outer cylinder) and M. sphincter ani; strengthened by two weaker muscles: M. transversus perinei superficialis and M. ischiocavernosus.

Function of the pelvic floor in labor. The flat pelvic floor layer is extended and telescoped in the second stage by the pressure from the head. The muscle layers, which were initially stacked on top of one another like roof tiles, lie edge to edge at the end of second stage. The anal sphincter muscle is stretched wide, so that the anus gapes when the fetal head extends the last part of the soft tissue canal (Fig. 7.17).

It must be clear that the soft tissue projection of the outer cylinder surrounds the last part of the inner cylinder, i.e., the vaginal part, because the outer cylinder does not begin until the pelvic floor; the outer cylinder is telescoped over the end part of the inner cylinder (Fig. 7.18). *Length.* The curved anterior wall extends from 3 to 5 cm, the posterior wall lengthens from 4 to 15 cm.

7.1.3 Force of labor, contractions

Definition. Expulsive forces or contractions, which only the corpus uteri (body of the uterus) is capable of producing.

Palpation. Contractions are assessed by placing a hand on the laboring woman's abdomen.

As the uterus hardens the following are felt: 1) onset and increase of the force of contraction (stadium incrementi); 2) climax of the contraction (acme, peak); 3) gradual abatement (stadium decrementi). At the beginning of the contraction the uterus rights itself and brings itself and its contents into the axis of the birth canal.

Characteristics of contractions. The following terms describe the forces of birth: strength, length and frequency of contractions, and the length of the interval between contractions.

Strength of contractions is judged at the bedside using hand contact.

Length of contractions and the **interval** between them are timed with watch in hand.

- Contraction length varies between 20–30–40–50–60 s and more; contractions < 20 s are short, > 45 s are long.
- Pauses vary greatly. In first stage they last 10 min and more, shorten gradually to 6 and 5 min, sometimes even to 3 min.

Contraction frequency is the number of contractions per time unit, e.g., per hour; expressed indirectly by information about the length of the interval.

Monitoring. Alongside palpatory assessment, an abdominal sensor (external tocometer) is available.

Types of contractions. There are 6 types of contractions.

1. 2 types of pregnancy contractions (Fig. 7.19):
   - Alvarez-waves are local uterine contractions of high frequency and low intensity.
   - Braxton Hicks contractions are tetaniform contractions at irregular intervals. They occur more frequently at the end of pregnancy. Depending on when they occur, they are also known as false labor or practice contractions (prelabor).
   - False labor. Pregnancy contractions which are more or less marked on "lightening", 3–4 weeks before the EDD.
   - Practice contractions/prelabor. Irregular contractions in the last weeks of pregnancy, occur quite often prenatally, 1–2 contractions/10min, intrauterine pressure (IUP) 40mmHg.
   - Engaging contractions. The practice contractions act as engaging contractions by engaging the head in primigravidae.
2. Active labor. Regular contractions bring about cervical dilatation. Initially 2–3 contractions in 30 min are registered, later 2–3 in 10 min, with a pressure of 40–50 mmHg.
3. Second stage contractions. The contractions in second stage have a frequency of 4/10 min and an IUP of 60 mmHg.
4. Expulsion contractions. The expulsion contractions at the end of second stage are far stronger than second stage contractions (IUP 200 mmHG).
5. Third stage contractions. Contractions of the uterus to bring about separation and expulsion of the placenta.
6. Afterpains. Contractions of the uterus to support uterine involution.

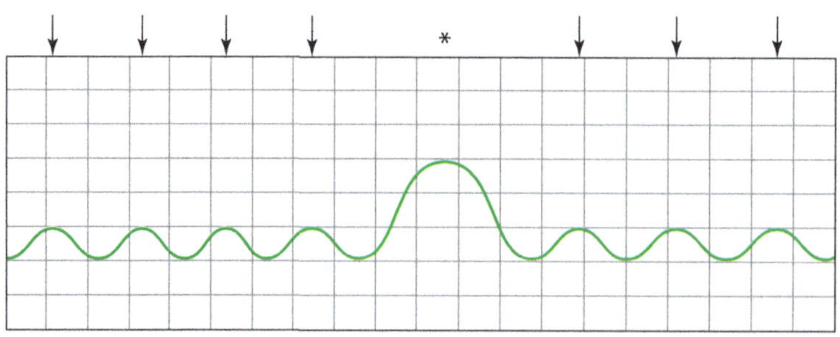

Fig. 7.19: External tocograph with both types of pregnancy contractions, Alvarez waves (arrows), Braxton Hicks contraction (asterix).

Uterine baseline tone. The intraamniotic pressure at rest, or IUP in the interval between contractions (baseline tone) increases from 6 to 12 mmHg during labor.

It is measured by a pressure-monitoring device and filled intrauterine catheter (→ internal tocometry).

Uterine function in labor. When labor commences, the uterus shows a functional bisection with a contractile ring.

- The upper, active segment is the corpus uteri, strong, contractile, and performing the work of contractions.
- The lower, passive segment, lower uterine segment, and cervix uteri (parts of the birth passage) is stretched (Fig. 7.20).
- These parts have nothing to do with the creation of contractions. They yield in every corpus uteri contraction, stretching and widening by transforming their tissues (cavernous transformation, increase of elastic fibers, swelling) in order to allow the entry and passage of the pressurized uterine contents.
- Retraction ring. The border between the upper and lower segments of the uterus is a physiological retraction ring (Bandl's ring) between the lower passive segment (lower uterine segment + cervix uteri) and the corpus uteri.

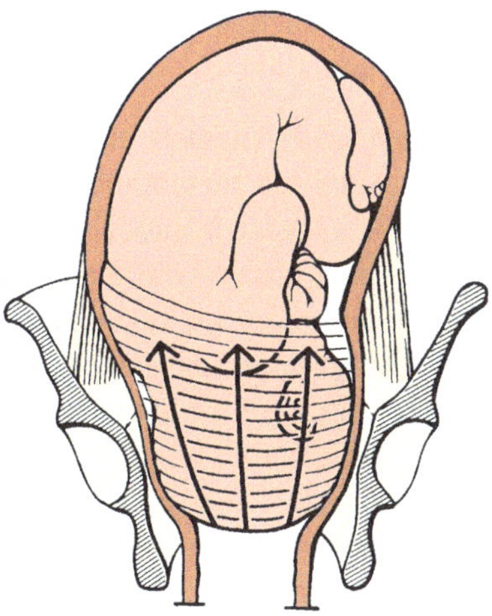

Fig. 7.20: Upper active and lower passive sections of the uterus (functional bisection of the uterus in labor).

Genesis of contractions. 1) Contraction. The muscles of the corpus contract, the muscle wall thickens. 2) Retraction (tightening). 3) Distraction. This causes a pull on the thinner lower uterine segment (and on the cervix); it is stretched and drawn out.

Contraction and retraction of the body of the uterus and distraction of the lower uterine segment have two effects:

- The cervical canal is opened as it is drawn up (mechanism I of the opening of the birth canal).
- The contents of the uterus (AF, fetus, placenta) are forced downwards by the pressure.

Internal pressure increase. Contraction and retraction of the corpus uteri reduce the size of the space enclosed by the corpus and increase the internal pressure.
If the body of the uterus were freely mobile, it would have to retract upwards over its contents, the fetus, at every internal pressure increase upon contracting and retracting and the fetus would not descend. The body of the uterus is held in place by an anchoring system, which cannot retract upwards. The increase in internal pressure affects the fetus as pressure, an expulsive contractile force driving it downwards in the direction of the place of least resistance (Sellheim), the internal os of the cervical canal.

- The uterine anchoring system which makes upwards retraction of the uterus over the fetus impossible is composed of 3 structures.
- Ligamentous. The round ligament of the uterus (ligamentum teres uteri).
- Attachment (Martin) Retinaculum uteri. Parametrial ligamentous attachment of the

cardinal ligaments, a tissue containing collagen and elastic-muscular fibers. The thin uterosacral ligaments does not play a role.
- Support (pelvic floor; see p. 146).

Amniotic sac, presenting fetal part. The first part to present is the amniotic sac with the forewaters. It is forced into the cervical canal, which is expanding according to mechanism I (upwards pull), when the uterine contents are expelled, and followed (after membrane rupture) by the presenting part of the fetus.
Result. Radial expansion/widening of the cervical canal from inside (mechanism II of the opening of the cervical canal) until it is wide enough for the head to pass through, which supports mechanism I.

Note. The (leading) head has the strongest expanding effect. The amniotic sac has a negligible widening effect.

When head or breech expand the cervical canal after premature or early ROM, it becomes clear that their effect is much stronger than that of the amniotic sac.
The anchoring system (see above) hinders the body of the uterus from retracting upwards. The attachment part of this anchoring system (see above), is set up so that it brings about descent of the uterus, draws it into the pelvis during the opening of the cervical canal. The muscular fibers of the parametrial ligamentous attachment are not only attached to the cervix, but spiral around the cervical canal and are thus interfused with wall of the cervical uterus on both sides.

7.2 Mechanism of labor

The trigger for labor is largely unexplained; a number of working hypotheses are in discussion. Induction of contractions mediates the interaction of intrauterine maturation of the fetus, hormonal and mechanical-neural factors. Directly before labor begins there is a rise in myometrial sensitivity to prostaglandins and oxytocin (accompanied by an increase in concentration of oxytocin receptors). In addition, it appears that the number of oxytocin receptors which stimulate prostaglandin synthesis in the decidua also multiplies. Furthermore, it is known that the fetal pituitary gland increasingly secretes oxytocin before labor begins. Moreover, the stress hormones cortisol and corticotropin-releasing hormone (CRH) play an important, contraction-triggering role.
It is possible that the maturation of the interaction between fetal hypothalamus and fetal pituitary gland is a signal for labor to begin, and if so, the fetus itself would initiate labor.

Hormonal factors. In this complex event particular significance should be afforded to estrogens in the triggering of contractions. Their increased activity leads to increased production of estrogen receptors and gap junctions. There are doubts today as to whether prenatal progesterone withdrawal should be attributed much importance in triggering labor. The local progesterone reduction in the decidua, however, appears important for prostaglandin synthesis.

The increased synthesis of prostaglandins in the decidua and membranes plays a critical role. This increase in production is explained by local progesterone withdrawal, immunological and noninfectious inflammatory reactions, in particular in response to bacterial irritation and the release of mediators such as Interleukin-1, Interleukin-6, Interleukin-8, and tumor-necrosis-factor (TNF). In addition, Interleukin-1 brings about the migration of leukocytes into the cervix, where the collagenase-protease effect is increased, which results in structural changes to cervical tissue.

Mechanical-neural factors. It has long been known that stress, e.g., shock, can trigger labor, probably via the neural-hormonal path. It has also long been known that stimulation of sensitive nerve-endings at the level of the internal cervical os can trigger or strengthen contractions. These nerve-endings lead to the paracervical (Frankenhäuser) ganglia in the uterovaginal plexus.

Uterovaginal plexus. Autonomic nerve plexus in the parametrium with fibers from the inferior hypogastric plexus, and innumberable ganglia; innervates uterus, vagina, Fallopian tubes, ovaries. Sympathetic and parasympathetic ganglia (Frankenhäuser ganglia) are spread over the lateral circumference of the cervix uteri in the parametrium. They appear to influence contractions in labor.

7.2.1 Signs, onset of labor, preparation for labor

Signs. The seven **signs of labor** are indications that labor is about to commence:

1. Lightening. 3–4 weeks before EDD, the fundus uteri, which had reached the height of the ribs at the end of week 36, drops markedly to the same height as at the end of week 32.
2. Pelvic engagement of the head in primigravidae. In the last 3–4 weeks, the head gives up its relaxed attitude and takes on a strongly flexed one (first rotation) and descends, occiput leading, into the pelvis.
3. Prelabor. Irregular tightening of the uterus in the last days, usually painless.
4. Repositioning of the longitudinal axis of the cervix in the direction of the axis of the birth passage.
5. Cervical ripening. The cervix becomes softer, flexible and suppler in the last weeks of pregnancy, it ripens. Experience has shown that the uterus is prepared for contractions when in addition, upon vaginal examination, the cervix is partially or completely effaced and dilated so that
   a) in nulliparae one finger may easily be inserted,
   b) in multiparous women two fingers may be inserted.
6. Appearance of blood. Discharge of bloody mucus from the vagina, expulsion of the cervical mucus plug. The blood comes from decidual vessels which were broken as the lower uterine segment stretched and the membranes attached to it detached.
7. Pressure on the bladder in the last weeks of pregnancy (and in labor) is explained by the proximity of the engaged and maximally flexed head to the bladder.

Signs of impending labor. Signs that labor is soon to commence are:

1. General appearance. Occasionally palpitations, headaches, general restlessness, rush of blood to the head, flushing, pain due to pressure on nerves (most commonly along the ischial nerve – N. ischidiacus – also in the true pelvis). Recurring backache, weight loss in the last days (see p. 33).
2. Gastrointestinal tract. Vomiting, diarrhea, loss of appetite, wind from pressure on the rectum.
3. Sexual organs. Increased vaginal discharge, feeling of fullness in the vulvar region.
4. Fetal movements are generally reduced shortly before birth, which the mother notices and reports if questioned.

Onset of labor

Labor has begun when at least 2 signs of active labor are present:

1. Regular contractions every 10 min over at least 30 min. The beginner must not confuse these with prelabor!

Practice tip. Prelabor can sometimes be so strong and persistent that these contractions are confused with active labor. They then abate and resume days later, stronger, to become active labor.

Vaginal examination reveals whether active labor has already commenced:
Nulliparae: cervix is partially or completely effaced, and dilated to the extent that at least the tip of a finger can be inserted (the cervix is usually further dilated when fully effaced).
Multiparae: cervix partially effaced and dilated so that 2 fingers can be inserted.

2. Membrane rupture, AF loss.

Practice tip. As soon as the membranes rupture, the woman is in labor, whether or not she has contractions.

Sometimes the membranes rupture and regular contractions take days, even weeks, to set in.

3. Mucus or appearance of blood: expulsion of the cervical mucus plug.

Preparation for labor. The midwife prepares the laboring woman for birth. A cleansing enema is offered to empty the bowels and stimulate contractions, or a bath or shower for relaxation and stimulation of contractions.
Shortening or shaving of pubic hair on admission is no longer routine.

7.2.2 History taking, examination, spontaneous vaginal delivery

Information about the birth situation must be gained as quickly as possible through history taking and examination.

Bedside history-taking during labor

First main question: Name, age, parity (see p. 19).

Second main question: Progress so far?

That is: amniotic sac? Temperature? At term? Contractions? Where is the head? Cervical dilatation? Auscultation or EFM?

Amniotic sac

- Have the membranes ruptured? Did the AF gush out? How much?
- If the membranes have ruptured: when (exactly) did this occur? How many hours have passed since then?
- Litmus test. If it is not clear whether or not membranes have ruptured, litmus paper is inserted into a pad which is placed in front of the vulva. After 30–60 minutes it will go blue if ROM has occurred.

Temperature

- The risk of infection begins once ROM has occurred. The longer the uterus is open, the greater the danger. With membrane rupture, the barrier between the germ-containing vagina and the germ-free uterine cavity is broken. Germs from the vagina ascend!

Is the laboring woman at term? Calculation see p. 20.
Contractions. When did regular contractions begin? Duration of labor (number of hours) so far (duration of labor see p. 208)?

Practice tip. Alongside PROM, prolonged labor is the primary cause of fever intrapartum.

Did the contractions weaken temporarily? How frequent are they? Are they strong? Do they last long? How long are the intervals between contractions?
Where (at what station) is the head (breech)?
Cervical dilatation?
How is the FHR or the cardiotocogram?

Third main question. Prior births?

- Ask multiparae: number of previous births? Age? Live or still births? Number of miscarriages and preterm births?
- Method of delivery – spontaneous or operative birth(s). If operative, forceps? Cesarean?
- Duration of labor? Spontaneous labor begin? Was labor augmented?
- Third stage. Blood loss? Was manual delivery of the placenta necessary?
- Puerperal period. Fever, bleeding, mastitis?
- Babies' birth weights.
- When was the last birth?
- Are the children still alive? Are they healthy?

External and internal examination during labor

Always wash hands and forearms beforehand with soap, warm water, and brush.

Practice tip. Always begin examination in the interval between contractions. The external examination can only be performed during this interval; the internal is continued during the contraction. It is more apparent during a contraction whether the membranes are still intact or have already ruptured, and how far the presenting part descends in the contraction.

External examination. Begin with the external inspection (see p. 23), followed by the external and internal examinations (see p. 31).

Practice tip. The four birth factors are evaluated in succession (ground rule of obstetrics!): 1) fetus, 2) pelvis, 3) contractions, 4) cervix. The sum of the factors (→ fetal head→ pelvis→ contractions→ cervical dilatation) has priority over individual factors! The possibility of spontaneous vaginal delivery (SVD) is tested in this way.

How labor will progress depends on to which degree the four main factors fetus, pelvis, contractions, and cervical dilatation deviate from the norm.

Fetus. The first main factor encompasses all obstetrical characteristics of the fetus: fundal height (see p. 23), fetal lie size (see p. 26), presenting part, and size of presenting part.
In addition:
Attitude (see p. 26), and presentation (see p. 26).
Station (see p. 162), and moldability see below.
Fetal condition (see p. 167).

Broad and hard skulls are not very flexible. The same is true for a skull in which the parietal bones are so close together that the sagittal suture cannot be palpated. These parietal bones will not be able to overlap to ease the passage of the head in to the pelvis.
Yielding skull bones and a narrow head adapt to the shape of the pelvis more easily if there are enough strong contractions to perform the remodeling work on the head.
The first main factor, the fetus, can be marginally influenced. In particular the size of the (living) fetus is an unchangeable factor. However, anomalies of position and presentation of the head can often be improved by positioning.

Pelvis. The second main factor can also be minimally influenced.

Operations to extend the bony birth canal, such as symphysiotomy, are hardly ever performed any more.
The main factor pelvis can be bypassed by abdominal delivery (cesarean section).
If the pelvis is narrow, the pelvic measurements are taken (particularly the external conjugate, see p. 31), and the vagina is explored in an attempt to reach the sacral promontory.
The soft tissue canal plays an almost equally important role to that of the bony birth canal (pelvis), in particular in its readiness to open up under the pressure of the advancing head.

Contractions. The third main factor can be influenced. The birth attendant can
- strengthen the contractions with physical measures and medicinal augmentation,

- reduce contractions with medication (p. 278),
- control the direction of the contractions by positioning (p. 184) and by directing the pressure of the contractions on to the fetal part which is to descend and lead.

Contractions are evaluated via abdominal palpation, and while doing so, the length of contractions and intervals are timed. Strength and length of contractions and the intervals are moreover registered with cardiotocography, p. 168.

Cervix. The fourth main factor is the external (Ostium uteri) and internal (Orificium internum canalis isthmi) os of the cervix.

Dilatation of the cervical canal and openings is often difficult because these tissues are too rigid or spastic. Oxytocic agents will not help in such cases, only spasmolytic agents. Incisions are only to be made in exceptional circumstances.

Note. Spontaneous vaginal delivery (SVD) is always desirable: if it happens naturally it works best! There are six conditions for spontaneous delivery: 1–3) the fetal head must not be too large, it must be easily configurable, and in a favorable presentation; 4) the pelvis must not be too narrow; 5) the contractions must be good (strong, regular); 6) the cervix must dilate quickly.

Internal examination. Neither the extent of cervical dilatation nor the leading presenting part can be adequately determined with external examination alone. Refined obstetrical diagnosis is based on the internal examination!

Vaginal examination. A routine examination in labor. Begin always in the interval between contractions. See below.

Technique. Examination in bed or on the gynecological chair.

Hand disinfection. Wash hands with soap and a scrubbing brush (clean nails!) for 3 min under running water. Surgical hand disinfection is not necessary. Sterile gloves should be worn. The labia are spread widely with one hand and the vaginal passage extended so that index and middle finger of the second hand do not touch the introitus and lower part of the vagina on insertion, to avoid introduction of bacteria from that area.

Arguments against examination: ascension of bacteria. Pathogenic bacteria from the vulva and vaginal passage are introduced to the germ-free part of the birth canal. In addition, foreign bacteria can be introduced into the birth canal.

Empirically it is known that bacterial ascension or the introduction of foreign bacteria plays a minimal role as long as aseptic conditions are maintained.
Examination is performed in the following order:

1. **Cervix**
   a) Dimensions? Condition: thick or partially effaced, sharp-edged, soft or rigid.
   b) Degree of cervical effacement? If unefaced: length, shape and consistency of the cervix? Cervical position: anterior, mid-position or posterior?

Practice tip. Diagnostic tool: Pressure on the cervical lip is painful; pressure on the presenting part is not.

---

2. **Amniotic sac**
   a) Intact?
   b) Ruptured? Wait for a contraction! The forebag tautens during a contraction and it is much easier to feel whether membranes are still intact.

Practice tip. Diagnostic tool: evidence that membranes have ruptured are edematous swelling (caput succedaneum) and skull configuration. If the presenting part is pushed upwards, amniotic fluid will flow if membranes have ruptured.

3. **Presenting part 4 questions: What? Where? How? Rotation?**
   a) Which part is presenting (head, breech, foot, shoulder, arm, hand)?
   b) Where is the presenting part? At what level: engaged in pelvic inlet, midpelvis, pelvic outlet, station in relation to the ischial spines (p. 164)? Subtract caput succedaneum (p. 166)!
   c) Main question: has the head passed through the terminal plane with its longest diameter (engaged; see p. 164).
   d) Position and presentation? Direction of the sagittal suture (facial line, frontal suture, hip diameter), position of the fontanelles? Resulting in which position and attitude?
4. **Pelvis**
   a) Is the sacral cavity empty or filled?
   b) Peculiarities of the pelvis. Is the sacral promontory reachable? Prominent/Inward-pointing tailbone? Prominent ischial spines? Particularly firm ligaments? Rigid soft tissues?

Palpatory findings

Cervix
- Cervix (almost) uneffaced: 2–3 cm.
- Cervix partially or 50 % effaced.
- Cervix completely or 100 % effaced.

External os (primigravidae)
- Cervix undilated.
- Cervix dilated to allow insertion of fingertip, thick.
- Cervix dilated to allow insertion of one finger.
- Cervix 2 cm dilated.
- Cervix 3, 6, 8 cm dilated.
- Cervical lip only palpable.
- Cervix no longer palpable, fully dilated; 10–12 cm.

The external os is already wide at the beginning of labor in multiparae.
The completely dilated external os is palpable in
- nulliparae as thin, sharp-edged and circular;
- multiparae as thick and often irregularly shaped.

Ultrasound examination
In addition to the external and internal examination during labor, transabdominal ultrasound should be performed, especially if findings are unclear. In this way, attitude and rotation of the head can also be followed. Further important information can be gleaned about the position of the fetal back by finding the fetal spine. Translabial ultrasound diagnosis can also be used – particularly in stage 2 – to determine fetal station.

Note. Intrapartal ultrasound is one of the most important diagnostic methods for following the progress of labor today. The large amount of information it can provide is rarely utilized.

7.2.3 Passage of the head through the birth canal

Note. Criteria for the behavior of the head are: 1) entering the pelvic inlet; 2) passage through the pelvic cavity; 3) exit through the pelvic outlet; 4) external rotation of the head.

1. Entering the pelvic inlet. Mechanism of entry (Fig. 7.23–7.25). The head enters the pelvic inlet with the sagittal suture transverse or slightly oblique (see Fig. 7.25).

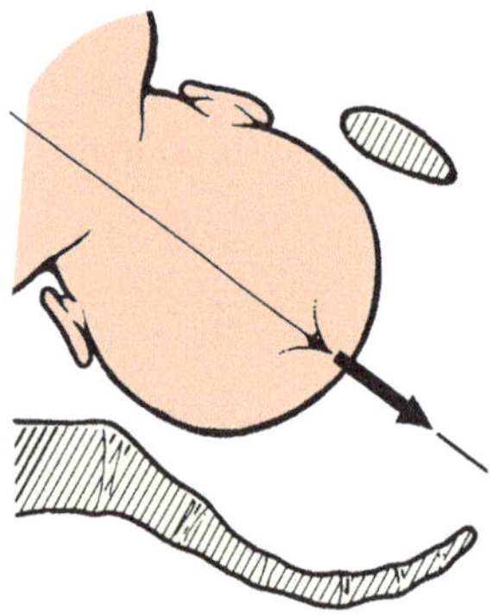

Fig. 7.21: Synclitic, axial alignment of the head in the pelvic inlet.

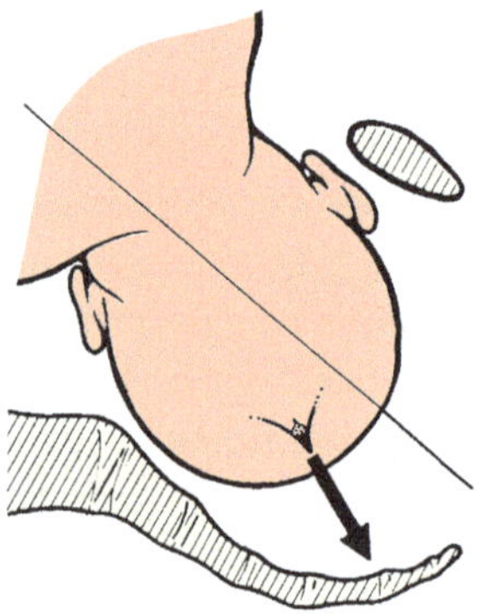

Fig. 7.22: Physiological anterior asynclitism, Naegele obliquity.

Figs. 7.23 to 7.25: Mechanism of entry, head enters the pelvic inlet (PI). The head enters the pelvic inlet in a transverse or slightly left oblique position. The sagittal suture is correspondingly positioned. The attitude of the head is still relaxed. The head is at this station, position and attitude by the last weeks of pregnancy in the majority of primiparae.

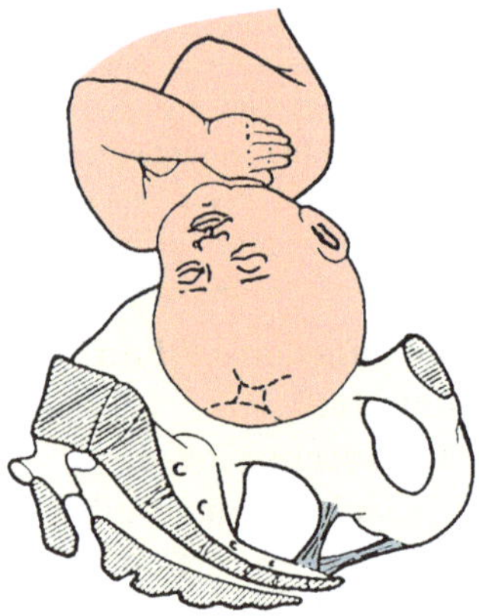

Fig. 7.23: From the side.

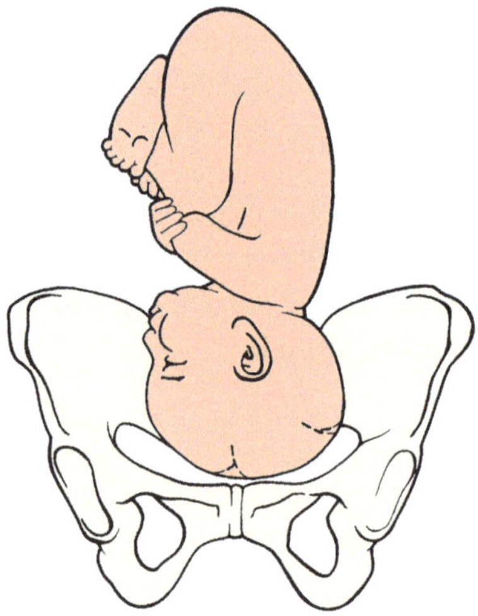

Fig. 7.24: From the front.

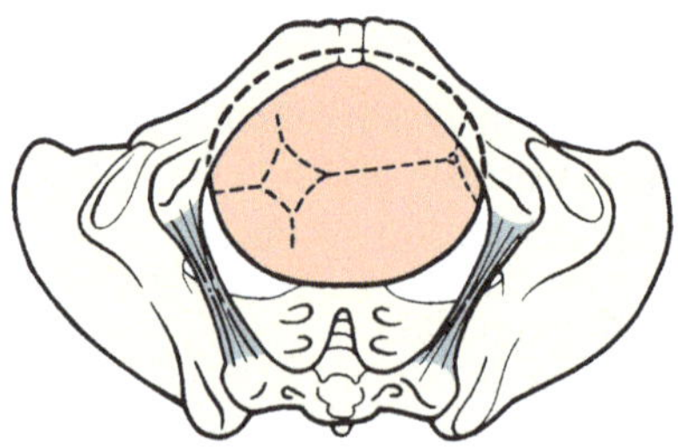

Fig. 7.25: Seen from below.

Reason. The head presents in each level of the pelvis in the way in which it best fits → Gauss' principle of least constraint. The pelvic inlet is oval; the transverse section of the fetal head is also oval. An oval object fits best through an oval opening by aligning both long and short diameters (principle of alignment as an expression of the principle of least constraint). The bones of the pelvic inlet force the head into a transverse position by their shape.

The attitude of the head is not under any pressure in the pelvic inlet: it is unconstrained, and it is neither flexed nor markedly extended (Fig. 7.24).

Synclitism (Fig. 7.21). Axial alignment of the fetal head; the sagittal suture of the partially or completely engaged fetal head lies in the transverse pelvic diameter, in alignment with the transverse axis of the pelvis.

Anterior asynclitism (Naegele's obliquity; Fig. 7.22). The head often presents with the sagittal suture unaligned with the axis of the birth canal, asynclitic and usually angled towards the sacrum.

This presentation is known as physiological anterior asynclitism, because the anterior parietal bone leads.
As there is no occipitoposterior presentation in the pelvic inlet, occipitoposterior positions are considered; only cephalic or vertex presentations are described.
The position in the pelvic inlet with transverse sagittal suture is taken on by the head in
- nulliparae in the last weeks of pregnancy,
- multiparae at onset of labor

Definitions for position, attitude, and presentation, see p. 26.

2. Passage through the pelvic cavity. Mechanism of passage (Fig. 7.26 to 7.28). The pelvic cavity is a pot-shaped space. The base is the pelvic floor, goal, and end of this passage. The pot is 8 cm deep from pelvic inlet (PI) to pelvic floor/outlet (PO); this is the distance which the head must cover on its passage through the pelvis.

The head must descend in order to cover the distance between PI and PO. It flexes in order to fit better into the space of the round pelvic cavity. In the PO, in order to achieve the most suitable starting position for negotiating the next level, the longitudinal PO, the descending head must rotate (90°), whereby the neck moves anteriorly towards the pubic symphysis.

Note. 3 movements of the head occur during the mechanism of passage:
- Descent (change in station).
- Flexion (change in attitude).
- Rotation (change in position).

Descent. The three movements are not performed successively; descent, flexion, and rotation occur concurrently: the head makes a twisting movement in the pelvic cavity.

Flexion. The occiput takes the lead; the posterior fontanelle is centered in the pelvic axis and becomes the lowermost point of the presenting part.

Occipitoanterior presentation. In this way, the occipitoanterior presentation has been created. The functional plane of the head during the passage is the suboccipitobregmatic plane, which has the smallest circumference (32 cm), and is thus the most favorable plane (it is almost circular). The anterior rotation of the neck means that the sagittal suture rotates from a transverse to an anteroposterior diameter in
- OA (see Fig. 7.28) from left occipitotransverse (LOT) over LOA to the anteroposterior diameter;
- Or from right occipitotransverse (ROT) over ROA to the anteroposterior diameter (OA).

Reason for the movement. The cross-section of the pot-shaped pelvic cavity is circular. Following the principle of least constraint, in which the head adapts to the form dictated by the birth canal, it must adapt to the round cross-section. This is achieved by adopting a flexed attitude, to the extent required for the longitudinal axis of the head to descend into

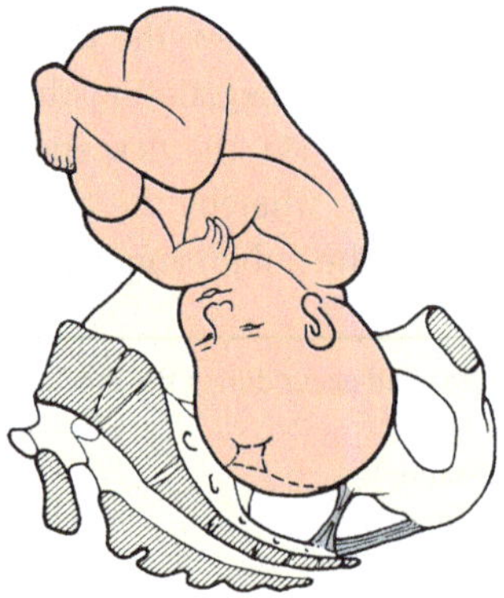

Fig. 7.26: From the side.

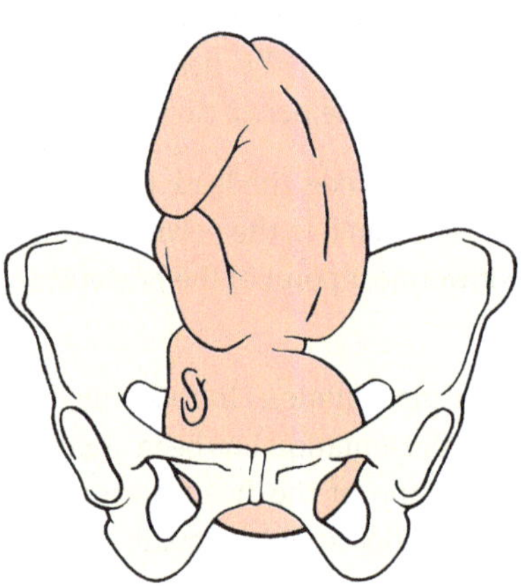

Fig. 7.27: From the front.

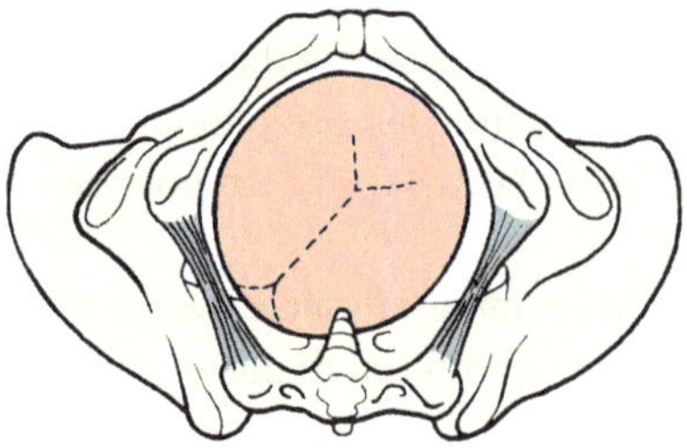

Fig. 7.28: Seen from below.

Figs. 7.26 to 7.28: Mechanism of passage, passage of the head through the pelvic cavity. The head has passed through the pelvic inlet with its largest diameter and is firmly engaged in the PI. The three (rotating) movements which the head makes simultaneously on traversing the pelvic cavity are: 1) descent; 2) flexion (the chin is well-flexed on the thorax); 3) rotation (position change, most recognizable by the rotation of the sagittal suture to the left oblique diameter). The posterior fontanelle is about to take the lead and become the presenting part.

the vertical axis of the pelvic cavity. Through flexion the occiput becomes the lowermost part and its circular suboccipitobregmatic plane, with a circumference of 32 cm, the plane of passage. Not only is this the only round plane of the head, but it is also the plane with the smallest and most favorable circumference. The mechanical aspect of this flexion occurs due to leverage between head and pelvic girdle.

The **anterior rotation of the neck** corresponds to the principle of the simplest alignment for two reasons:

- The vulvo-vaginal opening, which is passed through on crowning is longitudinal. The head will most easily pass through it if its longitudinal (anteroposterior) diameter is aligned with the longitudinal diameter of the opening.
- The head is forced (in the crowning movement still to be discussed) by the bend in the birth canal to curve around the pubic symphysis; it must make this turn in order to exit the birth canal.

The direction in which the head and neck generally most easily bend has been termed by Sellheim as

- facillimum of flexion (from Latin for easy: direction most easily flexed), and
- difficillimum of flexion (from Latin for difficult: direction most difficult to flex).

Every part of the baby has its own facillimum and difficillimum of flexion.

The difficillimum of flexion of the cervical spine is anterior, and its facillimum posterior:

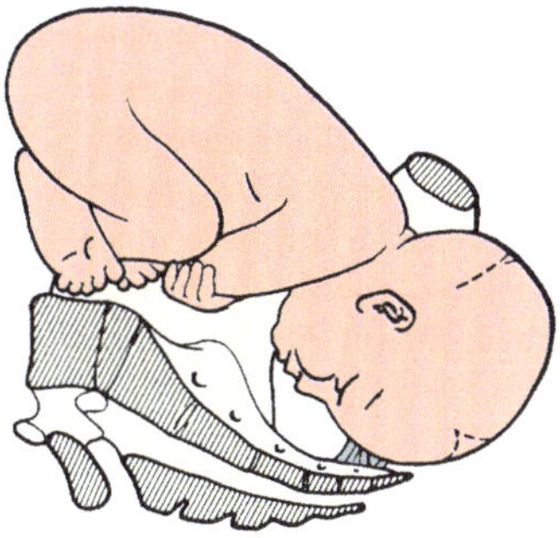

Fig. 7.29: From the side.

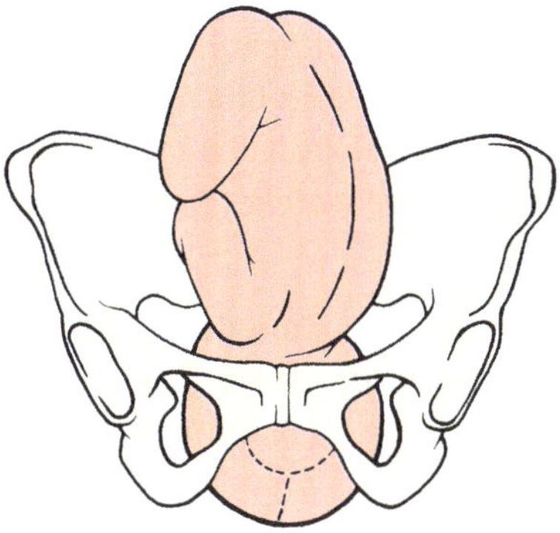

Fig. 7.30: From the front.

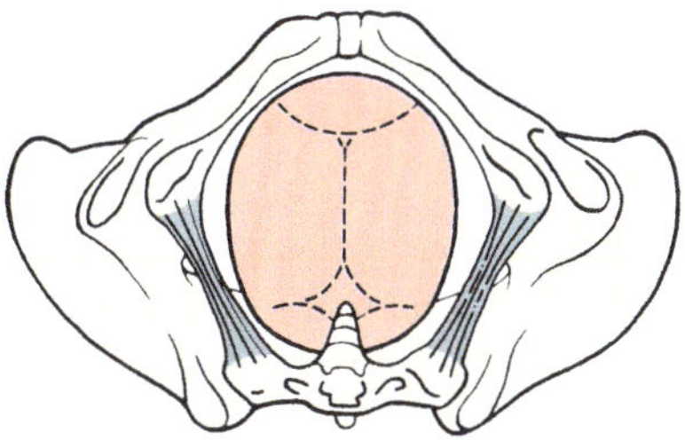

Fig. 7.31: Seen from below.

Figs. 7.29 to 7.31: Mechanism of expulsion, the head exits the birth canal (crowning), expulsion begins. In order to exit the birth canal, the head must negotiate the curve of Carus, which it does by arcing around the symphysis pubis, which it does by altering its attitude and extending from a well-flexed to a deflexed attitude. The expulsive movement is thus a simple alteration of attitude, whereby the posterior fontanelle leads and the base of the occiput functions as a hypomochlion against the inferior edge of the pubic symphysis, around which the rotation occurs. The sagittal suture is in the anteroposterior diameter. The shoulders enter the PI space transversely or slightly obliquely.

– The neck bends more easily backwards than forwards, flexion is more difficult (because the tissues are firmer) than extension, the movement in which the head is stretched backwards (something one can easily see on a newborn's head or on one's own).

If the neck is rotated anteriorly on passage through the pelvic cavity, this creates the only starting position from which the head can follow the prescribed curve of Carus, by bending backwards, following the facillimum.

Rotation mechanism. The sloped angle of the levator funnel, which ends in the longitudinal vulvo-vaginal opening, forces the head, approaching in the transverse diameter, to rotate into the anteroposterior diameter.

3. Expulsion from the birth canal, mechanism of expulsion (Figs. 7.29–7.32). The head is flexed for its entire journey through the pelvic cavity from PI to the pelvic floor. Now it has reached the pelvic floor, chin on chest, sagittal suture in the anteroposterior diameter, the occiput leading with the posterior fontanelle. In order to be born the head has to negotiate the curve of Carus, and to do this it must bend around the symphysis by moving from a sharply deflexed attitude to an extended (deflexed) one.

Note. The movement by which the head is born is extension, deflexion!

Attitude of the head is the only change required in order to exit the birth canal.

– The movement by which the head is born is thus simply an attitude change, whereby

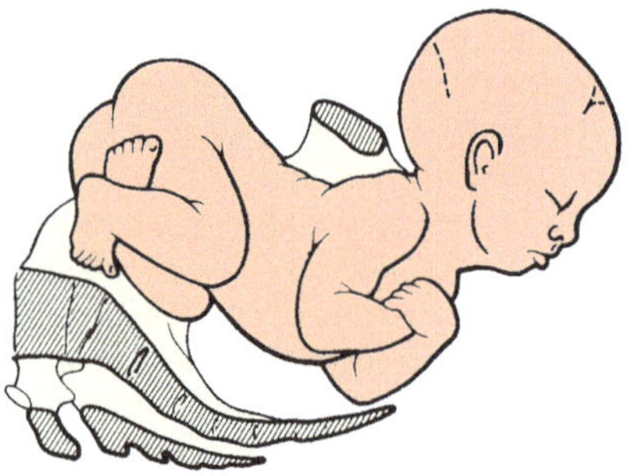

Fig. 7.32: From the side.

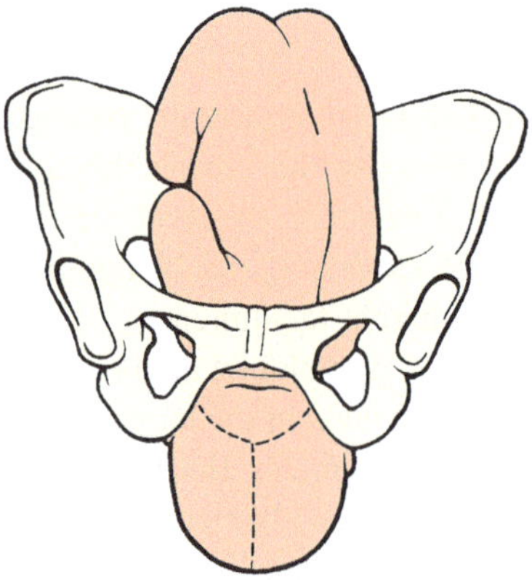

Fig. 7.33: From the front.

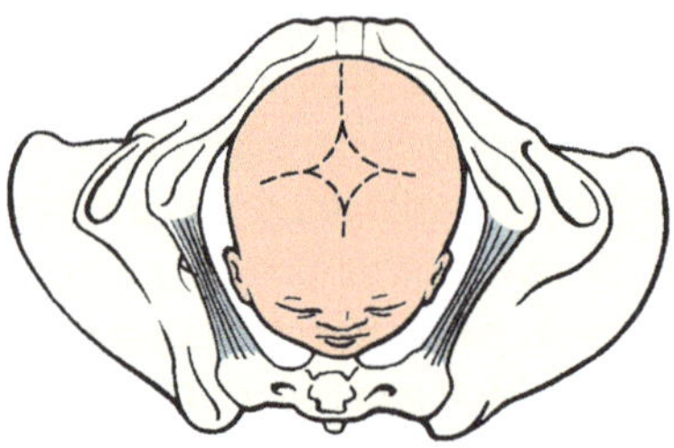

Fig. 7.34: Seen from below.

the suboccipital region functions as hypomochlion (or impinges) against the lower edge of the symphysis (Fig. 7.29), around which the rotation occurs.

- One after another occiput, sinciput, brow, face and chin are born over the perineum (Fig. 7.34).

Figs. 7.32 to 7.34: Expulsion completed, the head is born. The head has been completely expelled from the soft tissue canal. Occiput, sinciput, brow, and face have passed over the perineum consecutively. The deflexion led by the posterior fontanelle around the pubic symphysis has been concluded. The face is directed towards the bed, often at a slightly oblique angle (restitution).

External rotation of the head, restitution (Figs. 7.35–7.40). The head has been born from the soft tissue canal. It hangs out of the vulva, facing the bed (Fig. 7.34), often at a slightly oblique angle (either left or right lateral). After a short time the head makes a final movement: the external rotation. Hereby it turns to face the right or left thigh of the mother (Figs. 7.35 and 7.38).

As the head crowns, the **shoulders** (bisacromial diameter) enter the pelvic inlet in the transverse diameter (Fig. 7.33). During the birth of the head the shoulders rotate in the pelvic cavity (Fig. 7.36) into the anteroposterior diameter of the PO (alignment with the longitudinal vulvo-vaginal opening; Fig. 7.39). During the last part of this rotation the now fully born head is carried along and rotates externally. The anterior shoulder is born first, followed by the posterior shoulder.

Note. The mechanism of occiput anterior birth as described can be more simply depicted by five movements: 1) progression, 2) flexion, 3) rotation, 4) extension, 5) rotation.

Mechanism of labor with occiput anterior (OA) presentation

Rotation of the sagittal suture. When the head rotates, so does the sagittal suture. Practically, it is very important to understand the rotation of the sagittal suture for the second rotation. That is, the rotation of the head and neck from lateral to anterior (90°).

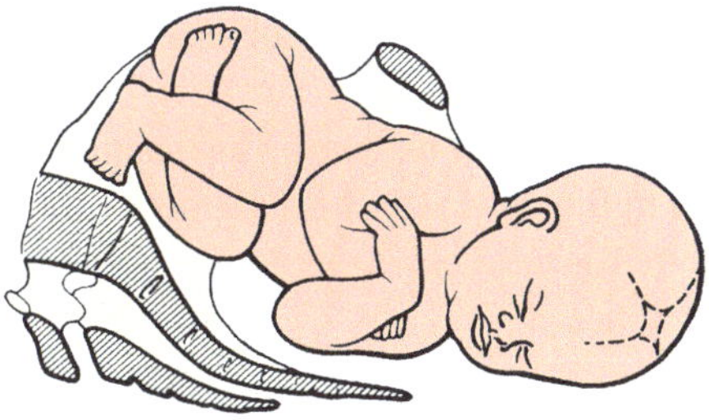

Fig. 7.35: From the side.

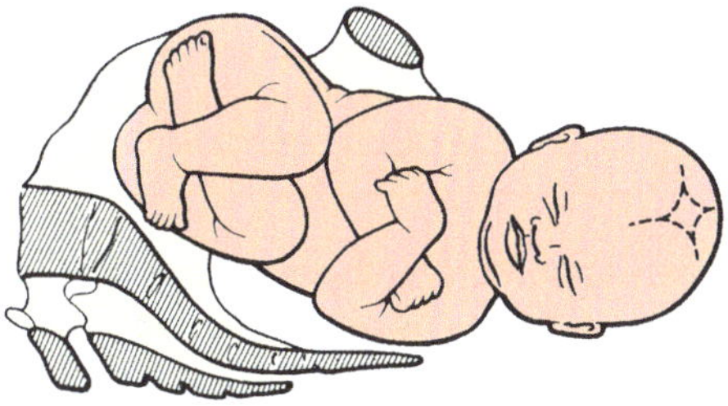

Fig. 7.38: From the side.

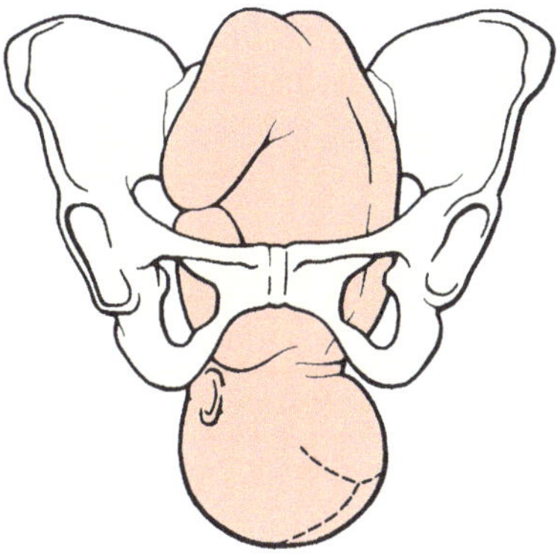

Fig. 7.36: From the front.

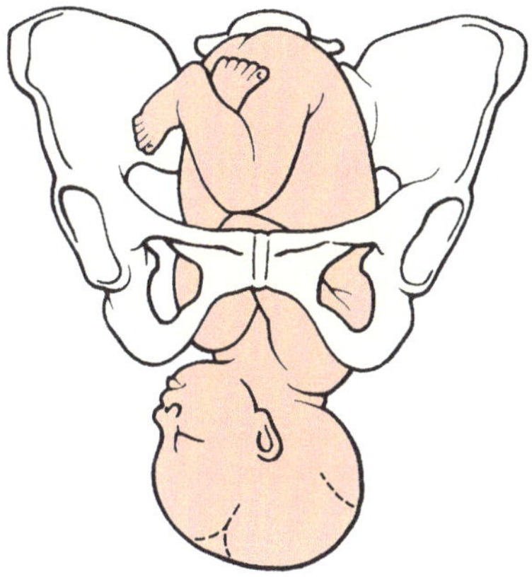

Fig. 7.39: From the front.

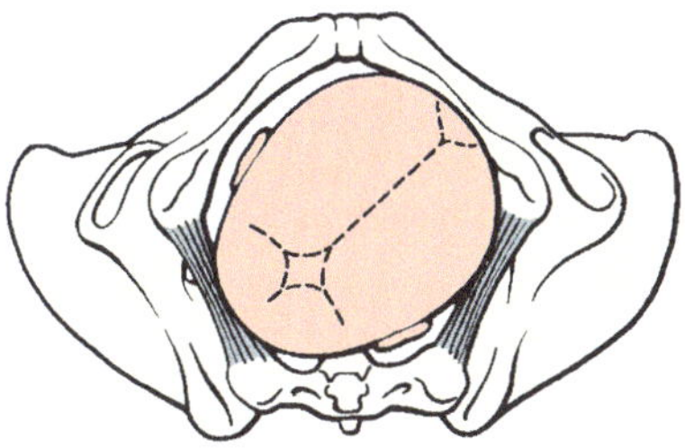

Fig. 7.37: Seen from below.

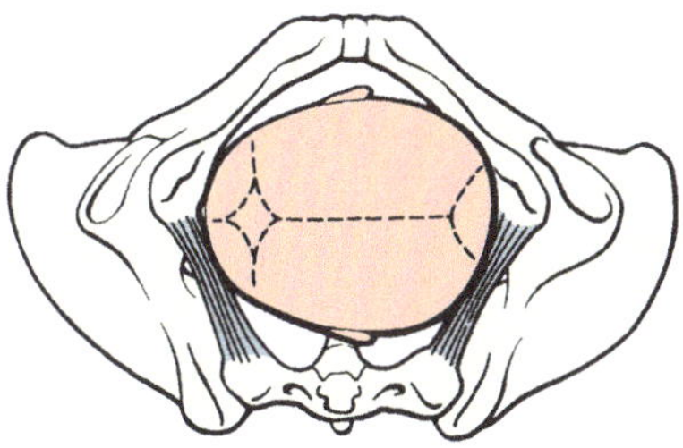

Fig. 7.40: Seen from below.

Figs. 7.35 to 7.37: External rotation of the head begins. During birth of the head, the shoulders, which have by now entered the pelvic cavity, have rotated over the oblique to the anteroposterior diameter of the PO (alignment with the longitudinal opening of the PO). The head follows the last part of this rotation and rotates externally. The anterior shoulder below the pubic symphysis is about to be born. It positions itself in the pubic arch.

Figs. 7.38 to 7.40: External rotation of the head is completed. In a left lie, the head faces the right thigh of the mother. The posterior shoulder has also swept the perineum.

Note. The head rotates from the transverse diameter over the oblique to the anteroposterior diameter of the pelvis. The sagittal suture rotates correspondingly.

The most important characteristics of the mechanism of labor in the normal occiput anterior presentation can be summarized as in the following overview:

Occiput anterior presentation

Lowermost part: posterior fontanelle.
Pivot point: base of occiput.
Head movement on crowning: extension.
Largest plane of passage: suboccipitobregmatic, circumference = 32 cm.

7.2.4 Station. Level of the head in the pelvis

Diagnosis of level of descent. The position of the head in the pelvis can be determined with the help of the external and internal (vaginal) examinations.

External examination for diagnosis of level of descent

Note. The **external examination** (see p. 153) often allows determination of the level of the head in the pelvis. It is also suitable for determining the station of the engaged head.

Head	Diagram	Determined with which external maneuver?
1. Freely mobile above PI (ballottable), (−4)	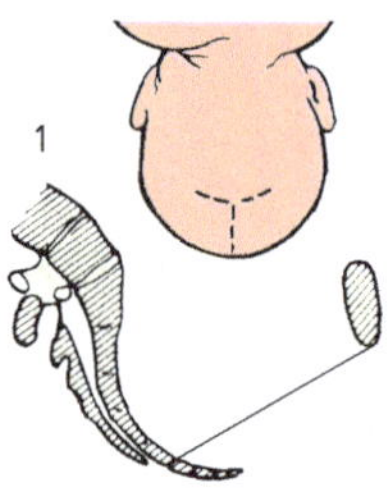 Fig. 7.41	Third Leoplod Maneuver (p. 24)
2. above the pelvis, (−3)	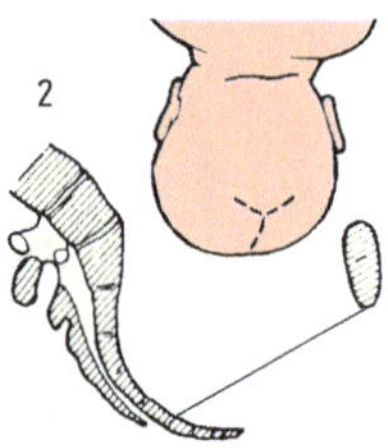 Fig. 7.42	Third Leoplod Maneuver (p. 24)
3. Minimally mobile in PI, (−2)	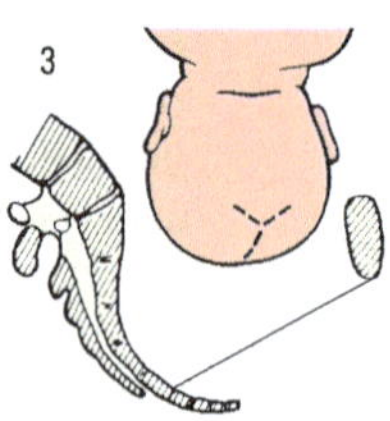 Fig. 7.43	Third and fourth Leoplod Maneuver (p. 24)

Head	Diagram	Determined with which external maneuver?
4. Fixed in PE, (–1)	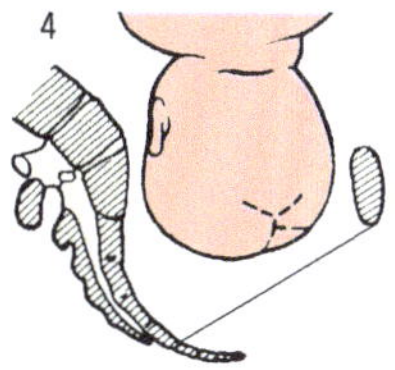 Fig. 7.44	Third and fourth Leoplod Maneuver (p. 24)
5. Engaged in PI, (Zero station)	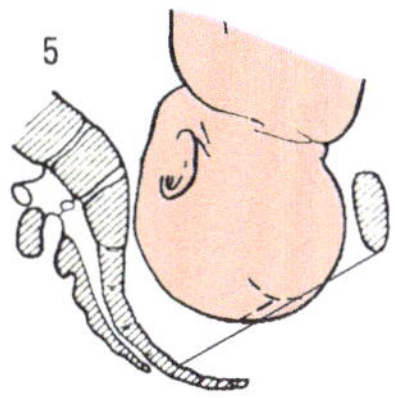 Fig. 7.45	Fourth Leoplod Maneuver (p. 24)
6. In Mid-pelvis, (+2)	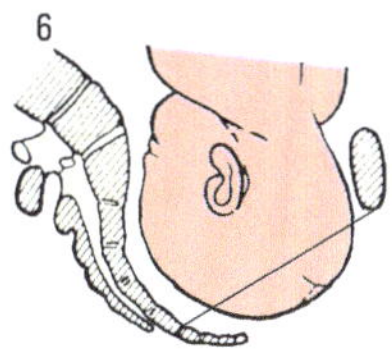 Fig. 7.46	It is not possible to determine the station in midpelvis externally, only with vaginal examination
7. On pelvic floor, (+4)	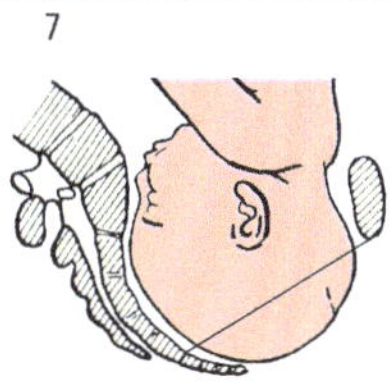 Fig. 7.47	Schwarzenbach maneuver, de Lee maneuver

Head at –4 station – freely mobile above PI (Fig. 7.41). The whole head is still palpable above the pelvis and can be easily moved. The head is ballottable (can be pushed back and forth) with the third Leopold maneuver. The fingertips can be inserted deeply between head and pelvic brim using the third Leopold maneuver.

Head at –3 station – above the pelvis (Fig. 7.42). The smallest segment of the head has entered the pelvis: it is beginning to engage. It is less mobile, progressing from freely mobile above the PI to minimally mobile in PI (level 3). A large part of the head is easily palpated externally.

Head at –2 station – minimally mobile in PI (Fig. 7.43). More of the head has entered the pelvis than in level 2. The head is still easily palpated externally. At this level in multiparae the head can easily be pushed out of the pelvis during vaginal examination; rarely in nulliparae.

Head at –1 station – fixed in PI (Fig. 7.44). A still larger part of the head has entered the pelvis; a smaller part is palpable externally.

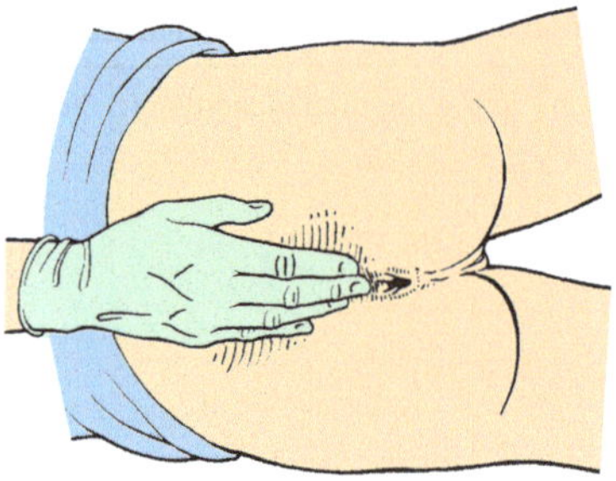

Fig. 7.48: Schwarzenbach maneuver. External maneuver: the head which has reached the pelvic floor is palpated between tip of tailbone and anus.

Internally. The lowermost part has not yet reached the inter-ischial plane.
The head is immobile in the PI but not: engaged, that is a different matter (see level 5). At level 5 the head has passed through the terminal plane with its greatest circumference, at level 4 this is not the case.

Head at zero station – engaged in PI → head has passed through the terminal plane with its greatest circumference (Fig. 7.45). Very little or none of the head is palpable externally. Due to the deep flexion of the head, the brow may be palpable with the fourth Leopold maneuver. The occiput is not palpable.

Internally. The lowermost part of the head has reached the inter-ischial plane at this level.

Practice tip. The head is only engaged in the PI when it is not at all or barely palpable externally with the fourth Leopold maneuver. As long as the head is palpable it is not engaged in the PI, but some distance above.

Head at +2 station – midpelvis (Fig. 7.46). This level cannot be determined externally but only on vaginal examination, as the head cannot be reached externally, from above or below.

Head at +4 station – has reached the pelvic floor (Fig. 7.47). The head fills the pelvic cavity completely and rests on the pelvic floor.

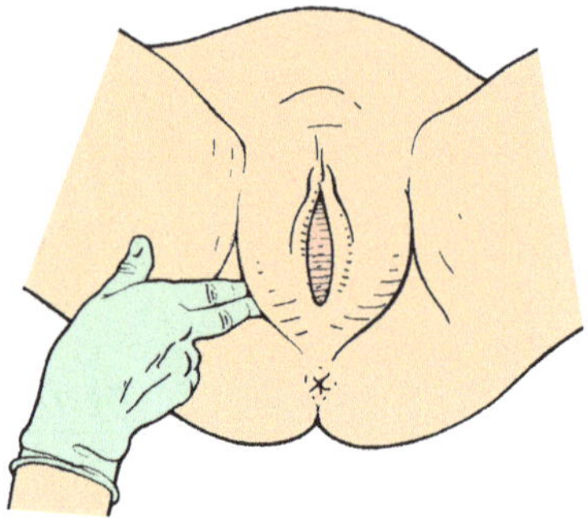

Fig. 7.49: de Lee maneuver. External maneuver: pressure from 2 fingers to the side of one of the labia majora in order to determine whether the fetal head has reached the pelvic floor.

Overview of external examination methods for determining station

Note. The head has reached the pelvic floor when it is palpable externally, which is possible with 2 maneuvers:

- Schwarzenbach's maneuver (Fig. 7.48). If one presses, with the four fingertips of one hand (coming from the sacrum), the area between the tip of the tailbone and the anus, the posterior perineum, one can feel the head on the pelvic floor as a broad, hard resistance.
- de Lee maneuver (Fig. 7.49). If one presses two fingers deeply at the side of one of the labia majora, one can feel the large, firm head if it has reached the pelvic floor.

Head at PO. The head is in the PO when it is visible in the vulva or vagina.

Internal examination for diagnosis of level of descent

Note. The descent of the head within the birth canal can be followed centimeter by centimeter using internal (vaginal) examination. The two most important questions during the internal exam are: Where is the lowermost part? Where, then, is the head (with its greatest circumference)?

Three defined pelvic stations

- Zero station; head engaged in the PI → head has passed the terminal plane with its greatest circumference.
- +3 station; head in midpelvis → head is in midpelvis with its greatest circumference.
- +5 station; head has reached the pelvic floor → head is pressing firmly on the pelvic floor.

Level of the leading part. The first two stations described are used to determine the level of the leading part (lowermost point of the presenting part in the axis of the birth canal, pelvic axis). They are defined by the level of the greatest head circumference, which is not directly accessible: the palpating finger cannot pass the lowermost section of the head! The real level of the head arises indirectly, as a result of known relationships, from the height of the leading part.

The height of the nonpalpable greatest head circumference is assessed according to the station of the section of the head which is directly palpable with a finger, the leading part. In order to do this, the corresponding station in the birth canal is related to a fixed bony point:
Interspinal line, line connecting the two ischial spines (Fig. 7.50).

Staion of fetal head (Fig. 7.51). From the simple ascertainment of the level of the leading part in relation to the inter-spinal line, the level of the greatest circumference of the fetal head is calculable according to the following specifications:

- **PI.** The head is engaged in the PI (at zero station) when the leading part of the head is palpable at the level of the ischial spines. At this level the head has passed the terminal plane with its greatest circumference.
- **Midpelvis.** The head is in midpelvis when the leading part is below the interspinal line.
- **Pelvic floor.** The head has reached the pelvic floor when it is not possible or almost impossible to insert a finger between head and pelvic floor. The ischial spines can no longer be reached.
- **PO.** The head has reached the pelvic outlet when it is visible in the vagina.

Practice tip. Serious consequences can arise for mother and baby when the level of descent has been misdiagnosed! The following three practice tips are therefore to be observed:

1. Inexperienced examiners regularly estimate the level of the fetal head as lower than it really is: the level of the head is only to be assessed when the finger examines directly in line with the pelvic axis! This is frequently not the case, and the examiner, usually examining too far anteriorly, not in the pelvic axis, reaches the head more easily and estimates it to be lower than it is.
2. The point of reference for the head is the leading bony part. If a caput succedaneum is present, it must be subtracted (Figs. 7.52, 7.53). It can be significant in labors which continue long after ROM, and severe if the pelvis is contracted.
   The caput can be visible in the vagina when the head has not yet entered the pelvic inlet with its greatest diameter!

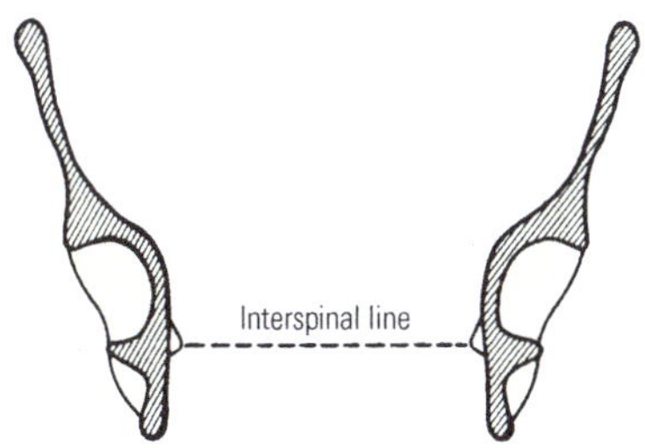

Fig. 7.50: Interspinal line, line connecting both ischial spines (spinae ischidicae).

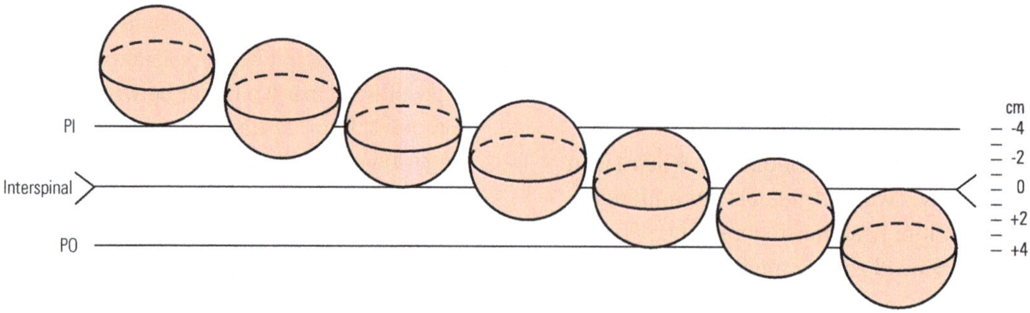

Fig. 7.51: Diagnosis of station of fetal head on vaginal examination by determination of the relationship between leading part and interspinal line.

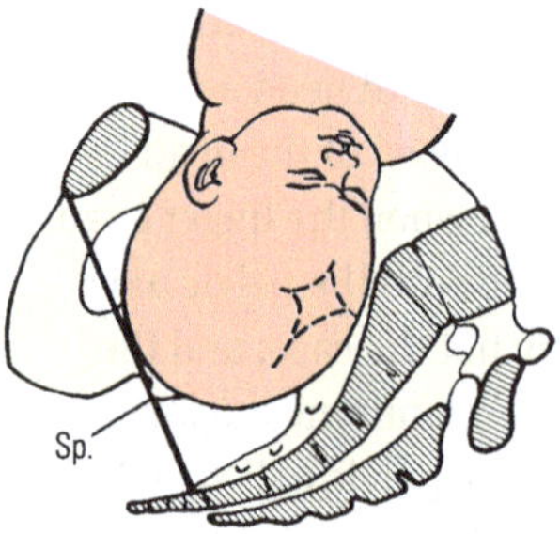

Fig. 7.52: Head without caput succedaneum. The leading part has reached the interspinal line, the greatest head circumference has passed the terminal plane: the head is engaged in PI at zero station.

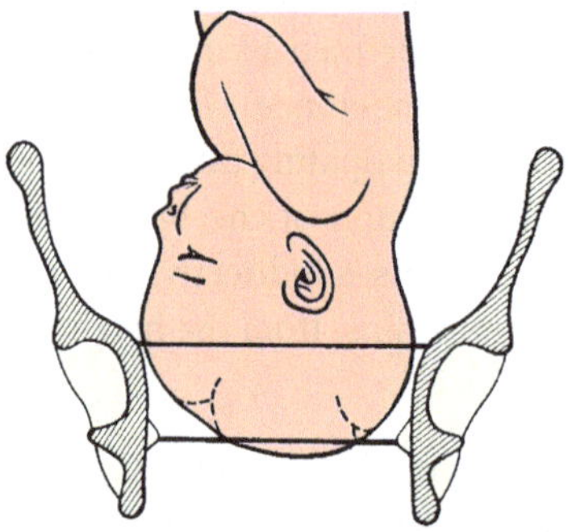

Fig. 7.54: The well-flexed head (normal occipitoanterior presentation) is engaged in PI (at zero station) when its lowermost point has reached the interspinal line.

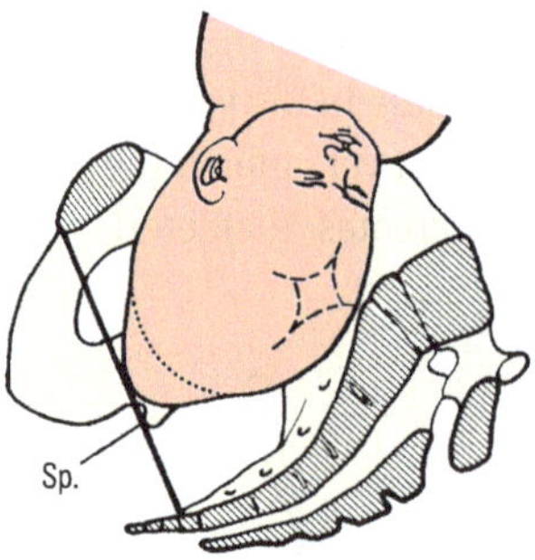

Fig. 7.53: Head with caput succedaneum. The leading part has not reached the interspinal line, the caput has. The greatest head circumference has not passed the terminal plane (after Beck).

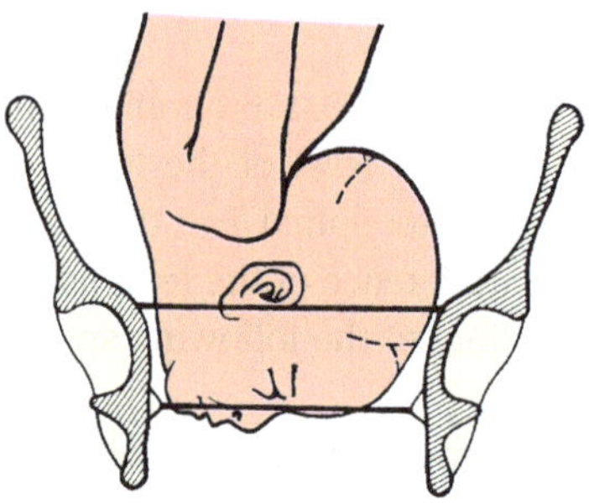

Fig. 7.55: The extended head (face presentation) is above the PI with its greatest circumference when its lowermost point has reached the interspinal line (after de Lee).

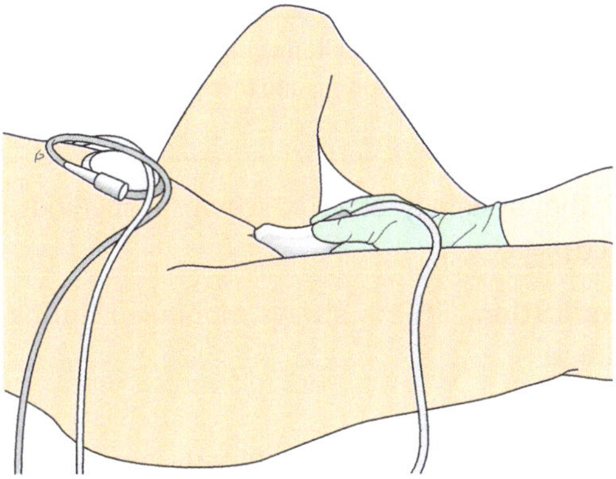

Fig. 7.56: Method of intrapartal transabdominal ultrasound examination (ITU) for determining level of descent.

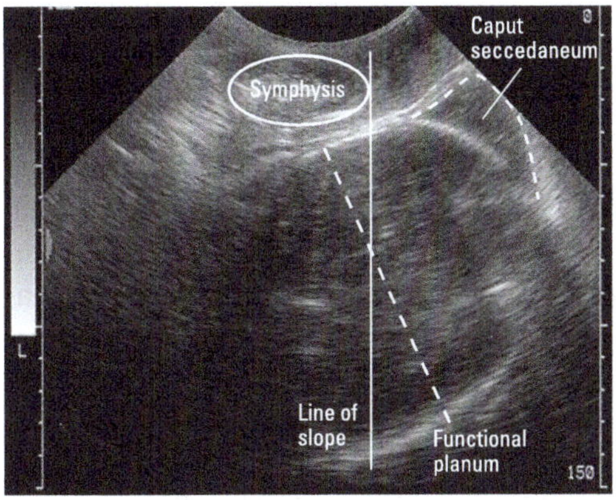

Fig. 7.57: ITU of a head at a station suitable for vacuum extraction.

3. The rules for diagnosis of the level of descent are only valid for flexed, not extended presentations (p. 220). In extended presentations, the head is only engaged (at zero station) when the bony leading part is 2 fingers below the interspinal line (Figs. 7.54, 7.55).

Ultrasound for diagnosis of level of descent

Intrapartum translabial ultrasound (ITU; Figs. 7.56, 7.57) assists in the assessment of the dynamic of stage 2 and the potential success of an operative vaginal delivery.

7.3 Examination of the fetus during labor

Intrapartal hypoxia. Hypoxia can cause intrapartal or neonatal death or permanent fetal damage. Fetal monitoring during labor is therefore very important!

Monitoring methods
- Auscultation, monitoring of fetal heart sounds.
- Observation of AF color.
- Fetal pulse oximetry .
- Fetal blood sampling (FBS) for evaluation of the fetal acid-base household.
- Cardiotocography, registration of fetal heart frequency, contractions.

7.3.1 Auscultation, amniotic fluid color

Auscultation

Normal heart sounds. 110–150/min (see p. 28).

Nonreassuring heart sounds (classical definition). Fetal heart rate (FHR) < 100/min in three consecutive contractions, without recovery! This signifies an acute fetal threat!

Practice tip. FBS has shown that only approximately one third of fetuses with decreased heart rate are at risk for intrauterine hypoxia. Nonreassuring heart sounds therefore mean: cardiotocography should be performed. Nonreassuring heart sounds → immediate termination of labor is an old rule for obstetricians who do not use cardiotocography. The combination of cardiotocography (p. 36, 168) and FBS are the most reliable methods for determining the exact degree of risk.

Warning signs for nonreassuring heart sounds. Acceleration of FHR > 150/min (advance signal) and FHR fluctuations of > 40 bpm.

Permanent acceleration, accentuation, extreme fluctuation above the physiological fluctuation (110–150), frequently with arrhythmia, and also FHR > 150 over a longer period are indicators of approaching danger.
Fetus at **risk**! Delivery desirable!

Practice tip. Decrease in FHR when the head enters the pelvis (entry effect acc. to Gauss) does not suggest risk. It requires, however, attentive monitoring of FHR.

Passage of meconium (in vertex presentations) → cardiotocography is indicated.

Color of amniotic fluid

Meconium-stained AF is an indication that the fetus is currently distressed, or was some time ago. Cardiotocography is indicated, as the danger (cord compression, disturbance of placental blood flow) may be repeated.
Green, formed meconium in AF (terminal meconium) is an advance signal! Meconium may have been passed some hours ago or just recently (hypoxia → carbon dioxide and lactic acid overload → acidosis → premature peristalsis; see p. 284).

Practice tip. Passage of meconium or leakage of meconium-stained fluid is not an indication for the termination of labor, but one for cardiotocography or FBS if FHR is nonreassuring or pathological.

Passage of meconium is an advance signal; nonreassuring FHR is an alarm signal!

7.3.2 Cardiotocography (CTG), electronic fetal monitoring (EFM)

Definition. Continual electronic registration and recording (cardiotocogram, CTG, or electronic fetal monitoring, EFM) of FHR and contractions in late pregnancy (antepartum EFM) and during labor (intrapartum EFM).

Note. Electronic fetal monitoring aids early recognition of fetuses at risk of hypoxia, and therefore avoidance of late complications.

Pathophysiology of FHR, technical methods: see p. 36.

Indication. FHR is always monitored during labor!

Pro and contra

Pro. The suggestion that EFM be performed only in risk situations appears inadequate as 17 % of fetuses have also been shown to be at risk in normal pregnancies.
Contra. On the other hand, prospective studies on the value of EFM compared to auscultation (McDonald 1985) did not demonstrate a lower incidence of compromised fetuses or cerebral palsy in the EFM group than in the group monitored via auscultation. Some clinics do not aim for continuous intrapartal EFM. The scientific dispute about the interpretation of these comparative studies continues. The recommendation in central Europe is currently for an acceptable concept of care for mother and baby which makes it possible to keep the number of compromised neonates down and thus the number of children with a greater probability of a potentially forensically reproachable cerebral palsy.

Practice tip. We practice a concept of care which consists of combined monitoring (EFM and FBS) of the fetus during labor.

Note. Absolute indication. Regardless of conflicting opinions, EFM is to be performed if the following pregnancy and labor risks exist:
- History. Stillbirth, perinatal brain injury.
- IUGR, preterm delivery.
- SIH.
- Carbohydrate metabolism disorder.
- Breech presentation.
- Induced labor, prolonged labor, administration of oxytocic agents.
- Multiple gestation.

- Bleeding in the second half of pregnancy.
- Antenatal diagnosis of birth defect, intrauterine infection.
- Postterm pregnancy, oligohydramnios, hydramnios.

Alternative to intrapartal EFM, standardized auscultation can be performed (every 15min in first stage, for at least 30 s after a contraction, in the second stage every 5 min) with documentation of time and frequency.

Minimum intrapartal EFM requirements
- Routine EFM on admission with accelerations.
- Auscultation every 15 min in first stage, 30 s after a contraction.
- EFM for 30 min after ROM, ARM.
- Immediate EFM in frequencies < 100 or > 150 bpm.
- EFM if oxytocic agents have been administered, meconium is stained, if bleeding has occurred, during the second stage.

Monitoring duration. The requirement for continuous fetal monitoring during labor has already been removed.

Intermittent EFM. It has been suggested that continuous EFM be replaced with intermittent if the pregnancy was normal and once admission EFM has been performed. This is understood to mean repeated EFM (e.g., every 30 min) over a number of minutes (e.g., 20 min) in the first stage.
This procedure is nonevaluable due to lack of scientific data.
Remote EFM (telemetry). Telemetric transmission of continuous EFM is a compromise between reduced maternal stress and safety of the baby.

Technique. How should electronic fetal monitoring be performed? Registration must be uninterrupted and easily interpretable. Such optimum monitoring is usually achieved using US cardiotocographs with autocorrelation. The method also allows restless laboring women to change position as desired and telemetric transmission. It is rare (in < 3 % of laboring women) that EFM is noninterpretable.

Direct (internal) fetal monitoring via fetal ECG (scalp electrode) is useful in such cases. Artificial ROM and possible lack of aseptic conditions result in a 1 % risk for infection.

Intrapartal heart rate pattern
Bradycardia caused by
- maternal circulatory disturbance, e.g., inferior vena cava syndrome (IVCS),
- fetal causes: cardiac (e.g., excitation or conduction disorder) or cerebral (e.g., anencephaly),
- disturbed placental gas exchange (Figs. 7.58, 7.59) or persistent cord complication. The response to short-term hypoxia is deceleration, to long-term hypoxia it is bradycardia (→ hypoxic bradycardia).

End- or second-stage bradycardia. If hypoxic bradycardia and absence of variability occur at the end of stage 2, it is often termed end-stage bradycardia.

Hypoxic bradycardia. Combined occurrence of hypoxic bradycardia and absence of variability (oscillations) is particularly threatening for the fetus.

Treatment
- Tocolysis if hypoxic bradycardia occurs in first stage or early second stage!
- FBS and summoning of operation team (→ cesarean alert!), if bradycardia persists for longer than 3min despite tocolysis.
- Immediate cesarean if pH sinks rapidly (p. 179).
- If pH increases expectant management.

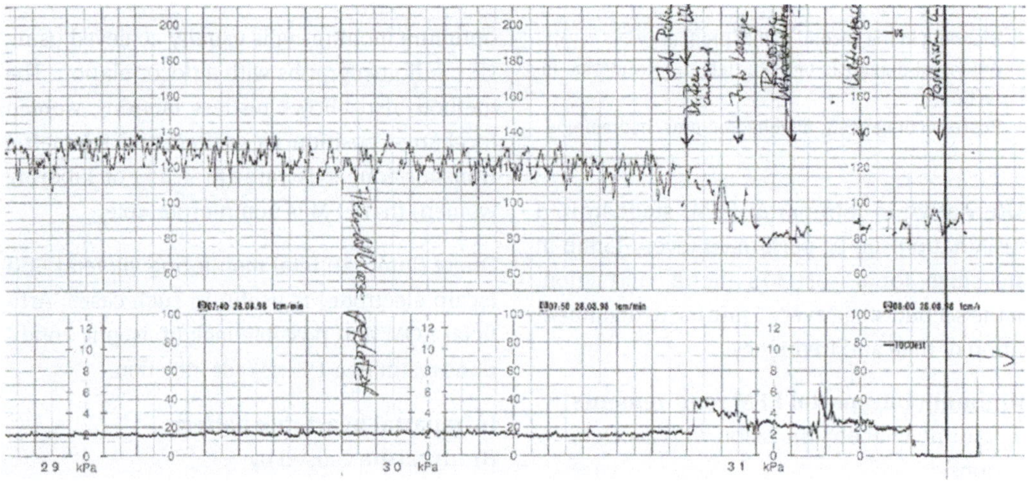

Fig. 7.58: FHR tracing, 29 year old para 2, week 32 + 6. Acute bradycardia due to placental abruption. Cesarean section, male, 1,955g, 43 cm, Apgar 4/7/7, umbilical artery pH 7.17, umbilical vein pH 7.23.

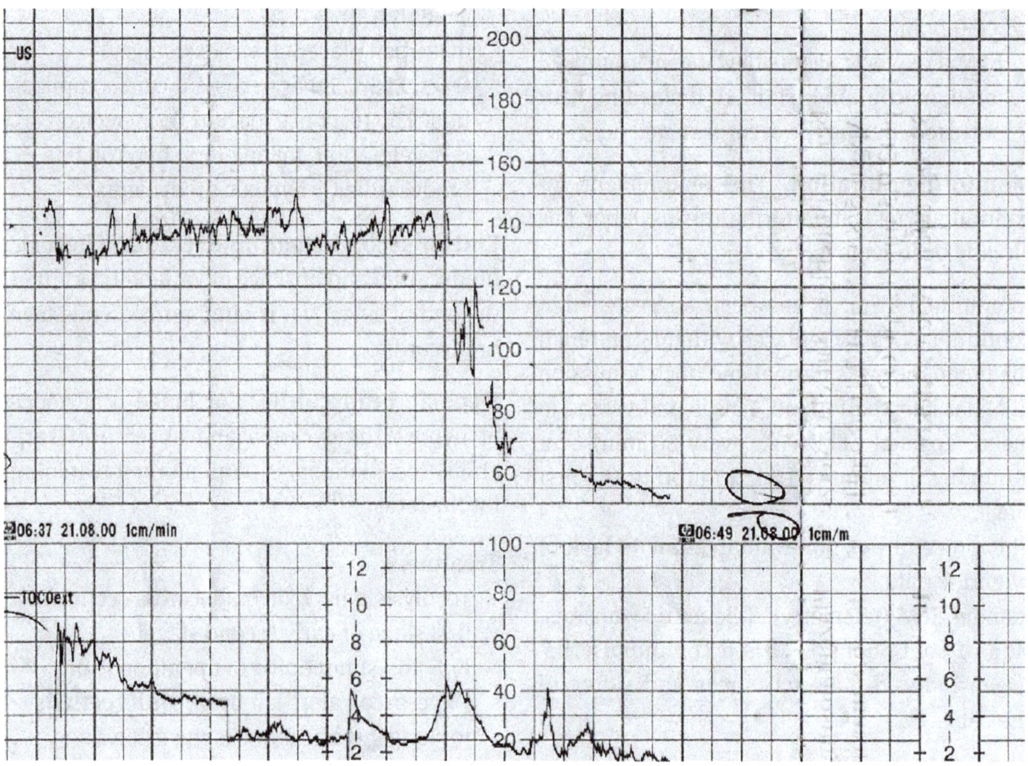

Fig. 7.59: Treatment-resistant acute fetal bradycardia, 32-year-old para 1, week 40 + 6. Nicotine abuse 7/day. Emergency cesarean section. Delivery of a female, thick meconium-stained liquor, 3,350 g, 50 cm long, 35 cm head circumference. Apgar 5/8/9, umbilical artery pH 7.16, umbilical vein pH 7.22, base excess –6mmol/l. Large incomplete placental abruption.

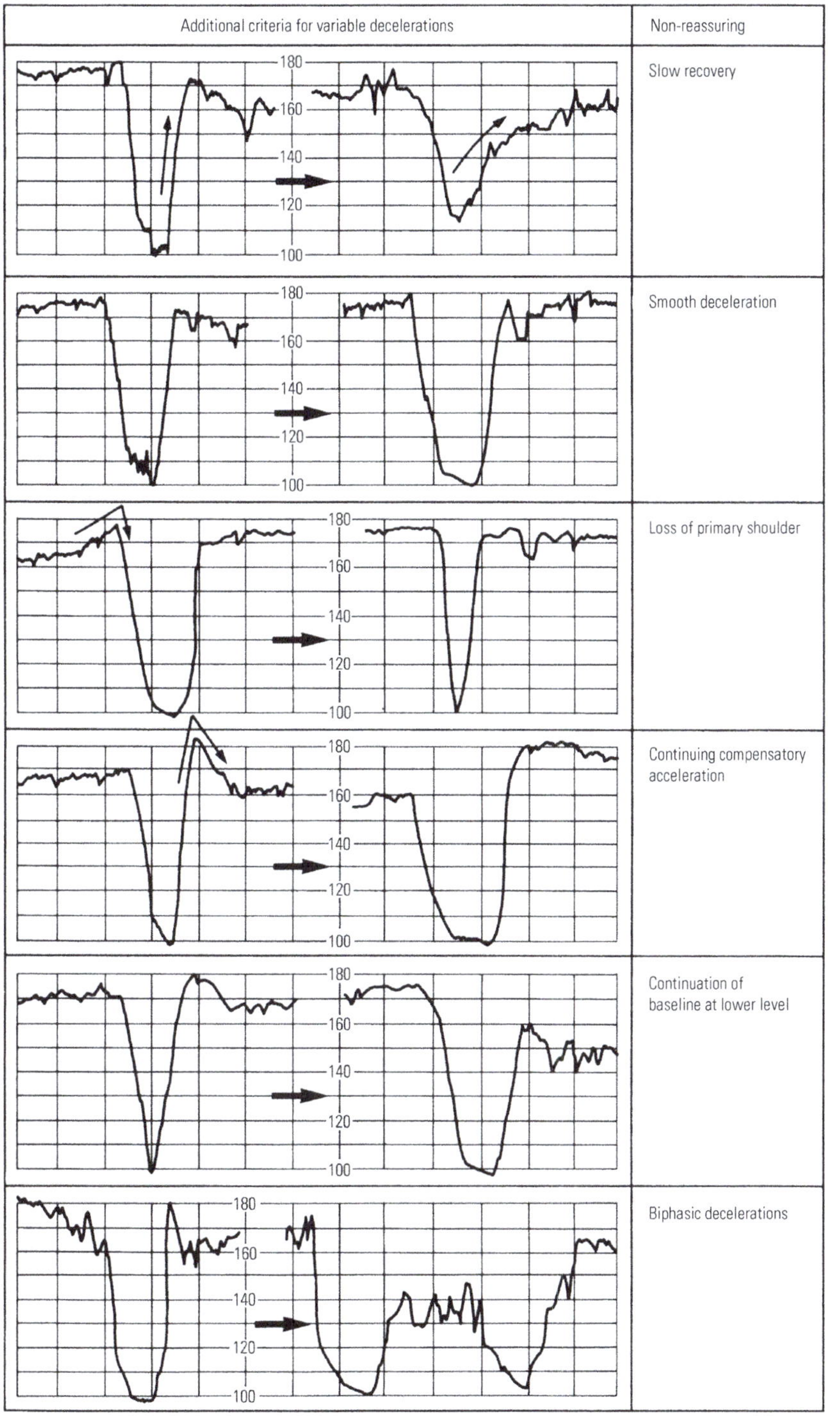

Fig. 7.60: Additional criteria for the evaluation of variable decelerations. Reassuring heart rates are shown on the left; nonreassuring on the right (after W.M. Fischer).

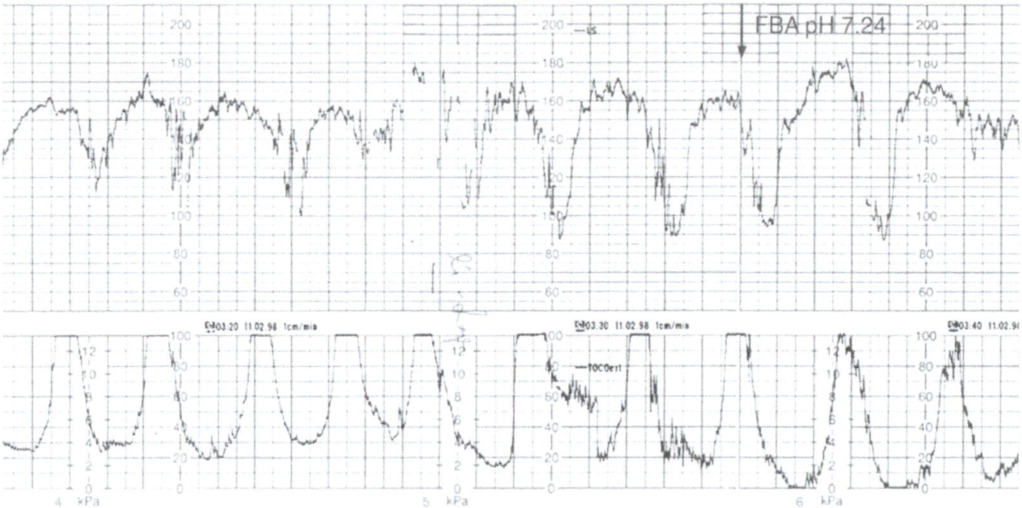

Fig. 7.61: FHR tracing with variable decelerations and FBS pH of 7.24; late first stage. 29-year-old para 1 at term; SVD, female, 3,260 g, 51 cm long, Apgar 7/8/9, umbilical artery pH 7.14, umbilical vein pH 7.28.

Practice tip. End-stage bradycardia is an indication for rapid termination of labor.

Decelerations

Early decelerations are the result of brief fetal episodes of cerebral ischemia due to mechanical causes (→ compression of the head!) which lead to vagotonic dominance. Incidence: 10 %, after ROM < 10 %. If heart rate patterns are otherwise normal there will be no consequences.

Variable decelerations (Figs. 7.61–7.63).

Causes are disturbances of umbilicoplacental circulation. The disturbance is in the placental capillary system or the umbilical cord.
Variable decelerations are registered during every second labor.
Three classifications are used (mild, moderate and severe) according to depth and duration, these are correlated with the pH values of fetal blood (Kubli). Moderate and severe decelerations are commonly linked with decreased pH.
Variable decelerations and additional criteria (Fig. 7.60). There are valid clinical guidelines for variable decelerations:

Treatment

- Change in maternal position (normalization of umbilical cord circulation).
- IV tocolysis: Fenoterol if heart rate pattern indicates hypoxia. Dosage: 2 mg Fenoterol in 500 ml electrolyte solution. Infusion speed: 20 drops/min until discontinuation or marked reduction of contractions.
- FBS if variable decelerations continue despite tocolytic agents. The result will determine the obstetrical procedure.

Late decelerations (Fig. 7.64) rarely occur during labor (5 %) and are most likely a sign that the fetus is at risk for hypoxia, whereby the pH value negatively correlates with the severity of the deceleration.

Nevertheless, FBS should determine procedure in first stage and early second stage!
Late decelerations in late second stage can be an indication for prompt operative delivery.

Tachycardia (Fig. 7.65, 66). The slow baseline increase commonly occurs in:

- Maternal fever or pharmacological cause.

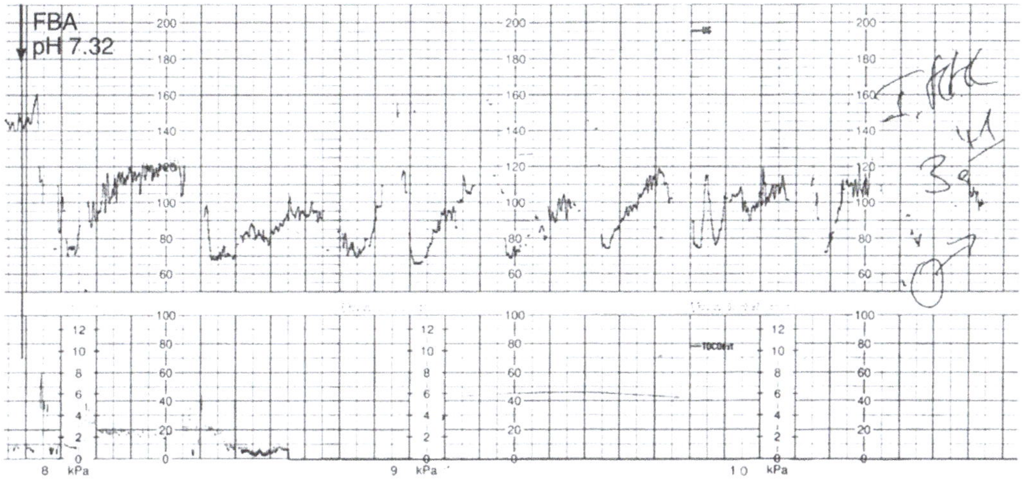

Fig. 7.62: FHR tracing with variable decelerations and four additional criteria in second stage: 1) slow recovery; 2) Smooth deceleration; 3) continuation of BL at lower level; 4) biphasic decelerations; SVD, male, 2,860 g, 50 cm long, Apgar 9/10/10, umbilical artery pH 7.12, umbilical vein pH 7.17.

- Transient fetal hypoxia. In this case, tachycardia demonstrates the compensatory ability of the fetal circulatory system.

Accelerations

Accelerations not associated with contractions occur in labor as a result of fetal movement, contact on vaginal examination, ARM, attachment of a scalp electrode, drawing of fetal blood; they are reassuring.

Accelerations associated with contractions can, however, be an indication of:

- Decreased uteroplacental perfusion synchronous with contractions.
- Cord compression only affecting the umbilical vein.

Practice tip. Accelerations associated with contractions can be an early warning signal for fetal compromise.

Fluctuation amplitude and frequency play a secondary role in fetal monitoring.

Amplitude and frequency are reduced by analgesics, sedatives, para- and sympathomimetics. Absent variability is a warning sign, if not caused by sleep or medication.

Practice tip. Reduced amplitude and frequency of fluctuations is a signal for a fetus at risk in the following constellation: tachycardia or bradycardia with reduced variability, or loss of variability at the nadir of the deceleration.

The American College of Obstetricians and Gynecologists recommended a three-tiered Fetal Heart Rate Interpretation System

Category I

Category I FHR tracings include all of the following:

- Baseline rate: 110–160 beats per minute.
- Baseline FHR variability: moderate.
- Late or variable decelerations: absent.
- Early decelerations: present or absent.
- Accelerations: present or absent.

Category II

Category II fetal heart rate (FHR), tracings includes all FHR tracings not categorized as Cat-

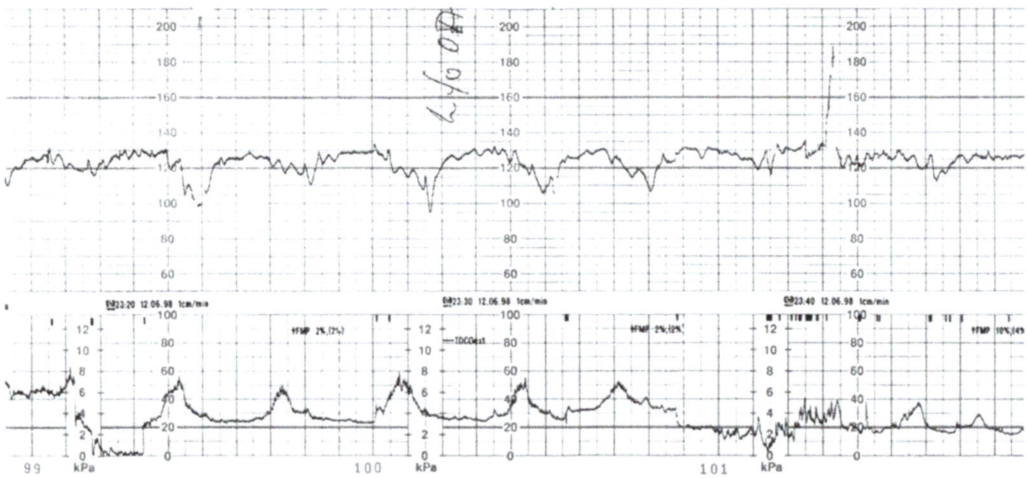

Fig. 7.63: Admission trace with decelerations and loss of variability suggestive of hypoxia; 27 year old para 3 at 35 + 0 weeks; cesarean delivery; male, 1,820g, Apgar 3/7/8, umbilical artery pH 6.74, umbilical artery BE – 23 mmol/l, umbilical artery lactate 14 mmol/l; umbilical vein pH 6.80, umbilical vein BE – 22 mmol/l, umbilical vein lactate 16 mmol/l.

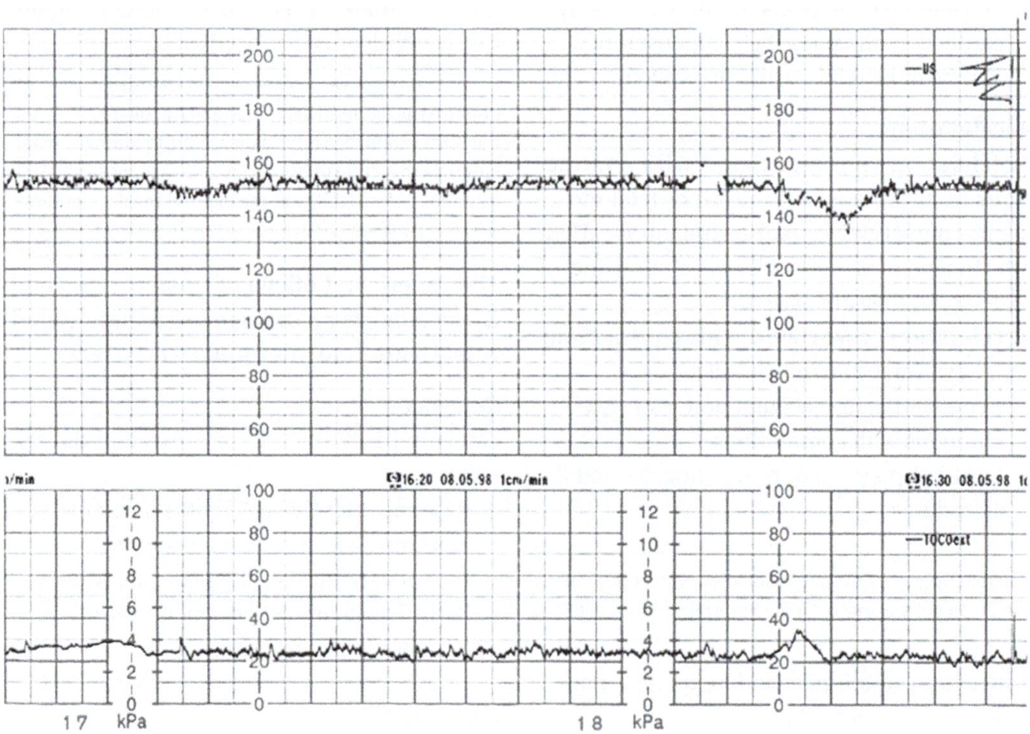

Fig. 7.64: Admission trace with late decelerations, 41-year-old para 3 at week 38 + 6 with known intrauterine hypotrophy. Cesarean section; male, 1,845 g, Apgar 2/8/9, umbilical artery pH 7.03, umbilical artery BE – 16 mmol/l.

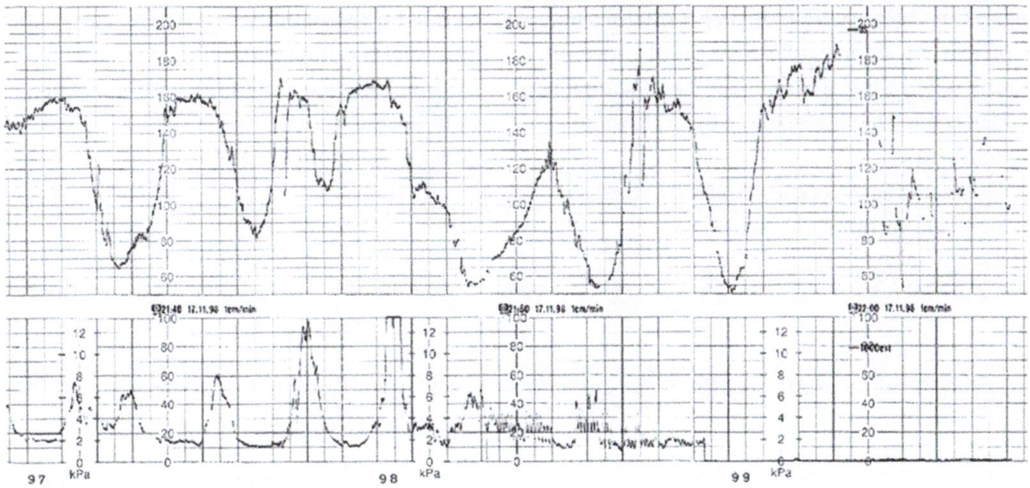

Fig. 7.65: Trace in late second stage showing progressive tachycardia and severe late decelerations; 36-year-old para 1 in week 41 + 6, vacuum extraction from mid-pelvis (leading part 3 cm below inter-spinal line) due to pathological CTG; mildly deflexed head, sinciput presentation; female, 3,620 g, Apgar 9/10/10, umbilical artery pH 7.22, umbilical vein pH 7.28.

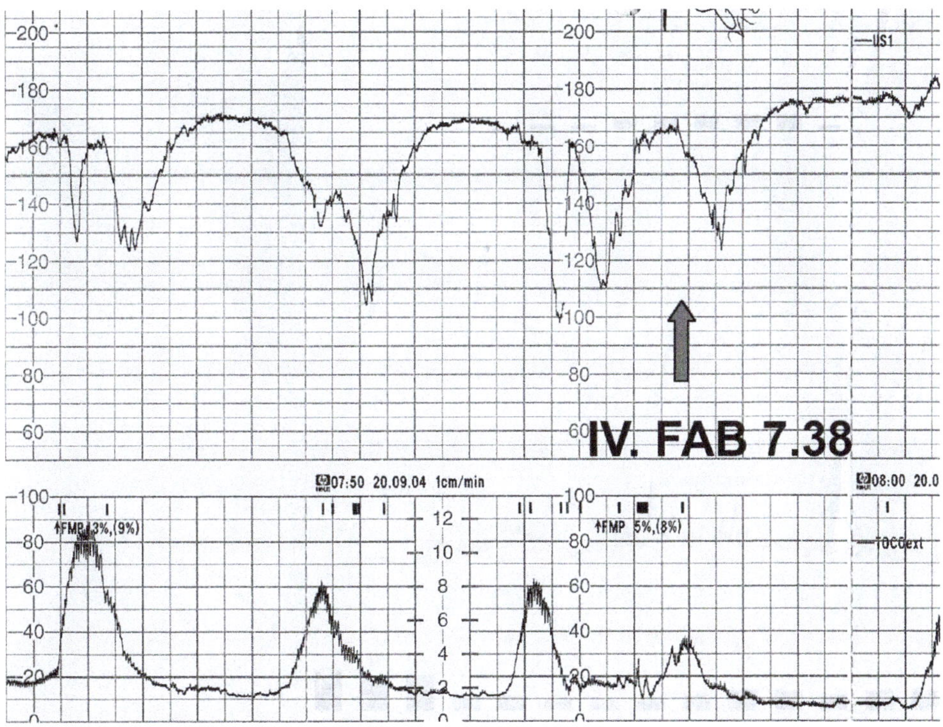

Fig. 7.66: Trace in late second stage, 40-year-old para 1; i.v. oxytocin 20 ml/h, on pressing presenting part descends to I + 3. SVD, reactive female from ROA, 3,260 g, 53 cm long, 36 cm head circumference; Apgar 8/10/10, umbilical artery pH 7.44, BE – 3.7 mmol/l. True cord knot and battledore cord insertion.

egory I or Category III. Category II tracings may represent an appreciable fraction of those encountered in clinical care. Examples of Category II FHR tracings include any of the following:

Baseline rate
- Bradycardia not accompanied by absent baseline variability.
- Tachycardia.

Baseline FHR variability
- Minimal baseline variability.
- Absent baseline variability with no recurrent decelerations.
- Marked baseline variability.

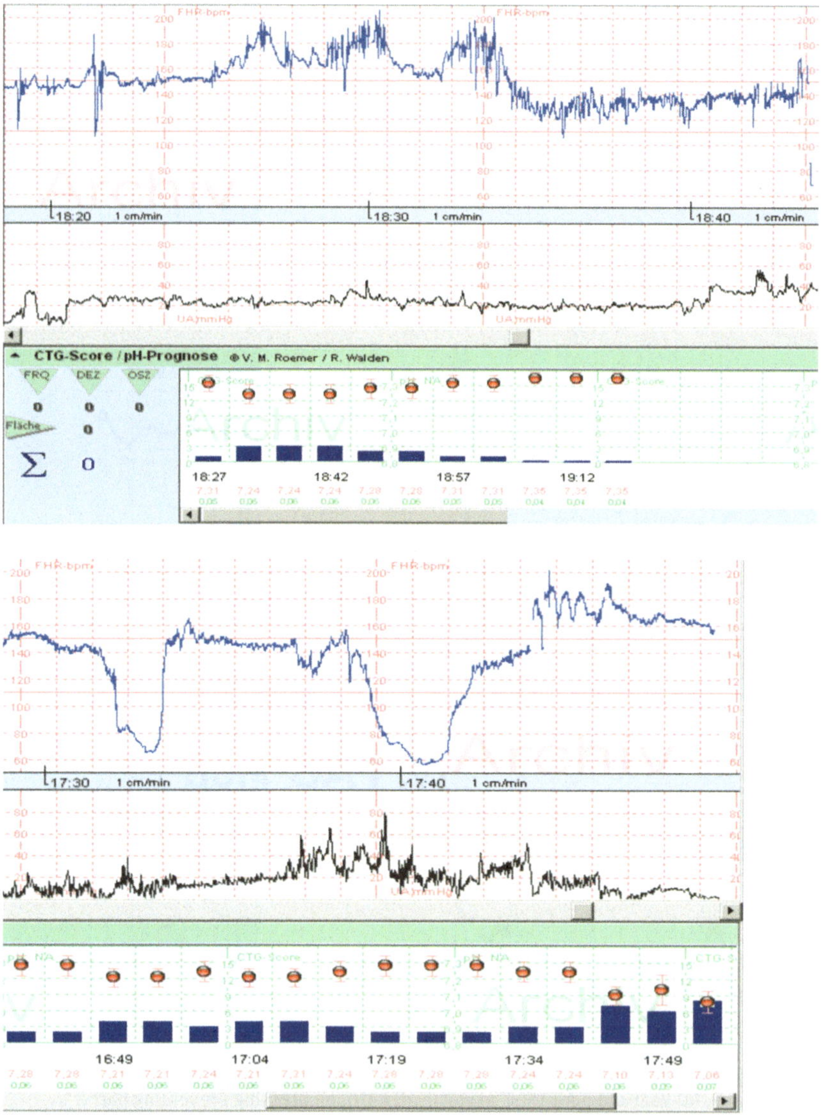

Fig. 7.67a,b: Electronic CTG evaluation with CTG score and pH prediction showing normal and pathological CTG.

Accelerations
- Absence of induced accelerations after fetal stimulation.

Periodic or episodic decelerations
- Recurrent variable decelerations accompanied by minimal or moderate baseline variability.
- Prolonged deceleration more than 2 minutes but less than10 min.
- Recurrent late decelerations with moderate baseline variability.
- Variable decelerations with other characteristics such as slow return to baseline, overshoots, or "shoulders".

Category III
Category III FHR tracings include either
- Absent baseline FHR variability and any of the following:
  - Recurrent late decelerations.
  - Recurrent variable decelerations.
  - Bradycardia.
- Sinusoidalpattern.

CTG evaluation by single examiners is unsatisfactory. Expert evaluations which differ on a day-to-day basis and between experts demonstrate the limits of this monitoring method. As a result, electronic CTG evaluation has long been a goal. Both the Dawes–Redman microfluctuation evaluation and Römer's evaluation strategy (Fig. 7.67a,b) are excellent examples of these efforts.

7.3.3 Fetal blood sampling (FBS)

Definition. Sampling of fetal scalp blood. Method of monitoring the fetus during labor (early recognition of preacidosis or perinatal acidosis) by drawing a few drops of blood from the skin of the presenting part of the fetus and determining the pH (Saling 1961).

The diagnostic value of FBS is recognized! The use of FBS is seen differently – too often, according to some obstetricians. Others do not use the FBS method at all. This is difficult to understand, because cardiotocography has a high false-positive rate for hypoxia and a complement is therefore necessary.
The use of FBS in 5 % of all deliveries (Huch and colleagues, 1994) appears reasonable.

Technique. Depending on the stage of labor, the presenting part is accessed either with an endoscope or a speculum.

Use of an endoscope is recommended until the cervix is fully dilated and the leading part has passed zero station.
If labor is further progressed, a speculum is used for FBS.
Endoscopic FBS (Fig. 7.68)
- *Position.* The woman in labor is in the lithotomy position or on her side. The external genitalia are cleaned with a disinfecting solution.
- *Instruments.* All instruments must be prepared before insertion of the endoscope: incision instrument with blade extending 2 mm (depth of incision), heparinized capillary tube, light device, swab clamp with swabs, paraffin oil.
- *Technique.* After vaginal examination, the endoscope with the largest possible diameter (16, 10, 33 mm) is inserted with obturator into the cervical canal. After the obturator has been removed and the light device attached, the presenting part can be seen. The scalp is swabbed dry. Sterile paraffin oil is spread thinly with a swab on the visible portion of the scalp to prevent the blood spreading. The blood collects in a droplet on this fatty layer after incision. The puncture-like incision is made in the upper visible section and the blood sucked up into

the capillary tube as quickly as possible without air intake.
- When the capillary tube contains sufficient blood it is passed on for examination.

FBS using speculum (Fig. 7.69)
- *Position.* The pelvis of the woman in labor is elevated in the bed using a pelvic cushion or by raising the pelvic section of the bed. After disinfection of the external genitalia it is covered by a drape with a hole in it.
- The speculum FBS procedure is the same as with the endoscope. An assistant is needed to hold the posterior speculum. The operator holds the anterior speculum in the left hand and handles the instruments with the free right hand.

Mistakes (Bretscher and Saling)
Biological causes. Difference between contraction and contraction-free interval, caput, fever.

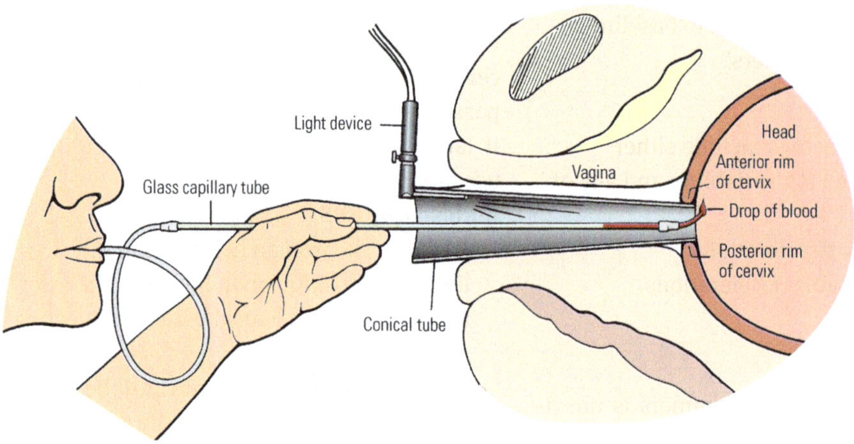

Fig. 7.68: Endoscopic fetal blood sampling (FBS).

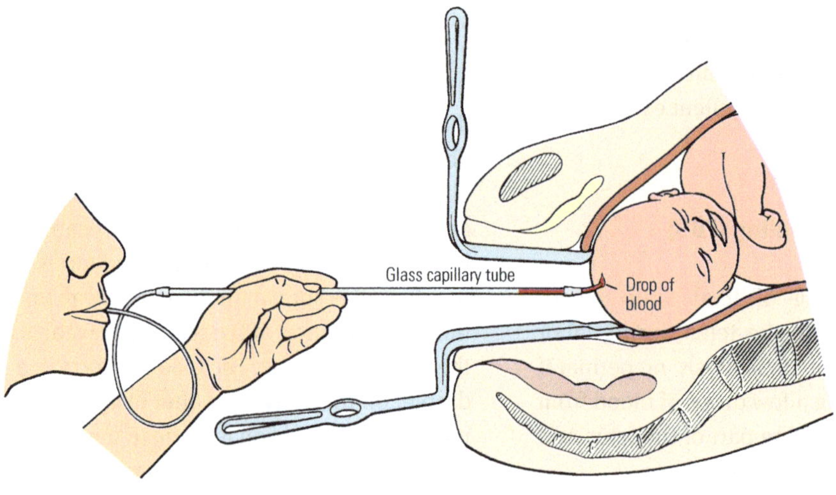

Fig. 7.69: Fetal blood sampling using speculum.

During blood sample collection. Contact with air, mixture of blood and air in the capillary.
During storage of the blood sample. Autooxidation, sedimentation.
In calculations for scientific questions. Addition of extremely differing pH values.

Disadvantages, risks. The effort required to extract a sample from the presenting part is a disadvantage. Risks (continued blood loss from the incision, infection of the incision) are reduced to a minimum if the correct technique is employed.

Note. Blood pH level. The pH level registers respiratory and metabolic hypoxic acidosis. If the pH is normal (≥ 7.25) there is no danger!

Increased acidity (decreased pH) in:
- pCO_2 increase due to respiratory acidosis → initial sign of acute hypoxia!
- fetal metabolic acidosis due to anaerobic glycolysis (→ progressive hypoxia).

Progression. Respiratory acidosis exists at the beginning of a respiratory disturbance. The longer hypoxia persists, the stronger the metabolic character of the acidosis, which can be estimated on further examination of the fetal blood sample: base excess, lactate content.

Stages of acidity. Saling suggested the following clinical stages:
- 7.24–7.20: pre-acidosis.
- 7.19–7.15: mild acidosis.
- 7.14–7.10: moderate acidosis.
- 7.09–7.00: advanced acidosis.
- 6.99 and <: severe acidosis.

Indication. Nonreassuring cardiotocographic FHR patterns give the indication for FBS:
- Bradycardia < 100 bpm immediately.
- Late or variable decelerations (3 and more consecutive contractions).

If the head has already reached the pelvic floor or outlet, an assisted delivery is performed without FBS!

Repeat FBS. If EFM is pathological, repeated blood sampling as soon as possible, perhaps three or four times, is recommended. If the pH levels remain normal no action need be taken.

FHR improves frequently as a result of the accompanying tocolysis or repositioning of the mother.
If the nonreassuring heart rate patterns persist, the FBS should be performed within 10 min, later at 15 min intervals. The intervals can become longer if the heart rate pattern remains consistent and the pH values do not continue to drop.

Contraindication. The examination is prohibited if the mother is HIV-positive.

While with an HBV-positive mother the use of FBS appears possible due to the active and passive immunization of the baby directly after birth, care should be exercised with HCV-positive mothers.

Conseqences

Note. Drop in pH: a steep decline in fetal pH values is a warning sign: acute fetal hypoxia!

Causes. Cord complications, placental insufficiency, reduced uterine perfusion, contractions too strong or too frequent.

Treatment
- Immediate tocolysis, as contractions increase hypoxia: Fenoterol infusion 50 μg/min IV in up to five single doses. Dosage is based on the effect of the tocolytic agent. This bridges the time until assisted delivery of the fetus.
- Variable decelerations with or without pH drop: change in maternal position. Occa-

sionally cord complications can be treated successfully in this way.
- If the pH level is sinking chronically, tocolysis should be administered. The primary goal is not to postpone the operation, but to make it unnecessary (→ intrauterine reanimation).

Practice tip. Temporary stoppage of contractions must not begin when pH levels are already too low; a pH between 7.23 and 7.27 is ideal. In some cases uncomplicated progression of labor is possible once contractions resume.

Maternogenic increase in acidity

Causes of the increased concentration of lactic acid in the maternal organism during labor are: pain-related hyperventilation due to increased exertion of the uterine and skeletal muscles, hunger, diabetic metabolism.

Pathophysiology. The response to the reduced pCO_2 (as a result of hyperventilation) is increased renal excretion of bicarbonate. This leads to decreased concentration of buffer bases, or rather a decreased base excess (BE). Concentration gradients of lactate and bicarbonate occur in both directions on the placental membrane between fetal and maternal blood. They are compensated for by transfer processes or cannot be balanced (decompensated). The transfer of lactic acid from maternal to fetal blood occurs at the same time as a bicarbonate transfer in the opposite direction.

Note. If the fetal pH is 7.25–7.30, the base excess in maternal capillary blood must be tested! If the BE values of mother and baby differ by ≤ 5 mval/l, this indicates a maternogenic fetal metabolic acidity increase.

The maternogenic increase in acidity does not appear to be as dangerous as the overload of acidic valencies caused by fetal hypoxia. Therefore, maternogenic acidity increase does not necessitate operative termination of labor to the same extent as threatened fetal hypoxia does.

Fetal pulse oximetry. Fetal pulse oximetry allows continuous transcutaneous monitoring of fetal oxygen saturation. The transducer is placed on the cheek or back of the fetus once the membranes have ruptured (usually). The value of this method in monitoring fetal status has not yet been conclusively decided. On the one hand, claims are made that when $fSpO_2$ is ≤ 30 % fetal acidosis increases, and when levels are > 30 % and EFM is pathological the number of FBS and operative deliveries can be reduced. On the other hand, the high predictive value in recognizing risk situations is disputed.

STAN. Continuous registration of fetal ECG via a scalp electrode and the electronic evaluation of the ST-segment allows recognition of fetal metabolic oxygen deficiency situations and makes the recognition of endangered fetuses with nonreassuring FHR traces possible, thereby reducing the rate of operative deliveries. The value of the method in monitoring the fetus has not yet been conclusively decided.

7.4 Management of labor

7.4.1 Management of first stage

Definition. First stage begins with the first regular contractions (birth contractions, true labor) and ends when the external cervical os is fully dilated.

Birth contractions

Characteristics
- Frequency > 2–3 contractions in 30 min with a regular rhythm.
- Dilatation of the cervical canal.
- Painful contractions, particularly in primigravidae. The pain of labor contractions is

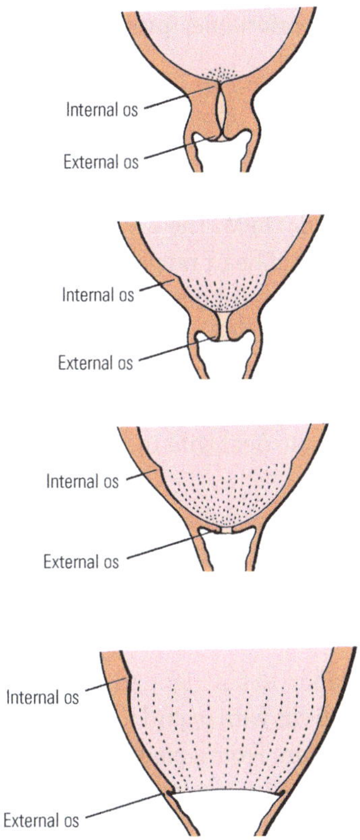

Fig. 7.70: Effacement and dilatation of the cervical canal in primiparae. It begins at the internal os and slowly incorporates the external os.

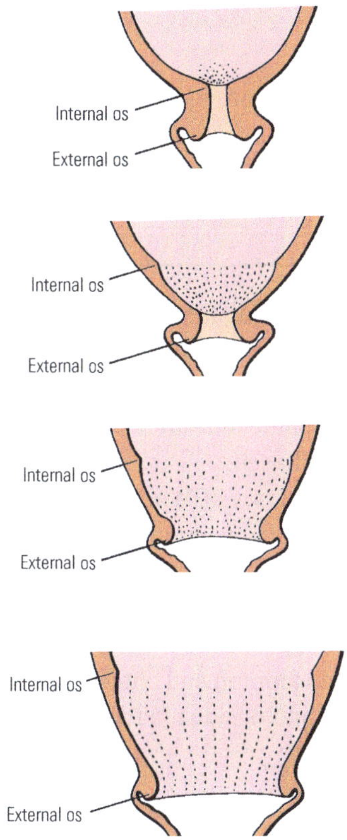

Fig. 7.71: Effacement and dilatation of the cervical canal in multiparae, which occurs in all parts simultaneously.

the pain of the stretching of the cervix and corpus.

Effect. The cervical canal is opened wide enough that the head can pass through it. In nulliparae the head is always forced down to the pelvic floor, in multiparae almost always.

Effacement and dilatation of the cervical canal. The cervical canal opens differently in nulli- and multiparae.

In **nulliparae** (Fig. 7.70), effacement begins at the internal os and progresses towards the external os, while the opening of the cervix remains closed. As soon as the cervical canal is fully effaced the ring of the external os gives in to the pull of the cervical walls and dilates around the advancing fetal part.

In **multiparae** it is very different (Fig. 7.71). The external os is 1–2 cm dilated in the last weeks of pregnancy. While the cervical canal effaces from the internal os during first-stage contractions, the already open external os does so at the same time.

All parts of the cervical canal efface and dilate at the same time. If the internal os is completely dilated the external os is also or almost completely effaced.

Rupture of membranes (ROM). The membranes rupture at the end of first stage, when the cervix is fully dilated → timely rupture!

Types of rupture
- Pre-labor ROM.
- ROM before labor begins.

Practice tip. Prelabor rupture of membranes means danger of ascending infection with fever in labor or puerperium.

- Early ROM – ROM during first stage.
- Timely ROM – ROM when cervix is fully dilated and effaced.
- Late ROM – ROM some time after cervix is fully dilated and effaced.
- Rupture of hindwaters – ROM above the cervix, the forewaters remain intact.
- Double ROM – After hindwater rupture the forebag in the cervix ruptures.
- False ROM – Leakage of fluid which has collected between amnion and chorion, or between chorion and decidua (a few milliliters).

Induced ROM. If the forebag becomes visible in the vulva it is ruptured with a sterile instrument.

This action is performed by the midwife or obstetrician.
Examination after ROM
- Immediate monitoring of FHR.
- Amount and color of fluid is noted.
- If FHR pattern is pathological directly or a few minutes after rupture cord prolapse (see p. 288) may have occurred; then
- Immediate vaginal examination.

Practice tip. The midwife should observe the bladder in first stage. The woman in labor should be asked to empty her bladder frequently: a full bladder inhibits contractions!

Monitoring, posture, birth positions, water birth

Monitoring. It is the responsibilty of the obstetrical team to suggest positions to the woman in labor which are comfortable, provide relief, and allow monitoring.

The fetus is continually monitored, whereby the method depends on the technical possibilities:
- Remote (telemetric) EFM. The wireless transmission of fetal heart rate and contractions using transmitter and receiver allows freedom of movement to a large extent, which suits most women in first stage: different positions can be adopted in order to find out how best to deal with the contractions.
- The use of the following objects: birth stool, rope (Fig. 7.72), sitting (Fig. 7.73), birth ball (Fig. 7.74), wall bars, or bathing in birthing pool or bathtub.

The woman in labor has a right to her own ideas and expectations with regard to **mobility** and **birthing position.** From a medical point of view – as long as monitoring indicates maternal and fetal wellbeing – the laboring woman should be allowed to choose regarding her position, the use of analgesics, and the length of first stage are reduced in upright positions.
If FHR is nonreassuring, further diagnostic or therapeutic measures (FBS, tocolysis) are required, which necessitate utilization of the bed.

Upright birthing position. Advantages:
- The fetal head is better accommodated by the maternal pelvic inlet.
- Strengthening of contractions and support of cervical dilatation and effacement due to the influence of gravity.
- Improved pressure on bearing down.
- Improved fetal circulation, or rather avoidance of inferior vena cava syndrome.
- Subjective labor relief, or rather pain relief.

Practice tip. Women laboring in upright positions have a significantly shortened second stage!

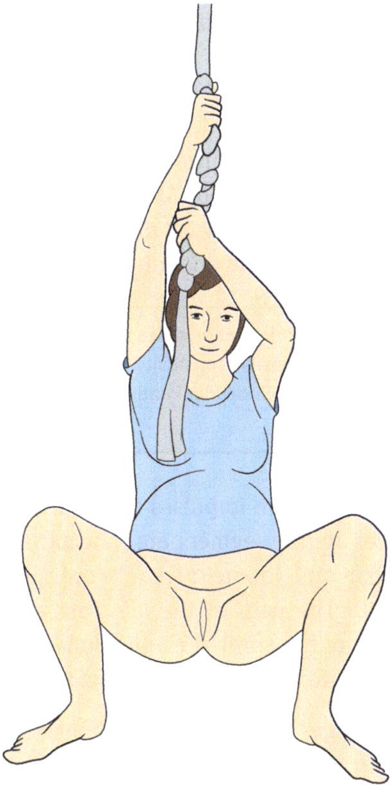

Fig. 7.72: Holding on to a rope during first stage.

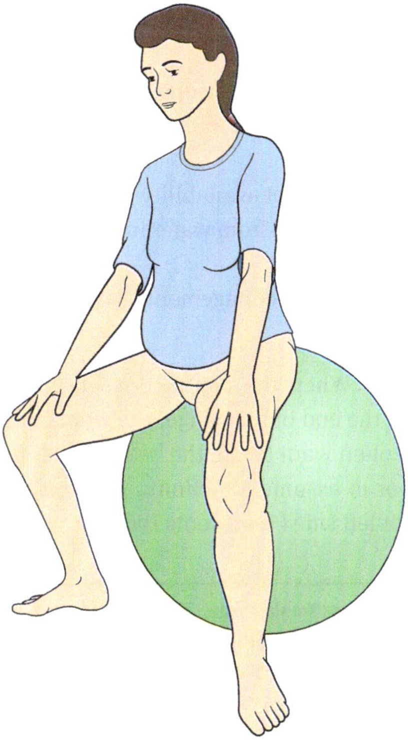

Fig. 7.74: Sitting on the gymnastic ball during first stage.

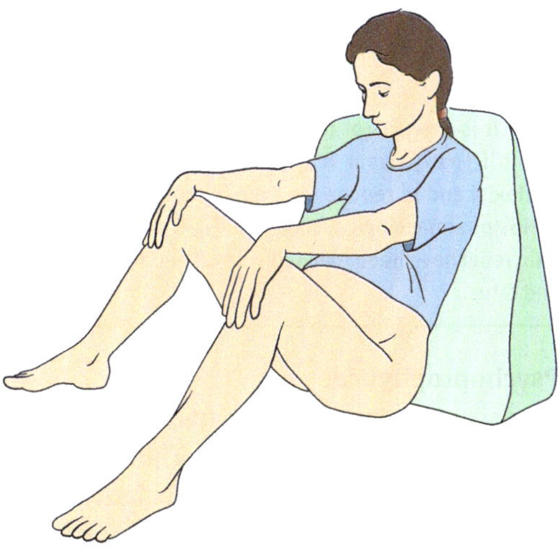

Fig. 7.73: Supported sitting position during first stage.

Relaxation bath. Bathing during the first stage is done because it not only relaxes, but reduces pain. The standpoint on continuous monitoring (p. 167) should be taken into account.

Water birth. Water birth has gained supporters amongst midwives, obstetricians, and parents in central Europe as an alternative to technologized birth (→ type of gentle birth).

Scientific studies are not available, so no judgment will be made here, also with regards to potential risks or lack thereof.

Guidelines (acc. to Eldering 1999)

- Only normal births.
- Contraindication: malpresentation, multiple gestation, preterm birth, chorioamnionitis, epidural block, medication which

affects the CNS, maternal infection (hepatitis, HIV).
- Only if requested by the woman.
- Intensive support from midwife and obstetrician.
- Permanent, prompt availability of a second person for removal from water in case of problems.
- Same monitoring management as with "dry" births.

Positioning. When the contractions become stronger at the end of first stage, the woman in labor will often want to use the bed in order to sit down or to assume a reclining position on her back or left side (→ prevents IVCS).

Note. Obstetric positioning rule. The laboring woman lies on her side towards which the part of the head which is to take the lead should descend and rotate anteriorly.

Monitoring by the physician

- Heart tones (see p. 167), or rather cardiotocography (see p. 167)

Practice tip. Heart tones are to be heard every 15 min in the first stage, immediately after ROM, after each contraction if they are strong and frequent.

- Cervical dilatation and effacement (see p. 152).
- Level of the head (buttocks) in birth canal (see p. 162) with presentation, attitude, descent.
- Contractions (see p. 147).
- Amniotic fluid (see p. 167).

Birth pain, pain relief

Definition. Birth pain is an intensive pain which increases with cervical dilatation, duration of labor, distension of pelvic floor. Pain can cause a prolonged, complicated birth.

Etiology. Birth pain in the first stage is caused by the distension of cervix and lower uterine segment, or rather cervical dilatation and effacement. The pain in the late first stage and second stage is caused by distension of the soft tissue canal and pelvic floor. During delivery the pain increases with cervical dilatation, duration of labor ,and pelvic floor distension.

Practice tip. The pain during labor varies with the progress of labor and in intensity; sensitivity to pain varies greatly from individual to individual and must be dealt with sensitively.

Pain transmission. Pain impulses from the cervix and lower uterine segment are transmitted to the lumbar and thoracic spinal cord segments L1–T10. The pain of the late first and second stage are transmitted via the pudendal nerve to the sacral vertebrae S2–S4 (Fig. 7.75).

Pathophysiology. Birth pain is physiological; however fear and pain increase the contractions and can potentially compromise the fetus.

For example, maternal hyperventilation due to the pain of contractions can lead to hypocapnia, alkalosis, and decreased uteroplacental perfusion.

Note. It is the task of the obstetrician to ease the fear of birth (→ expectant fear) and tension (→ psychoprophylaxis) and to reduce the pain of labor (acupuncture, TENS, pharmacological pain relief). The limitations of pain relief have been reached when it endangers mother and fetus.

Psychoprophylaxis

Fear-spasm-pain syndrome (model of explanation for birthing disorders). The woman in labor perceives the pain as particularly strong because she fears the birth (Read). Fear is linked with tension and causes muscular tension (→ spasms cause pain), breathing disorders (→ hyperventilation) and vasoconstriction

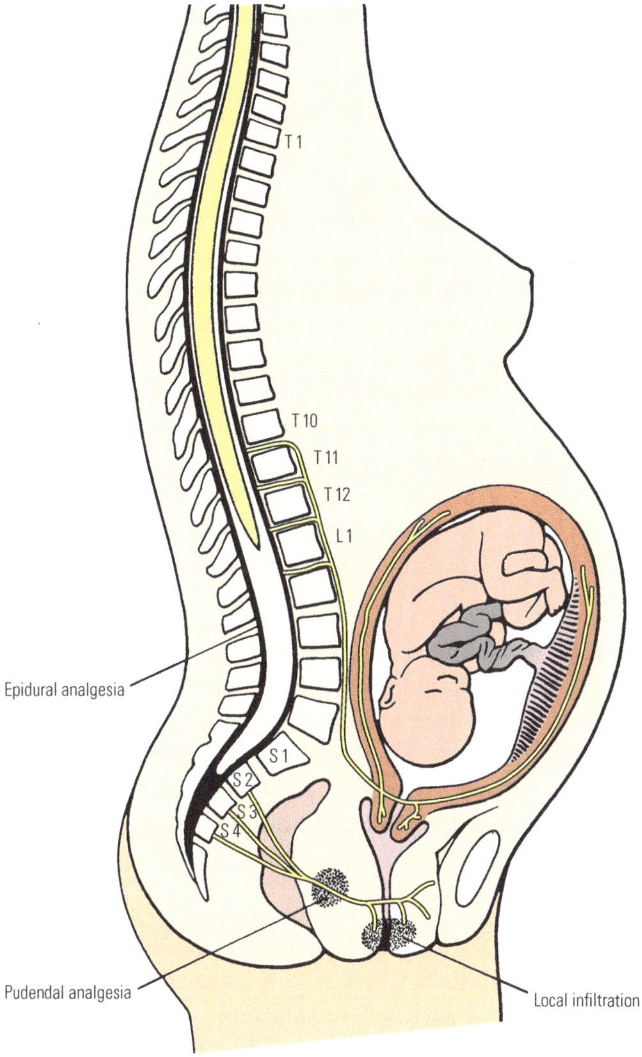

Fig. 7.75: Pain conduction and blockage (modified; after Baumann and Huch).

(→ intensify spasms) as well as affective oversensitivity (circulus vitiosus, vicious circle).

Note. Prophylaxis. Systematic antenatal preparation with education, exercises, relaxation exercises and breathing techniques.

Education

- 1–2 talks about birth and the reason for the prophylaxis, film presentation.
- Introduction of women who have recently given birth and can report on experiences.
- Discussion with the pregnant woman, answering of questions. Demonstration and practicing of different birth positions.

Practice tip. Exaggerated promises about the success of psychoprophylaxis are to be avoided. Goals: reduction of fear, perception of birth as individual, active process, aim for satisfactory birth experience.

Antenatal exercises. Loosening exercises have priority throughout the pregnancy. Goal: improved muscle control so that relaxation can be more easily achieved.

Contraindication. Women with a history of miscarriage or preterm delivery.

Practice tip. Women in late pregnancy should not perform strenuous exercises.

Relaxation exercise based on autogenic training (I.H. Schulz) with birth-related methodology.

- Breathing technique in first stage.
  - Until 4 cm dilatation: relaxed, deep breathing, with abdominal breathing in the intervals between contractions.
  - Between 5 and 10 cm dilatation: breathe in for 4 s, out slowly for 12–15 s. Complete relaxation during contractions as previously practiced with a certain amount of concentration on the breathing technique.
- Breathing technique in second stage. Bearing down in a supine or lateral position is only demonstrated, not practiced by the pregnant woman. One can, however, have the women lie on their backs, legs slightly drawn up (hands behind knees), take a deep breath and hold it for as long as possible. Practicing of panting for crowning.

Note. Women are to be cautioned that the contractions could become unbearable despite psychoprophylaxis, that despite all good intentions pharmacological pain relief (e.g., also for a cesarean) may be necessary. Some women have feelings of failure if they cannott manage a natural birth. The more successful the psychoprophylactic preparation the less pain medication is administered.

Gentle birth (according to Leboyer) does not have the goal of easing birth for the mother, but is expressly focused on the baby before and directly after birth. These considerations have been taken on by many obstetricians. A peaceful atmosphere in the delivery room, dimmed lighting at birth, and promotion of the mother-baby unit while still in the delivery room are consequences.

Positive conditioning (according to Lamaze) is implemented in many psychoprophylactic lessons in its original or adapted form. Relaxation and concentration on breathing exercises with the involvement of a birthing partner provide distraction from pain.

The success of psychoprophylaxis is dependent on:

- Motivation of the mother to learn.
- Opportunity to apply learnt techniques.
- Motivation and sensitivity of personnel.
- Normal course of labor.

Acupuncture, TENS

Acupuncture is used successfully for non-pharmalogical pain relief in the first stage; it is reserved for experienced practitioners who have completed additional training. Women are to be cautioned despite acupuncture there coule be severe contractions and analgesics be then be necessary.

TENS, transcutaneous electrical nerve stimulation. TENS is a noninvasive mechanical method which stimulates sensory skin receptors via electrostimulation. The intensity of the impulses can be regulated by the woman herself. Success in early first stage has been reported. Analgesic use is reportedly reduced in this time period if TENS is employed.

Pain relief drugs

Principle. Allowances must be made for the physiological adaptation of the organism in pregnancy and labor with regards to pain relief and anesthesia: disruption of feto-maternal gas exchange and uterine or placental perfusion are to be avoided. The fetal pharmacological metabolism is to be taken into account.

Analgesics (pain relief medication, painkillers) are classified according to the region affected (earlier mistakenly classified as central or peripheral analgesics), effectiveness (strong or weak analgesics, also incorrect, as dependent on indication) or according to the type (currently preferred):

- Nonopioid analgesics have a partly peripheral effect (inhibition of synthesis of inflammatory mediators such as prostaglandins, with nonsteroidal antiinflammatory drugs – NSAIDs), and work partly via central mechanisms; frequently with additional antipyretic and anti-inflammatory effect (metamizole and paracetamol do not have an antiinflammatory effect).
- Opioid analgesics act partly on 3 opiate receptors (δ-, χ-, μ-receptors and their subtypes, see below) of pain neurons in brain and spinal cord. The prototype is morphine.
- Special analgesics. Certain types of pain need special treatment: glyceryl trinitrate for angina attacks and sometimes abdominal colic (see below), pilocarpine for glaucoma, sumatriptan for migraine.

Note. The majority of pain relief in labor is provided by: opioid analgesics, of which pethidine/meperidine is preferred; nitrous oxide analgesia and regional anesthesia: epidural block, patient-controlled epidural anesthesia (PCEA), combined spinal-epidural anesthesia (CSE), pudendal block.

Pethidine/meperidine is a synthetic opioid analgesic which acts on the μ-receptors.
Indication. Maternal pain in labor, promotion of cervical dilatation.
Dosage. If contractions are regular 50 mg IM, may be repeated after 4 hours. Maximum daily dose 100 mg. Mechanism of action. Morphine-like agonist, primarily on the central and spinal μ-receptors, spasmolysis of the birth canal, rarely constipation.
Pharmacokinetics. Effect after 4–10 min, maximum effect after 1 h, effective for 3–5 h, elimination half-life 3–4 h. Norpethidine is a metabolite which causes convulsions (tremor, cramps) with a longer half-life (> 15 h)
Side effect. Increased risk of fetal acidosis, in particular if CTG is pathological. The effect of respiratory depression on the neonate is dependent on the interval between administration of pethidine and birth, dosage and method of application.

Practice tip. Neonatal respiratory depression is highest 2–3 h after administration of pethidine.

Further side effects. Dysphoria, mild tachycardia (increased myocardial oxygen consumption), histamine release (frequently causes wheals at injection site and along the vein), rarely full-blown allergic reaction with shock, bronchospasms.
Sedatives and **tranquilizers** (e.g., benzodiazepine derivatives) should not be used for pain relief due to multiple side effects: respiratory depression and drinking difficulties of the newborn, floppy infant.

Inhalation analgesia with nitrous oxide. Laughing gas (N_2O) or enflurane in oxygen, or methoxyflurane in air are easy to use (selfadministration with inhalation mask). Rapid action!

The inhalation timepoint must be considered: begin N_2O inhalation 50–60 s before contraction peaks!

Conduction anesthesia

Definition. Nerve or transmission block; form of local analgesia with perineural anesthetic application along the path of the nerve. Most common are:

- Epidural block, continuous lumbar epidural anesthesia (→ central nervous blockade).
- Pudendal block (→ peripheral blockade).

Continuous lumbar epidural block (Fig. 7.76). Intervertebral puncture between L_3 and L_4 or L_2 and L_3 and introduction of an epidural catheter.

Note. Freedom from pain occurs after administration of anesthesia (dosage: 10ml 0.175 % ropivacaine, with 40 µg fentanyl), also for vaginal assisted delivery and cesarean section (dosage: 20–30 ml 0.75 % ropivacaine, with 30–50 µg fentanyl).

Positioning. The spread of the anesthetic in the epidural space is dependent on the maternal position, which varies in labor, in order to reach the relevant spinal sections (see Fig. 7.76):
- In first stage a supine position is required.
- In second stage a semisitting position.

Contraindications for epidural block are: infection at the injection site, clinical signs of a coagulation disorder, allergy to local anesthetic, severe hypotension, and hypovolemia. Neurological or cardiac disorders can be relative contraindications, they require individual assessment.
Indications for epidural block:
- Pain relief.
- Prolonged labor due to cervical dystocia.
- Anesthesia for vaginal operative procedures (vacuum extraction, forceps, manual exploration of the uterus), cesarean.
- Improvement of placental perfusion in hypertension.
- Multiple birth.
- Breech delivery.
- Preterm delivery.

Note. The continuous epidural block is the most effective method of pain relief in labor and has positive effects on maternal breathing and uterine perfusion due to the reduction of painful contractions.

Side effects. Arterial hypotension, loss of pelvic floor tone in cephalic births with malpresentations, and deflexed attitudes.

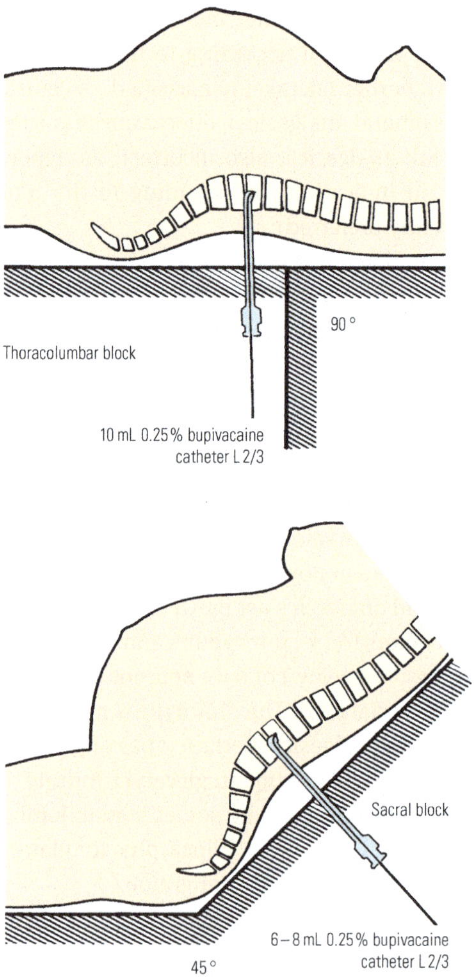

Fig. 7.76: Epidural anesthesia, above in first stage, below in second stage (after Dick and colleagues).

These effects can largely be avoided by prior administration of 500 ml electrolyte infusion, or rather a dose reduction in the second stage. Prospective studies have shown an insignificant lengthening of labor duration of approximately 30 min; an increase in the rate of cesarean sections or assisted vaginal births was not found.

Post-dural headache. In 1–2 % of epidural blocks the dura is accidentally punctured. The resulting headache may require treatment postpartum. It should, however, be borne in mind that 30 % of women complain of headaches after SVD.

Treatment:
- The commonly prescribed bed rest and increased oral fluid intake are not convincingly effective in treatment of post-dural headache.
- Nonopioid analgesics have been proven to be effective, (500 mg oral paracetamol, up to 4 x daily) or 300 mg oral caffeine.
- If headache is severe, an epidural blood patch (EBP) is indicated (10–20 ml of autologous blood is injected into the epidural space at the level of the dural punction or one segment lower).

Epidural block modifications are PCEA and CSE.

PCEA. Patient-controlled epidural anesthesia is a further development of the epidural block: the laboring woman self-administers fractional doses of the analgesic.

CSE. The combined spinal-epidural block, walking epidural, fulfills the requirements of pain relief in labor outstandingly:

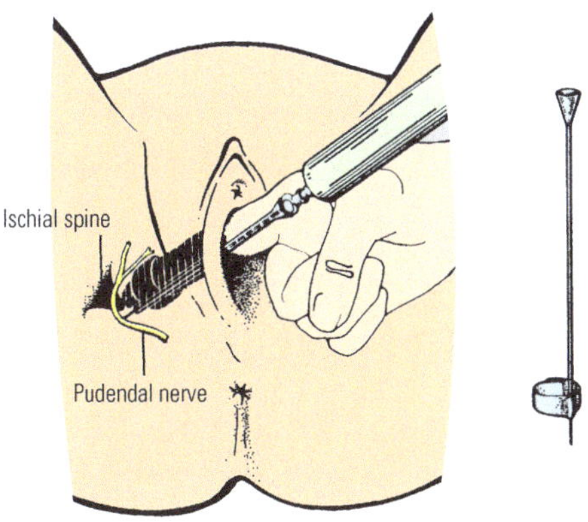

Fig. 7.77: Vaginal pudendal block.

- Rapid reduction of the pain of contractions.
- No influence on contractions.
- The laboring woman can get out of bed and ambulate.

Procedure. The epidural space is found, and then an atraumatic spinal needle is inserted through the epidural needle into the subarachnoid space. After administration of opioids (e.g., 5–10 µg sufentanil or 10–25 µg fentanyl) the spinal needle is removed and the epidural catheter inserted.
Pain relief occurs within 5 min, analgesia lasts 2–3 h. If further analgesia is required epidural anesthesia is provided with bupivacaine or ropivacaine.
Pudendal block (Fig. 7.77). In this pudendal vaginal anesthesia, 10 ml of a 1 % mepivacaine solution are injected with a long needle into the loose tissue on both sides of the vagina 1 cm caudal (towards the vulva) from the ischial spines, i.e., immediately below the palpated spinae. Aspiration must be attempted before each injection to exclude intravascular infusion.

Note. Indications. Spontaneous vaginal delivery, forceps and vacuum delivery, episiotomy and perineal suturing.

7.4.2 Management of second stage

Definition. Second stage begins with complete dilatation of the external os and ends with the birth of the baby; the last part of second stage is characterized by the active participation of the woman in labor (bearing down).

The following are discussed in order: laboring woman in second stage, fetus in second stage, perineal support.

The laboring woman in second stage: bearing down contractions, birth position, bearing down, breathing

Expulsive period with bearing down or second stage contractions. The work of delivery is now, in addition to the uterine contractions (smooth muscle of the corpus uteri), performed by the trunk (abdominal or secondary) muscles, striated muscles of the torso, defecation muscles. At the end of first stage, the leading part (head, buttocks) has filled the upper part of the soft tissue canal (lower uterine segment, cervical canal).

In the second stage, the leading part is expelled from the upper sections of the soft tissue canal into and through the lower sections (vagina, pelvic floor, perineum, vulva, extension of the soft tissue canal), whereby these parts are simultaneously distended.

Note. Effect of bearing down contractions. Expulsion of the head which has reached the pelvic floor in a curve around the pubic symphysis with distension of the extension of the soft tissue canal (see above) so that the head may pass through it.

Trigger for bearing down contractions. The contractions can be voluntarily initiated as long as the head has not reached the pelvic floor. On descent of the head they are triggered reflexively by spinal nerve pathways, are thus no longer subject to the will of the laboring woman.

Bearing down or pushing becomes an irresistible urge. The bearing down contractions become increasingly powerful; in the end the woman is pushing extremely hard using the muscles of the entire body, so that her whole body trembles.

Practice tip. Do not allow to bear down too early, not until the irresistible urge is there. Midwife question: Is there rectal pressure? Multiparae in particular tend to bear down early, which is not a good idea.

Conditions. Bearing down is allowed under the following conditions:

- Cervix is fully dilated.
- Membranes have ruptured.
- Head has descended, in the best case has reached the pelvic floor (maneuvers p. 164).

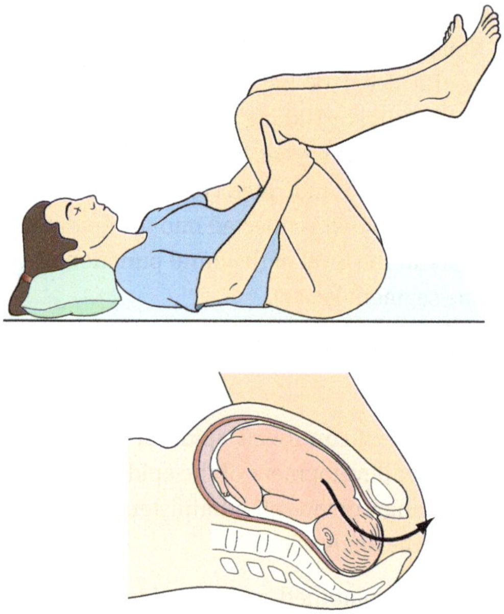

Fig. 7.78: Posture and birth route during second stage in a supine position. The baby is born around the pubic symphysis.

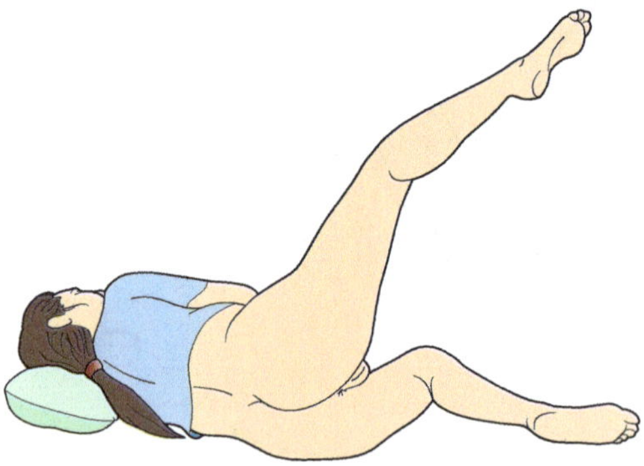

Fig. 7.79: Lateral position of the laboring woman in second stage.

- Sagittal suture is in the anteroposterior diameter.

Complications of bearing down too early:
- Head rotation is impaired → delivery is delayed, possible persistent occipitotransverse presentation.
- Unnecessary tiring of the laboring woman.
- Spontaneous cervix laceration (rare!).
- Pinched cervical lip.

Options for birthing positions during expulsive contractions
- Supine (Fig. 7.78), also semirecumbent, knees drawn up, back must not be overarched, sacrum and lumbar spine should lie flat.
- Left lateral position (Fig. 7.79), right leg is held or supported.
- Lithotomy position.
- Standing, supported from behind by partner, possibly holding on to a rope or wall bars.
- Squatting (Fig. 7.80), a birthing stool may be used.
- Kneeling.
- On all fours (Fig. 7.81).
- Knee-chest position (Fig. 7.82) on the birthing bed or a mat; the midwife stands or kneels behind the woman. She covers the anus with a cloth in one hand and regulates descent of the head with the other.

Supine birth position. Advantages:
- Delayed passage of the head with better adaptation of the perineum.
- Familiar and relaxed position for the woman.
- Good possibility for intervention for the obstetrician.

Disadvantages:
- Possible feeling of impotence and lack of self-determination.

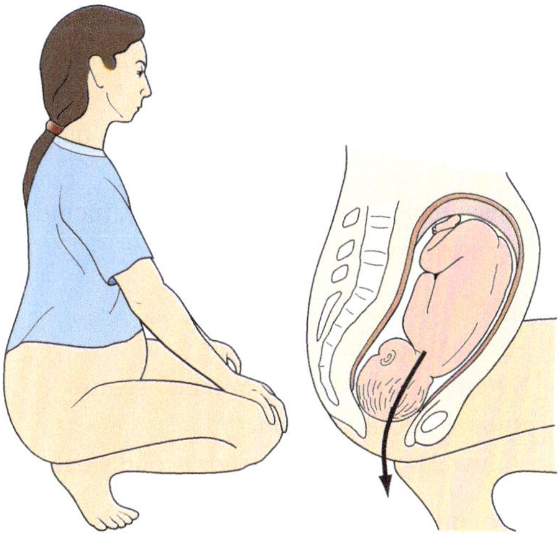

Fig. 7.80: Posture and birth route during second stage in a squatting position. The baby is born with gravity.

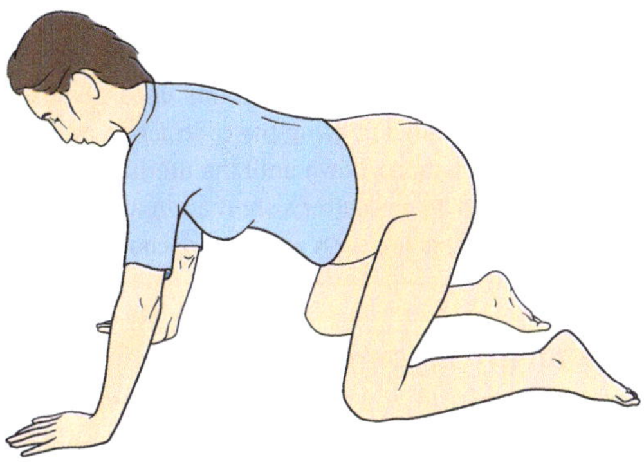

Fig. 7.81: Laboring woman on all fours.

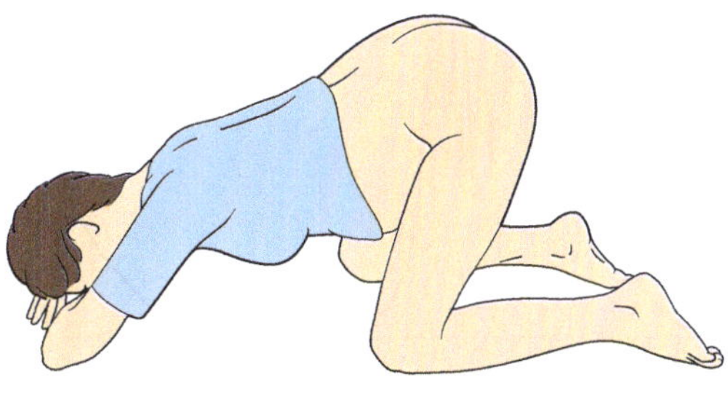

Fig. 7.82: Laboring woman in knee-elbow position.

Upright birth position. Advantages:
- Utilization of gravity and acceleration of second stage.
- Laboring woman feels she has had a natural birth.
- Lower incidence of perineal injury, including episiotomy.

Disadvantages:
- Perineal protection difficult.
- Strenuous for laboring women because unused to this position.
- Vulvar edema in prolonged second stage.

Active bearing down (Fig. 7.83). The force exerted by bearing down is dependent on the timepoint at which it supports the lapsing uterine contraction.

Practice tip. Active bearing down is not begun (arrow in Fig. 7.83) until the peak (acme) of the uterine contraction has been reached. Most women do this unconsciously correctly; this is called utilizing the contraction properly: do not allow bearing down until the uterine contraction has reached its peak after a short approach. Others begin bearing down too soon and require coaching.

Breathing. The correct, practiced breathing technique minimizes the abdominal cavity and provides a firm resistance which the laboring woman can work against.

Breathing technique. At the beginning of the contraction a deep breath is taken, then at the height of the contraction the breath is held, mouth closed, and instead of breathing out the head is bent (chin to chest) and all strength is put into bearing down (like straining at bowel movement).

Coaching. The midwife instructs the woman regarding active bearing down: not to scream or bear down without bending her head; how to utilize the contraction correctly and not to begin bearing down until the uterine contraction is at its peak.

The fetus in the second stage, caput succedaneum, cephalhematoma

Practice tip. The second stage is a vulnerable period for the fetus: cardiotocography is now essential! If cardiotocography is not used, the heart tones are to be auscultated after every contraction until the head has been fully born.

Caput succedaneum

Definition. Cap-like swelling of the skin and loose cellular tissue of the fetal part which led in labor (leading part). The result of serous (and bloody) infiltration of the tissue between galea and periosteum = supraperiosteal edema or serous hematoma (Fig. 7.86).

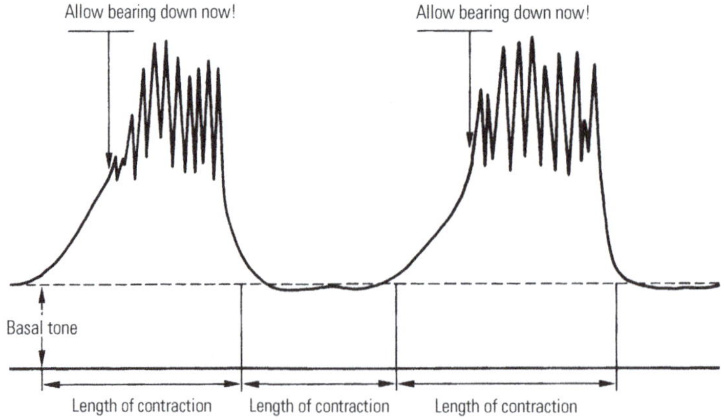

Fig. 7.83: Active bearing down, arrow (↓) indicates when to begin bearing down.

Cause. The loss of the membranes results in the head being constricted by the soft tissues of the birth canal. Extreme forces and counterforces are hereby applied: the head is forced towards the pelvic outlet, the rim of the cervix works against this by binding the head and holding it back, slowing its descent.

Circular tourniquet. The soft tissues are applied to the head as a girdle, a 1–1.5 cm wide contact girdle. The effect of this soft tissue ring is known as the tourniquet effect; it compresses the head firmly with three consequences:

1. Parietal bones, which till now lay next to one another, are forced on top of each other (overlapping, molding):
   a) In LOA the left below the right (Fig. 7.84).
   b) In ROA the right below the left (Fig. 7.85).

Since the right parietal bone is anterior, and thus somewhat inferior, and hereby leading in LOA (and the left in ROA), it can be seen that the posterior, superior parietal bone is forced under the anterior and inferior parietal bone. Or: what was once anterior (and leading) remains anterior and leading.

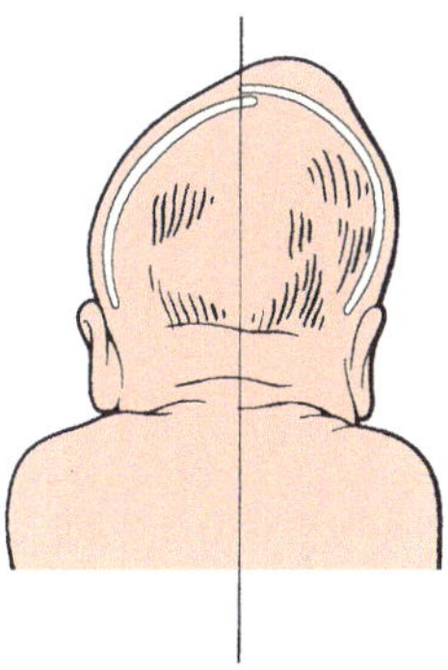

Fig. 7.84: Molding of the skull and development of caput succedaneum in LOA: left parietal bone is forced under the right.

The part of the head below the tourniquet of the soft tissue ring is under less pressure than the rest of the head above the tourniquet ring. Two changes occur in the area of lower pressure, that is on the cap of the head born into the vagina; consequences 2 and 3 of the circular tourniquet.

2. Puckering of the skin. The skin is pushed together below the soft tissue ring, it puckers and develops folds.
3. Development of the caput succedaneum. Veins are occluded in the scalp below the soft tissue ring, while the tourniquet effect is not sufficient to obstruct the arteries. Consequence:
   a) Venous congestion, venous hyperemia with serous exudation into the part of the scalp which lies in the vagina

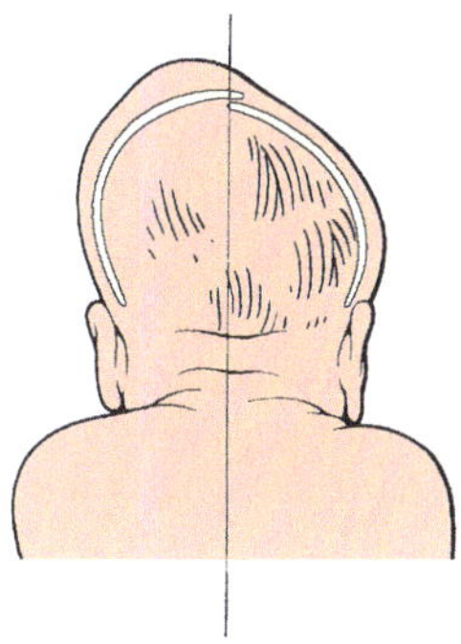

Fig. 7.85: Molding of the skull and development of caput succedaneum in ROA: right parietal bone is forced under the left.

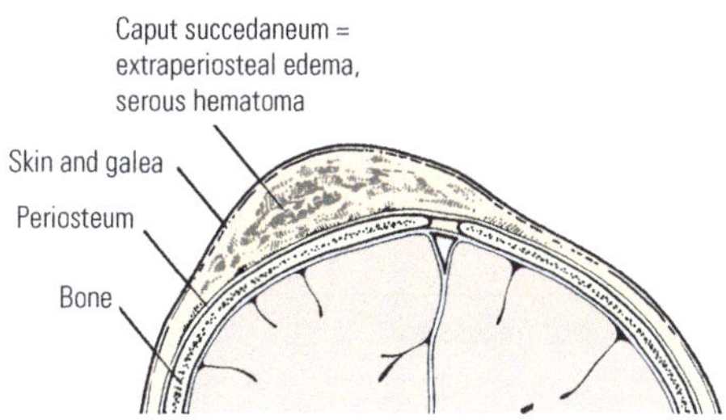

Fig. 7.86: Caput succedaneum.

below the soft tissue ring. This is the lowermost presenting part, the leading part.

The exudation of serum into tissues, which during prolonged labor is also linked with tissue laceration and hemorrhage, causes the formation of a cap-like swelling, the caput succedaneum.
The caput occurs on the anterior and therefore inferior portion of the presenting part:
- In a **left** cephalic presentation (LOA) near the posterior fontanelle on the right parietal bone.
- In a **right** cephalic presentation (ROA) near the posterior fontanelle on the left parietal bone.

Size. Two factors determine the extent of the caput: duration of labor after ROM, in addition to strength and duration of contractions. This means the size is the same in: long labor and weak contractions, short labor and strong contractions.

Practice tip. A caput succedaneum is the watch of the obstetrician: prolonged labor and strong contractions cause a rapidly growing and particularly large caput. Slow progress in labor despite strong contractions damages the fetus!

Cephalhematoma

Definition. Hematoma between the periosteum and the bone, subperiosteal hematoma which raises the periosteum; markedly fluctuating, pigeon- to hen's-egg sized, semicircular pathological swelling on the skull in newborns (Fig. 7.87, Tab. 7.3).

Incidence. Much rarer (0.5 % of births) than caput succedaneum!

Cause. Tearing of blood vessels between periosteum and bone during passage of the head in labor as a result of displacement of the soft tissues on the flat skull bones (pressure difference between parts of the head below and above the tourniquet).

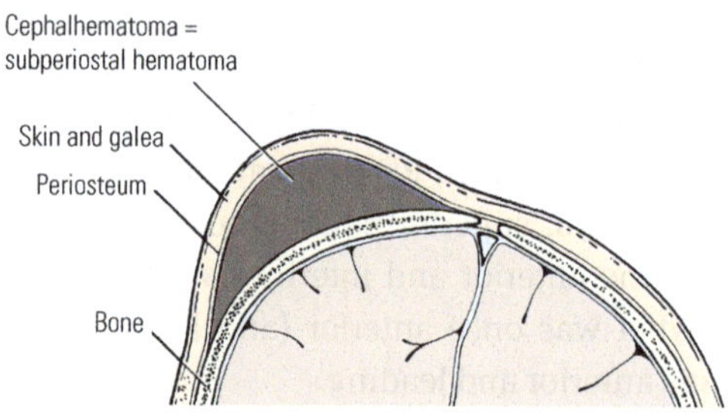

Fig. 7.87: Cephalhematoma.

Tab. 7.3: Differential diagnosis between caput succedaneum and cephalhematoma.

	Caput succedaneum = **supra**perisoteal edema, Fig. 7.86	**Cephalhematoma = sub**periosteal hematoma, Fig. 7.87
Extent	Diffuse spread across sutures (Caput is caused by the mechanics of labor, see above)	Never crosses the sutures (anatomically impossible, see above)
Consistency	**Doughy**, edematous	**Fluctuating**, cystic
Size and Development	Largest at birth, usually goes down within a day	Develops to full size within the first days of life and remains unchanged for 8–16 weeks
Treatment	Not necessary	No special treatment necessary. If skin damaged, sterile bandage. Vitamin K to increase serum Prothrombin levels = stops further hemorrhage

Note. In contrast to the caput succedaneum, the cephalhematoma cannot cross the sutures, as the periosteum is attached to the bone at the sutures; it is restricted to one bone!
Puncturing of caput succedaneum or cephalhematoma is **contraindicated.** Puncture can lead to abscess → life-threatening for the infant.

Guarding the perineum

Definition. Maneuvers to regulate the speed of crowning and birth of the head and to prevent perineal laceration on birth of the head.

Practice tip. Perineal protection must not be attempted too early, or crowning will be hindered!

Preparation. Disinfection of hands and lower arms as prescribed, sterile gloves.

Note. Main goal is slowing down the birth of the head; guarding the perineum brakes the head (!).

The head should pass over the perineum slowly, over the course of several contractions, to allow the perineal tissues sufficient time to stretch.
The head should be born with the smallest possible circumference (most favorable plane), which is the suboccipitobregmatic plane in occipitoanterior presentations: 32 cm circumference.
Birth of the head is less favorable in all other presentations.

- In anteroposterior presentations the broad, firm occiput must be born over the perineum.
- In deflexed attitudes the plane of passage is also greater than in anteroposterior presentations.
- Brow presentation is the least favorable with the occipitomental plane: 35.5 cm circumference.

Practice tip. The plane of passage can only be minimally influenced with perineal protection maneuvers.

Indication. Readiness to protect the perineum in:

- Primiparous women when the head appears for the first time in the labia in the depths of the vagina, but recedes once the contraction has ended.
- Multiparous women when the head has reached the pelvic cavity.

The perineum is protected when the head crowns, that is, when it does not recede after the contraction but remains in the vulva.

Technique (Fig. 7.88). If the birthing woman is in a supine position, the midwife stands on her right. The legs are to be spread apart and drawn up firmly. The pelvis is raised with a firm cushion or by raising the height of the pelvic section of the bed.

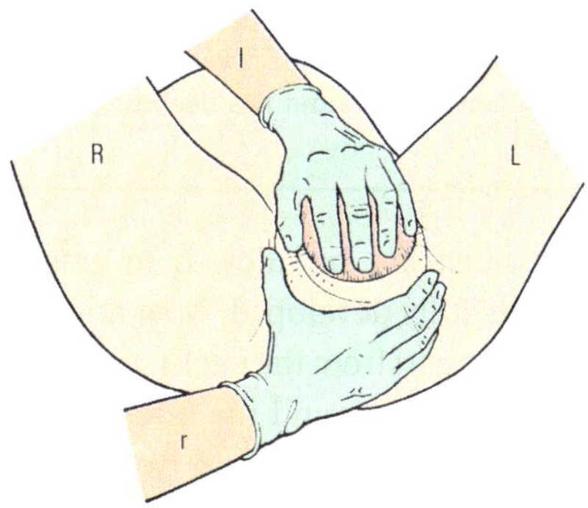

Fig. 7.88: Perineal guarding (the drape is not pictured).

Note. The **head** is to be held in such a way that the speed of passage and birth can be controlled.

The **left hand** lies on the part of the head which is being born and controls (with the right hand) the speed of birth. At the same time, it is also

responsible for ensuring that the head passes through in the smallest possible plane.
The fingertips hold the brow back or, to the same end, press the occiput towards the perineum away from the symphysis pubis until the occiput has emerged from under it (→ prevention of premature extension) and the suboccipital region can impinge against it.

Right hand. Thumb, second and third finger are spread over the perineum. The aim is to palpate the frontal tubercles of the head, which should be easily palpated through the well-stretched perineum.

The perineum is not directly touched; a sterile cloth is used. The edge of the perineum is never to be covered up; at least 1 cm must be uncovered.
The **right hand supports the left** in slowing the speed of delivery: the fingers are spread and placed on the frontal tubercles and exert a firm counterpressure on the forehead during every contraction.

Practice tip. The forehead remains covered by the edge of the perineum until the occiput has been born under the pubic arch.

The occiput must not be allowed to emerge freely until it is fully developed. Now no other part of the head apart from the neck (suboccipital region) can pivot around the inferior edge of the pubic symphysis; the head can only be born in the most favorable plane, the suboccipitobregmatic plane (32 cm circumference).

Note. The perineal protection maneuvers serve primarily to slow down the speed of passage of the crowning head, to ensure it stays well-flexed and is brought millimeter by millimeter into the furthermost extension of the soft tissue canal, so that it can then be allowed to make the necessary exit movement (extension only in anteroposterior presentation).
Perineal protection is not, however, written in stone!

Episiotomy. If the muscular soft tissue canal is of unfavorable width or elasticity (perineum too high, thick or rigid, narrow vulvo-vaginal opening, narrow pubic arch, particularly in older primiparous women) an episiotomy can be performed.

Practice tip. The perineum becomes pale immediately before laceration occurs.

It does not depend on the perineum, but on the pelvic floor! Someone with a good perineal protection technique is definitely capable of guarding the high, rigid perineum of an older primipara. It does not depend so much on the perineum, but rather on the pelvic floor. As a result of extremely long-lasting and unbearable tension of the pelvic floor muscles and fascia, unnoticed subacute lacerations occur (with intact perineum), substantial vaginal tears are not infrequent. At the very least the shanks of the bulbocavernosus muscle, the deep transverse perineal muscle and particularly the anterior part of the levator ani are extremely overdistended, and can tear at the point of attachment on the pubic arch, even tear off completely.
Birth of the head is often drawn out. The expulsive phase is overlong, which endangers the fetus. Cause is usually a slowing down of expulsive contractions.

Hastening the birth of the head. The woman is asked to bear down without a contraction. If this does not work, one of the following maneuvers is used:
- Ritgen maneuver = posterior perineal maneuver (Fig. 7.89). Posterior perineum: area between the tip of the tailbone and anus. One hand lies on the visible part of the head, as for perineal protection, the other is placed on the posterior perineum and the chin, which is usually easily palpable, is found. Pad or cloth on the anus! By

exerting a strong, pushing pressure on the chin the head is slowly pressed out of the soft tissue canal. An assistant can perform the Kristeller maneuver at the same time if necessary.

- Kristeller maneuver, transfundal pressure (expulsion of the baby). The assistant stands at the side of the laboring woman, waits for a contraction or stimulates one by carefully rubbing the fundus. Then the fundus is gripped with one or both hands and slowly increasing pressure is exerted in the direction of the pelvic axis. This maneuver is not to be performed with extreme force. Even the correct application is controversial; the hoped-for shortening of second stage could not be demonstrated. The maneuver is **not indicated** in cases of prior uterine surgery (e.g., cesarean section).

If the head has still not reached and passed over the perineum, the following methods can be considered:

- Speculum delivery, forceps, vacuum extraction. When performed with gentle, skilled hands, these methods damage mother and baby less than expectant management and prolonged bearing down in second stage.

Delivery of shoulders, trunk, hips

Delivery of the shoulders. Protection of the perineum is not concluded with delivery of the head. The shoulders need to be delivered. The perineum is in acute danger if it is not performed correctly.

Expectant management is called for between delivery of the head and delivery of the shoulders: birth of the trunk should occur spontaneously with one of the next contractions.
If the baby is hypoxic or the interval between contractions lasts too long, the shoulders are to be delivered immediately.

Shoulder delivery in two acts (Fig. 7.90). The head has performed its fourth or external rotation: it has turned to face the mother's thigh (in LOA the right, in ROA the left).

The anterior shoulder is delivered first (act 1), which corresponds to the natural mechanism of birth (see Fig. 7.90): the hands are placed flat on the parietal bones and cheeks with the thumbs pointing towards occiput or sinciput and in this hold the head is pressed towards the perineum, that is downwards, until the anterior shoulder appears under the pubic arch.

Practice tip. Do not pull. Press downwards!

The pelvis must be raised in order to be able to lower the head sufficiently: pelvic cushion, raised pelvic section of the birthing bed.
Delivery of the posterior shoulder (see Fig. 7.91) is act 2. The head is carefully raised towards the pubic symphysis, with continued transfundal pressure, until the posterior shoulder has been born over the perineum.

Note. All movements are slow, gentle and made with a light hand and no abrupt movements. Increased risk of perineal laceration.

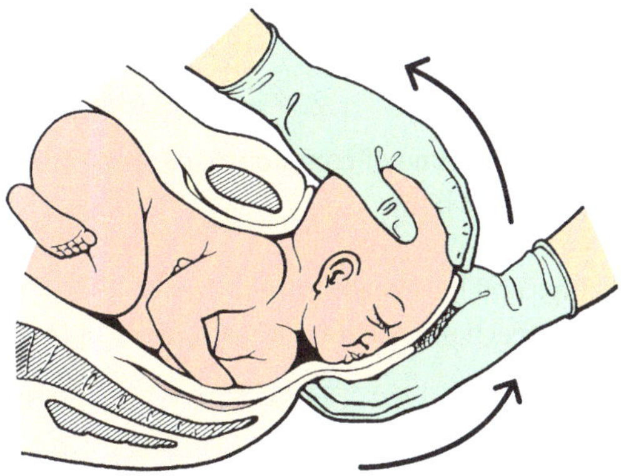

Fig. 7.89: Ritgen maneuver.

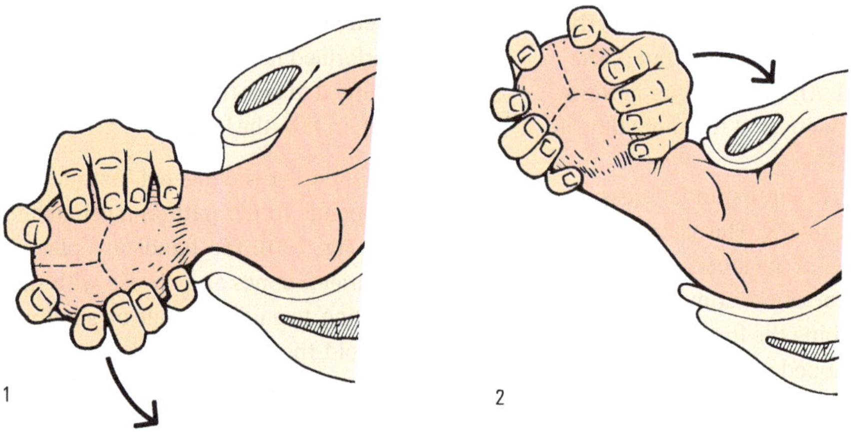

Fig. 7.90: Delivery of the shoulders. Acts 1 (anterior shoulder) and 2 (posterior shoulder).

Delivery of the trunk. Fixation. Cautious traction is applied in the direction of the extended pelvic axis. After the first shoulder has been released, one finger is placed in the axilla from behind, the same after delivery of the posterior shoulder, in order to have a better grip on the baby (Stoeckel).

Delivery of hips and legs. The trunk is lowered in order for the anterior hip to emerge from under the pubic symphysis, and then the posterior shoulder is allowed to pass over the perineum by raising the trunk (taking care of the perineum!).

Birth time, cutting the cord, signs of maturity

Birth time

Definition. Time of complete separation from the mother's body:
- In vertex presentations after delivery of the hips and lower extremities.
- In breech presentation after delivery of the head.

Cutting the cord

Definition. Aseptic severance of the umbilical cord, a hand's width from the baby's umbilicus after the cord has been clamped on either side of the planned cut.

Note. Timing of aseptic cord severance: immediate, early and delayed.

Immediate. Cutting of the cord as soon as possible, directly after the baby is delivered.

Indication. Hemolytic disease of the fetus. Prevents antibody transfer from placental blood to the baby. If the mother is only Rhesus negative immediate severance is not indicated.

Early. Cutting of the cord after initial care of the newborn (aspiration of mucus from mouth and throat): 1–1.5 min after birth.

Indication. Normal method with mature baby.

Delayed. Cutting of the cord after transfer of blood from the placenta (→cord has stopped pulsating) until 5 min after birth.

This results in an increase of the total blood volume of the newborn by one quarter to one third because placental blood is transferred (a hydrostatic concentration gradient between the site of placental attachment and the newborn must be present).

Indication. Babies at risk of anemia: preterm babies, multiple gestations.

Note. The transfusion of placental blood due to late clamping can lead to hypervolemia, respiratory disorders and hyperbilirubinemia.

Blood from umbilical artery and veins. The ascertainment of the pH level and blood gases in umbilical artery and veins is a part of the assessment of the neonate's condition alongside the Apgar score. The procedure is strongly recommended as a method of obstetrical quality control.

Technique. Blood for blood gas analysis is drawn from both cord blood vessels directly after birth and clamping of the cord. Interpretation see p. 436.

Signs of maturity

Definition. Criteria of maturity of a neonate:

Note. The mature neonate is rosy, cries loudly immediately, moves actively, and can suck powerfully.

External characteristics of the mature neonate:
- Length. 49–52 cm (length from crown to heel). Measurement is best made using a measuring tray (orthopedic surgeons advise against the earlier method of measurement by hanging the baby upside-down from its calves!). Length is an important sign of maturity.
- Weight 3,000–3,500 g.
- Nails extend beyond the tips of fingers or toes.
- The skin of preterm babies is bright red (erythema neonatorum), as subcutaneous fatty tissue is missing.
- Umbilicus lies in the middle between symphysis and xiphoid process.
- Testes are in the scrotum. Descensus testis is concluded.
- Labia majora close the vulva; labia minora and clitoris are completely covered.

The diameters and circumferences of the mature baby listed on p. 141 are very important indicators of its maturity and need to be evaluated as such.

7.5 Management of third stage

Definition. Time from birth of the baby until expulsion of the placenta, which separates from its site of attachment.

Note. Main goal is avoidance of unnecessary blood loss during placental separation and emptying of the uterus.

Mechanisms of placental separation

Note. Placental separation is based on area displacement (reduction of the inner surface of the uterus) as a result of uterine contraction and retraction.

X-ray examinations have shown that separation begins at the end of second stage in some cases, during expulsive contractions.

Normally, however, placental separation does not occur until the baby has been born, with contractions. The placenta is completely separated after the first or second strong contraction. The site of placental attachment on the uterus wall becomes smaller with every separation contraction. The placenta, which cannot contract and can therefore not reduce its size, becomes to a certain extent too large, and it is sheared off the uterine wall.

Decidua basalis is the layer within which placental separation occurs. Separation occurs in the maternal part, decidua spongiosa, the part of the decidua basalis which is the most loosely constructed and offers the least resistance to separation.

Grey outer layer. A part of the decidua basalis remains as a grey outer layer on the maternal side of the separated placenta, outermost tissue layer of the maternal placenta.

Physiological separation bleeding, retroplacental hematoma. When the placenta separates from the decidua spongiosa, blood vessels are torn off and open: blood flows into the free space between the wall of the uterus and the detached surface of the placenta. The thus created retroplacental hematoma becomes progressively larger due to continuing blood flow and thus supports the detachment of the placenta from its site of attachment. Some of the blood flows out of the vagina during or after placental separation, the remainder is attached to the maternal side of the placenta as clot. Blood loss on vaginal delivery 200–400 ml.

Increased blood loss on placental separation. Blood loss > 400 ml (nonmedicated third stage).

Separation mechanisms. The mechanism by which a placenta separates depends upon its location: central, lateral or eccentric separation.

Schultze mechanism (Fig. 7.91; obstetrician in Jena, Germany, 1827–1919). Separation begins in the center (central separation); most common mechanism: 80 %! The center of the placenta detaches first, leads, and appears first in the vulva.

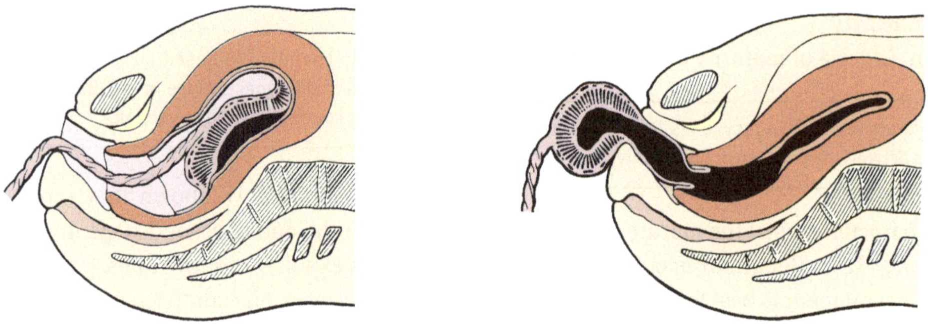

Fig. 7.91: Central placental separation, Schultze mechanism.

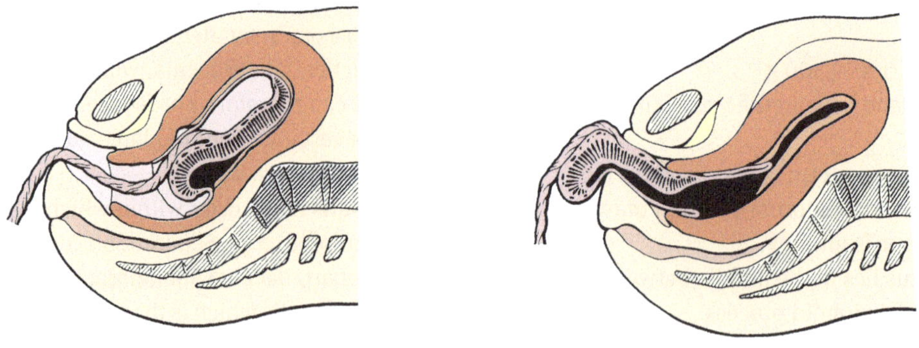

Fig. 7.92: Lateral placental separation, Duncan mechanism.

Duncan mechanism (Fig. 7.92; obstetrician in Edinburgh, Schottland, 1826–1890). Separation begins at the lower margin (lateral or eccentric separation) and continues from bottom to top. The lower edge of the placenta is born first. Incidence 20 %.

Note. Bleeding is continuous throughout separation in the Duncan mechanism. The volume of blood lost is greater than with the Schultze mechanism of placental separation.

Once separated, the placenta lies in the uterine cavity and is expelled into the birth canal by further contractions.

Duration. Placental separation and expulsion take 10–20 min if pharmacological prophylaxis is not administered.

Hemostasis on the site of attachment. Once the placenta has been expelled, two factors play a role in hemostasis. If one of these mechanisms fails, blood loss will be greater and last longer:

Uterine contraction with muscular ligature of the vessels. The muscle fibers intertwined around the blood vessels clamp the vessels and pull them closed (muscular ligature). As uterine contraction and relaxation alternate, a second mechanism is necessary.
Clots are formed in the openings to the blood vessels of the site of placental attachment.

Practice tip. Hemostasis does not occur in coagulation disorders (hypofibrinogenemia, afibrinogenemia, p. 377); even if the uterus is firmly contracted and maximum muscular ligature has been achieved!

Note. The goal of active management of third stage is to reduce blood loss by emptying the uterus early and removal of the placenta. Methods of choice are: pharmacological prevention of hemorrhage and birth of the placenta using controlled cord traction.

Pharmoacological prophylaxis. Directly after birth until delivery of the placenta:
- Rapid infusion (500 ml/h) oxytocin solution (6 IU in 500 ml basic solution) or
- 1 ampule (1ml) methylergometrin IM (in common use, but poor controllability).

Average blood loss in the third stage and the postplacental period is lower, and high blood losses are reduced.
At the same time, there is controversy as to whether this prophylaxis should be administered routinely or upon indication.

Controlled cord traction (CCT). As soon as the first marked uterus contraction occurs, the placenta is removed by applying cord traction.

CCT method. Controlled cord traction requires some practice. One quickly develops a feeling as to whether the placenta will be extracted easily or not:
- The woman remains in the birthing position with legs drawn up and knees bent. Midwife or obstetrician places the left hand flat and without pressure on the fundal region directly after birth of the baby and checks the status of uterine contraction.
- At onset of the first strong contraction (the classical signs of placental separation are not waited for), the hand lying on the abdomen presses the abdomen lightly above the symphysis pubis and thus pushes the uterus towards the back and up (correcting the curve of the birth axis).
- At the same time, light, even traction is applied with the right hand, around which the cord has been wrapped 2 or 3 times, in line with the birth axis, which causes the placenta to be expelled. The placenta follows cord traction immediately, when traction is applied at the right time. The right time means that traction is begun as soon as the first strong uterine contraction is felt by the hand lying on the abdomen. Other-

wise there is a risk that the placenta will be retained due to a spasm of the internal os.
- 24 minutes lie between birth of the baby and the first uterine contraction (if pharmacological prophylaxis is used).

Complications. Placenta does not follow the pull of traction, torn cord, increased bleeding (p. 380), and uterine inversion.

Placenta does not respond to traction. A second and a third contraction are waited for and the maneuver is repeated. If the placenta does not respond to traction, it is either not separated, or incompletely separated (separation normally occurs with the first or second contraction after birth of the baby), or the placenta has separated and is retained due to a cervical spasm.

Procedure. If the classical separation signs are absent, they are waited for and the procedure repeated.

Note. Two signs of placental separation: uterine and umbilical cord signs.

Uterine sign (Schroeder's sign; Fig. 7.94). The uterus rises and the transverse diameter is reduced.

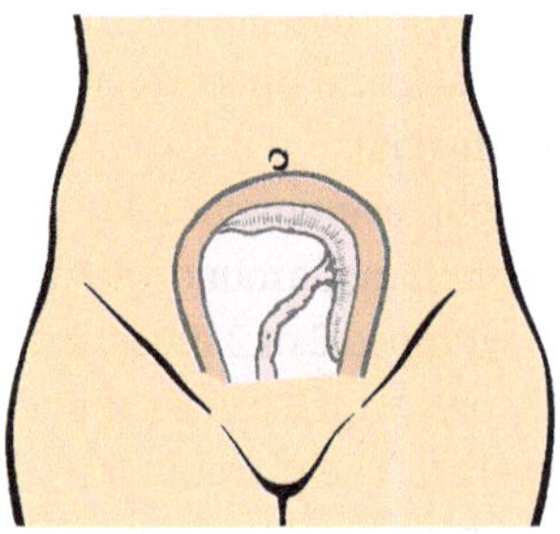

Fig. 7.93: First station of the uterus. The upper edge of the fundus is at navel height, or a number of centimeters lower or higher after birth of the baby. The uterus is round and midline.

If the placenta has separated and been expelled into the birth canal, the uterine fundus is to be found 2–3 cm above (usually to the right of) the navel. The uterine diameter is hereby markedly reduced: it has become narrower, angular, and at the same time firmer.

Cord sign (Küstner's sign; Fig. 7.97). The cord retracts towards the vagina if the placenta has not yet separated when the fingers are pressed deeply into the abdomen above the symphysis pubis.

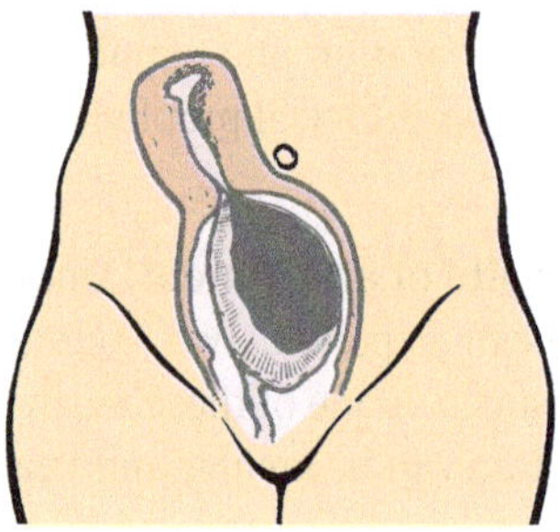

Fig. 7.94: Second station of the uterus in third stage. The placenta is completely separated and lies in the lower uterine segment. The uterus has risen above the placenta to the right, is 3–5 cm up to a hands' width above the navel. It is narrow, firm, angular.

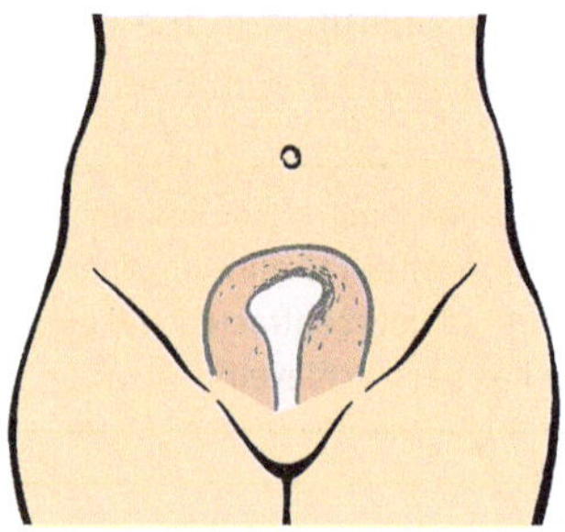

Fig. 7.95: Third station of the uterus in third stage. The placenta has been expelled. The uterus is once again midline. The upper edge of the fundus is to be found in the middle between symphysis pubis and navel.

Practice tip. The uterus can also rise above the navel if the placenta has not detached, when hemorrhaging into the uterine cavity occurs because the placenta has not separated or is only partially separated.
In such a case, the transverse diameter of the uterus has not been reduced; that is, it is not firm, narrow, and angular, but thicker, larger, and fuller than before, and in particular it is not angular!

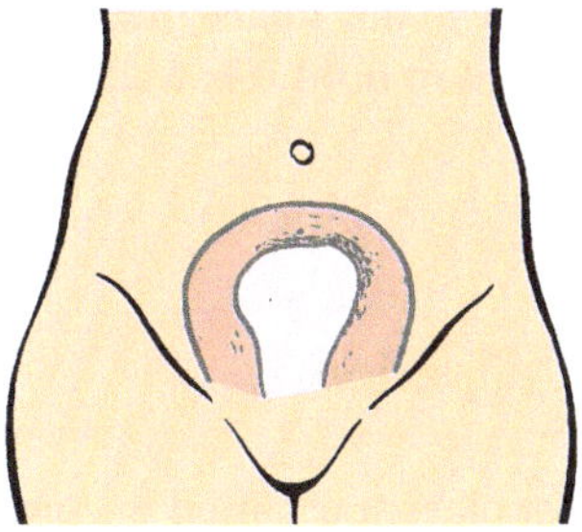

Fig. 7.96: Fourth station of the uterus. The uterus rises somewhat in the first 24 hours. The upper edge of the fundus is 2–3 cm below the navel.

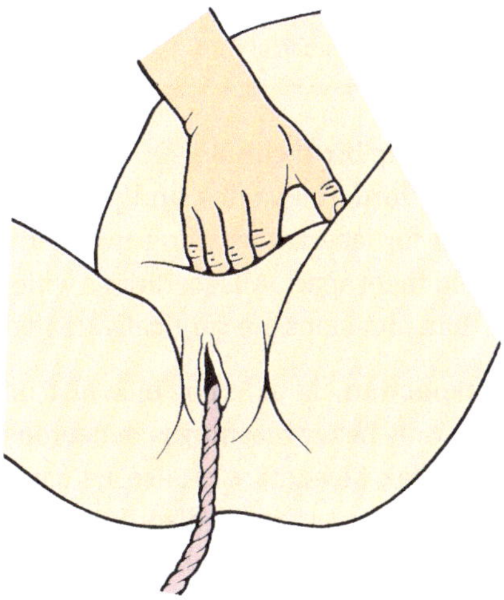

Fig. 7.97: Küstner's sign. The hand pressed towards the sacral promontory between uterus and symphysis pubis moves the uterus upwards. If the umbilical cord retracts hereby, the placenta is not yet detached. Very reliable sign! Recommended for beginners in particular due to its simplicity.

The signs of separation are not always present concurrently. Also, neither of the signs are definite.
X-ray examinations have shown that placental separation occurs before clinical signs are observed.

Note. Separation is delayed if none of the clinical signs are present within 30 min.

Delayed placental separation is treated as follows:
- 3 IU oxytocin IV if uterus is atonic.
- Gentle performance of the Credé maneuver (see below).
- If unsuccessful: manual removal of the placenta (p. 380).

Credé's maneuver (Fig. 7.98; Karl S. C.; obstetrician, Leipzig Germany, 1819–1892). After the bladder has been emptied, the uterus is brought to the center, a contraction is stimulated with light massage, and one hand grasps the uterus and pushes it in line with the birth canal towards the pelvis, whereby the placenta can be expelled.

If hemorrhaging occurs follow procedure outlined on p. 380; in cases of cervical spasm see p. 380.

Torn cord. If the placenta cannot be delivered by applying cord traction, increasing the force of traction is of no use. The cord could tear or be broken. An indication that the cord is about to tear is that it becomes conspicuously pale.

The following recommendations apply if the cord tears:
- Wait for signs of separation.
- Credé's maneuver (see above); if unsuccessful:
- Manual removal of the placenta (p. 380).

Uterine inversion. Inversion of the uterus (uterus is turned inside-out), whereby the uterine corpus lies in the vagina or in front of the vulva with the mucosal layer outwards.

Very rare occurrence, even rarer as a result of cord traction than due to forced Credé's maneuver.
Acute inversion is inversion in the third stage.
Manual repositioning (reinversion) in deep narcosis (Fig. 7.99). The whole hand is inserted into the vagina, the fingertips surround the inversion ring, and the inverted uterus lies in the palm of the hand. Steady pressure is applied to push the uterus in the direction of the navel. The reinversion is supported by the pull of the parametrial ligaments and the round ligament, which are tensed on reinversion.

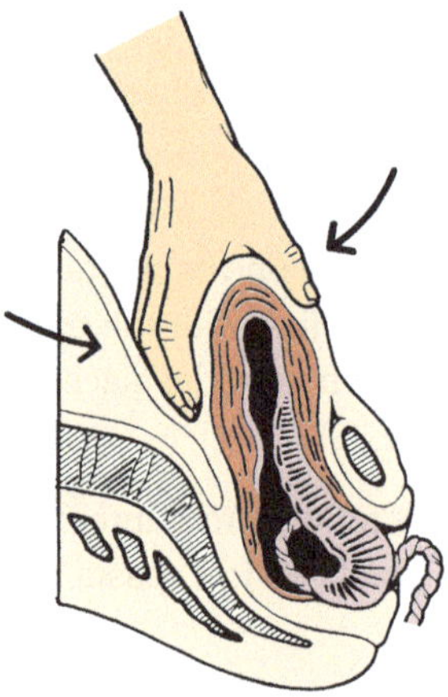

Fig. 7.98: Credé's maneuver.

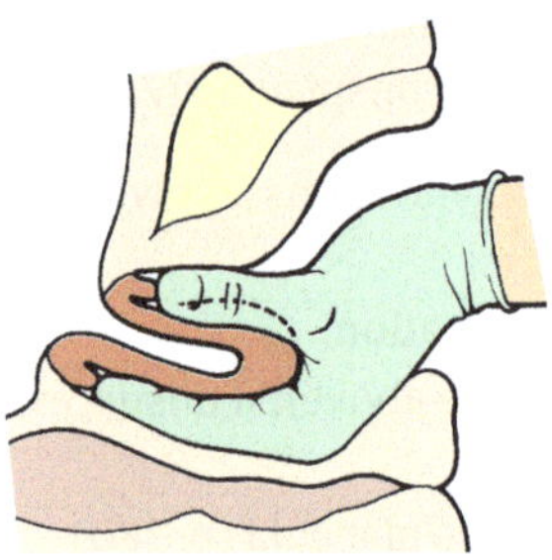

Fig. 7.99: Manual repositioning of the inverted uterus (after Johnson).

If the inversion is diagnosed immediately, repositioning is usually simple.
The placenta which is still attached to the uterine wall must not be separated before repositioning. Hemorrhaging can occur as the inverted uterus cannot contract. If repositioning proves difficult, separation of the placenta beforehand is recommended, whereby hemorrhaging is to be expected. After conclusion of the repositioning, an oxytocin infusion is necessary. The internal hand holds the repositioned uterus in position until it is well-contracted.

7.6 Postplacental period

Definition. The post-placental period encompasses the first 2 hours after delivery of the placenta.

Note. The puerperal woman must be monitored closely in the first hours postpartum because of the risk of hemorrhage. Duties are: inspection of the birth canal, placenta and membranes, umbilical cord.

Inspection of the birth canal
Initial inspection. The vagina and perineum are inspected for lacerations using two sterile swabs to hold them apart. All lacerations which are worse than abrasions are surgically treated.

Second inspection. Is external bleeding occurring? Not only heavy bleeding is dangerous, continuous weak bleeding can also be cause for concern, as coagulation disorders often begin as weak, continuous trickling bleeding.

Fritsch's position (Fig. 7.100). The woman is placed in Fritsch's position in order to monitor blood loss: a clean absorbent cloth is placed under the woman, her buttocks are stroked downwards and the legs crossed. A sterile pad is placed in front of the vulva. Blood from the vagina can thus collect in the small bowl-like area between vulva and thighs which holds 500 ml.

In case of hemorrhage the cervix must be inspected using ring forceps. All larger lacerations must be surgically repaired, even if not bleeding heavily.

Monitoring of the uterus. Is it well-contracted, between symphysis pubis and navel? It is to be noted that the consistency varies as a result of the afterpains. If it is poorly contracted uterotonics are given. If pharmacological prophylaxis was practiced in third stage uterotonics are required less often.

Observation of facial color, pulse (slow, strong), **respiration** (particularly after narcosis), **temperature.**

Check bladder. A full bladder inhibits contractions and afterpains. Women often do not recognize the urge to urinate postpartum, although the bladder fills rapidly due to diuresis setting in. If spontaneous elimination is not possible despite numerous attempts catheterization must be performed.

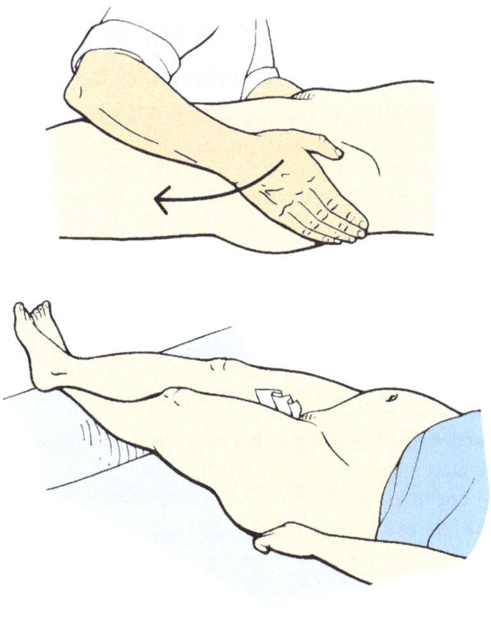

Fig. 7.100: Fritsch's position: the buttocks are stroked downwards and the legs are crossed.

Transfer to postnatal ward. The woman is transferred 2 h after delivery of the placenta after standard hygiene measures have been performed.

Inspection of the placenta

Note. The placenta is a disk, 2–3 cm thick. Diameter 16–20 cm. Weight: 500–700 g. The size is related to the size of the baby, this relationship varies greatly, however.

Pathological placenta

- Overweight placentae are found in diabetes mellitus, hemolytic disease of the newborn, syphilis; underweight in cases of chronic placental insufficiency.
- Placenta membranacea, a very thin placenta, which can be the cause of reduced fetal supply of oxygen and nutrients.
- Bipartite or bilobate placenta. The placenta divides when the conceptus implants in a corner of the uterus, the placenta grows on the anterior and posterior walls and two (or more) interconnected lobes develop.
- Placenta anularis. The ring-shaped placenta develops because the central tissue has atrophied.
- Extrachorial placenta: circummarginate and circumvallate placenta. The membranes do not continue to the edge of the placenta, but leave an area free all or partway around the periphery. A small strip of fibrin is recognizable at the margin of the chorionic plate (placenta marginata or circummarginate placenta). The edge often appears folded (placenta circumvallata or circumvallate placenta). The cause is unknown. Peripheral detachment and recurrent bleeding can occur more easily in

pregnancy and labor in the area where the villous tissue is exposed. Fetal mortality is twice as high as normal.

Inspection. The placenta should be thoroughly macroscopically examined, weighed and measured postnatally. Even when a placenta is macroscopically reassuring it should be histologically examined if there is suspicion that the baby is ill, as some defects can only be histologically detected (placental insufficiency, infections).

Note. Examination of the maternal (decidual) side of the placenta for completeness, infarctions, chorangioma.

Completeness. The placenta is spread on a large, flat plate, with the maternal side uppermost. Old, usually firmly attached clots are signs of placental abruption, or if found on the margin, bleeding from the ruptured marginal sinus. They are carefully washed away under running water:
- Are all of the lobes (cotyledons) covered with the thin gray layer (decidual covering)?
- Is any placental tissue missing?
- Can the lobes be neatly positioned next to each other, and is a gap apparent?

Practice tip. If a fragment of placenta has been retained (bean-sized or larger), a manual exploration of the uterine cavity must be performed, regardless of whether or not there is bleeding, whether or not the uterus is contracted, and whether or not the woman has a fever!

There are four dangers if placental tissue is retained in the uterus:
1. Postpartum hemorrhage (PPH) due to atonic uterus.
2. Hemorrhage in the puerperium (so-called secondary hemorrhage).
3. Life-threatening puerperal infection (septicemia).
4. Transformation of the remainder into a trophoblastic tumor (p. 360).

Note. Manual examination of the uterine cavity must be performed if, despite thorough examination, the completeness of the placenta is doubtful, even when bleeding is normal. Even if the placenta is pronounced complete, manual examination can still be indicated by PPH.

Infarctions. Firm white scars can be attributed to placental infarctions, which occur in PIH; they are not real infarctions, simply intervillous spaces blocked by fibrinous clots, which causes necrosis of the villi and their fetal blood vessels.

In cases of widespread infarctions, fetal growth is delayed: IUGR (p. 107).

Chorangioma. Circumscribed, tumor-like hyperplasia of the chorionic vessels (→hematoma), a further cause of IUGR. Incidence: 1% of all placentae.

A chorangioma can be associated with polyhydramnios and cause hypertrophy of the fetal heart. Other tumors of the placenta are rare.

Inspection of the membranes

Procedure. The placenta is held up by the cord in one hand so that the membranes hang upside down like a sack: are they complete or torn somewhere on the very margin of the placenta?

Incomplete membranes do not necessitate manual examination; they are expelled in the first few days postpartum, can however cause raised temperature! Documentation whether membranes have been retained or not. Uterotonics should be administered postpartum.

Practice tip. If membranes are torn, check the margin of the placenta or membranes for large, gaping blood vessel openings →indicator for succenturiate (accessory) lobe retained *in utero!*

Main question. Do torn vessels end on the margin of the placenta (Fig. 7.101, 2) or membranes (Fig. 7.101, 3)? Can best be assessed if held up

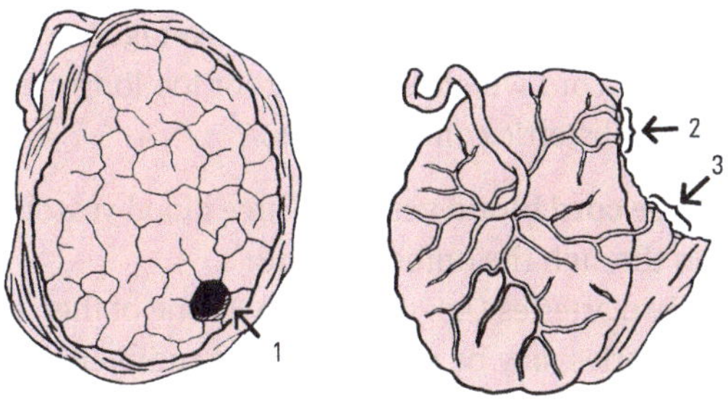

Fig. 7.101: Examination of the placenta for completeness, 1. Missing placental fragment, 2. Torn blood vessels at the margin of the placenta, 3. Torn blood vessels at the margin of the membranes.

to the light after the amniotic sac has been torn open.

Succenturiate lobe vs. aberrant vessel. A torn marginal vessel does not always mean that an accessory lobe has been retained. Aberrant blood vessels are more likely (vasa aberrantia); vessels which pass from the cord insertion over part of the placenta into the membranes and back to the surface of the placenta. They are insignificant.

Practice tip. If gaping blood vessel openings are found on the edge of placenta or membranes a manual exploration of the uterine cavity must be performed to remove the accessory lobe. It is irrelevant whether or not there is bleeding, whether or not the uterus is contracted, and whether or not the woman has a fever!

Cord insertion (Fig. 7.102 to 105). Membranous or velamentous insertion is important; it is common in multiple gestations.

Is the amnion stained? The amnion is greenish yellow if meconium has been passed and in cases of hyperbilirubinemia (hemolytic disease of the newborn).

Are the membranes clear, transparent or opaque?
Opaque. Cause is a bacterial infection, e.g., if birth was delayed after PROM, prolonged labor, in which leukocytes migrate from the umbilical and placental blood vessels →milky cloudiness, in some cases with fetid odor (→ chorioamnionitis).
The maternal signs of intrauterine infection are foul-smelling discharge, often purulent, fever, increased pulse and leukocytosis with left shift, less often: fever in puerperium.
The intrauterine infection causes fetal tachycardia and in particular bronchopneumonia due to aspiration of the purulent exudate, septicemia.

Examination of the umbilical cord

Note. Length, thickness, blood vessels and knots are examined.

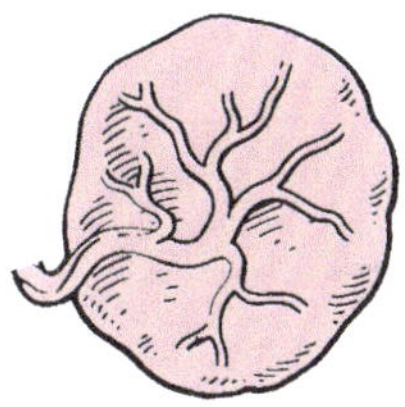

Fig. 7.102: Central insertion of the umbilical cord.

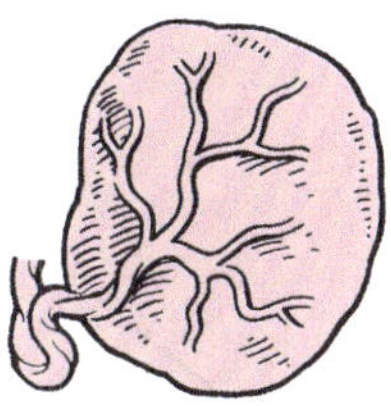

Fig. 7.103: Lateral (eccentric) insertion of the cord.

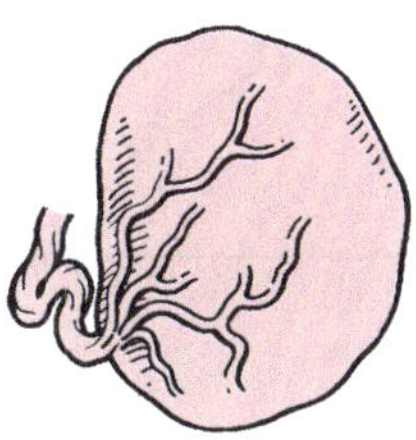

Fig. 7.104: Battledore (marginal) insertion of the cord.

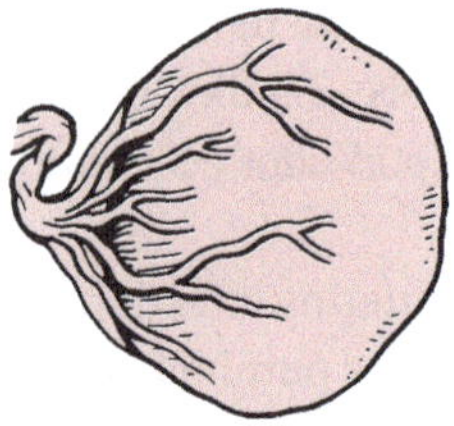

Fig. 7.105: Velamentous insertion of the cord.

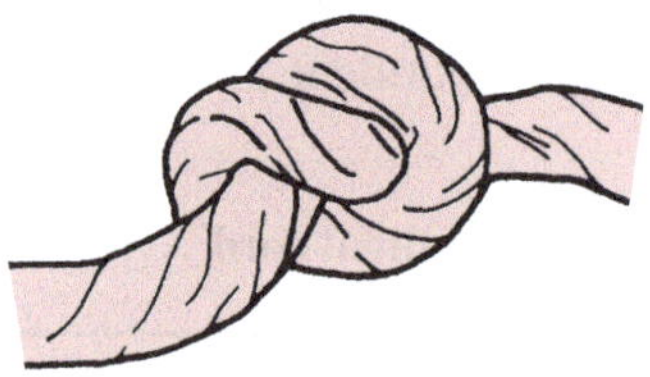

Fig. 7.106: True cord knot.

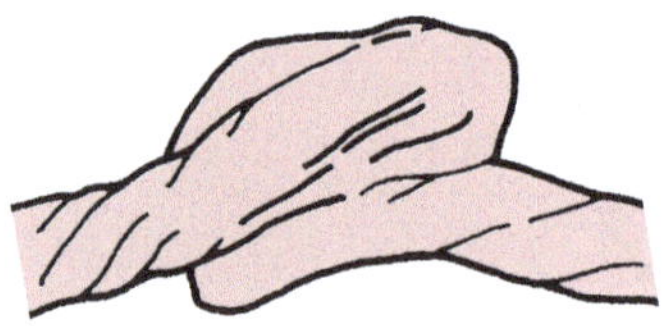

Fig. 7.107: False cord knot.

Length. The umbilical cord is on average 50 cm long. A cord which is too short or too long can cause obstetric complications.

Three cord blood vessels. Three blood vessels run through the umbilical cord:
- Two arteries (Aa. umbilicales). One of the arteries may be missing or only rudimentarily present, which may be associated with malformations.
- One vein (Vena umbilicales); easily recognized due to its broad lumen!

Knots (Fig. 7.106, 7.107).

7.7 Duration of labor

Definition. Time from begin of active labor and birth of the baby.

Average lengths. Primiparous women 6–7, multiparous 4 hours

First stage primiparous women 5, multiparous 3.5 hours.

Second stage primiparous women 1, multiparous 0.5 hours.

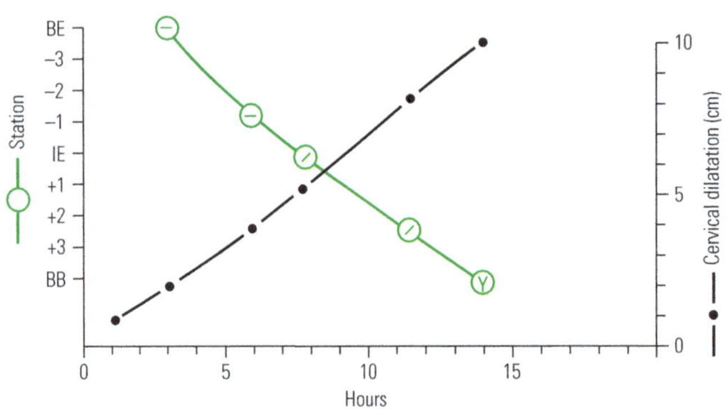

Fig. 7.108: Partograph of a primiparous woman; station of the bony leading part and cervical dilatation with sagittal suture and fontanelle are depicted.

Maximum labor duration. The labor of a primiparous woman should not last longer than 12–14 hours, of a multiparous woman not longer than 8–9 hours!

In some cases it will be possible to exceed these times, however, as long as the mother is not disadvantaged and the fetus not in any direct danger. Today's possibilities allow recognition of any risk to the fetus.

Labor progress. More important than the duration of labor is the labor progress.

Criteria:
- Cervical dilatation.
- Station of the presenting part (usually the head).
- Course of the sagittal suture monitored.

Practice tip. General rule for labor progress: cervical dilatation at a rate of 1 cm per hour.

Partogram (Fig. 7.108). Graphical documentation of examination results is more informative for management of birth. The line of cervical dilatation crosses that of descent of the presenting part in a normally progressing labor.

Dangers of prolonged labor

For the mother
- Infection (after ROM), rise in temperature, fever.
- Signs of pressure. Edema of a cervical lip (→necrosis), bloody urine, vulvar edema, vesicovaginal fistula, vesicocervical fistula, rectovaginal fistula.
- Exhaustion.

For the fetus. Acidosis (p. 284) due to placental insufficiency, particularly when potentially damaging conditions such as PIH, maternal diabetes, postterm labor, rhesus incompatibility are involved; chorioamnionitis from ascending infection.

Late primiparous women (> 35 years) may have prolonged labor (greater soft tissue resistance, primary or secondary uterine inertia). Age alone is no indication for a cesarean section however. Daily experience shows that first births of women between 40 and 45 can go smoothly.

Precipitate birth (Partus praecipitatus) is, as the name says, an unusually fast birth, in which the baby is born for example with a single expulsive contraction. Observed in multiparous women with very strong contractions and lax soft tissues.

A forensically relevant form of birth is when the baby falls from the birth canal to the floor or for example into the toilet. The cord is usually torn off. It is not necessarily a precipitate birth.

References

Akmal S, Tsoi E, Kameras N, et al.: Intrapartum sonography to determine fetal head position. J Matern Fetal Neonatal Med 2002; 12:172

American College of Obstetricians and Gynecologists: Intrapartum fetal heart rate monitoring: Nomenclature, interpretation, and general management principles. Clinical management Guidelines for Obstetrician-Gynecologists No. 106, July 2009

American College of Obstetricians and Gynecologists: Management of intrapartum fetal heart rate tracings. Clinical Management Guidelines for Obstetrician-Gynecologists No. 116, November 2010

Barbera AF, Pombar X, Perugino G, et al.: A new method to assess fetal head descent in labor with transperineal ultrasound. Ultrasound Obstet Gynecol 2009;33:313–319

Chen H-Y, Chauhan SP, Ananth CV: Electronic fetal heart rate monitoring and its relationship to neonatal and infant mortality in the United States. Amer J Obstet Gynecol 2011;204:491–2

Clark SL, Nageotte MP, Garite TJ, et al.: Intrapartum management of category II fetal heart rate tracings: towards standardization of care. Amer J Obstet Gynecol 2013;207:89

Dudenhausen JW, Luhr C, Dimer JS: Umbilical artery blood gases in heathy term newborn infants. Inter J Gynecol Obstet 1997; 57:251

Dückelmann AM, Bamberg C, Michaelis SAM, et al.: Measurement of fetal head descent using the ‚angle of progression' on transperineal ultrasound imagimg is reliable regardless of fetal head station or ultrasound expertise. Ultrasound Obstet Gynecol 2010;35:216–222

FIGO: Guidelines for the use of fetal monitoring. Int J Gynaecol Obstet 1987; 25:159

Henrich W, Dudenhausen JW, Fuchs I, et al.: Intrapartum translabial ultrasound: sonographic handmarks and correlation with successful vacuum extraction. Ultrasound Obstet Gynecol 2006; 28:753

Hutchon D: A view on why immediate cord clamping must cease in routine obstetric delivery. The Obstetrician & Gynaecologist 2008; 10:112–6

Le Ray C, Audibert F, Goffinet F, Fraser W: When to Stopp pushing; effects of duration of second stage expulsion efforts on maternal and neonatal outcomes in nulliparous women with epidural analgesia. Am J Obstet Gynecol 2009; 201:361. e1–7

Luttkus A, Callsen TA, Stupin JH, Dudenhausen JW: Pulse oximetry during labour – does it give risk to hope? Value of saturation monitoring in comparison to fetal blood gas status. Europ J Obstet Gynec Reprod Biol 2003; 110:132

Luttkus AK, Stupin JH, Calllsen TA, Dudenhausen JW: Feasibility of simultaneous application of fetal electrocardiography and fetal pulse oximetry. Acta Obstet Gynec Scand 2003; 82:443

Macones GA, Hankins GD, Spong CY, Hauth J, Moore T. The 2008 National Institute of Child Health and Human Development workshop report on electronic fetal monitoring: update on definitions, interpre- tation, and research guidelines. Obstet Gynecol 2008;112:661–6.

National Institute of Child Health and Human Development Research Planning Workshop: Electronic fetal heart rate monitoring. Research guidelines for interpretation. Am J Obstet Gynecol 1997; 177:1385

Nizard J, Haberman S, Paltieli Y, et al. : How reliablbe is the determination of cervical dilatation? Comparison of vaginal examination with spatial position-tracking ruler. Amer J Obstet Gynecol 2009;200:402

Nizard J, Haberman S, Paltieli Y, et al.: Determination of fetal head station and position during labor: a new technique that combines ultrasound and a position-tracking system. Amer J Obstet Gynecol 2009;200:404

Parer JT, Ikeda T: A framework for standardized management of intrapartum fetal head rate patterns. Amer J Obstet Gynecol 2007;197: 26

Rosenberg K, Trevathan W: Birth, obstetrics and human evolution. Br J Obstet Gynaecol 2002; 109:1199

Sosa CG, Buekens P, Hughes JM, et al.: Effect of pethidine administered during the first stage of labor on the acid-base status of birth. Eur J Obstet Gynecol Reprod Biol 2006; 129:135

Vintzileos AM, Nochimson DJ, Antsaklis A: Comparison of intrapartum electronic fetal heart rate monitoring versus intermittend auscultation in detecting fetal acidemia at birth. Am J Obstet Gynecol 1995; 173:1021

Wolfberg AJ: The future of fetal monitoring. Reviews Obstet Gynecol 2012; 5:132–6

Wong CA, et al.: The risk of cesarean delivery with neuraxial analgesia given early versus late in labor. NEJM 2005; 352:655–65

Zhang J, Landy HJ, Branch DW, et al.: Contemporary patterns of spontaneous labor with normal neonatal outcomes. Obstet Gynecol 2010; 116:1281–7

8 Pathological labor

8.1 Malpresentations and malpositions of the occiput

Occipital malpositions and malpresentations are: persistent occipitotransverse position, high anteroposterior position, occipitoposterior position and deflexed or overextended (mal)presentations: sinciput, brow or face presentation.

8.1.1 Persistent occipitotransverse position (POT)

Definition. Malposition. Abnormal development in labor. The head has reached the pelvic floor and the sagittal suture is transverse, which delays delivery due to missing flexion and rotation of the head if the occiput transverse position persists for a longer period (30–60 min).

In a normal birth the head often reaches the pelvic floor with the sagittal suture in the transverse diameter, where rotation into the anteroposterior diameter occurs. This can therefore only be called a malposition when the resulting delay in delivery is included in the definition.

Incidence. 1 % of all cephalic presentations.

Classification
Persistent left occipitotransverse position (Fig. 8.1): posterior fontanelle and back on the left.
Persistent right occipitotransverse position (Fig. 8.2): posterior fontanelle and back on the right.

Etiology. Internal rotation of the small, round heads does not occur if the soft tissues of the pelvic floor are not firm and the skull does not encounter any counterpressure on descent. In contrast, internal rotation of a large head can also be hindered when it encounters too much counterpressure (friction) from soft tissues and bony pelvis.

Secondary hypotonic contractions are the main cause. The possibly only semi-developed uterine musculature has driven the head down on to the pelvic floor. Now, when the powerful expulsive contractions which would force the head to rotate should set in, the body fails, exhausted from first stage: the rotation of the occiput does not occur, the sagittal suture remains in the transverse diameter. Pelvic shape. In the rare funnel-shaped pelvis, the transverse narrowness of the pelvic outlet impedes the internal rotation of the head on the pelvic floor.

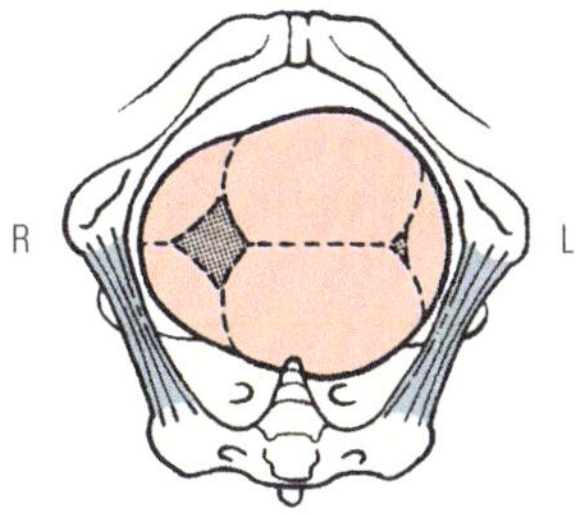

Fig. 8.1: Persistent left occipitotransverse position.

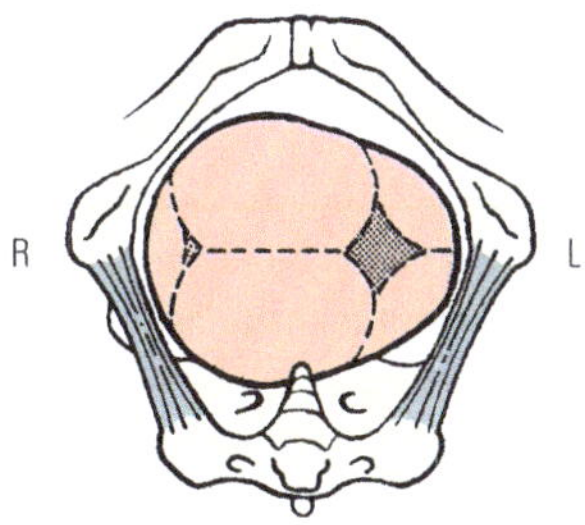

Fig. 8.2: Persistent right occipitotransverse position.

Clinical manifestation. Cervix fully dilated, ischial spines can no longer be palpated. A finger can no longer be inserted between head and pelvic floor.

Persistent left occipitotransverse position:
- Head has reached the pelvic floor; sagittal suture in the transverse diameter, posterior fontanelle on the left, anterior on the right, almost at the same level (Fig. 8.1).

Persistent right occipitotransverse position:
- Head has reached the pelvic floor; sagittal suture in the transverse diameter, posterior fontanelle on the right, anterior on the left, almost at the same level (Fig. 8.2).
- Both fontanelles are palpable: malposition (sagittal suture in transverse diameter), malpresentation (light deflexion instead of normal flexed attitude).
- The failed flexion explains why the head can't complete the internal rotation: the head doesn't rotate because it isn't flexed.

Practice tip. Persistent occipitotransverse position means arrested labor at the pelvic outlet, delivery impossible!

Spontaneous delivery is only possible when the head has rotated internally into the anteroposterior diameter. Exceptions confirm the rule: the head lies transverse to the longitudinal pelvic soft tissue outlet, contractions force it against the lateral pubic bones and the longitudinal strands of the bulbocavernosus as if against a barrier.

Practice tip. Intervention occurs far too often and far too early! Method of choice: expectant management (wellbeing of mother and fetus is a prerequisite); initially this is not an indication for operative birth termination.

Expectant management

Therapeutic repositioning of the laboring woman! Even when the head has reached the pelvic floor, position change (alteration of the fetal axis) can affect the presentation of the head.

General positioning rule. The laboring woman lies on the side on which the part of the head lies which is to take the lead, descend and rotate anteriorly. The occiput should lead with the posterior fontanelle. In persistent left occipitotransverse position the woman should lie on her left side, and in persistent right occipitotransverse position the woman should lie on her right.

Example. In persistent left occipitotransverse position the woman lies on her left side. The uterus sinks to the left as it is heavier on the left. The line of pressure of the fetal axis runs diagonally from the upper left down to the right. This pushes the sinciput against the right pelvic wall, and the occiput with the posterior fontanelle distances itself from the left wall of the pelvis. It is free and mobile, can follow the pressure and descend. It is simplest to remember:
- The head always moves in the opposite direction to the buttocks. The neck is the pivot.

The head flexes on descent (see etiology) and, if contractions are adequate, completes the internal rotation.

Treat hypotonic contractions (see p. 278)!

Practice tip. Delivery is assisted if the head has not rotated after 30 min in a lateral position with good contractions.

Assisted birth: forceps, vacuum extraction

Vacuum extraction

Vacuum extraction (see p. 332) is the method of choice because the head will rotate spontaneously under the pressure of extraction.

Practice tip. The cup is placed eccentrically on the occiput (not on the leading part), which brings about flexion (therapy for the malpresentation) and rotation of the head (therapy for the malposition).

Forceps (Naegele) delivery

Forceps application is difficult for the beginner. It is technically impossible to apply the Naegele forceps biparietal (the anterior blade cannot move under the symphysis pubis) or the pelvic curve of the forceps would lie at a right angle to the curve of the pelvic axis.

Standard application of the Naegele forceps, that is, in the transverse diameter, is also impossible, as they would lie over face and occiput.

In order to grasp the head, the forceps are placed obliquely on the head and in the pelvis: in persistent left occipitotransverse position one assumes that the sagittal suture already lies in left oblique diameter (which is not the case) and applies the forceps in the left occipital diameter (Fig. 8.3). In persistent right occipitotransverse position one assumes that the sagittal suture already lies in the right oblique diameter and applies the forceps in the right occipital diameter (Fig. 8.4).

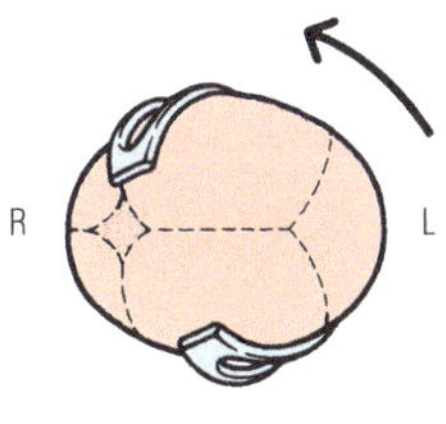

Fig. 8.3: Forceps application in persistent left occipitotransverse position, the blade is inserted in the right oblique diameter.

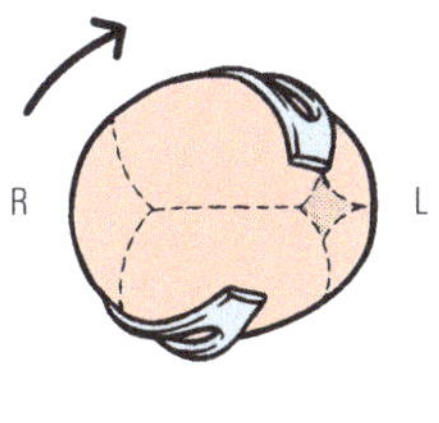

Fig. 8.4: Forceps application in persistent right occipitotransverse position, the blade is inserted in the left oblique diameter.

Forceps application in persistent left occipitotransverse position. Cervix fully dilated, head has reached pelvic floor, sagittal suture in transverse diameter, posterior fontanelle left and anterior fontanelle right.

The head must be rotated counter-clockwise until the posterior fontanelle comes toward the front (anterior). The forceps is applied as if the sagittal suture already lies in left oblique diameter, that is, it comes in the right oblique diameter. As always, the left blade is inserted first, posteriorly on the left. The right blade, which comes to the right, anteriorly, must migrate. It is introduced posteriorly on the right, and moved laterally towards the front. The forceps are locked and a check is made. Traction is applied in the direction of the handles with simultaneous rotation counterclockwise until the sagittal suture is in the anteroposterior diameter (APD). Extraction continues in the usual manner.

An exception is made and the head is not grasped transversely, but obliquely. The situation often changes when the forceps are locked however, in that the head rotates between the blades into the APD, so that the forceps are applied transversely before extraction is begun.

This forceps operation on the oblique head is technically speaking an exceptional case. It is recommended that the anterior blade is moved far to the front and the posterior blade far towards the back, so that the application is between the oblique and the anteroposterior diameter.

Forceps application in persistent right occipitotransverse position. Finding as above, difference: the posterior fontanelle is to the right, the anterior to the left (Fig. 8.4).

In order to bring the posterior fontanelle towards the front, the head must be rotated clockwise. The forceps are applied as if the sagittal suture lies in right oblique diameter, that is, they are placed in the left oblique diameter. The left blade, which must be on the left front, must migrate. It is introduced first posteriorly on the left and brought far towards the front. Then the right blade is applied, posteriorly on the right. The forceps are locked and traction applied with simultaneous clockwise rotation.

Practice tip. In persistent right occipitotransverse position, experienced practitioners prefer to insert the right blade first, not the left, contrary to the normal method. Advantage: the head is rotated in the right oblique diameter on application of this blade. Disadvantage: insertion and movement of the left blade is more difficult, as is locking the forceps.

8.1.2 High anteroposterior head

Definition. Malposition of the head at the beginning of labor: the sagittal suture is almost in the anteroposterior diameter (normal: oblique or transverse) of the pelvic inlet.

From a mechanical point of view, the malpositioned high anteroposterior head is the counterpart to the persistent occipitotransverse position.

Incidence. 0.5 % of all births.

Classification:
- Occipitoanterior (Positio occipitalis pubica). The occiput is anterior, towards the pubis (Fig. 8.5).
- Occipitoposterior (Positio occipitalis sacralis) The occiput is posterior, towards the sacrum (Fig. 8.6).

The occipitoanterior AP malposition is more common (2 : 1 to 3 : 1). The cause is thought to be the maternal spine, which does not often allow posterior positioning of the fetal back and forces the head to rotate anteriorly.

In the occipitoposterior AP malposition, the posterior occiput remains posterior (Fig. 8.6). The back is forced to a left or right lateral position by the spine: high occipitoposterior position.

Etiology. Long pelvis, contracted pelvis (round pelvic inlet), cephalopelvic disproportion; rare causes: placenta previa, uterine malformations, myoma, prolapsed hand/foot, deformity, functional disorder.

Findings, diagnosis

3rd Leopold maneuver. Head feels conspicuously narrow because the fingers do not grasp the occipitofrontal diameter as usual but:
- In the occipitoanterior AP the biparietal diameter (9.5 cm; see Fig. 8.7, 8.8).
- In the occipitoposterior the bitemporal diameter (8 cm). In particular in these cases, many small parts are also palpated.

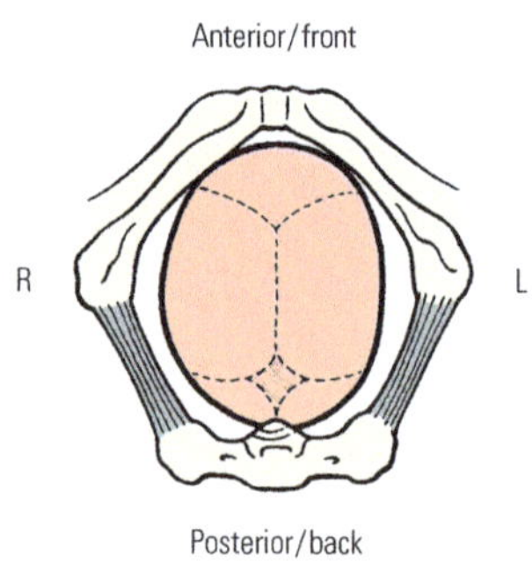

Fig. 8.5: Occipitoanterior high anteroposterior position.

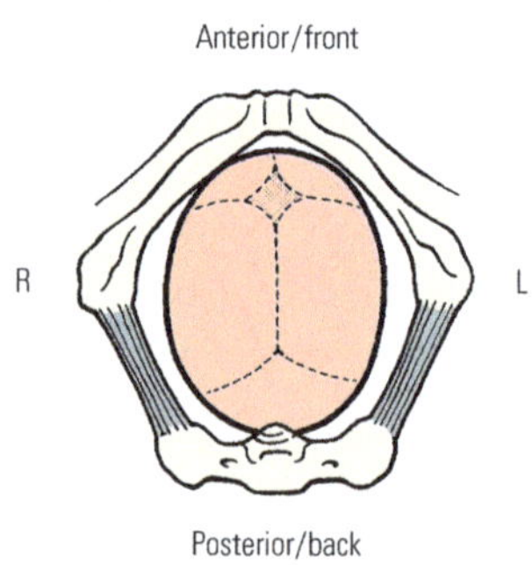

Fig. 8.6: Occipitoposterior high anteroposterior position.

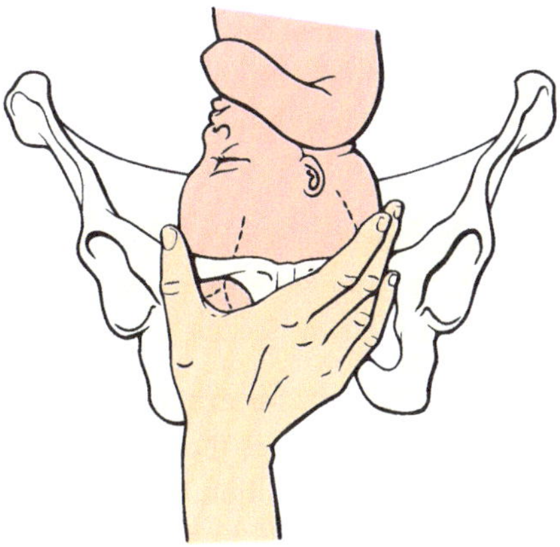

Fig. 8.7: Normal palpatory finding.

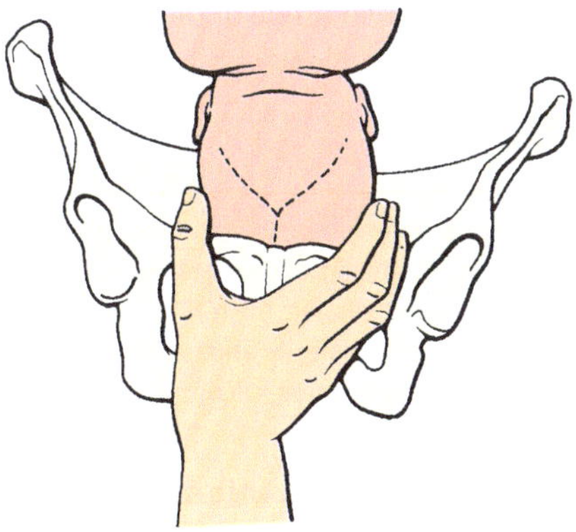

Fig. 8.8: In the high AP positions the head feels conspicuously narrow.

Vaginal examination (Figs. 8.5, 8.6). Palpatory findings are shown in the figures.
Sonography. Clarifies!

Course of labor, prognosis. Birth is impossible if this malposition isn't resolved spontaneously or with assistance.

Every second laboring woman with high AP position experiences a spontaneous delivery, whereby the sagittal suture only deviates from the anteroposterior diameter (APD) briefly in order to pass around the sacral promontory with light zigzag movements, in effect passing through all levels of the pelvis in the APD.
Labor is prolonged, as extensive molding of the skull is necessary.
Narrow, long pelvis. If the cause is a narrow or long pelvis, it is questionable whether spontaneous delivery will be possible. Labor is usually arrested and uterine rupture threatens if cesarean section is not performed.

Treatment

- Expectant management, lateral supine positions on alternating sides and tocolysis to promote spontaneous entry and passage of the head.
- Manual repositioning (→ Liepmann's bowling ball maneuver) if cervix is fully dilated:
  - The whole hand is inserted into the vagina, the head is grasped and turned to the left or right in the oblique diameter into which it most easily rotates. Once the head has been brought into the transverse diameter, external pressure is exerted to press it downwards into the pelvis.

Cesarean section is usually necessary!

8.1.3 Occipitoposterior position

Definition. Malposition. The fetal back is positioned posteriorly (LOP or ROP positions see Figs. 8.9 and 8.10) and the head is in the normal occipital attitude: chin on chest. In the occipitoposterior positions the occiput (lowermost part of the head) leads (as in the normal occipitoanterior position). It is, however, posterior, towards the sacrum, and the brow is directed towards the symphysis pubis.

Incidence. 1 % of all cephalic presentations.

Etiology, occurrence. Dorsoposterior or occipitoposterior positions. Normal-sized fetuses position themselves in occipitoposterior positions only in multiparous women with lax soft tissues. This malposition is otherwise only found in small fetuses, as well as preterm deliveries and dead babies.

Findings, diagnosis. Arrested labor when head has reached the pelvic floor, sometimes also in midpelvis.

- The finger searches for the sagittal suture, which is in an oblique or anteroposterior diameter. When it is followed anteriorly in search of the posterior fontanelle, the anterior fontanelle is found, to the left front, right front or in the middle below the symphysis pubis.
- The posterior fontanelle is posterior (towards the sacrum): left, LOP (Fig. 8.9), right, ROP (Fig. 8.10) or at the back in the middle. It is hard to palpate because a caput develops here.
- The head is often so well flexed that the anterior fontanelle is not reachable. The leading part in the birth axis is the posterior fontanelle or the parietal region between anterior and posterior fontanelle.
- Ultrasound examination shows the fetal spine to be posterior, towards the maternal spine and the fetal eyes to be directed anteriorly.

LOP is much more common than ROP:

- Occipitoposterior position with sagittal suture in the left oblique diameter → ROP (Fig. 8.9).
- Occipitoposterior position with sagittal suture in the right oblique diameter → LOP (Fig. 8.10).

Explanation. In all occipitoposterior positions the posterior fontanelle is to be found posteriorly to the left or right if the sagittal suture is in one of the oblique diameters. The position of the posterior fontanelle is also that of the back. Occipitoposterior position with sagittal suture in left oblique diameter (which runs from left anterior to right posterior): the posterior fontanelle and the back must be right posterior. Therefore if the sagittal suture is in the left oblique diameter it is a right occipitoposterior position.

Differential diagnosis. Occipitoposterior positions are not easy to diagnose; in particular quick examiners are easily deceived.

The sagittal suture is felt, for example, in the left oblique diameter and it is thought to be a normal occipitoanterior position. The sagittal suture is followed anteriorly and a v-shaped fork is felt, which is assumed to be the posterior fontanelle. On closer examination, a hard bony plate is not felt, but rather an indentation with a soft base; the rear angle of the diamond-shaped anterior fontanelle was palpated.

Course of labor

Note. Two birth variations are possible: the occiput rotates anteriorly: occipitoposterior changes into a normal occipitoanterior. Occiput rotates posteriorly: occipitoposterior remains occipitoposterior and is developed as such (persistent occiput posterior – POP).

Variation 1 occiput rotates anteriorly

The occiput usually remains posterior until it reaches the pelvic floor, where the anterior rotation takes place.

In ROP the sagittal suture rotates over 135° from the left oblique diameter over the transverse and the right oblique into the anteroposterior diameter (Fig. 8.11).

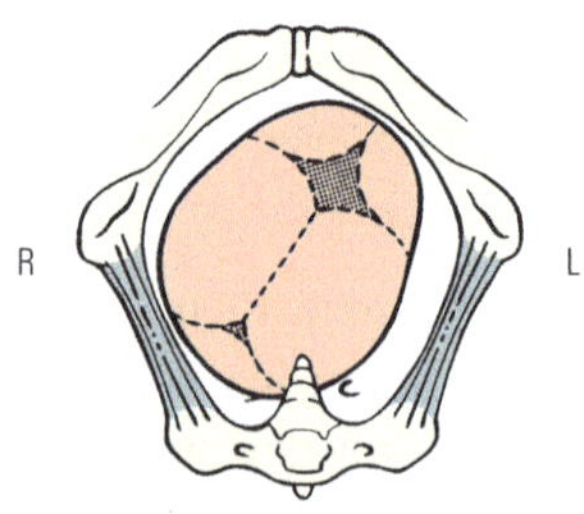

Fig. 8.9: Right occipitoposterior (ROP) presentation.

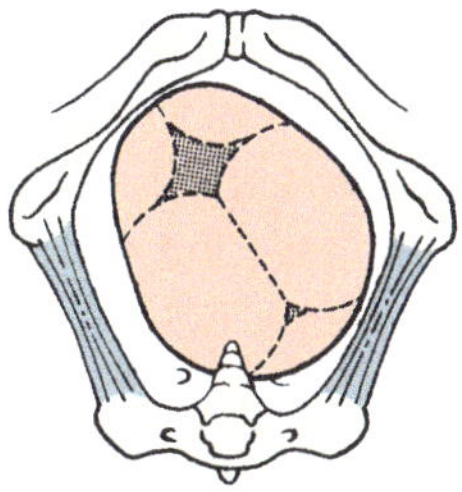

Fig. 8.10: Left occipitoposterior (LOP) presentation. (palpatory findings), leading part is the posterior fontanelle to parietal region.

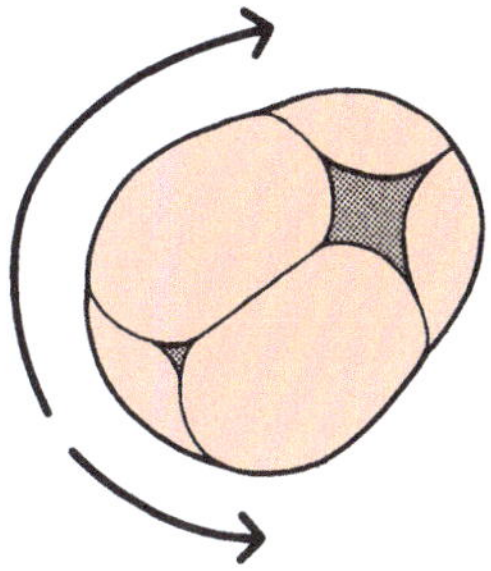

Fig. 8.11: Two birth variations for occipitoposterior presentations.

Crowning movement is via extension only, as in occipitoanterior positions (p. 162).
The occipitoanterior rotation occurred in 50 % of 415 assessed occipitoposterior positions (Dawson).

Variation 2 occiput does not rotate anteriorly, it remains posterior (POP).

Note. Overview. Crowning possibility.
- Leading part. Posterior fontanelle to parietal region.
- Pivot point. Area from anterior fontanelle to hairline (brow).
- Birth of head. First strong flexion then mild extension.
- Largest plane of passage. Suboccipitobregmatic plane (32 cm).
- Characteristics. Plane of passage in occipitoposterior and occipitoanterior positions are identical (32 cm).

On the pelvic floor the sagittal suture rotates from the oblique diameter with the posterior fontanelle towards the back into the anteroposterior diameter; this route amounts to only 45° rotation.
The flexed head is positioned with the sagittal suture in or almost in the APD, the posterior fontanelle posterior and the anterior fontanelle anterior. When the head crowns from this attitude (flexion!) and position (occiput posterior!), that is, in order to curve around the pubic symphysis, it can only do so by attempting to adapt the head-neck to the curve axis of the exit passage. The existing flexion is increased (Fig. 8.12), whereby the chin is pressed with great force into the breastbone region.
The force required to bring about the posture dictated by the shape of the birth canal causes much greater friction between the soft tissue walls of the birth canal and the skull. The increased frictional resistance between head and soft tissue canal markedly increases the length of second stage, the fetus is at risk.
Crowning (Fig. 8.13) is only possible if flexion is increased (arrow 1 in Fig. 8.13). The occiput is born over the perineum in this attitude. The anterior fontanelle is the hypomochlion, and braces itself against the lower edge of the symphysis pubis. Once the occiput has been born and the neck is free the forced head flexion ends; the head goes from flexion into a mild extension (arrow 2 in Fig. 8.13), whereby sinciput, brow and face can be born from under the symphysis pubis (i.e., face to pubis).
The plane of passage is the same as for the occipitoanterior position, the suboccipitobregmatical (circumference 32 cm).
Birth of the head occurs when the occiput has rotated into the APD (second variation), via 2 opposing movements (Fig. 8.13):

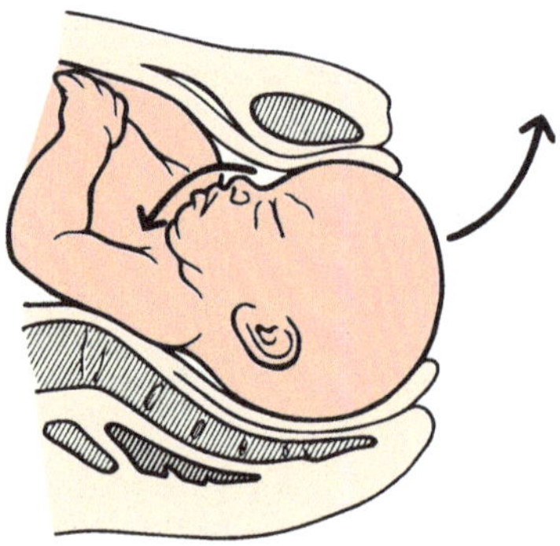

Fig. 8.12: Extreme flexion on birth of the head (occipitoposterior presentation).

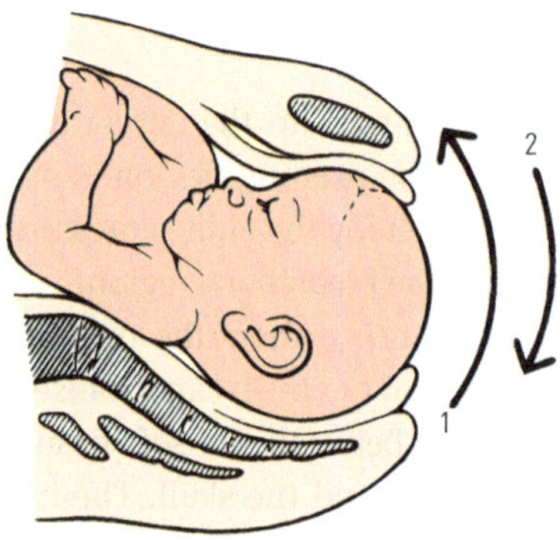

Fig. 8.13: Crowning movement in OP presentation: 1) extreme flexion, 2) moderate extension.

- Flexion (strengthening the attitude of flexion).
- Extension.

Second stage

Second stage is prolonged in AGA fetuses! There are 3 definitive reasons:

- The main reason is the maximum flexion required of the head in order to negotiate the curve of Carus and exit the birth canal. This causes increased friction between the head and the soft tissue canal, which makes second stage in particular more difficult.
- The broad occiput must pass over the perineum, not the narrow sinciput. This results in far greater transverse perineal distension and stretching (→ increased transverse strain on the perineum).
- The narrow, well-fitting occiput (as in normal OA delivery) does not function as hypomochlion in the angle of the pubic arch, instead the much broader sinciput must. This means that the full depth of the pubic arch cannot be utilized, and the head is forced lower, towards the perineum, so that it is also under more sagittal strain. This is a further reason for the increased frictional resistance and thus prolongation of labor.

Practice tip. Perineum and levator shanks are more endangered in OP than in OA presentations: deep vaginal lacerations, lacerations of the levator ani muscle! Marked perineal distension calls for generous episiotomy.

Note. Treatment. Occipitoposterior positions are to be managed expectantly, operative delivery is not indicated!

Expectant management

Lateral positioning (→ on the side of the occiput).

Oxytocics if contractions are inadequate.

Operative treatment. If the occiput does not rotate or arrested labor with sagittal suture in APD necessitates active assistance the birth is operatively terminated:

Note. Vacuum extraction should be given preference over forceps or VE plus forceps!

Vacuum extraction (see p. 332) is the method of choice. The cup is attached to the leading part (anterior fontanelle!). The head usually rotates spontaneously to an anterior position.

POP forceps. Forceps (Naegele) delivery only when the head has reached the perineum! Forceps deliveries are difficult, often cause tissue lacerations and require great strength and skill.

The three concrete dangers of forceps delivery for the mother are: deep perineal and vaginal lacerations, levator ani shank detachment, and atony.
The fetus is at risk due to the force exerted by the operator to gain traction and the duration of extraction.
Method. A generous episiotomy is a prerequisite. In an occipitoposterior position the forceps are applied exactly as for an occipitoanterior position: the head is grasped transversely. As always, the tips of the blades are directed towards the leading part, which in this case is the posterior fontanelle or parietal region.
Applying Naegele forceps (see Fig. 8.14, 15):
- Example 1. Sagittal suture in APD, posterior fontanelle directly posterior: blade is inserted laterally and applied transversely.
- Example 2. Sagittal suture in ROD, posterior fontanelle left posterior, LOP (Fig. 8.14): forceps is inserted in LOD.
  - Left blade is inserted left, posteriorly and moved towards anterior.
  - Right blade is inserted right, posteriorly.
- Example 3. Sagittal suture in LOD, posterior fontanelle right posterior, ROP (Fig. 8.15): forceps is inserted in ROD.
  - Left blade is inserted first, left, posteriorly.
  - Right blade is inserted right, posteriorly and moved towards anterior.

The **extraction technique** depends on whether the head can be rotated anteriorly (variation 1) or posteriorly (variation 2).
Method in 3 stages
This applies to examples 2 and 3. If, as in example 1, the head has reached the pelvic floor with the sagittal suture in the APD, it must be extracted as per the exit mechanism of the second variation: extreme flexion followed by moderate extension.

1. Horizontal traction (in the direction of the handles) until the leading part appears in the vulva (Fig. 8.16). After locking the forceps and checking manually, both hands are used to apply traction horizontally and slightly upwards in the direction of the handles.
   Traction is applied until the posterior fontanelle, or rather the crown, is visible in the vulva. This brings the pivot point anterior fontanelle (to hairline - brow) under the edge of the symphysis pubis, against the lower edge of which it can brace itself as the head is born around its curve.
   If the sagittal suture was in an oblique diameter (examples 2 and 3), the forceps (if the manner of rotation described on p. 217, Fig. 8.11 is to be copied) must be cautiously and slowly rotated during traction so that the anterior fontanelle comes towards anterior.
   Simultaneous rotation in
   a) LOP (Fig. 8.9) clockwise,
   b) ROP (Fig. 8.10) counterclockwise.
2. Elevation of the forceps handles to deliver the occiput (Fig. 8.17), perineal protection:

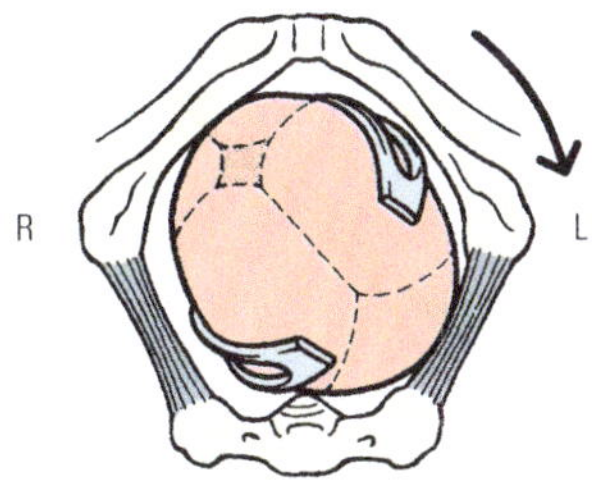

Fig. 8.14: Forceps application in LOP.

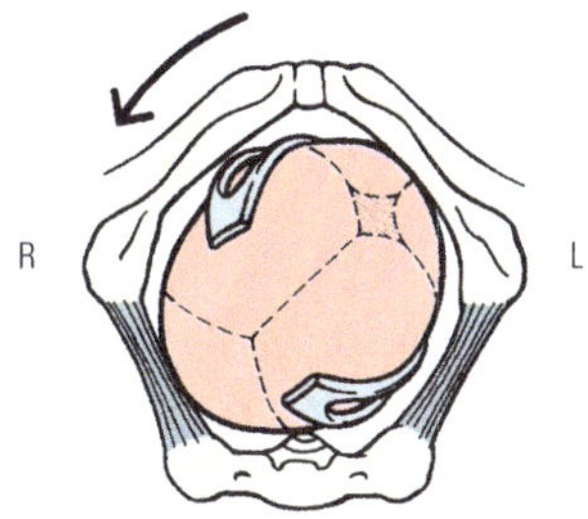

Fig. 8.15: Forceps application in ROP.

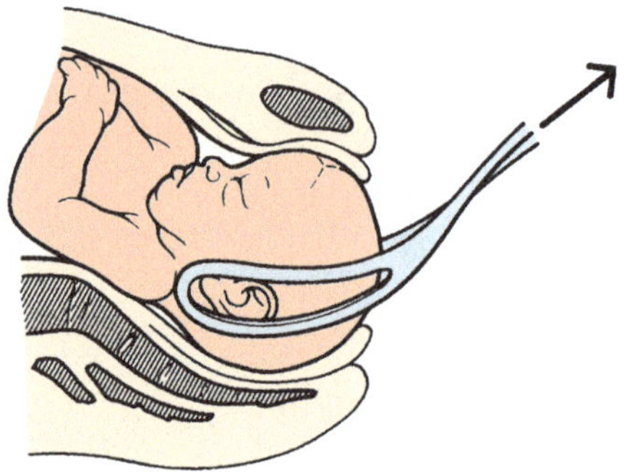

Fig. 8.16: Forceps in OP (1) traction in the direction of the handles.

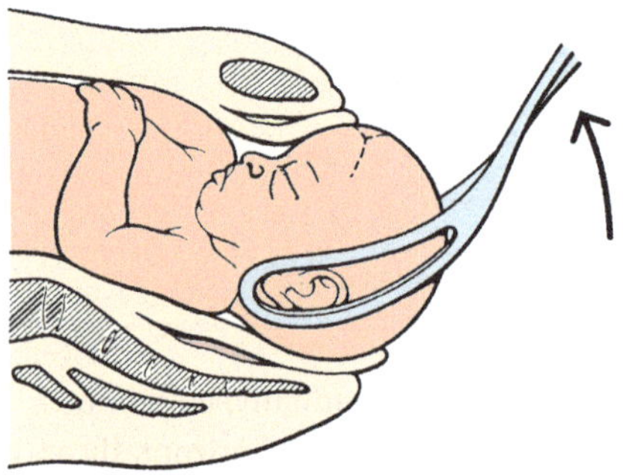

Fig. 8.17: Forceps in OP (2) elevation of the handles.

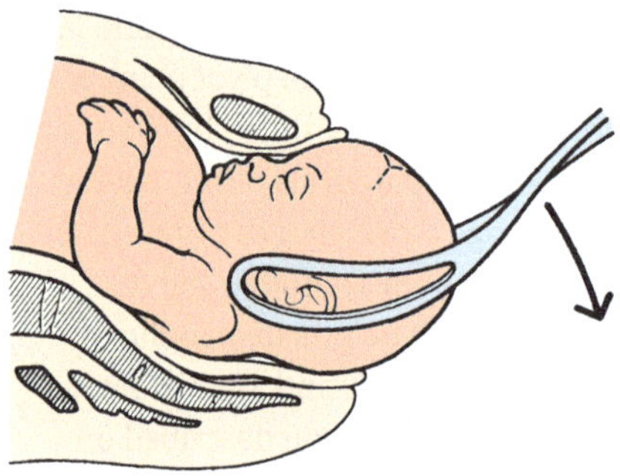

Fig. 8.18: Forceps in OP (3) lowering of the handles (reverse movement).

change of position and hand! Position change: move to the left of the woman. Hand change: the right hand holds the forceps alone; the left is moved to the perineum. The right hand grasps the lock, not the handles (far too much leverage!). Traction is no longer applied, the handles are simply elevated (Fig. 8.17). Initially carefully and slowly until vertical, then further in the direction of the maternal abdomen. Millimeter for millimeter, as slowly as possible, the broad occiput is delivered over the perineum.
All movements which are too abrupt or too fast can lead to perineal or levator ani laceration or levator ani detachment. The left hand protects the perineum and remains there continuously; this must never be neglected because the perineum is overstretched. As with the OA forceps delivery, the danger of severe perineal laceration in OP forceps delivery is high.

3. Lowering of the handles (reverse movement) for delivery of brow and face (Fig. 8.18). The handles are lowered towards the perineum, in order to deliver sinciput, brow and face under the pubic arch, also only using one hand (the right). The left hand continues to guard the perineum.

8.1.4 Extended presentations

Definition. Malpresentations (anomalies of attitude, position); extended presentations; extension of the fetal head during labor from the normal flexed attitude (see Figs. 8.22 to 8.24). Classification according to fetal presenting part (and leading part): 1. Sinciput presentation (anterior fontanelle), 2. Brow presentation (brow), 3. Face presentation (face).

Normal vertex presentation. Before the head enters the pelvis it is found in a relaxed neutral attitude midway between flexed and extended (Fig. 8.19) above the pelvic inlet. In normal vertex presentations the chin sinks to the chest at the onset of labor (→ 1st rotation) and the head is forced through the birth canal to the pelvic floor in this flexed attitude (Fig. 8.20). The back is on the right or left, anterior. 92 % of all births occur in this attitude and position.

Extended or deflexed attitude. Flexion does not occur in some cephalic presentations, the head adopts an extended or deflexed attitude, whereby the chin distances itself from the chest. These presentations are called extended presentations (Fig. 8.22 to 8.24).

Extended presentations have two characteristics:
The head is extended (anomaly of attitude).
The back is posterior (malposition).

Extended presentations are dorsoposterior presentations.

The head faces the ceiling on birth. Dorsoanterior extended presentations are rare.

Not all dorsoposterior births can be called extended presentations. Occipitoposterior presentations are also dorsoposterior, but not extended presentations; occipitoposterior presentations demonstrate only the dorsoposterior malpositioning, not the characteristic anomaly of attitude typical for the extended presentations, the extended head; on the contrary, in occipitoposterior presentations the head is extremely well-flexed.

Classification. According to the leading part, this is determined by the degree of extension: anterior fontanelle, brow, face:
1. Sinciput presentations (Fig. 8.22).
2. Brow presentations (Fig. 8.23).
3. Face presentations (Fig. 8.24).

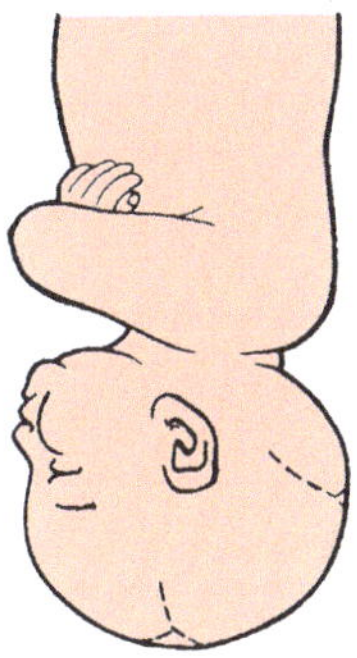

Fig. 8.19: Relaxed attitude of the head before entering the pelvis.

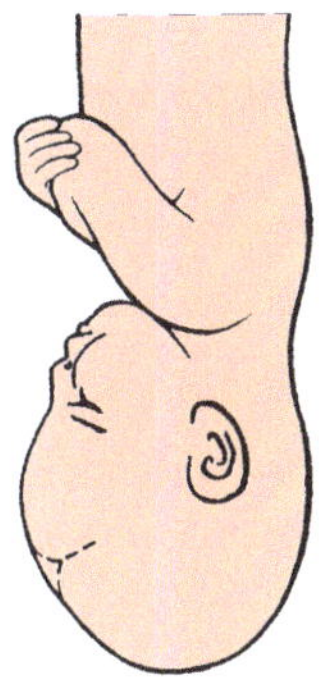

Fig. 8.20: Normal vertex presentation (flexed attitude)on entering the pelvis.

Normal (oa) vertex presentation

The 3 extended presentations

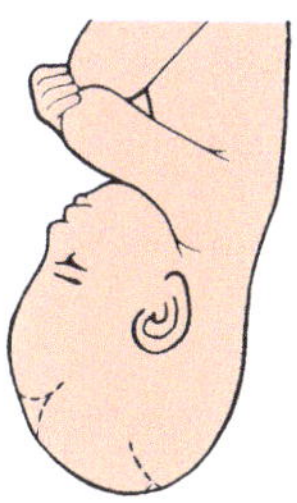

Fig. 8.21: Flexed attitude in normal vertex presentation.

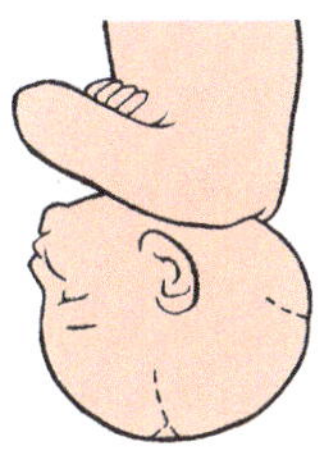

Fig. 8.22: Sinciput presentation.

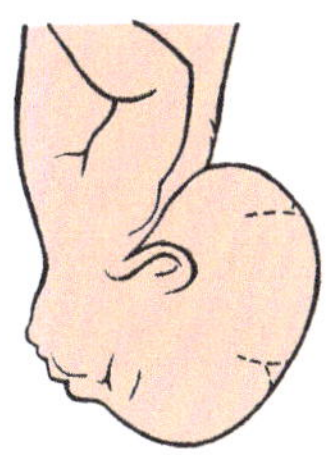

Fig. 8.23: Brow presentation.

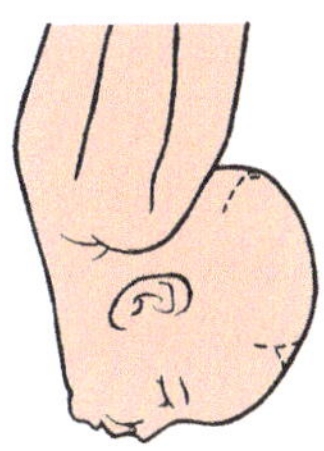

Fig. 8.24: Face presentation.

Sinciput presentation

Definition. Extended presentation with the least extension, dorsoposterior birth (back posterior). Leading part is the anterior fontanelle (sinciput).

Etiology. Occurs in preterm births and stillbirths or in term babies:
- In congenital head malformation (brachycephalus, short head; which causes presentation of the anterior fontanelle).
- In changes to atlanto-occipital joint.
- In cephalopelvic disproportion: buttonhole mechanism on entry of the head (see p. 298). In order to better pass through the pelvis, the narrower sinciput descends into the narrow pass: the anterior fontanelle descends; it is the lowermost point in the birth axis, and thus the leading part. Sinciput presentation also results from compound presentation, low-lying placenta, and tumor.

In over half of the cases no explanation is found for the abnormal attitude of the head. This is also true for the other extended presentations.

Clinical manifestation
- Prolonged labor.
- Endangered perineum in term deliveries.

Diagnosis
- The finger examining in the birth axis reaches the leading part, the anterior fontanelle (recognition see p. 143); the posterior fontanelle is difficult to reach or unreachable.
- If the posterior fontanelle is reached, it is found posteriorly, to the left, right or in the middle: in all cases its pelvic station is higher than that of the leading part.
- The caput is felt near the anterior fontanelle.
- The sagittal suture is found in an oblique diameter or more rarely in transverse diameter; later (in the curve of Carus) it rotates into the APD.
  - Sagittal suture in LOD → right sinciput presentation.
  - Sagittal suture in ROD → left sinciput presentation (Fig. 8.25; explanation see OP, p. 215).
- Ultrasound shows that the fetal back is directed posteriorly towards the maternal back and the fetal eyes are directed anteriorly.

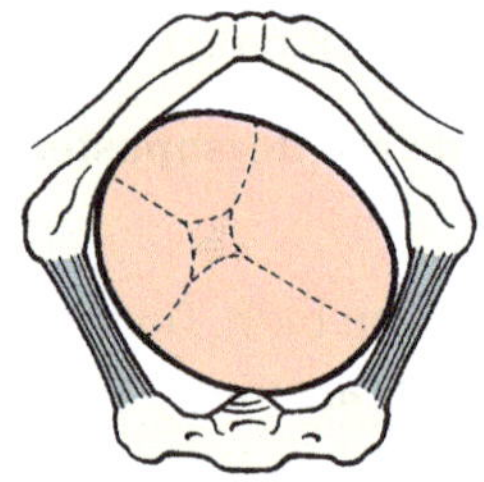

Fig. 8.25: Left sinciput presentation.

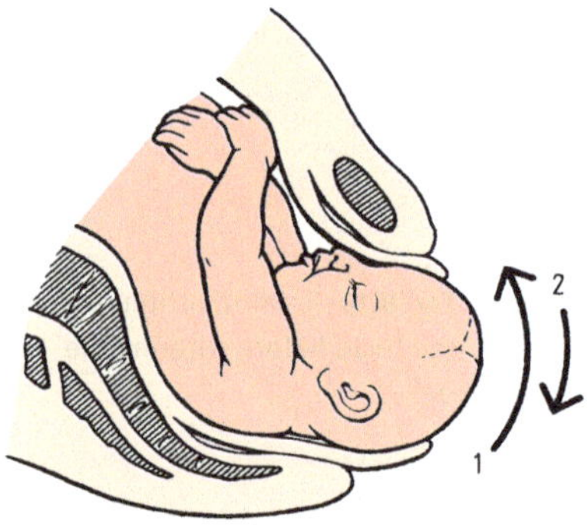

Fig. 8.26: Crowning movement in sinciput presentation: 1) greater flexion; 2) milder extension.

Course of labor

Note. Leading part. Anterior fontanelle.
Pivot point. Area slightly below the frontal hairline.
Birth of head. First flexion then extension.
Largest plane of passage. Occipitofrontal plane, 34 cm.

On entering the true pelvis, the anterior fontanelle takes the lead. The back is angled posteriorly (oblique position), the sagittal suture in an oblique diameter.
At the curve of Carus the face is rotated towards the symphysis pubis and with that, the sagittal suture in the APD and the posterior fontanelle posteriorly.
The **birth mechanism** encompasses flexion (Fig. 8.26, arrow 1) and extension (Fig. 8.26, arrow 2).

Flexion. Sinciput, parietal region and occiput (that is, only part of the head) are born over the perineum. The brow acts as pivot point (hypomochlion), impinging against the pubic arch.

The largest plane of passage is the occipitofrontal plane with 34 cm (larger than the normal vertex presentation with 32 cm circumference in the suboccipitobregmatic plane).

Extension. The extension which follows results in the birth of brow and face under the symphysis pubis.

Characteristics. Term deliveries are much slower than normal vertex presentations. The length of labor (primiparous women 12, multiparous women 8 h) is always exceeded.

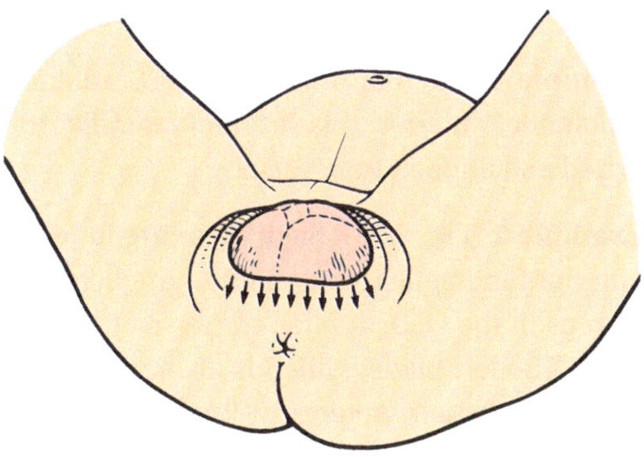

Fig. 8.27: Greatly increased pressure on the perineum in sinciput presentation.

The reason is the larger plane of passage, the occipitofrontal plane, which makes the passage of the head through the birth canal difficult. This plane causes a greater frictional resistance in the birth canal than the plane of passage of the normal vertex presentation with smaller circumference.

Second stage. Slow progress in second stage characterizes the sinciput presentation.

Even if the contractions are good and the laboring woman young, the head is often visible in the vagina for a long time and the woman does not have the strength to push it out on her own. This is caused by the increased strain on the soft tissue canal, in particular the perineum:
- In all directions, due to the larger plane of passage (see Fig. 8.27).
- Transversely. Similar to occiput posterior positions, instead of the narrow sinciput (in normal vertex presentations) the broad occiput encounters the perineum and can only pass over it by distending it transversely: increased transverse strain on the perineum.
- Sagittally. Instead of the narrow neck in a vertex presentation, which fits well into the pubic arch, the much broader brow must act as hypomochlion and brace itself against the pubic arch. This forces the skull posteriorly deeper into the perineum.

Note. The perineum is much more at risk in sinciput presentation than in normal occipitoanterior presentation!

The **fetus is more at risk** than in normal vertex presentation due to prolonged second stage: EFM is essential in second stage!

Rapid birth. Every birth attendant knows that a sinciput presentation delivery can be unusually fast if it is a preterm fetus with a small head, as they often present in this manner.

Differential diagnosis. Occipitoposterior presentation. In practice it is often mistakenly diagnosed as occipitoposterior presentation. OP and sinciput presentation have a common position: the fetal back is posterior (dorsoposterior), the posterior fontanelle also, the anterior fontanelle is palpable anteriorly. Both have prolonged labor at term.

The differences in attitude are:
- OP presentations are flexed, chin on chest.
- Sinciput presentations are in a deflexed or mildly extended attitude..
- The differences in leading part.
- Sinciput presentation. Anterior fontanelle.
- OP presentation. Posterior fontanelle or (often) the parietal region between posterior and anterior fontanelle.

Practice tip. A large caput often hinders diagnosis. The attitude is not determined until after birth by the location of the caput: sinciput presentation → anterior fontanelle; OP presentation → occiput-parietal region.

Treatment. Treatment is conservative if maternal and fetal conditions allow, not initially an indication for operative treatment. In sinciput presentations every unnecessary and premature intervention worsens the prognosis.

Expectant management
Conservative management is the method of choice for as long as possible.

Positioning rule. The woman lies on the side on which the part of the fetal head which is to descend and rotate anteriorly lies.

Positioning on the side of the occiput (posterior fontanelle) if the sagittal suture is oblique, so that the sinciput may become a normal occipitoanterior presentation.
Positioning on the opposite side if after some time (despite good contractions), the occiput has shown no tendency to rotate anteriorly.
This positioning is also valid for the common occurrence that, despite excellent contractions, the head, which is visible in the vagina, cannot be expelled. The sagittal suture rotates quickly into the APD and the head crowns.
Treat **hypotonic contractions** if necessary (p. 278)!

Operative delivery: VE, Naegele forceps.
Vacuum extraction. The VE is the method of choice in sinciput presentations. The cup is attached over the anterior fontanelle.

Delivery with forceps is to be avoided in sinciput presentations!
Midforceps should never be performed as it is extremely difficult due to the immense frictional resistance between head and birth canal! It is also better to wait until it is in the APD if the sagittal suture is oblique.
Risk of deep soft tissue lacerations on rotation of the head under traction!
Episiotomy. A generous episiotomy is necessary due to the extreme overstretching and associated high risk to the perineum (third degree laceration!).

Method
Insert forceps as for normal vertex presentation. The tips point towards the anterior fontanelle, the head is grasped transversely. As forceps are not used if the sagittal suture is in the transverse diameter there are 3 variations:

Example 1. Sagittal suture in APD, anterior fontanelle anterior: blades are laterally inserted and applied transversely.

Example 2 (Fig. 8.28). Sagittal suture in ROD, anterior fontanelle right, anterior. Application: forceps in the LOD, applied transversely to the head. The left blade, which is always inserted first, belongs left, anteriorly. It must therefore be inserted left posteriorly and moved towards anterior; the right blade is inserted right posteriorly.

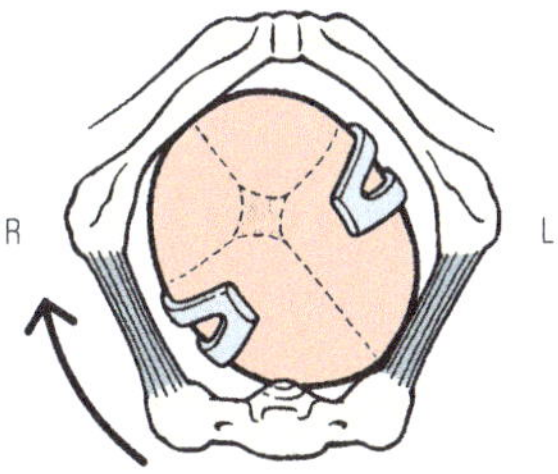

Fig. 8.28: Forceps application in left sinciput presentation.

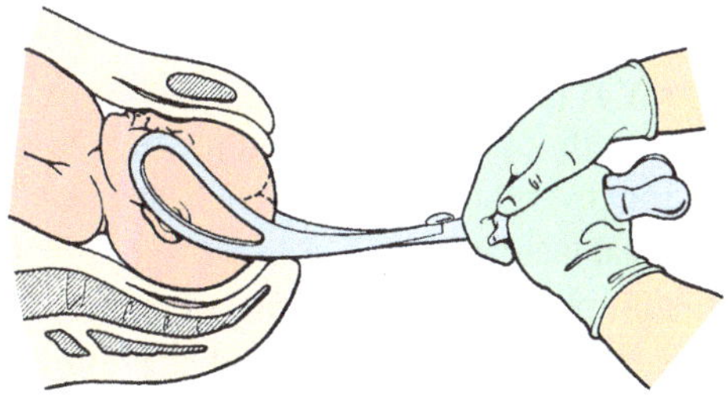

Fig. 8.29: Forceps in sinciput presentation (1) first, horizontal traction.

Example 3. Sagittal suture in LOD, anterior fontanelle left, anterior. Application: forceps in the ROD, applied transversely. The left blade is inserted first, links posteriorly; the right blade needs to be right, anterior, and is therefore inserted on the right, posteriorly and moved towards anterior.

Low Naegele forceps **extraction** (from pelvic floor) in direct sinciput anterior presentation (example 1) differs from that of the normal vertex presentation because the head (see course of labor) needs first to be brought into flexion, then extension.

Method (3 steps)

1. Traction in the direction of the handles for delivery of the sinciput (Fig. 8.29). The forceps are locked and a manual check is performed, then traction is applied horizontally and slightly upwards.
   Horizontal traction is applied until the anterior fontanelle is visible in the vulva. The hypomochlion (the area below the hairline of the brow) has reached the pubic arch, and can impinge upon it on the further delivery of the sinciput and occiput around the symphysis pubis.
   In examples 2 and 3 (see above), the forceps must be rotated simultaneously to bring the anterior fontanelle towards the symphysis pubis: in left sinciput presentation clockwise, and in right presentation counterclockwise.

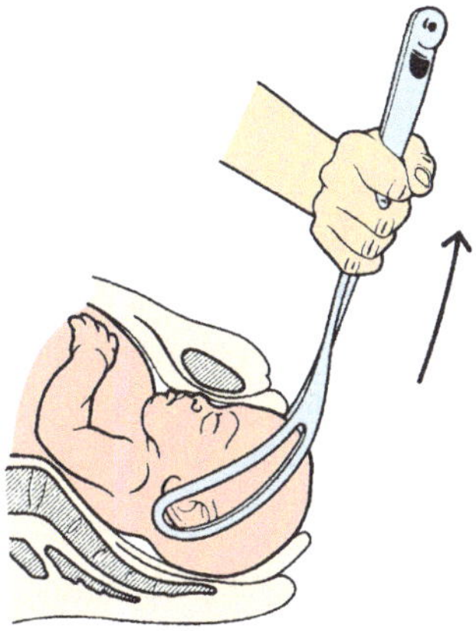

Fig. 8.30: Forceps in sinciput presentation (2) elevation of the handles.

2. Elevation of the forceps handles for delivery of the sinciput and occiput (Fig. 8.30). Position and hand change, perineal protection!
   Position change
   To the left side of the woman
   Hand change
   The left hand goes to the perineum and remains there in order to protect it; this must never be neglected because the perineum is overstretched. The danger of third degree perineal laceration is extremely high in sinciput anterior forceps. Gradual elevation of the forceps with the right hand alone. Note: the right hand encircles the lock (Fig. 8.30), not the handles

(far too much leverage!) and delivers as slowly as possible, millimeter for millimeter, the sinciput and then the broad occiput over the perineum (greatest risk of perineal laceration!).
All abrupt or rapid movements of the forceps threaten to end in perineal laceration.

3. Lowering of the forceps (reverse movement) for delivery of brow and face (Fig. 8.31).
Only the right hand lowers the forceps. The left hand remains on the perineum to protect it.

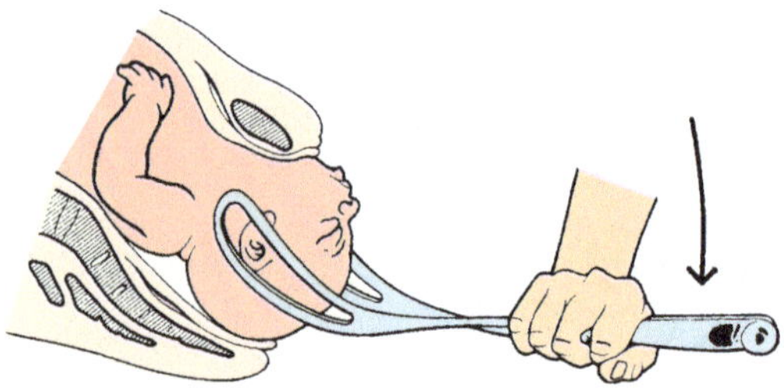

Fig. 8.31: Forceps in sinciput presentation (3) lowering of the handles, reverse movement. The left hand (not depicted) guards the perineum.

Brow presentation

Definition. Next degree of extension after sinciput presentation; brow takes the lead until the head is born. The plane of passage is the largest (35–36 cm; as opposed to normal OA with a plane of passage of 32 cm). Rare and dangerous (see below).

Incidence. Very rare, 1 : 2,000–3,000 births.

Note. Brow presentation is the least favorable and most dangerous of all cephalic presentations with the possibility of vaginal delivery: maximum circumference, molding of the brow is not possible.

Etiology. The main causes are contracted pelvis and oxycephalic (pointed) head shape.

Clinical manifestation, diagnosis

External examination

- Findings similar to face presentation: heart sounds on the side of the extremities (chest lies closer to the uterine wall than the back).

Vaginal examination

- On the one side the anterior fontanelle is palpated, on the other the eyebrows and root of the nose, the face (Fig. 8.32). The mouth is reachable, the chin, however, is not.

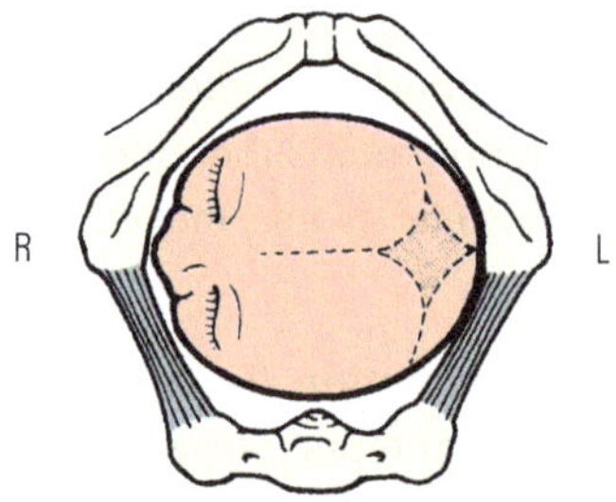

Fig. 8.32: Left brow presentation.

- If the chin is reachable, it is not a brow but a face presentation.
- The suture which runs from the anterior fontanelle towards the nose is the frontal suture. It is to be found mostly in transverse, more rarely in an oblique diameter.
- On ultrasound examination the fetal spine is shown to be posterior, towards the maternal spine.

Nomenclature. Brow position: if this finding is made when the head is still mobile in the pelvic inlet or even higher, it is called a brow position, a transitory position which develops into a face presentation (most face presentations begin as brow position).

Brow presentation. Not until the head has descended and retained its position after rupture of the membranes can it be thus termed.

Course of labor

Note.
Leading part. Brow (glabella).
Pivot point. Maxilla or malar bone.
Birth of head. First flexion then extension.
Largest plane of passage. Maxilloparietal (or zygomaticoparietal). > circumference 35 - 36 cm!

Leading part is the middle of the frontal suture or lower, the glabella: the hairless space between the eyebrows. Until the curve of Carus and the pelvic floor, the frontal suture is palpable in a transverse diameter (Fig. 8.32). Rotation occurs on the pelvic floor over the oblique to almost or direct anteroposterior diameter (occiput posterior!). Accordingly, the cheekbone (malar bone) or the middle of the maxilla present as pivot point against the lower edge of the symphysis pubis.
Similar to OP or sinciput presentation, birth occurs in 2 movements (see Tab. 8.1): flexion, whereby the parietal region and occiput sweep the perineum and extension so that the face may be born under the pubic arch.
The largest crowning circumference is the maxillo- or zygomaticoparietal with 35–36 cm!
Vaginal delivery is not possible from the dorsoanterior, nasoposterior brow presentation (brow doesn't rotate anteriorly, but posteriorly) or from the mentoposterior presentation!

Treatment. Spontaneous delivery is possible if the head is small or the pelvis spacious, which applies in 30–40 % of all cephalic presentations.

Cesarean section is the method of choice.
VE is preferred by other authors. It is possible to bring the high head (pelvic inlet) into an attitude of flexion and then an OA presentation by applying the extractor twice.
Forceps delivery is contraindicated because the forceps become a dangerous instrument! Brow presentation forceps is the forceps delivery with the worst prognosis: fetal mortality is shockingly high and the maternal risks are not minor.

Face presentation

Definition. Complete extension. Presenting part is the face, leading part the chin (mentum). Circumference of the plane of passage: 34 cm.

Incidence. One mentoanterior face presentation in 200–300 births; the mentoposterior face presentation (back anterior!) is rare.

Classification. Mentoposterior (dorsoanterior) face presentation: chin posterior, vaginal birth impossible if the fetus does not rotate; mentoanterior (dorsoposterior) face presentation: chin anterior.

Etiology. Dolichocephalic skull (long, thin skull), CPD, e.g., due to goiter, hygroma. According to Kneer, the permanent contraction of the neck muscles plays a particular role; it occurs in brain defects and also in normal fetuses. In tumors of the birth canal, cervical myomas in particular cause the head to take on the extension or face presentation.

Clinical manifestation, diagnosis (Fig. 8.33). Vaginal examination: chin, mouth, nose, eyebrow area are palpated.

Differential diagnosis. Breech presentation. Should not be mistaken for other presentations

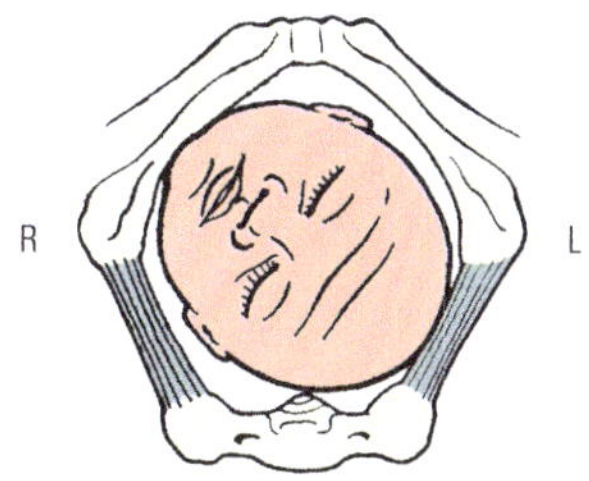

Fig. 8.33: Findings on internal examination of right mentoanterior presentation.

on vaginal examination. Inexperienced examiners can mistake the mouth for the anus and diagnose a breech presentation; if a large caput is present differentiation is difficult:
- Characteristics of the mouth: the finger can be inserted easily; hard gums, tongue, and sometimes sucking movements are felt. The fetus often becomes restless on insertion into the mouth.
- Characteristics of the anus: the finger cannot be inserted into the anus of a living fetus, or only with force. If successful, the finger is meconium-stained.

Mechanism of labor

Note.
Leading part. Chin (mentum).
Pivot point. Hyoid bone.
Birth of head. Flexion only.
Largest plane of passage. Hyoparietal, circumference 34 cm

Brow position of the face presentation in the pelvic inlet, brow becomes the leading part, the face looks to the right or left side:
- Face → left: back right, right mentolateral.
- Face → right: back left, left mentolateral.

The axis of the face (line from the frontal suture over nose and mouth to chin), which corresponds to the sagittal suture in OA presentations, is in the transverse pelvic diameter, the chin laterally to the left or right.

After the first strong contractions the extension increases and the head enters the pelvis. The occiput is hereby forced even further towards the back, which at the same time forces the brow out of its leading position as the face takes the lead and enters the pelvis (secondary face presentation).

Descent continues in this maximally extended attitude with the facial axis in the transverse diameter until the head reaches the pelvic floor.

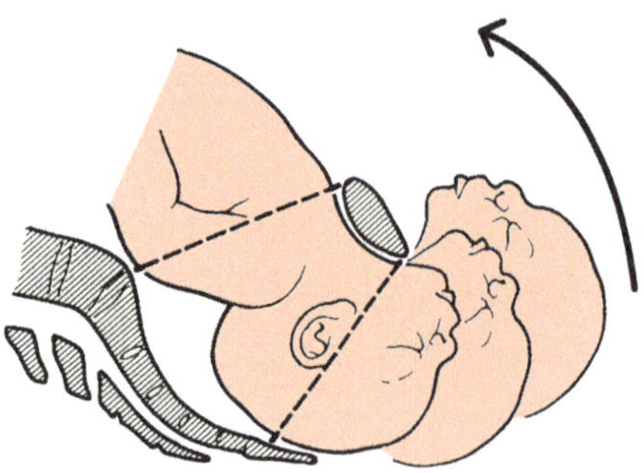

Fig. 8.34: Crowning movement: in a face presentation the curve of Carus is negotiated via extension only.

Crowning mechanism. The position of the facial axis changes once the pelvic floor has been reached.
- Left mentolateral presentation over the left oblique diameter (Fig. 8.33).
- Right mentolateral presentation over the right oblique diameter.

Hyperextended head. In order to negotiate the curve of Carus, the completely extended head must become flexed. The attitude of extension persists until chin, mouth, nose, and eyes have been born in that order.

Then the hypomochlion of the face presentation, the hyoid bone, impinges against the pubic arch and flexion of the head begins so that it may follow the birth canal around the symphysis pubis: sinciput, then occiput are born slowly over the perineum (Fig. 8.34).

Plane of passage. Hyo- or tracheoparietale, circumference 34 cm. Of note is that in face presentations the hypomochlion is outside the head, on the hyoid bone.

The **caput** occurs on the face, mostly on the presenting cheek. In
- left face presentation on the right cheek,
- right face presentation on the left cheek.

Facial disfigurement, stretch marks. As a result of the facial deformation, which also affects mouth and eyes, the face presentation baby looks disfigured for a few days. Hyperextension also remains for a number of days. Stretch marks are visible on the neck.

Practice tip. The mechanism of labor in face presentation is the opposite to that of a normal vertex presentation. This fact is helpful in understanding the course of labor in face presentation (Tab. 8.1).

Characteristics of the course of labor. Labor is often longer than in normal vertex presentation. There are 3 reasons for this:
- larger plane of passage: hyoparietal plane,with 34 cm (instead of 32),
- the face as presenting part is less suitable for widening the soft tissues,
- the extreme force due to hyperextension.

Tab. 8.1: Normal vertex presentation versus face presentation.

Pelvic entry, exit	Normal vertex pres.	Face pres.
On entering the pelvis	Maximum flexion	Maximum extension
On exiting	Extension only	Flexion only
Pivot point (in both cases not on the head)	Neck hairline at the back of the neck	Hyoid bone at the front of the neck
order of birth over the perineum	Occiput sinciput brow eyes nose mouth chin	Chin mouth nose eyes brow sinciput occiput

It is possible to imagine the strength of force necessary to uphold this enforced attitude if one tries to force the head of a newborn lying on a table into this hyperextended attitude, the exact attitude in which the head must pass through the birth canal. The same force is exerted on the soft tissue padding of the birth canal, which leads to a severe increase of frictional resistances.

In addition, the perineum is extremely distended on crowning by the passage of the posterior occiput, which necessitates active perineal protection.

Prognosis. Most face presentations run a spontaneous course without artificial assistance if the chin rotates anteriorly (threat of perineal laceration!)

Obstructed labor occurs when the chin does not rotate into a mentoanterior but rather a mentoposterior presentation (Fig. 8.35) on reaching the pelvic floor. Vaginal delivery is impossible from a mentoposterior presentation:

The head is hyperextended with the posterior chin on the pelvic floor. In order to negotiate the curve of the birth canal so that the head may be born in a curve around the symphysis pubis, the head would need to be further extended, overextended. This degree of overextension is impossible, as the occiput has already reached its maximum extension, is forced as far as possible backwards.

Treatment (→mentoanterior face presentation). Strict expectant management, as with all

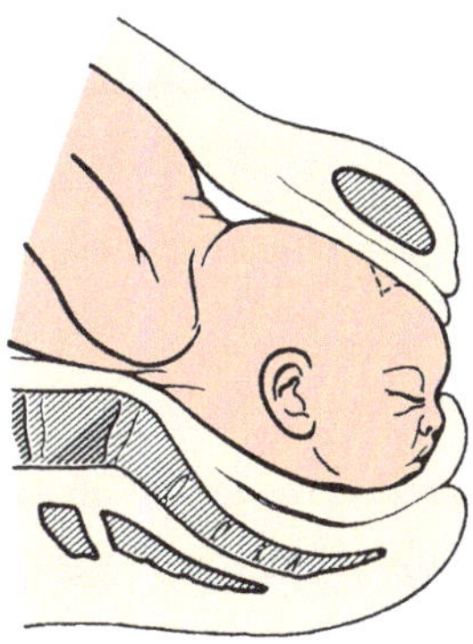

Fig. 8.35: Mentoposterior face presentation, spontaneous delivery impossible.

extended presentations (exception: brow presentation); operation is an exception!

Conservative treatment

Positioning. Correct positioning is necessary so that a brow position at the onset of labor does not develop into a brow presentation!

The woman is to lie on the side of the chin, which under favorable circumstances will thus be released and enter the pelvis.

Operative treatment

Note. Cesarean section is the method of choice at the onset of labor to terminate labor in midpelvis.

Forceps should be avoided if possible! Indication: fetal hypoxia or pathological CTG.
Wait until the facial axis is in or close to the APD of the pelvic outlet. The chin must be anterior. If it is posterior, delivery of the head is impossible!
Forceps delivery is contraindicated as long as the facial axis is in or close to the transverse diameter. Forceps delivery of a head in an unfavorable plane of passage (sinciput, face or brow presentation) is not recommended. The head circumference is increased with forceps application, and rotating under traction is particularly difficult and dangerous, whereby deep laceration of the maternal soft tissue canal can result.

Practice tip. Face presentation forceps is extremely difficult. It is a dangerous procedure for mother and fetus if the head has not yet reached the pelvic floor or outlet and the facial axis is not in the anteroposterior diameter!

Method

Example 1. Head has reached the pelvic floor, facial axis in APD, chin anterior below the symphysis pubis.

The tips of the Naegele forceps must always point towards the chin. Both blades are inserted laterally as for normal vertex presentation with sagittal suture in the APD (Fig. 8.36; see general rules, p. 322).
The forceps are not closed, but the disarticulated handles are first elevated (Fig. 8.37) and then locked.
If the forceps were closed after insertion as usual, the occiput would not be grasped, but rather the face and neck, and the tips would injure the neck.
The occiput, to which the blades are to be applied, lies deeply posterior in the sacral cavity. In order to grasp it, the unlocked handles must be lifted up high before locking.

Extraction in 2 steps:
Horizontal traction until the chin is born. If uncertain about the direction of traction, the

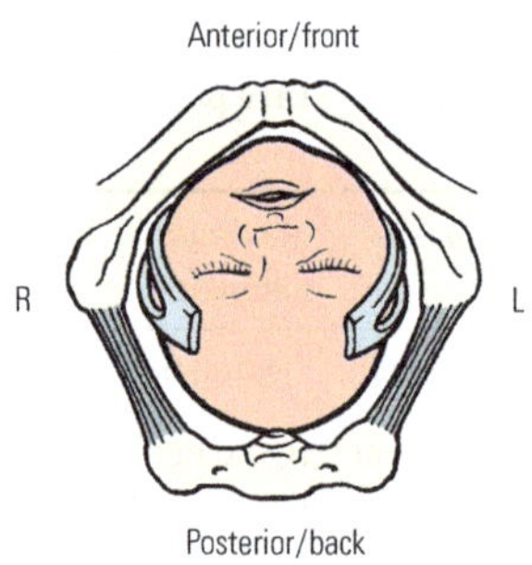

Fig. 8.36: Face presentation forceps. Apply when facial axis is in the anteroposterior diameter.

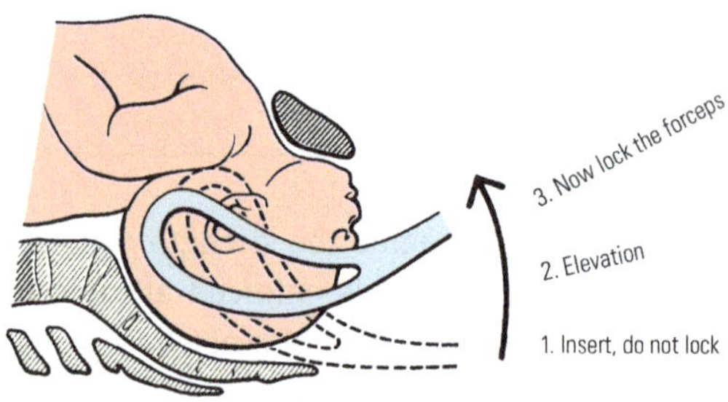

Fig. 8.37: After insertion of the forceps (1) they are not closed, the unlocked handles are elevated (2), and then locked.

operator only needs to let go of the handles briefly:

1. if the forceps have been correctly applied, the handles will always point in the direction in which traction is to be applied. In particular, the manner in which the face presentation forceps must be held in order to avoid losing grip;
2. both hands hold the handles, whereby the Busch finger rest is between index and middle finger of the hand closest to the blades (right).

Once the chin is visible the pivot point (hyoid bone) is below the pubic arch, which leads to:
- position and hand change (Fig. 8.38), move to the left side.

Only the right hand is now holding the forceps, encircling the lock, and it brings about flexion of the head with the forceps in order to negotiate the curve around the symphysis pubis. The forceps are hereby slowly elevated towards the maternal abdomen.

- The left hand is always on the perineum: active perineal protection!

Do not perform face presentation forceps without a generous episiotomy!

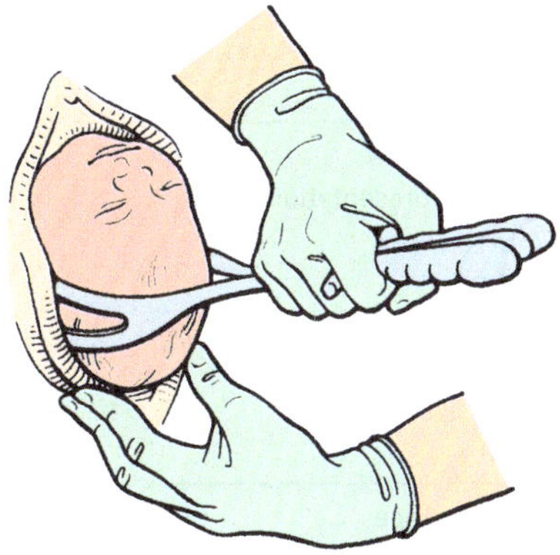

Fig. 8.38: Extraction, face presentation (example 1). Once the chin has been born, only the right hand holds the forceps, at right angles to the handles, encircling the lock. Left hand on the perineum (modified; after Stoeckel).

Tab. 8.2: Overview of normal vertex presentation, malpresentations and malpositions.

Diagram	Diagnosis	Leading part	Pivot point (hypomochlion)	Crowning	Largest plane of passage	Circumference
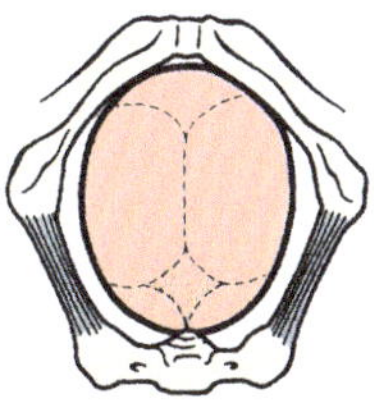 Fig. 8.39	Normal vertex (occipitoanterior) presentation	Posterior fontanelle	Occiput	Extension	Suboccipitobregmatic	32 cm
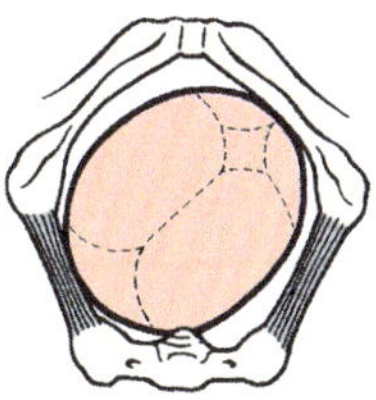 Fig. 8.40	Occipitoposterior presentation	Anterior fontanelle–parietal region	Anterior fontanelle–brow hairline	First extreme flexion then extension	Suboccipitobregmatic	32 cm

Diagram	Diagnosis	Leading part	Pivot point (hypomochlion)	Crowning	Largest plane of passage	Circumference
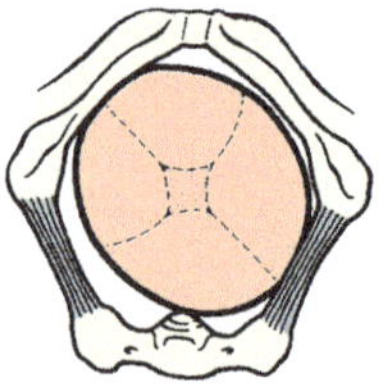 Fig. 8.41	Sinciput presentation	Anterior fontanelle	Brow hairline to root of nose	First flexion then extension	Occipitofrontal	34 cm
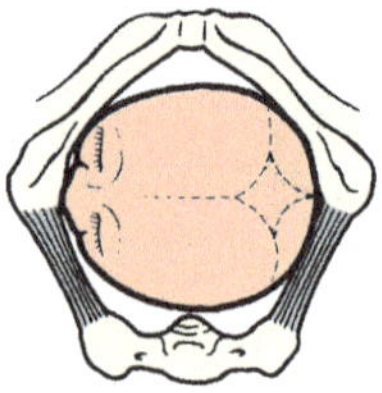 Fig. 8.42	Brow presentation	Brow	Maxilla (usually) or malar bone (zygoma)	First flexion then extension	Maxillo- or zygomaticoparietal	35–36 cm
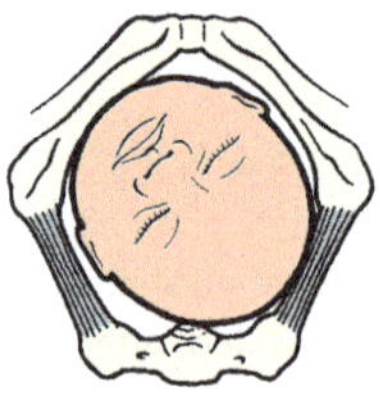 Fig. 8.43	Face presentation	Chin	Hyoid bone	Flexion only	Hyo- or tracheoparietal	34 cm

Diagram	Diagnosis	Findings
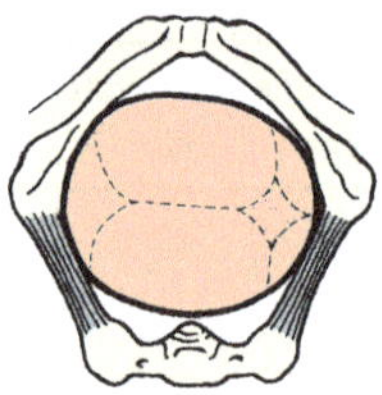 Fig. 8.44	Persistent occipitotransverse presentation	Head on pelvic floor, transverse sagittal suture, posterior fontanelle left (or right) lateral, anterior fontanelle right (or left) lateral.
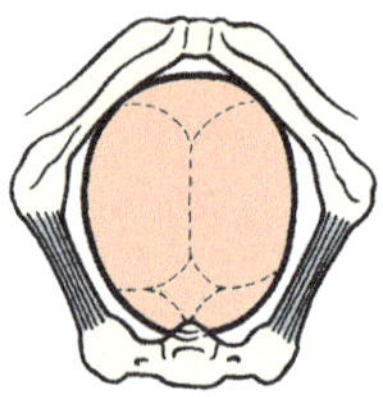 Fig. 8.45	High anteroposterior head	Head above pelvic inlet, sagittal suture in anteroposterior diameter, posterior fontanelle at symphysis pubis (or sacral promontory), anterior fontanelle at sacral promontory (or symphysis pubis).

Practice tip. To be internalized for face presentation forceps:
- After insertion the forceps are elevated and then locked (Fig. 8.37).
- The forceps are to be held in both hands at right angles to the handles in the first step of extraction, the head can only be born only via flexion (see Fig. 8.38). There is no reverse (extension) movement in face presentation forceps. The reverse movement belongs to the forceps technique in: OP, sinciput, and brow presentations.

Example 2. The head has almost reached the pelvic floor, chin left anterior, root of nose right.

Treatment (→ mentoposterior face presentation).

Lateral positioning. If the fetus is in a high (pelvic inlet, midpelvis) lateral to posterior presentation, an attempt is made to encourage the chin to move anteriorly.

Positioning on the side of the chin.
Vaginal delivery impossible. If the head has reached the pelvic floor and the chin is palpable direct posteriorly, there is no longer any possibility that the chin will rotate anteriorly. This finding is one of the rarest in obstetrics. The chin cannot rotate spontaneously into an anterior position, and neither can it be brought into one with forceps. Delivery of the head is impossible when the chin is posterior because the head would need to overextend further in order to be born. Vaginal delivery is therefore impossible.

Cesarean section. If lateral positioning is unsuccessful and the head is high or midpelvis, a cesarean section is performed.

The use of **forceps** is contraindicated because success is not possible. Instead, severe vaginal tissue lacerations may be caused.
Expectant management is now contraindicated, because the mother is at risk:
- Fever intrapartum → septicemia.
- → vesicovaginal fistula.

Immediate termination of labor, because mother and fetus are at risk. If contractions are strong uterus rupture is a danger. Termination with
- living fetus by cesarean section,
- stillbirth by perforation of the head with cranioclasm (see p. 343), best via mouth or frontal bone (frontal suture).

8.2 Breech presentation

Definition. Longitudinal lie in which the buttocks are the leading part. Classification according to the presenting part (see below).

Incidence. 5 % of all births, over half affecting nulliparous women; more common in preterm deliveries (Tab. 8.3).

Etiology. The cause in unclear in about 80 % of cases.

Influencing factors are:
- Preterm delivery; breech delivery is more common the more premature the delivery. Around 1/3 of all breech deliveries are preterm babies.
- Deformity. Hydrocephaly, anencephaly, tumors of the caudal end of the body make fixation of the fetal head at the pelvic inlet

Tab. 8.3: Fetal presentations (in percentages) according to gestational age (Scheer and Nubar 1976).

Gestational age	Cephalic presentation	Breech presentation	Transverse presentation
21–25 weeks	55	33	12
25–29 weeks	62	28	10
29–33 weeks	78	14	8
33–37 weeks	89	9	3
37–40 weeks	92	7	1

difficult or alter the head/trunk weight ratio so that the lighter head remains in the fundus.
- Uterine cause. Distended uterus of the multiparous woman, bicornuate or subseptate uterus, which obstruct fetal rotation; furthermore hydramnios. Result: increased fetal mobility, hampering fixation of the head; oligohydramnios (→ rotation is not possible!)
- Contracted pelvis with restricted fetal mobility, also in twins, cervical tumors.
- Deformity. Hydrocephaly, anencephaly, tumors of the caudal end of the body.

8.2.1 Classification, diagnosis, differential diagnosis

Classification. Depending on the attitude of the lower extremities, the types of breech presentation are frank, complete, footling, or kneeling (rare):

Presenting part is:
- Buttocks: Frank breech (Fig. 8.46). Legs are extended along the fetal abdomen.
- Buttocks, two feet: Complete breech (Fig. 8.47).
- Buttocks, one foot: Single footling breech (Fig. 8.48).
- Both feet: Double footling breech (Fig. 8.49).
- Both knees: Kneeling breech (rare).
- One knee: Incomplete kneeling breech (rare).

Clinical manifestation, diagnosis

External examination. Breech presentations are usually recognized by external examination. Examination is more difficult in cases of obesity, firm abdominal muscles, and hydramnios.
- The back is on one side, the extremities (small parts) on the other. The back is usually anterior, on the left or right. Head in fundus.
- The head is ballottable. If the abdominal wall is not too thick, the head can often be grasped quite easily between thumb and two fingers and moved back and forth (see Fig. 8.50).
- The head is palpable in the fundus as a firm, round, mobile mass.
- The breech is palpable above the pelvic inlet.

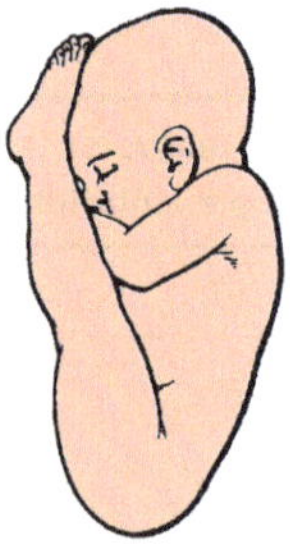

Fig. 8.46: Frank breech (extended legs).

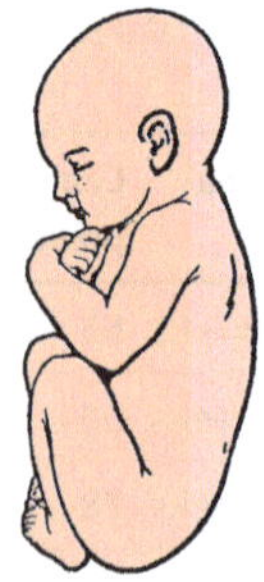

Fig. 8.47: Complete breech.

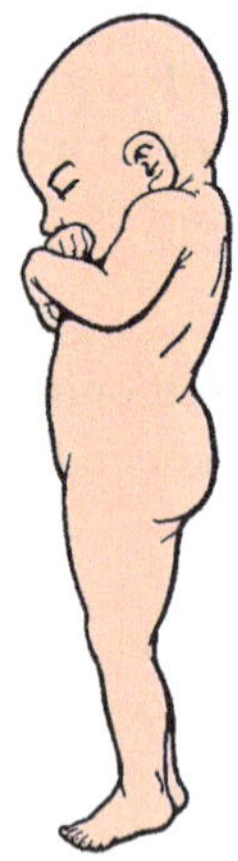

Fig. 8.48: Double footling breech.

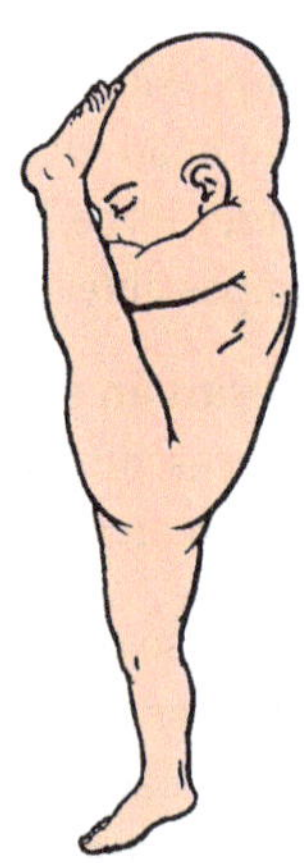

Fig. 8.49: Single footling breech.

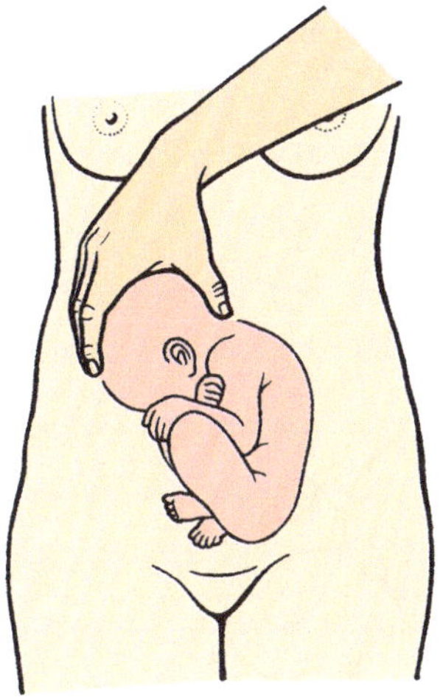

Fig. 8.50: Ballottement of the head.

Note. Third and fourth Leopold maneuver (head maneuver) demonstrate that the head is not being palpated.
The "head feeling" is missing due to the four negative signs: the presenting part is not as large, hard, evenly round, or ballottable as the head.
The four positive signs on grasping the presenting part are: a smaller part, softer, alternating soft and firm parts, and irregular shape.

Sonography confirms the diagnosis!

Vaginal examination. As soon as the presenting part has entered the pelvis, an irregular and primarily soft fetal part is felt; here a bony protrusion is felt, there a bony ridge.

Three negative signs of breech as opposed to head: not evenly firm, no sutures or fontanelles.

Practice tip. If the cervix is fully dilated and the presenting part has descended the following are felt: ischial tuberosities, sacrum, and hip joint. The main characteristic is the crista sacralis media(na), the medial sacral crest, which is felt to the left or right. This marked bony ridge is not overlooked! If the buttocks are still high, they are pushed from above deep into the pelvis.

Anus. Sometimes the anus is felt in the longitudinal groove between the buttocks (caution:

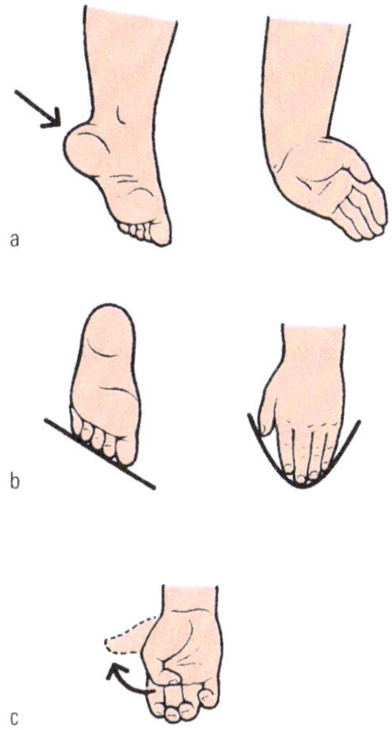

Fig. 8.51: Differentiation between hand and foot; a) heel sign; b) toe sign; c) thumb sign.

sphincter injury if penetrated roughly!), the scrotum is also often felt (→ predictions as to gender should be avoided; the supposed scrotum often turns out later to be a caput).

Diagnosis of footling presentation. Internal examination is simple when a single foot presents. However, one must beware of confusion between foot and hand, resulting in misdiagnosis of a breech presentation instead of the correct and life-threatening for mother and baby: transverse lie (prolapsed arm is much rarer in cephalic presentations).

Foot vs. hand (Fig. 8.51). The birth attendant must know the characteristics of foot and hand very well:

- Heel sign (Fig. 8.51a). The heel (heel bone, calcaneus) is the most important characteristic of the foot. At the junction between calf and foot the pointy heel is felt, the junction is angular! The junction of arm and hand is flat; the hand is the straight extension of the lower arm.

- Toe sign (Fig. 8.51b). Toes are shorter than fingers, of equal length; fingers are not (thumb!).
- The line of the toes is straight, the finger line is bent
- Thumb sign (Fig. 8.51c). The thumb can be opposed, the big toe cannot.

Diagnosis of kneeling breech. Rare subtype of breech presentation. The mobile patella must always be distinguished from the immovable olecranon. If uncertain, the smaller part of the extremity is followed with the finger until a hand or foot is encountered.

Differential diagnosis. Face presentation. The frank breech presentation can only be confused with the face presentation. Transverse presentation, hydrocephalus. Occasionally there has been confusion with a transverse presentation (shoulder!), and a hydrocephalus, when the cervix was only minimally dilated.

Differentiation between mouth and after (see p. 227) becomes difficult if a large caput is present.

Note. Diagnostic signs are:
First Leopold maneuver. A large, hard, round ballottable mass is felt in the fundus.
Third and fourth Leopold maneuver. The correct "head feeling" is missing (p. 25).
Heart sounds slightly above the navel.
Vaginal examination. Irregularly shaped, mostly soft fetal part with bony protrusions and ridges; medial sacral crest, leg(s), foot (feet) or (rare) knee(s).
Confirmation. Ultrasound.

8.2.2 Mechanism of labor

Frank breech presentation (Fig. 8.52–8.75)

It is not possible to understand management of a breech presentation delivery or the rules of operative intervention without knowledge of

Fig. 8.52–8.75: Mechanism of labor in breech presentation (frank breech in RSA).

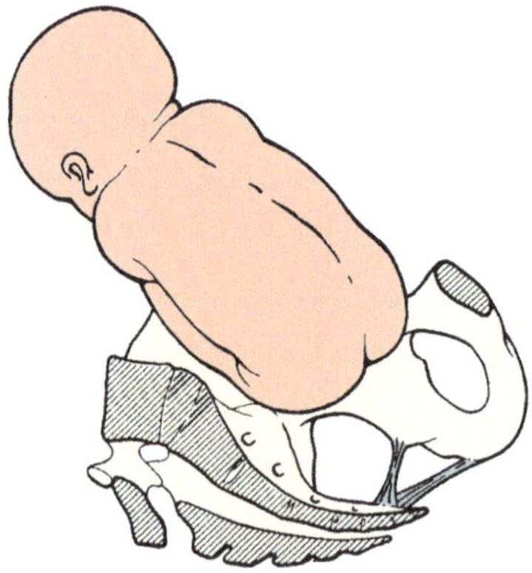

Fig. 8.52

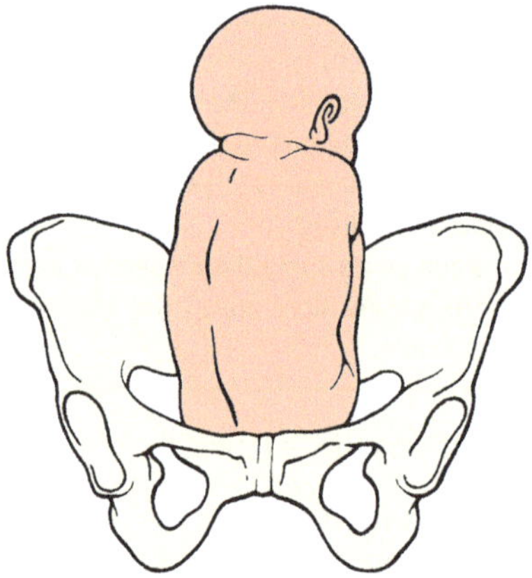

Fig. 8.53

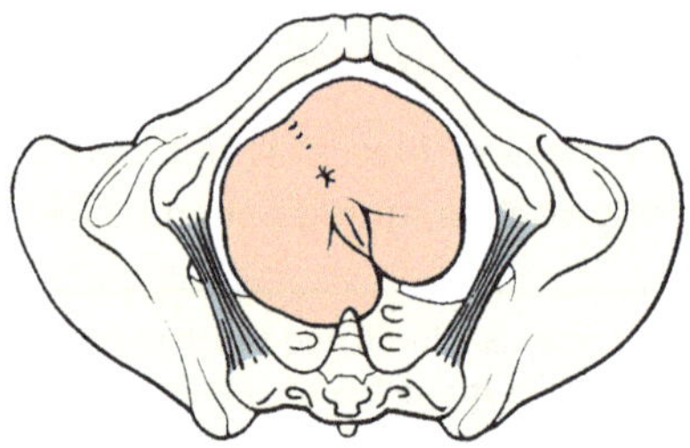

Fig. 8.54

Fig. 8.52–8.54: The breech enters the pelvic inlet (Figs. 8.52–8.54). The breech as presenting part usually engages in an oblique diameter. In a right sacroanterior presentation (RSA) the bitrochanteric diameter is in the left oblique diameter: Fig. 8.52 from the side, Fig 8.53 the same from the front, Fig. 8.54 the same seen from below.

the birth mechanism. For didactic reasons, the birth mechanism is divided.

Note. Five stages of the birth mechanism:
1. Breech engages and descends to the pelvic floor.
2. Negotiation of the curve of Carus and birth of the buttocks.
3. Birth of the trunk.
4. Birth of the shoulders.
5. Birth of the head.

The breech engages and descends to the pelvic floor. The breech as leading part usually engages in the pelvis with the bitrochanteric diameter (largest diameter) in an oblique diameter (Fig. 8.52–8.54):
- The back is anterior, therefore:
- Back (sacrum) left anterior: Left sacroanterior (LSA), bitrochanteric diameter in right oblique diameter.
- Back (sacrum) right anterior: right sacroanterior (RSA), bitrochanteric diameter in left oblique diameter (Fig. 8. 54).
- The beginner can best understand this using a model.

Rarely the bitrochanteric diameter engages in the transverse or anteroposterior pelvic diameter.

Negotiation of the curve of Carus and birth of the breech. Once it has reached the pelvic floor (Figs. 8.55–8.57) the breech has entered the curve of Carus. In order to progress, it must negotiate the curve around the symphysis pubis; the breech rotates onto its side which enables it to then bend sideways (lateral flexion).

Two possibilities for negotiating the curve of Carus:
- Rotation of the bitrochanteric diameter of the breech from the oblique into the anteroposterior diameter. The bitrochanteric diameter passes most easily through the longitudinal vulvo-vaginal opening if it is in the APD.
- The more anterior hip rotates towards the symphysis pubis:
  - In left sacroanterior the left hip.
  - In right sacroanterior the right hip (Fig. 8.54).
- The back (sacrum) moves into a lateral position (Figs. 8.55–8.57).
- Lateral flexion (Figs. 8.58–8.60), bending sideways. The fetus which is on its side in the APD must now bend laterally (lateral flexion), in order to adapt to the curve of Carus; the fetus is in a forced flexion.

Both negotiation possibilities belong together as a process of adaptation. The fetus rotates in the direction into which the following section of the body (in this case, the lumbar spine) can most easily bend (facillimum of flexion) in order to best fit into the birth canal.
As long as the legs, in particular the thighs, are extended on the abdomen, the spine can most easily bend to the side. In preparation for delivery, the breech best fits into the curve of Carus by rotating into the APD and flexing laterally (Figs. 8.52–8.57).
The anterior hip braces itself as hypomochlion against the pubic arch and becomes the pivot point around which the posterior hip rotates on delivery (Figs. 8.58–8.60).
First the anterior buttock becomes visible in the vulva and remains there; then the posterior also appears. The posterior hip sweeps the perineum first, and after the rest of the pelvis has rotated out the anterior buttock emerges and the anterior hip is born under the pubic arch and the breech has been born.

Birth of the trunk. Once the breech has been born, the trunk follows with extreme lateral flexion of the thoracic spine (Figs. 8.61–8.63). The back rotates anteriorly (towards the symphysis pubis, Fig. 8.65) as soon as the legs have slipped out. The breech and the part of the trunk which has already been born are steeply angled upwards in the extension of the birth axis (Figs. 8.64–8.66).

Why does the back rotate anteriorly (towards the symphysis pubis)?

- The shoulders have entered the pelvis. The shoulders, which have descended to the pelvic inlet, can only pass through it with the bisacromial diameter (greatest shoulder diameter) transverse or oblique. This forces the back to rotate anteriorly.
- Altering of the facillimum of flexion, utilization of the easiest direction of flexion. The

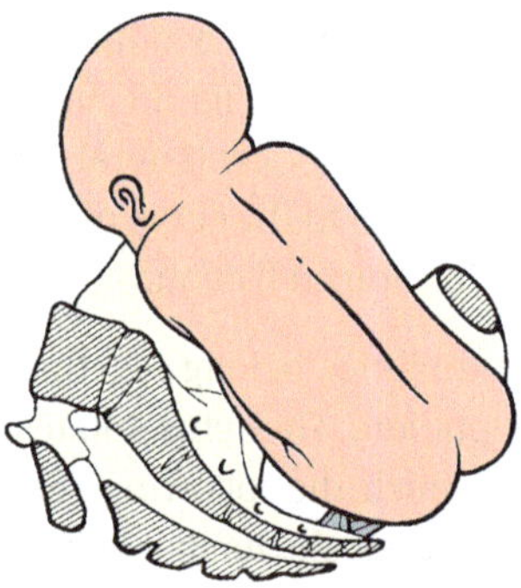

Fig. 8.55

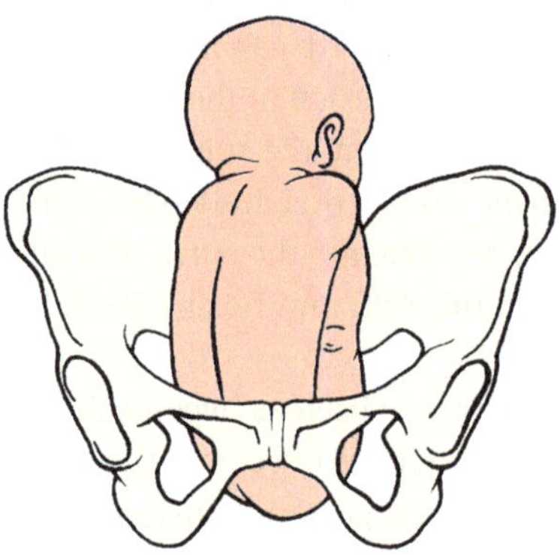

Fig. 8.56

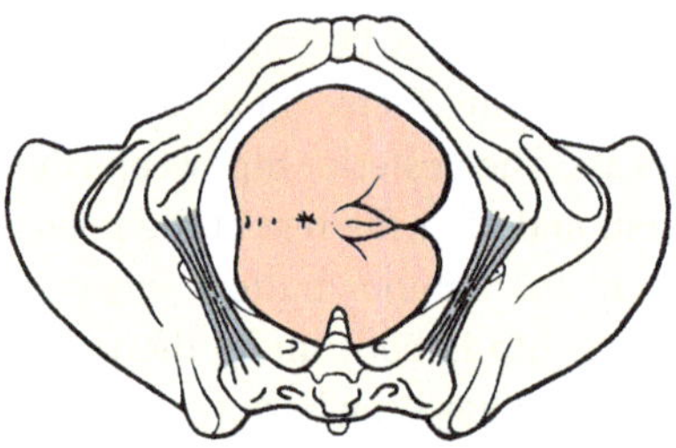

Fig. 8.57

Fig. 8.55–8.57: The breech has reached the pelvic floor (Fig. 8.55–8.57). Having reached the pelvic floor, the curve of Carus, the breech rotates from the oblique into the anteroposterior diameter: Fig. 8.55 from the side, Fig 8.56 the same from the front, Fig. 8.57 the same seen from below.

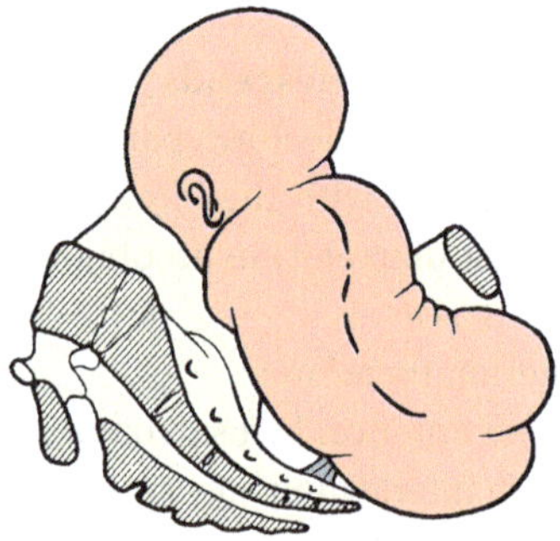

Fig. 8.58

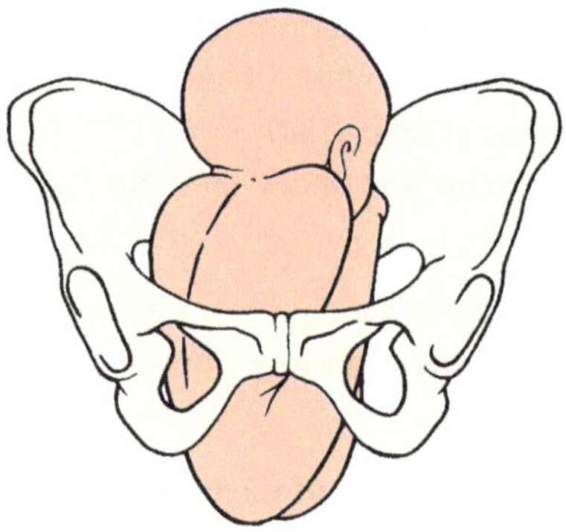

Fig. 8.59

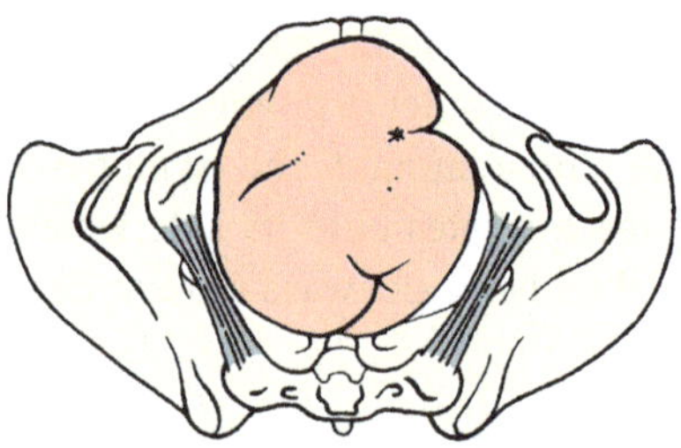

Fig. 8.60

Fig. 8.58–8.60: Mechanism of expulsion of the breech (Fig. 8.58–8.60). The lumbar spine must undergo lateral flexion in order to negotiate the curve of Carus once the bitrochanteric diameter has rotated into the APD: Fig. 8.58 from the side, Fig 8.59 the same from the front, Fig. 8.60 the same seen from below.

facillimum of flexion of the thoracic spine, that is the easiest direction of flexion, depends on whether the legs are extended onto the trunk.

– – Extended legs act as a splint for the trunk: the thoracic spine can bend more easily to the side as to the back. Once the legs have been born (splinting is removed) the thoracic spine can be bent backwards more easily. This is why the back rotates after the legs have been born in such a way that it can be bent backwards, that is, from the birth canal anteriorly towards the symphysis pubis.

Birth of the shoulders. The shoulders have now reached the pelvic floor. In order to be able to pass through the longitudinal open-

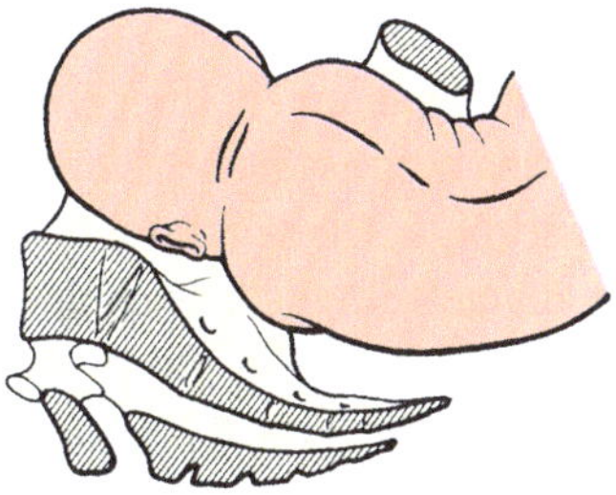

Fig. 8.61

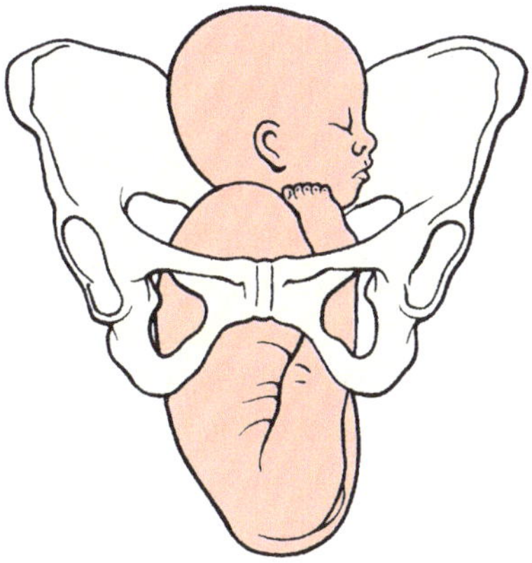

Fig. 8.62

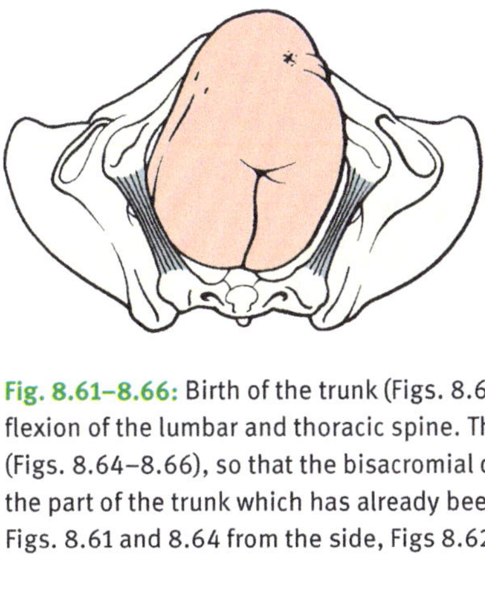

Fig. 8.63

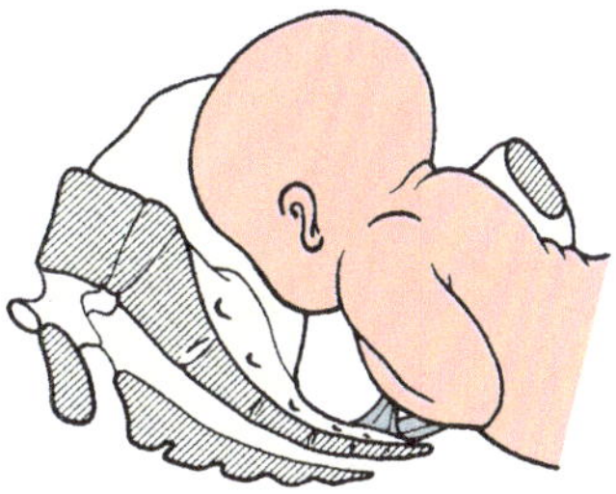

Fig. 8.64

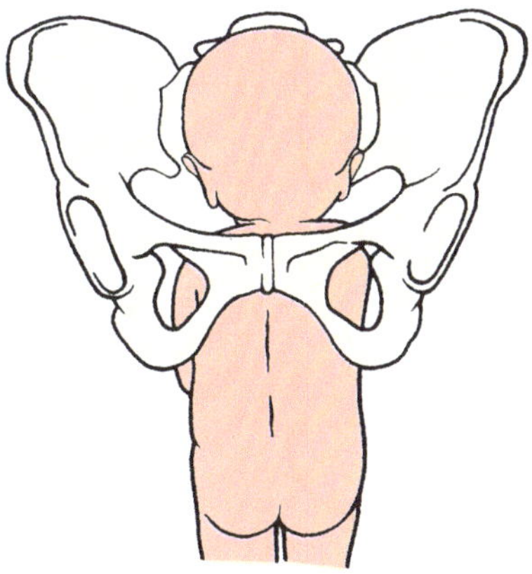

Fig. 8.65

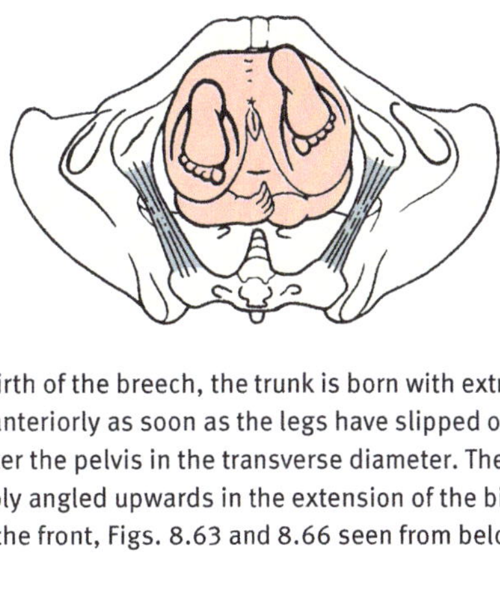

Fig. 8.66

Fig. 8.61–8.66: Birth of the trunk (Figs. 8.61–8.66). After birth of the breech, the trunk is born with extreme lateral flexion of the lumbar and thoracic spine. The back rotates anteriorly as soon as the legs have slipped out (Figs. 8.64–8.66), so that the bisacromial diameter can enter the pelvis in the transverse diameter. The breech and the part of the trunk which has already been born are steeply angled upwards in the extension of the birth axis: Figs. 8.61 and 8.64 from the side, Figs 8.62 and 8.65 from the front, Figs. 8.63 and 8.66 seen from below.

ing of the pelvic outlet, the shoulders position themselves in the APD. With that, the back rotates and returns once more to its original side (Figs. 8.67–8.69).

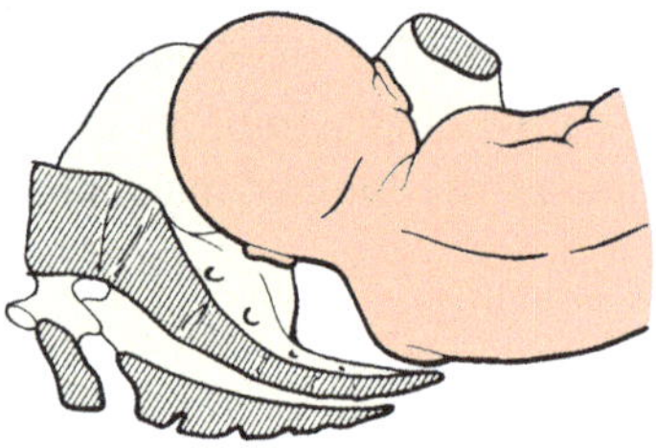

Fig. 8.67

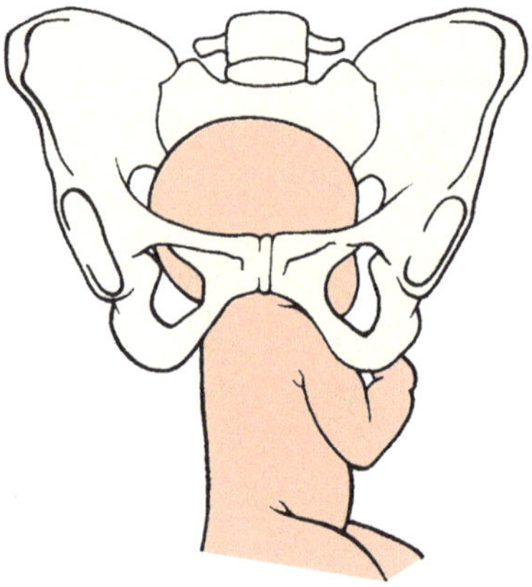

Fig. 8.68

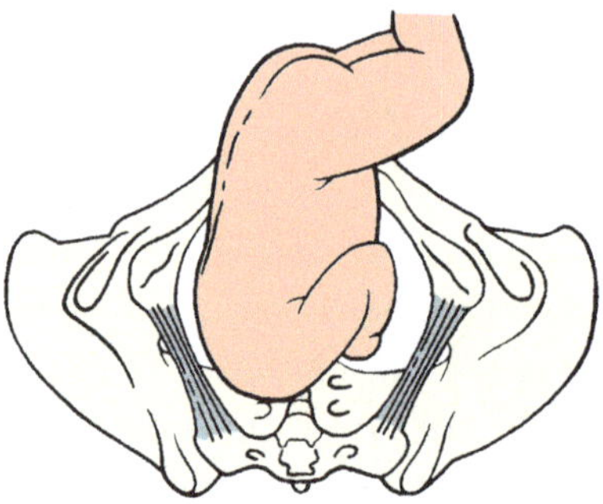

Fig. 8.69

Fig. 8.67–8.69: Birth of the shoulders (Fig. 8.67–8.69). The shoulders position themselves with the bisacromial diameter in the APD on the pelvic floor in order to be able to pass through the longitudinal vulvo-vaginal opening. The anterior shoulder is born first (under the symphysis pubis), later the posterior sweeps the perineum: Fig. 8.67 from the side, Fig 8.68 the same from the front, Fig. 8.69 the same seen from below.

If the birth continues spontaneously, which is not uncommon in multiparae, the anterior shoulder, that is, that closest to the symphysis pubis, will be born first, followed by the posterior shoulder, that closest to the perineum.
The bisacromial diameter is in the transverse or oblique diameter in the pelvic inlet, in the oblique in midpelvis and in the pelvic outlet in the anteroposterior. The bisacromial diameter descends through the same diameters as the bitrochanteric diameter before it.

Birth of the head. The head enters the pelvis when the trunk has been born as far as the lower edge of the anterior scapula. The sagittal suture is in the transverse diameter in the pelvic inlet, in midpelvis in the oblique and in the pelvic outlet in the APD of the pelvis (Figs. 8.70–8.72).

The occiput rotates anteriorly on the pelvic floor; the facillimum of flexion is in the cervical spine, towards the back. Now it is the head which rotates in the easiest direction which lines up with the axis of the birth canal.

- Hypomochlion is the suboccipital hairline, as in a normal vertex presentation (Figs. 8.70 and 8.73). Chin, mouth, nose, brow, sinciput, and lastly the occiput are born one after another over the perineum.
- The most favorable plane of passage is the suboccipitofrontal: 32 cm.

Note. The back (sacrum) rotates laterally twice (Figs. 8.77, 8.79) and twice anteriorly (Figs. 8.78, 8.80) on its passage through the birth canal.

Footling presentation

The **double footling breech** is to be managed as a frank breech, just that here the feet and legs are born first.

Single (incomplete) footling breech. If the anterior leg leads, birth is similar to that of the frank breech. If the posterior leg is in the lead, the fetus must rotate 180°, so that the posterior leg rotates anteriorly and the birth then progresses as when the anterior leg is leading.

Note. Complications: there are five dangers to the fetus in breech presentations.

1. Hypoxia, danger of asphyxiation as soon as the breech has been born.
2. Intracranial hemorrhage due to tentorial laceration as a result of birth trauma.
3. Soft tissue injury.
4. Premature rupture of membranes.
5. Cord prolapsed.

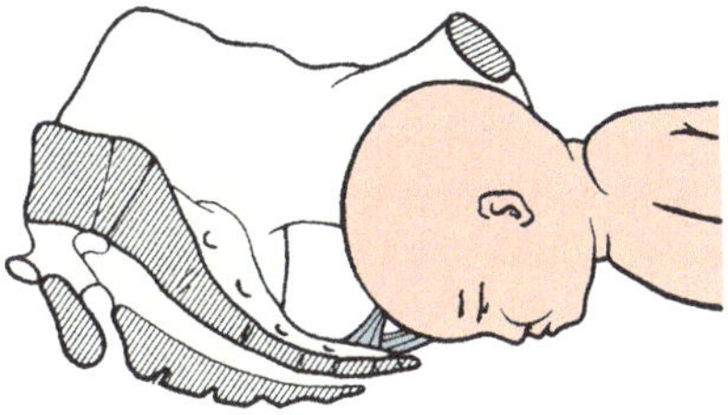

Fig. 8.70

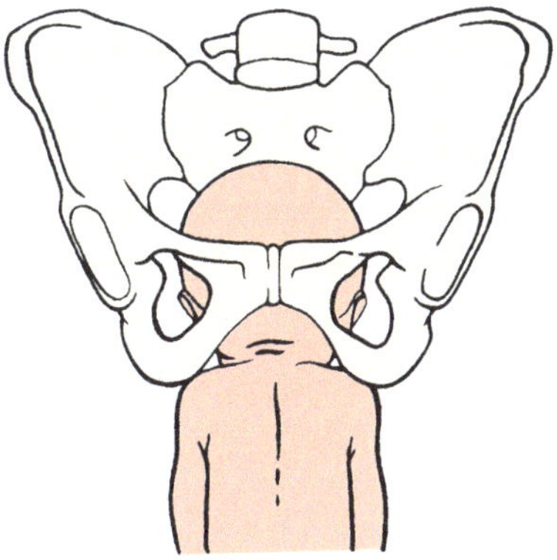

Fig. 8.71

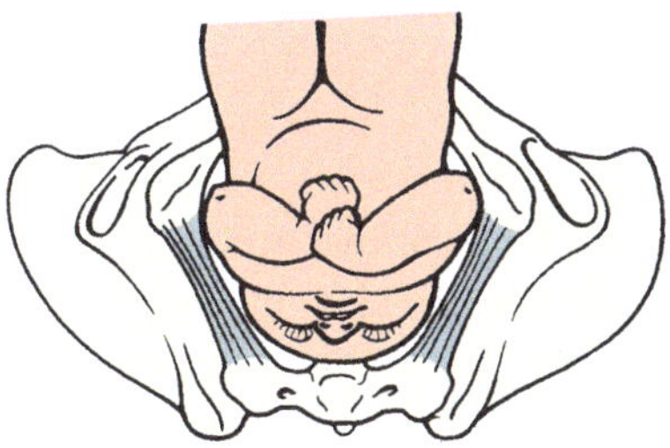

Fig. 8.72

Hypoxia occurs shortly before and during the birth of shoulders and head.

Practice tip. The baby's life is in danger when the breech is born.

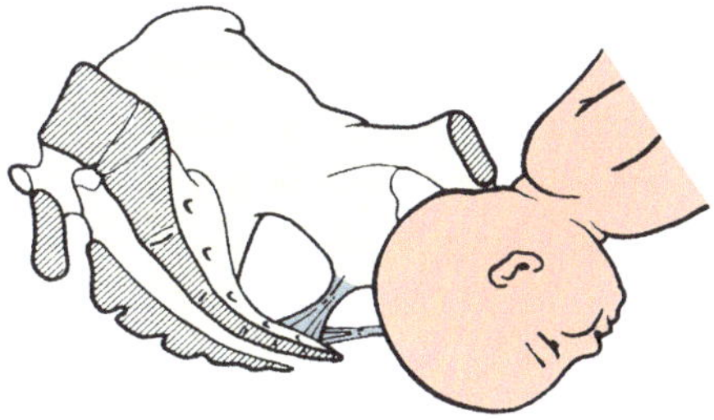

Fig. 8.73

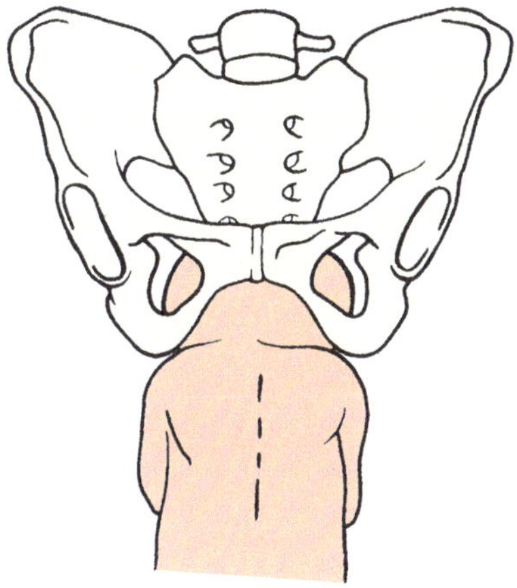

Fig. 8.74

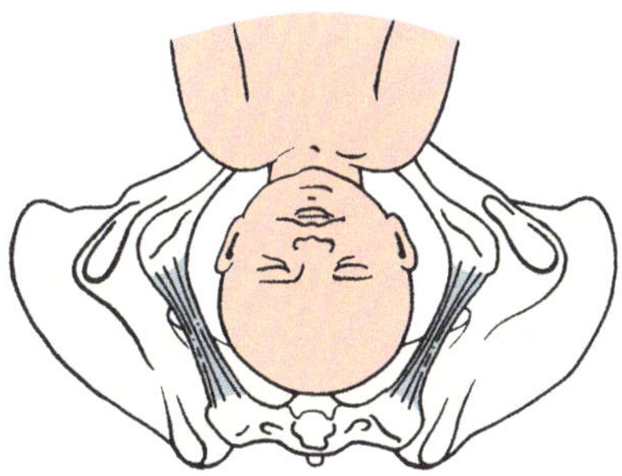

Fig. 8.75

Fig. 8.70–8.75: Birth of the head (Fig´s. 8.70–8.75). The occiput rotates anteriorly on the pelvic floor, the sagittal suture therefore in the APD. The hypomochlion is, as in the normal vertex presentation, the suboccipital region (Figs. 8.70 and 8.73). Figs. 8.70 and 8.73 from the side, Figs. 8.71 and 8.74 from the front, Figs. 8.72 and 8.75 seen from below.

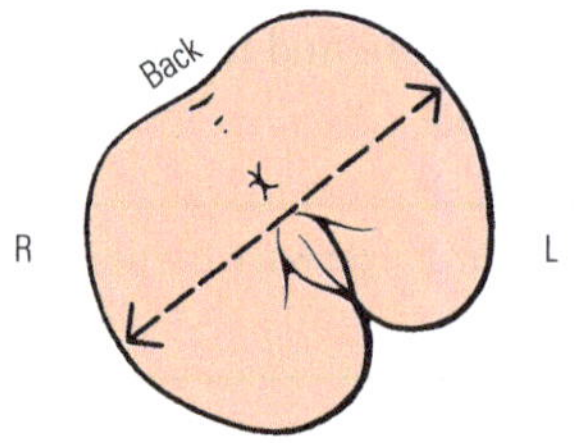

Fig. 8.76

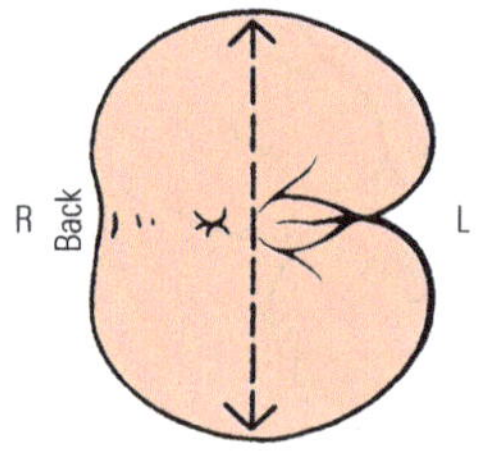

Fig. 8.77

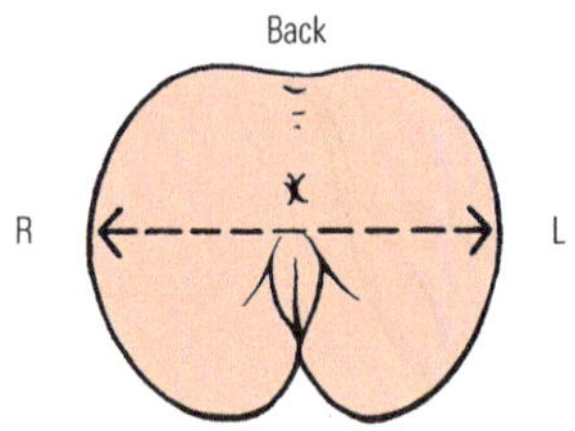

Fig. 8.78

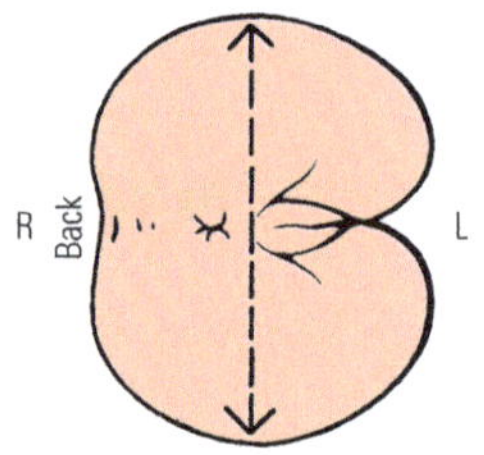

Fig. 8.79

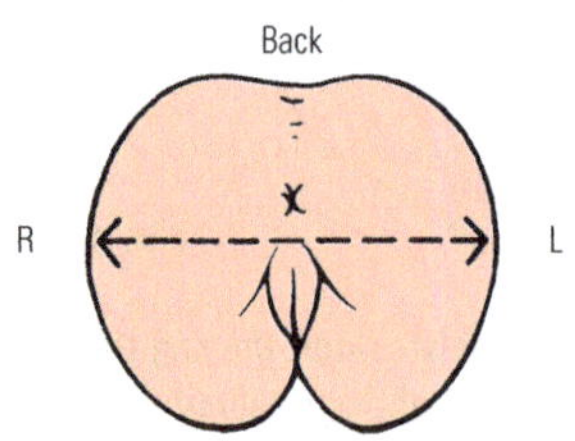

Fig. 8.80

Fig. 876–8.80: Fig. 8.76: Breech presentation. Positions of back (sacrum) and bitrochanteric diameter. Entering the pelvis: In the PI the back is lateral, anterior, the bitrochanteric diameter in an oblique diameter. Here, in RSA presentation, in LOD. Fig. 8.77: Birth of breech and trunk. On the pelvic floor the breech rotates anteriorly so that the bitrochanteric diameter is in the APD. This is the start position for the lateral flexion with which the breech and part of the trunk is born. At the beginning of the lateral flexion the back is directly lateral for the first time. Fig. 8.78: The shoulders enter the pelvis. The shoulders must enter the pelvis once the breech has been born. This is only possible if the bisacromial diameter can pass through the PI at a transverse or slightly oblique angle. The bitrochanteric diameter rotates correspondingly from the APD over the oblique diameter, in which it has already been into the transverse diameter. When the shoulders enter the pelvis the back is directly anterior for the first time. Fig. 8.79: Birth of the shoulders, the head enters the pelvis. In order that the shoulders can pass through the longitudinal soft tissue opening of the PO they must rotate into the APD. This results in the back rotating to the side again, back into the same position it took on for the lateral flexion for the birth of the breech and trunk. The back has thus rotated anteriorly a second time. The position of back and bitrochanteric diameter is also the same as that in which the head enters the PI with the sagittal suture in the transverse diameter or slightly oblique. Fig. 8.80: Birth of the head. Once the head has reached the pelvic floor, it must rotate anteriorly in order that it can pass through the longitudinal soft tissue opening of the PO. In this way, the back is rotated anteriorly for the second time.

Causes. There are two causes for hypoxia.
- Reduction of the placental attachment site. Once the breech and part of the trunk have been born, the uterus retracts and contracts over the head, which is in the cervical canal and vagina. This means that no space remains between the head and the inner wall of the uterus (Fig. 8.81). This reduces the area of the placental attachment site → first cause of hypoxia!
- Cord compression. When the head enters the pelvis (the lower margin of the anterior scapula becomes visible), the umbilical cord

which lies next to it becomes completely compressed; blood circulation ceases and with it the oxygen supply during passage through the pelvis. Hypoxia ends as soon as the mouth has been born. The baby suffocates if the head is not born within 3–5 minutes → second cause of hypoxia!

Note. More than 3–5 minutes must not pass between the time at which the lower margin of the anterior scapula becomes visible and the birth of the head. If it does, the baby will die or be seriously damaged!

Intracranial hemorrhage due to tentorial laceration after birth trauma is the other major risk; as cause of death in breech presenting babies it is at least as common as asphyxiation. Cranial hemorrhage has become rare in term breech deliveries because traumatizing vaginal operative methods of delivery are avoided.
The rate of intracranial hemorrhages appears to be higher in preterm breech babies than in cephalic presentations; whereby preterm babies born by cesarean section appear to have a lower incidence of intracranial hemorrhage than those born vaginally.

Soft tissue difficulties, inadequate soft tissue distension. The breech is softer; it distends the soft tissues more slowly than the firm head. The breech is not as bulky as the head, therefore the soft tissues and in particular the cervix are inadequately stretched.

As the hard part, the head, comes last in a breech presentation, its passage through the inadequately dilated cervix is often difficult. This is not the case in the complete breech, the greatest circumference of which is approximately the same as the plane of passage of the normal vertex presentation (32 cm).
The double-footling breech presentation is the one worst prepared to deal with the head coming afterwards.

Circumference of the presenting part:
- Head in normal vertex presentation: 32 cm.
- Breech in complete breech: 32 cm.
- In frank breech: 27 cm.
- In single footling breech: 25.5 cm.
- In double footling breech: 24 cm.

Note. The passage of the head is greatly delayed in double-footling breech, with the smallest circumference of 24 cm. Cord compression lasts longer; the danger of asphyxiation is greater than in frank and complete breeches. Footling breech, in particular the double footling presentation, is the most dangerous breech presentation for the baby!
The risk is higher for primiparae (unprepared, rigid soft tissues), in particular those of late age at first birth (rigid soft tissues), contracted pelvis, and large head.

Premature rupture of membranes. The lower pole of the membranes is particularly at risk in footling presentations. Those with experience understand the importance of intact membranes in breech presentations.

Note. In breech presentations the membranes are to remain intact until the cervix is fully dilated!

Cord prolapsed. Also most common in footling presentations. Cord prolapse is not a particularly alarming occurrence in breech presentations. As long as only legs and breech are in the birth canal the cord will not be compressed.

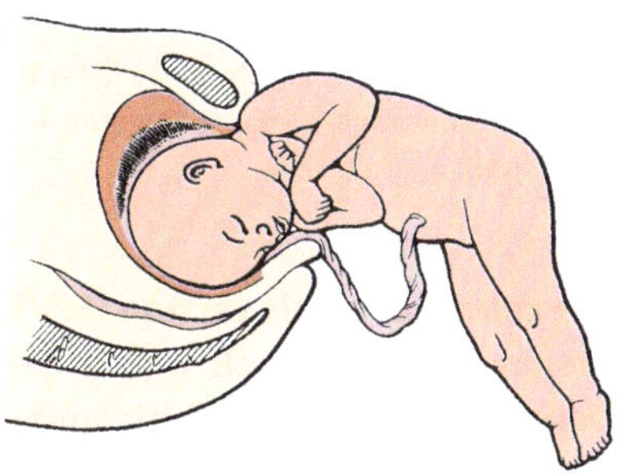

Fig. 8.81: Fetal asphyxia threatens once the breech has been born.

8.2.3 Antenatal counseling

Diagnosis of a breech presentation at 35 weeks is important for counseling a pregnant woman and her partner. Birth management options must then be discussed and a course of management agreed upon. The pelvic exam and evaluation of the size and proportions of the fetus are important for this consultation.

The clinical pelvic exam is performed by an experienced obstetrician (for details see p. 29). Diagnostic imaging for pelvimetry (Fig. 8.82) is usually unnecessary.

On **sonographic examination** it is important to make a weight estimate as well as to check the proportions between head and abdominal circumference.

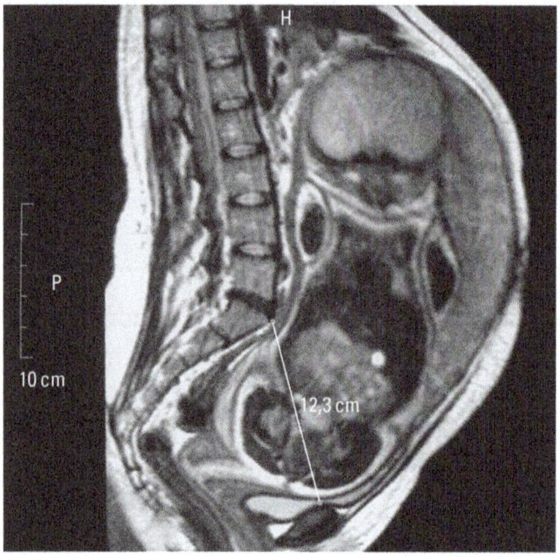

Fig. 8.82: Magnet resonance tomography close to term in breech presentation showing the true conjugate (Conjugata vera obstetrica) of 12.3 cm.

Prophylactic external cephalic version (ECV)

External version from a breech into a cephalic presentation under tocolysis near term. ECV avoids the complications of a vaginal birth for the fetus and the risks of cesarean section for the mother.

The ECV (8 weeks before EDD, Ranney) or close to the EDD (Psychrembel) in combination with tocolysis was publicized in the 1970s by Saling. Advantages:

- If complications arise, the term fetus can be delivered operatively.
- Unnecessary ECVs are avoided, as the incidence of breech presentations is lower at 37 +0 weeks than earlier in the pregnancy.
- The rate of spontaneous version back into a breech presentation is low.

Contraindications

- PROM-
- Vaginal bleeding of unclear origin-
- Placenta previa.

Method. After 30 min of EFM in a lateral position, a 10 min infusion of Fenoterol (5 mg/min) is administered under blood pressure control. Legs are bent and slightly adducted to reduce tension in the abdominal muscles, the pelvis is elevated. One person attempts to rotate the fetal breech out of the maternal pelvis from above the symphysis pubis. The hands of the second person are spread over the fetal skull; the version is attempted as a backward somersault. If this is not successful a forward somersault is attempted. EFM is resumed directly after the procedure. Blood is drawn from Rh-negative women 30 min after the attempted ECV and Hb-F determined. If necessary, anti-D immunoglobulin is administered. Tocolysis is not used in cases of heart defects or heart rhythm disorders (arrhythmia).

Result. 50–60 % of breech presentations are converted to cephalic presentations!

Complications

- Reversible, nonreassuring FHR patterns are observed after 25 % of attempted ECVs.
- Vaginal bleeding occurs in 4 % without further consequences.
- Cesarean section must be performed in 2 % due to pathological or persistent nonreas-

suring FHR patterns directly after or in the hours following ECV.

8.2.4 Mode and management of delivery

The mode of delivery has been controversially discussed since Kubli recommended routine cesarean for breech presentations in 1975. The Term Breech Trial Collaborative Group, whose results have been reflected in renowned guidelines, has caused a marked preference for abdominal operative delivery. On the other hand, significant deficits in the study have been pointed out. The results of the follow-up examinations of the children also relativized the study results. In spite of year-long studies, discussions, and consensus conferences, the hard debate on the extensive indications for cesarean section has still not been concluded.

Indications for elected cesarean section

The absolute indications for cesarean section are undisputed:
- Suspected cephalopelvic disproportion/contracted pelvis/maternal pelvic anomaly.
- Cord prolapsed.
- Placenta previa.
- Fetal macrosomia.

Relative indications are:
- IUGR < 10th percentile.
- Sonographically estimated weight of > 3,800 g.
- LBW fetus of < 1,800 g.
- Fetal disproportion: head circumference >> abdominal circumference.
- Double footling breech.
- PROM and unripe cervix.
- Maternal diabetes mellitus.

The question of the mode of delivery in preterm breech presentations is the subject of continuing debate. Preterm vaginal breech births have a higher perinatal mortality rate than those of the same age born by cesarean section. For this reason, cesarean section is indicated in preterm births before 34 weeks after exclusion of severe fetal defects. No clear recommendation can be given for extreme preterm babies from a breech presentation with an estimated birth weight < 1,500g, as neither mortality nor early morbidity rates have been shown to be related to the mode of delivery.

Indications for emergency cesarean section

In addition to the indications for emergency cesarean section which also exist for cephalic presentation births, the indication for cesarean section in breech presentations – also in delayed labor – must be generously made. Cervical dilatation in breech delivery also proceeds at an average rate of 1–2 cm/h. If dilatation is slower, the indication for cesarean section should be made. Delayed first stage in vaginal breech delivery, calculated from 3 cm cervical dilatation, is linked with increased early infant morbidity. 30–40 % of the breech presentation deliveries which begin as vaginal deliveries end in emergency cesarean sections.

Practice tip. In counseling the pregnant woman and her partner, the diagnosis of a breech presentation at around 35 weeks and a referral for ECV are important. Obstetrical institutions which take on pregnant women with breech presentations should have both organizational and personnel expertise ready for ECV, vaginal breech delivery: the possibility that a cesarean section may suddenly be necessary and neonatologists and anesthetists should be available. The obstetrical team should regularly practice their knowledge of assisted breech and breech extraction on an obstetrical model.

Management of breech presentation delivery

After risk assessment vaginal birth of a breech presentation at term can continue to be performed as a safe and gentle mode of delivery. Management is divided into two phases, which require opposing behavior from the birth attendant:

- A long first phase of calm, expectant management, in which labor is allowed to progress naturally.
- A short second phase of prompt action.

Phase I. Period of expectant management until the breech has been born, to be exact: until the lower margin of the anterior scapula has become visible; following the principle of expectant management as long as maternal and fetal wellbeing is assured. This applies to all breech presentations!

The birth attendant needs patience and time in phase I!
The following are prohibited: applying traction to foot, leg, breech, trunk (see rules below) in order to hasten delivery. The opposite is achieved, delayed delivery, baby's life is endangered:
- The arms, which are lying on the chest, extend, which makes arm extraction difficult.
- The circumference of the presenting part is reduced and passage of the head is made more difficult!
- The head will adopt an extended attitude. Arm extraction in phase II will be difficult.
- The worst consequence: the back may rotate posteriorly. In phase II there are only 3–5 minutes for the arms, shoulders, and head to be born.

Only emergencies (e.g., fetal acidosis) necessitate intervention by the birth attendant. Manipulated delivery of a breech presentation before the breech has been born is termed breech extraction; for details see p. 255.

Phase II. Period of prompt action, once the breech has been born and the lower edge of the shoulder blade is visible (→ phase II begins!) Danger of acute asphyxia (reduced size of placental attachment site, cord compression, see p. 243). A maximum of 3–5 min remain for action, for manual assistance!

Management of phase II can, however also be expectant until spontaneous delivery occurs if the mother changes position (on **all fours**).

Assisted breech. The arms are extracted, shoulders and head delivered. The maneuvers must be performed not only quickly, but gently, sensitively and carefully in
- primiparae always (if the baby is alive),
- multiparae it may be possible to wait and see whether the arms and shoulders or head are born spontaneously with the next contraction.

Assisted breech: arm extraction, delivery of shoulders, head

Definition. Procedure of assisting delivery of arms, shoulders and head once the breech has been born. Not to be confused with manual extraction of breech presentation!

Aim. Removal of the risk of asphyxia which threatens every breech baby. To be performed in all breech births for delivery of arms, shoulders and head.

Breech births may proceed spontaneously in multiparae. If the baby is not born spontaneously with the next contraction once the lower edge of the anterior scapula has become visible, manual assistance must also be used to finish this birth.

Note. Five methods can be chosen from: 1) Bracht maneuver, 2) Mueller arm extraction maneuver plus Smellie–Veit or Mauriceau maneuver for delivery of the head, 3) Bickenbach arm extraction, 4) Loevset arm extraction, 5) classical arm extraction.

Prerequisite
- The trunk must be born as far as the lower margin of the anterior scapula. Caution: never begin before the lower margin of the anterior scapula is visible. Exception: the

Bracht maneuver is begun once the umbilicus has been born.
- Performed with the woman in the lithotomy position.

Suprapubic pressure! In order for any of the methods of manual assistance to succeed, it is crucial that an assistant exerts strong pressure through the abdomen on the head, which is still in the PI, pushing it with both hands into the pelvis. The assistance of the midwife is very important:
Sometimes in multiparae this pressure is all that is required for spontaneous birth, so that manual assistance is no longer necessary.
The suprapubic pressure on the head is not begun until the breech is emerging from the vulva.
Why is suprapubic pressure on the head so important?

1. **Main reason.** The arms are not extended over the head!
2. The head remains in the normal flexed attitude and is not extended.
3. Manual assistance is easier and faster.

Preparation. The obstetrician begins scrubbing up when the breech appears in the vulva (primipara), on ROM (multipara).

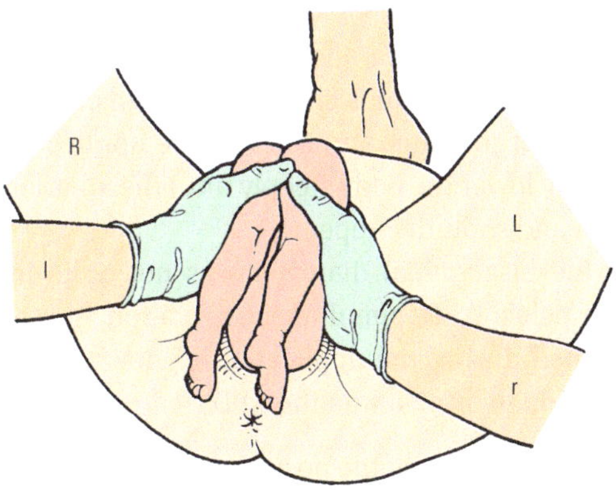

Fig. 8.83: Bracht maneuver (I). The breech is encircled with both hands.

Anesthesia. Epidural!
Episiotomy. Manual assistance begins in primiparae with an episiotomy, performed once the anterior edge of the shoulder blade has become visible and directly before manual assistance.

Bracht arm extraction and delivery of the head (Figs. 8.83 and 8.84)

The **Bracht maneuver** is begun once the umbilicus has been born (earlier than with all other methods).
Method. The breech is encircled with both hands so that the baby's thighs are pressed against the abdomen by the operator's thumbs (Fig. 8.83). The other fingers are placed on the sacrum and lumbar regions of the baby.
In this position the baby is slowly elevated, but no traction is applied!
The breech is slowly elevated in an arc around the maternal symphysis pubis towards her abdomen (→ rotation around the symphysis pubis).
Hereby the baby must continually be held in the same position and moved in such a way that the back is bent anteriorly. Constant suprapubic pressure is applied with adequate but not excessive force.
The rotation around the symphysis pubis is performed slowly and evenly. Pressing the breech vigorously onto the maternal abdomen (Fig. 8.85) leads to spontaneous delivery of the arms and shoulders.

Practice tip. The operator does nothing more than hold and guide the baby! The main work is performed by the assistant from above! Traction is prohibited! Danger to the cervical spine otherwise.

Further pressure is applied to the breech and the head is born spontaneously. The operator must take care that it is not expelled too rapidly from the vagina. The speed of birth is regulated

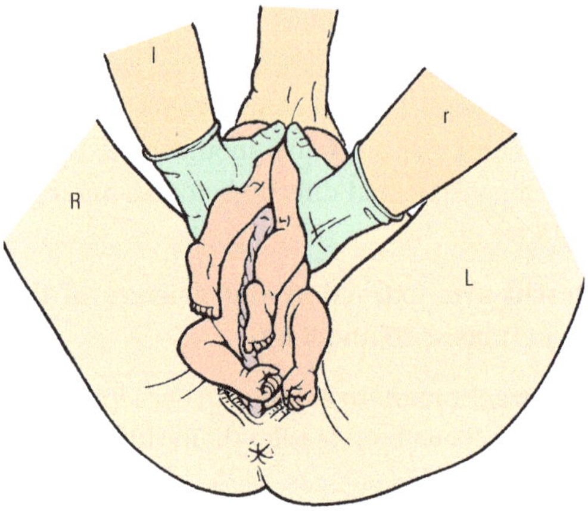

Fig. 8.84: Bracht maneuver (II). Slow elevation, traction is not applied.

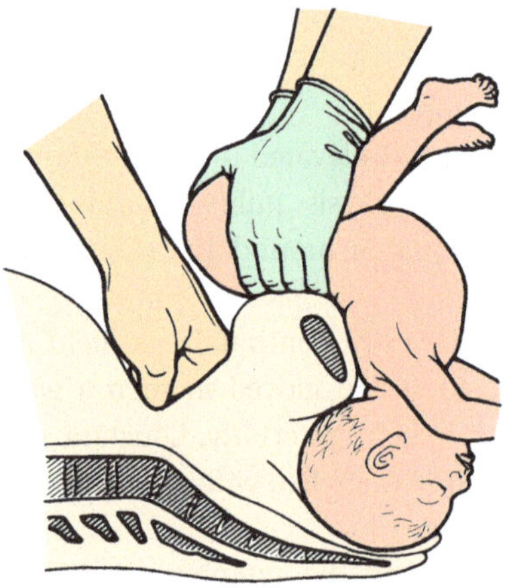

Fig. 8.85: Bracht maneuver (III). The breech is slowly rotated around the symphysis pubis. The breech is pressed firmly onto the maternal abdomen. Suprapubic pressure.

with one or both underarms, or the midwife takes on the task of perineal protection.

Suprapubic pressure must be applied with controlled pressure directed by the obstetrician from the beginning until the whole baby has been born. The importance of the application of suprapubic pressure by an assistant is often not properly appreciated by beginners, which is the main reason for unsuccessful Bracht maneuvers.

Practice tip. Suprapubic pressure is responsible for the entry of the head into the pelvis, its descent to the pelvic floor, and birth over the perineum!

Note. Advantage of the Bracht method: arms, shoulders, and head are delivered without it being necessary to go into the vagina. In the Mueller, Bickenbach, and Loevset maneuvers (see below) the arms and shoulders are also delivered with external maneuvers, but it is necessary to insert a hand into the vagina for delivery of the head (see below).

If the Bracht maneuver is not effortlessly successful, or if the slightest complication arises, it must be immediately discontinued and another method (→ Mueller arm extraction maneuver) must be employed!

Mueller arm extraction maneuver

Arm extraction begins once the lower edge of the anterior scapula becomes visible. Suprapubic pressure! Episiotomy is usually performed on primiparae. First the anterior, then the posterior arm is extracted; two steps:

Step 1. Delivery of the anterior arm: baby is firmly grasped at the base of the pelvis (Fig. 8.86).

The thumbs lie parallel on the buttocks; the fingers of both hands encircle the thighs. Even, constant pressure and traction are applied to slowly lower the body steeply until the anterior arm and shoulder appear.

If the bisacromial diameter was not quite in the pelvic APD, simultaneous rotation is performed during the application of downwards traction to bring it into the APD.

Step 2. Delivery of the posterior arm (Fig. 8.87).

The trunk is elevated in the opposite direction, steeply upwards, and pressed firmly against

the mother's abdomen until the posterior arm slips out and the posterior shoulder appears.
Often one or other of the arms doesn't deliver spontaneously, but remains stuck in the vulva. In this case 2 fingers are inserted carefully into the vagina and the arm gently removed.
When the head follows, it must then be delivered immediately with the Mauriceau or Smellie–Veit maneuver unless it follows spontaneously due to suprapubic pressure, which sometimes occurs.

Bickenbach arm extraction maneuver
Arm extraction begins once the lower edge of the anterior scapula becomes visible. Suprapubic pressure! First the posterior, then the anterior arm is extracted; two steps:

Step 1. Delivery of the posterior arm: baby is firmly grasped at the base of the pelvis. The thumbs lie parallel on the buttocks; the fingers of both hands encircle the thighs. Even, constant pressure and traction are applied to slowly move the body anteriorly and steeply downwards until the posterior arm and shoulder appear.

Step 2. Delivery of the anterior arm (Fig. 8.87); traction is applied in the opposite direction, posteriorly and downwards, until the anterior shoulder and arm appear below the symphysis pubis.

Often one or other of the arms doesn't deliver spontaneously, but remains in the birth canal. In this case 2 fingers are inserted into the vagina and the arm delivered.
The head following after must then be delivered immediately with the Mauriceau or Smellie–Veit maneuver (p. 253).

Loevset arm extraction maneuver
Arm extraction begins once the lower edge of the anterior scapula becomes visible. Suprapubic pressure! Episiotomy is usually performed on primiparae. First the posterior arm is extracted.

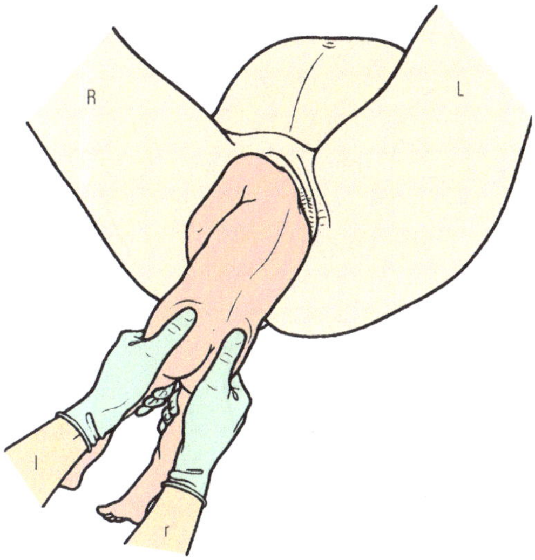

Fig. 8.86: Mueller arm extraction (I).

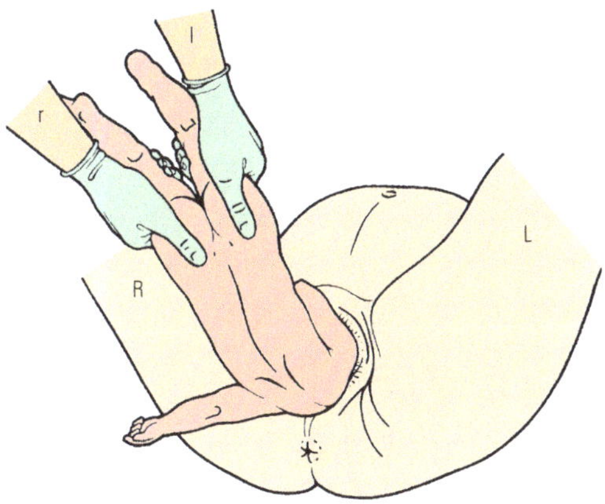

Fig. 8.87: Mueller arm extraction (II).

The operator grasps the baby's pelvis as for the Mueller maneuver (Fig. 8.88): thumbs lie on the buttocks, fingers encircle the thighs.
In this hold, the baby's body is rotated around its longitudinal axis. Two steps:

Step 1. Delivery of the posterior arm. With the pelvis thus grasped, downward traction is applied and the baby is simultaneously rotated 180°: in left breech presentation counterclockwise, in right breech (Fig. 8.89) clockwise.

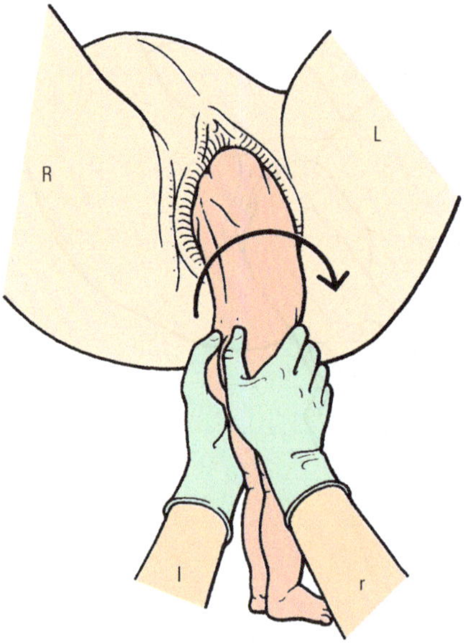

Fig. 8.88: Loevset arm extraction. Step 1. The baby's pelvis is grasped, downwards traction is applied while simultaneously rotating 180° anteriorly.

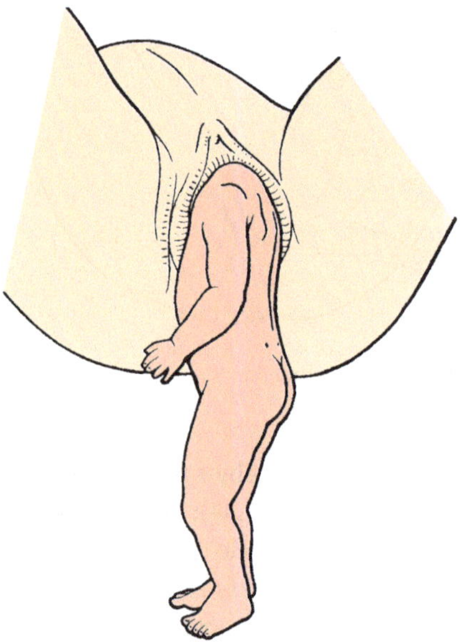

Fig. 8.89: Loevset arm extraction. Step 1.End position after performing step 1, start position for step 2.

This brings the posterior shoulder (in left breech presentation the right, in right breech presentation the left; Fig. 8.88) forwards and outwards from the sacral cavity,
in front of the symphysis pubis (Fig. 8.89), whereby the arm usually slips out spontaneously. If not, it can easily be removed after splinting with 2 fingers.

Step 2. Delivery of the arm which has been brought posteriorly. The baby is rotated back 180°; the shoulder which was rotated anteriorly in step 1 is rotated the same way back again. The back is uppermost (towards the symphysis pubis) once again.

The back is rotated anteriorly both times; the fetal back is rotated upwards, towards the symphysis pubis.
Afterwards the head is delivered immediately with the Mauriceau or Smellie-Veit maneuver (p. 253).

Practice tip. If the Bracht maneuver is unsuccessful, a switch is made to the Mueller (p. 248), Bickenbach or Loevset maneuvers without delay. If they are not immediately successful the classical arm maneuver (see below) must be performed.

Classical arm extraction maneuver

Arm extraction begins once breech has been born and the lower edge of the anterior scapula becomes visible. Suprapubic pressure! Episiotomy is usually performed on primiparae.
As opposed to the four methods described above, in this maneuver the operator manually delivers the arms.
The arm extraction must always be performed in the spacious sacral cavity as only here is there sufficient room for the operator's hand. This means that the arm to be found in the sacral cavity, that is the posterior arm, must be delivered first. It is always within easy reach, whereas the anterior arm is unreachable.

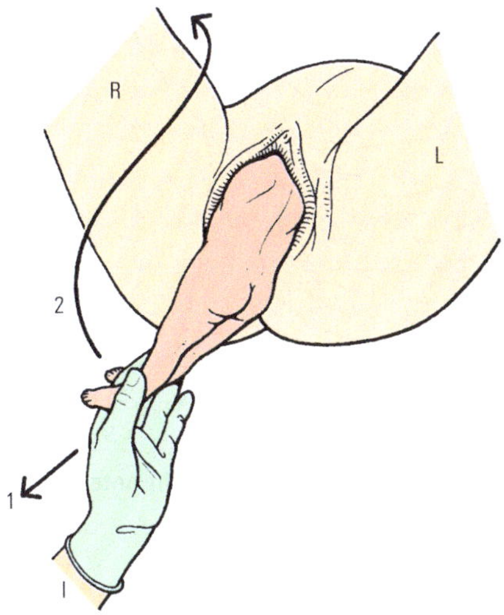

Fig. 8.90: Feet are grasped around the ankles and the baby is firmly stretched downwards (towards the floor).

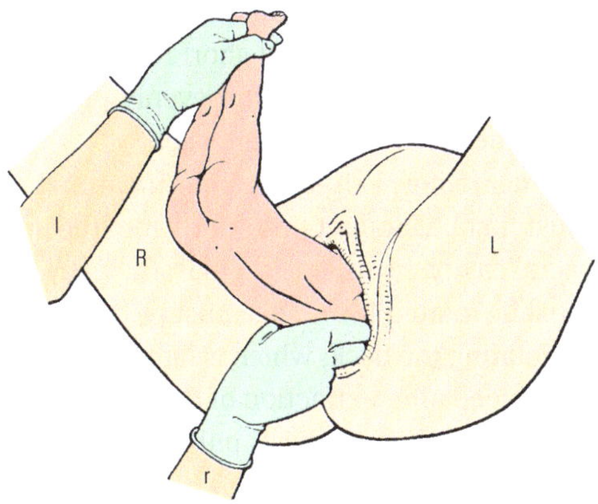

Fig. 8.91: The legs are pushed firmly into the corresponding inguinal region. At least two fingers of the internal hand pass over the shoulder onto the upper arm to be extracted.

Practice tip. Ground rule of the classical arm extraction is that the posterior arm, which is to be found in the sacral cavity, is always delivered first!

Both hands are used: one hand holds the feet and uses them to elevate the trunk; the inner hand is inserted into the vagina to extract the arm.

The hand corresponding to the side the baby's abdomen is on always holds the feet (Fig. 8.90): in a left breech presentation the left hand, in a right breech the right hand.
The other hand is inserted into the vagina, the same hand as the arm which is to be extracted (Fig. 8.91).

Practice tip. In order to extract the posterior right arm (left breech presentation) the right hand is inserted, in order to extract the posterior left arm (right breech presentation) the left hand is inserted.

---

3 step procedure for left breech presentation:

Step 1. Release of the posterior arm in the sacral cavity. Always begin by grasping the feet.
- The left hand grasps the feet firmly near the ankles from behind with thumb and second and third fingers (Fig. 8.90). The baby is stretched firmly downward, that is, traction is applied to the legs in the direction of the floor: this brings the shoulders and arms deeper which makes them easier to release.
- Next the baby's trunk is elevated, pulled somewhat to the side and placed in the mother's groin. This opens up the introitus so that the hand may be inserted. Sometimes the posterior arm slips out of its own accord on this movement; if not:
- At least 2 fingers of the right hand are inserted to the left and posteriorly into the vagina (Fig. 8.91). The fingers are moved towards to the baby's shoulder. The more fingers that can be inserted into the vagina, the easier and less dangerous the arm extraction is. One always attempts to insert the whole hand into the vagina with multiparae!
- Now, under constant upwards oblique traction on the feet, the trunk of the baby is pushed as firmly as possible further into the mother's right groin!

Practice tip. The more energetic the legs are brought into the woman's groin, the more firmly the traction away from the operator is exerted, the deeper the posterior shoulder and with it the arm to be extracted move, and the easier the extraction is. If the trunk is only elevated halfway without pushing the legs firmly into the groin, the extraction is needlessly made far more difficult.

During this energetic elevation and stretching of the trunk with the external hand, at least two fingers of the internal hand, which were already on the shoulder, pass over it (Fig. 8.92) to the upper arm which is to be extracted and are stretched out along it, to "splint" it. If possible, the lower arm ((Fig. 8.90. 8.91)) is included and then drawn down over the chest and out until it is in front of the vulva (Fig. 8.92). The posterior arm has now been extracted.

Practice tip. The operator's fingers must never be placed at right angles to the baby's arm. Grasping the upper arm by hooking it is also not permissable.

Note. This would cause an arm fracture. For the same reason it is prohibited to take hold of the upper arm with only one finger!

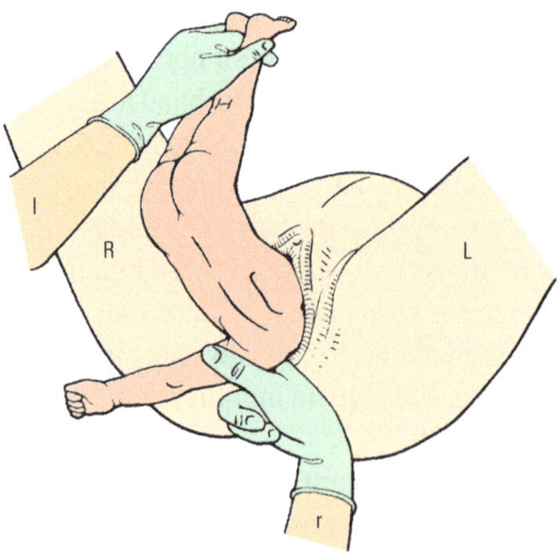

Fig. 8.92: The upper arm is "splinted" with at least two fingers, drawn over the chest and swept out.

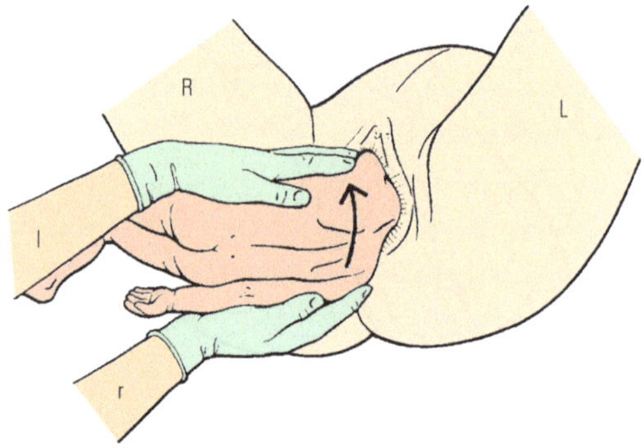

Fig. 8.93: Plugging movements to bring the anterior arm posterior and into the sacral cavity.

Step 2. The baby is rotated 180° with plugging movements.

Plugging movements. The baby is not rotated 180° in a single movement (this is not possible), but with a number of short rotations, in which the trunk is briefly and evenly pushed towards the sacrum and pulled back.

- In order to now extract the anterior arm, it must first be brought posteriorly into the sacral cavity. In order to do that, the baby must be rotated 180°. This must be done by rotating the back, which is laterally positioned after extraction of the posterior arm, below the symphysis pubis to the other side.
- The trunk is held as shown in Fig. 8.93: both hands lie flat with fingers spread like splints on the sides of the trunk. The arm which has already been delivered is held against the body.
- It is also possible to encircle the thorax (please note, only the chest, never the abdomen → liver rupture → exitus letalis) with both hands: the thumbs on the scapulae, the 4 fingers on both sides of the chest.

Step 3. Extraction of the (second) arm which has been brought back to the sacral cavity with the same technique as for the first arm, but with reversed roles: right hand holds the feet, left hand is inserted into the vagina for extraction of the left (same sided) arm.

After extraction of the arms the head must be delivered immediately with the Smellie-Veit maneuver. The forceps (see below) are within reach.

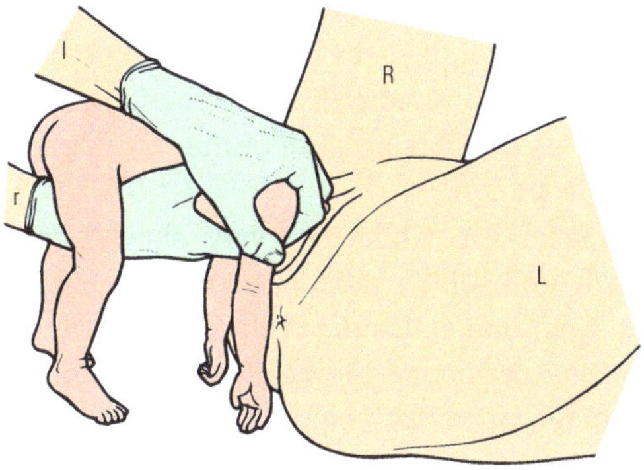

Fig. 8.94: Smellie-Veit maneuver (I). Pull rapidly downwards until the hairline is visible.

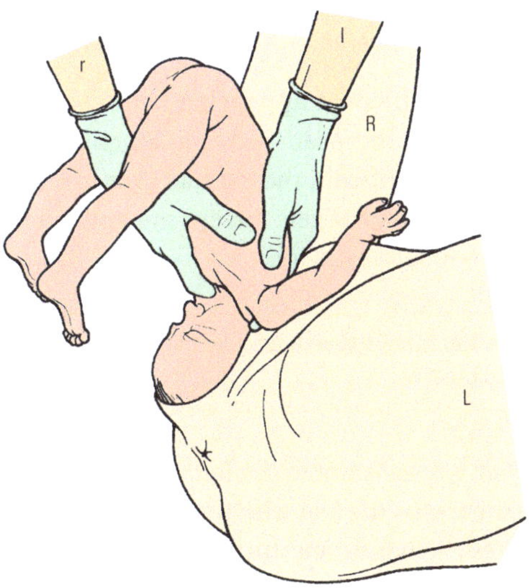

Fig. 8.95: Smellie-Veit maneuver (II). From now on exaggerated slowness!

Smellie–Veit maneuver

Delivery of the head coming afterwards (Figs. 8.94, 8.95). After extraction of the arms the back is to one side, oblique. The head, which is still in the pelvis, is at an oblique angle.

- The hand towards which the face is directed, or, as one can also say, the one which is on the same side as the baby's abdomen (both head and trunk are at an oblique angle, so both face the same hand) is inserted into the vagina.
- The external hand is that which corresponds to the baby's back. It is in a forked grip over the shoulders (Fig. 8.94).

The arm of the operator corresponding to the baby's abdomen is placed under the baby's extremities so that the baby rides on this arm (Fig. 8.94). The hand belonging to this arm (the internal hand) is inserted into the vagina.
The index finger feels for the mouth, which is usually to the right or left, and is inserted into it. Must not be inserted into the eye! Penetration of the mouth must not be too deep (risk of injury!)
The finger in the mouth directs the baby's head and maneuvers it into the desired presentation and attitude.
The internal hand has two duties. It rotates the head into the pelvic APD. The head is usually in an oblique diameter. As it must under no circumstances be allowed to pass over the perineum at an oblique angle (→ perineal laceration), it must be rotated beforehand into the APD, (that is, with the mouth towards the back!) The sagittal suture is in the APD when the mouth is directly posterior.
It pulls the head to the chest, that is, it flexes the head until the chin touches the chest and holds the head in this position during the following maneuver until it has been completely delivered.
If the head is to pass over the perineum with the smallest, most favorable plane of passage,

the suboccipitobregmatic plane (32 cm), it must be brought into and remain in this well-flexed attitude (birth mechanism).

The de Lee speculum maneuver. A very valuable maneuver which allows the baby to breathe immediately, during the Smellie–Veit maneuver. Two variations:

- After the operator has inserted a finger into the baby's mouth, an assistant inserts a large, broad obstetric speculum into the vagina and exerts downwards pressure to pull the rear wall of the vagina and perineum away from the baby's mouth and nose.
- If the vagina is wide the same effect can be brought about using 2–3 fingers.

Note. If extraction of the head is difficult, the de Lee speculum maneuver can be life-saving. Once the speculum has been inserted posteriorly, the time can be taken to perform the maneuvers unhurriedly.

In the meantime, the second and third fingers of the operator's free hand have the shoulders in a forked grip (Fig. 8.94). The hand lies on the baby's neck. The fingers must never be hooked, however, as pressure easily causes injury to the brachial plexus (Erb's palsy). This hand now quickly brings the body downwards until the neck hairline is visible (birth mechanism!) under the symphysis pubis. Under constant tension, the neck hairline remaining in sight constantly, the arm of the operator which is lying under the baby is slowly elevated towards the symphysis pubis (Fig. 8.95).
Never begin elevation before the neck hairline is clearly visible!

Beginner's mistakes. Two typical mistakes of the inexperienced are:

- The arm the baby is riding on is elevated too early, before the neck hairline is clearly visible.
- The operator brings the neck hairline properly into sight, but lets it slip back up under the symphysis pubis again. Enough tension must be applied, however, that the neck hairline remains constantly in sight.

Danger of perineal laceration. The perineum is at greatest risk of lacerating when the chin has been born over the perineum and the mouth is visible in the vulva because the perineum will be maximally distended in the next seconds and as both hands are in use, neither is free to guard it (Fig. 8.95).
Change in speed. From now on, deliberate slowness! From the moment the mouth has been born and the baby is no longer in danger, every further movement must be performed as slowly as possible because of the risk of perineal laceration.
Millimeter for millimeter, very slowly, cautiously and gently, maxilla, nose, brow, sinciput, and finally also the occiput are delivered over the perineum; the head is slowly rolled out of the vulva like a ball.
Three speeds determine the mechanism of birth in breech presentations: slow, fast, slow! 1) Slow until the anterior scapula has been born. 2) Fast, from then on until the mouth emerges in the vulva. 3) Very slow until the head has been completely delivered.

Forceps on the post-appearing head

If delivery of the head with the Smellie–Veit maneuver is difficult, the manual procedure is abandoned and Naegele forceps are applied to the post-appearing head.

Practice tip. Always have forceps within reach at every assisted breech!

Method. An assistant to the left of the laboring woman grasps the feet with the right hand and elevates the hands and trunk of the baby with the left hand. The head is now accessible and the forceps are applied transversely, as usual. The Naegele model has proven to be suitable.

Delivery of the head is simple and performed without difficulty by the experienced. Traction is applied in the direction of the handles.

Breech extraction

Definition. Complete extraction; manipulative termination of birth in breech presentation before the birth of the breech. Expectant management has been waived, cesarean section is not indicated (for list of indications see p. 245). Not to be confused with assisted breech; see p. 246.

Four conditions:
- The cervix must be completely dilated.
- The pelvis must not be too narrow; the head must be able to pass through it easily.
- The baby must be living.
- The membranes must have ruptured. If not, amniotomy.

The extraction can be a difficult procedure and strenuous for the obstetrician. It is particularly difficult in primiparae, on whom it is not willingly practiced, due to the unyielding, rigid tissues. If it is unavoidable, a generous episiotomy is first performed, to remove pelvic floor resistance.

Note. Breech extraction is the most dangerous obstetrical procedure for the baby due to the time required and the extreme traction exerted by the operator! (The most dangerous vaginal obstetrical operation for the mother is the combined version.)

Indication. Necessary termination of labor of the second twin in breech presentation. In a singleton no longer necessary, in contrast to earlier practice.

Technique. The operation depends on the type of breech presentation:
- Single footling presentation, anterior foot presenting.
- Single footling presentation, posterior foot presenting.
- Double footling presentation.
- Complete breech.
- Kneeling breech (rare).
- Frank breech.

Anesthesia. Method of choice is epidural anesthesia; general anesthesia if time is not sufficient for application of the epidural anesthesia or it is contraindicated.

Transfundal pressure. Main requirement here is also that the traction from below is actively supported by pressure from above.

The assistant must be encouraged to apply vigorous transfundal pressure with both hands (→ Kristeller maneuver). If this is done, the extraction proceeds much more easily and the arms cannot extend.

Single footling breech (anterior foot presenting)

Index and middle finger grasp the calf above the ankle and draw it out of the vulva.

Traction is applied to the anterior presenting foot/leg (Fig. 8.96); the other foot must never be prematurely pulled down.

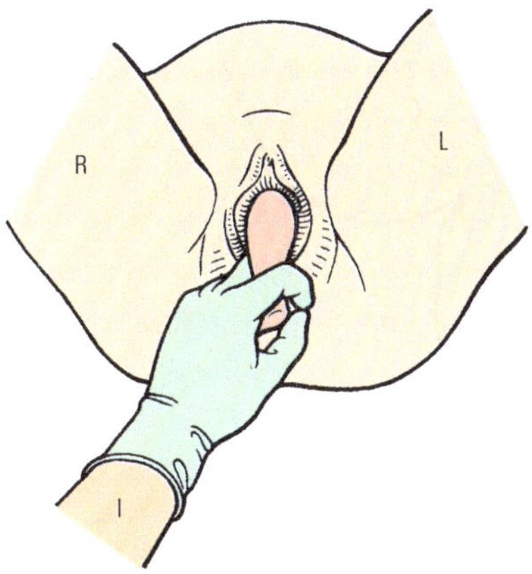

Fig. 8.96: Breech extraction (I). The presenting foot is grasped and drawn out through the vulva.

As soon as the calf has been delivered, the whole hand grasps it: thumb is always placed on the calf (caudal side, flexor muscles; Fig. 8.97).

Practice tip. Care must be taken that the calf (flexor-caudal side) faces anteriorly or is rotated anteriorly from the beginning, to avoid the unwelcome posterior rotation of the back.

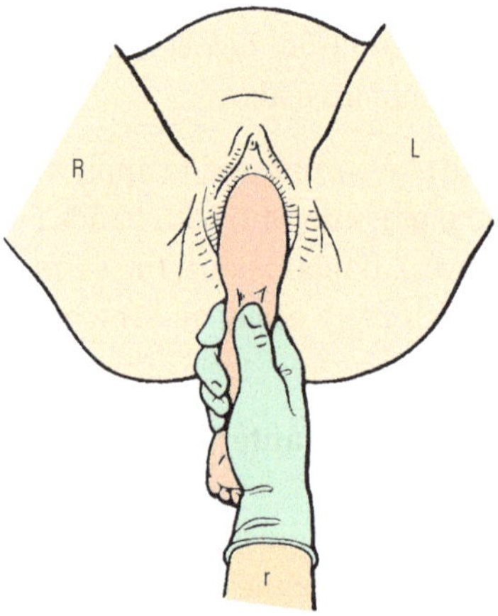

Fig. 8.97: Breech extraction (II).The calf is grasped with the whole hand. Downwards traction is applied to the breech.

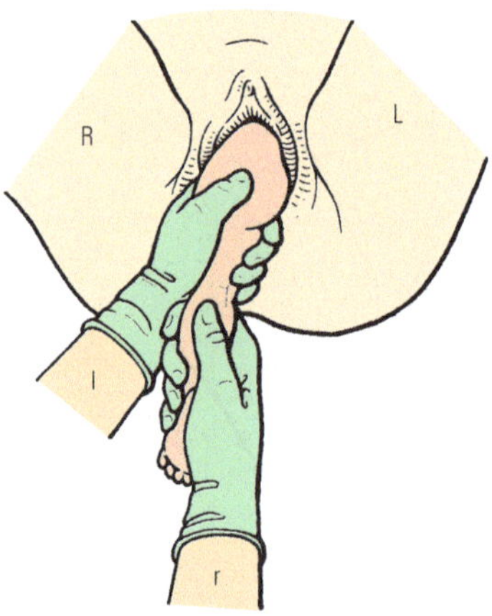

Fig. 8.98: Breech extraction (III). Grasp successively higher! The corresponding hand of the same name must be highest on the thigh. Steep downwards traction until the anterior hip is delivered.

The remaining fingers encircle the lower leg firmly and completely. The most important thing is that traction is applied in the right direction.

- Steep downwards traction! Vertical traction towards the floor!
- Successively higher sections of the leg are grasped with alternating hands, placing the hand close to the vulva and climbing from the calf to the thigh, whereby the thumb remains on the flexor side.

Practice tip. Grasp as high as possible. The hand which is placed highest on the thigh must be the same as the thigh (left hand on left thigh; Fig. 8.98). This rule is crucial for the continuing smoothness of the procedure: the same hand must be placed on the thigh of the same name.

- The thumb of this hand is placed on the buttock next to the sacrum; the other fingers completely and firmly encircle the thigh.
- Continued downward traction is applied until the anterior hip is completely delivered (Fig. 8.98). The skin is usually slippery due to its covering of vernix caseosa. In order to have a better hold a sterile cloth is used.

After the anterior hip has been born the direction of traction changes.

- Traction is applied to the leg in the opposite direction, upwards, following the axis of the birth canal, in order to bring the posterior hip over the perineum. As soon as the posterior hip is within reach (Fig. 8.99), the index finger is hooked into the posterior groin (in Fig. 8.99 the free hand is the left, the right continues to hold the thigh). Never insert 2 fingers into the groin or femur fracture!
- The thumb is placed on the posterior buttock so that the thumbs lie parallel next to the sacrum (Fig. 8.99).

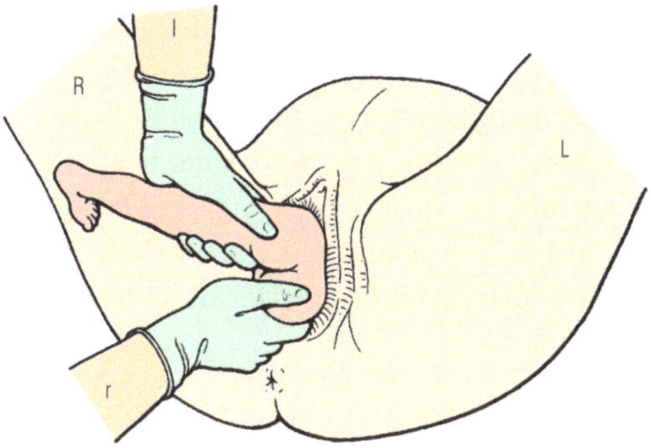

Fig. 8.99: Breech extraction (IV). The index finger of the "free" hand is hooked into the fold of the posterior hip as soon as it is within reach.

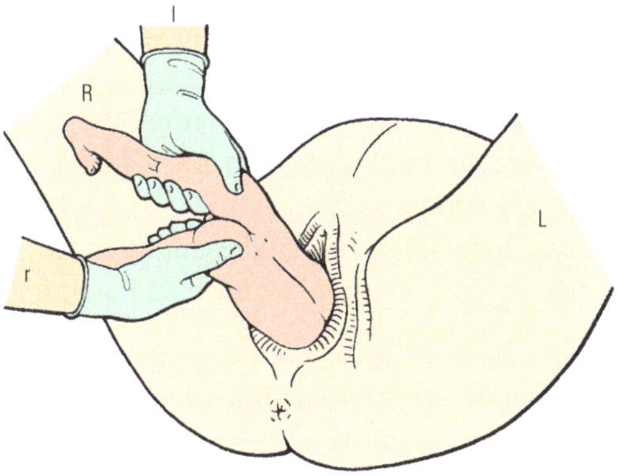

Fig. 8.100: Breech extraction (V). Steep upwards traction with both hands until the lower margin of the anterior-lying shoulder blade is visible.

- Both hands remain in this position while strong upwards traction is applied, whereby the second leg slips out. Both hands now encircle the thighs (Abb. 8.100) and continuing traction is applied in the same direction until the lower margin of the anterior scapula is palpable (Fig. 8.100).

Practice tip. The arm is extracted with at least 2 fingers! Only 1 finger is to be inserted into the posterior groin! Insert into the posterior groin in:

- Left breech presentation the right index finger (→ the right index finger is inserted into the right groin).
- Right breech presentation the left index finger (→ the left index finger is inserted into the left groin).

Thumbs are placed on the buttocks of the same name.

Practice tip. If the extended posterior foot doesn't slip out but remains in the vagina when the lower margin of the anterior shoulder blade appears, traction must never be applied to one leg. A simple maneuver can be applied to make it emerge: the baby's back is pressed laterally towards the mother's thigh which it is closest to.

Afterwards classical arm extraction and delivery of the head (Smellie–Veit maneuver), see p. 253.

Common beginners' mistakes. Downwards traction is not steeply enough applied initially, and later the upwards traction is not steeply enough applied. Only these two directions of traction are used!

Extraction is more difficult if the thigh is grasped with the wrong hand:
- The corresponding hand of the same name must always be placed on the thigh! If the opposite hand is used, the other hand cannot reach the posterior groin properly; the **hands get in each other's way.**

Practice tip. Supposedly in order to be able better exert traction, the second (extended) foot is often extracted: a serious mistake!
The circumference of the lower trunk section is 25.5 cm; in a double footling presentation only 24.5 cm (see p. 244). The soft tissue of the birth canal is therefore less distended by the presenting part in a double than in a single footling presentation. The passage of the aftercoming head is unnecessarily made more difficult!

- Only insert the index finger, never 2 fingers into the groin, or a femur fracture or dislocated hip may result.
- Arm extraction is often begun too early! Do not begin until the lower margin of the anterior shoulder blade is visible.
- The beginner, concentrating on performing the maneuver, frequently forgets to ask for an assistant to apply vigorous transfundal pressure with both hands. Having once experienced how much easier the whole maneuver is when combined with transfundal pressure; it will never again be forgotten. In addition, transfundal pressure ensures that the arms will not extend upwards.
- The baby's abdomen must never be touched in any of the maneuvers.

Single footling presentation (posterior foot presenting)

Traction is applied to the presenting posterior foot. Never pull the other foot down prematurely!

Method. As for the single footling presentation (anterior foot presenting). Here, the posterior hip is delivered first. The steep downwards traction must be applied until the anterior hip has also emerged. Continue as for the single footling presentation with anterior foot presenting.

If upwards traction is applied earlier, the anterior buttock or hip must remain behind the symphysis pubis.
Afterwards classical arm extraction and delivery of the head (Smellie–Veit maneuver); see p. 253.

Double footling breech. Traction is applied to both feet! The hands hold the corresponding feet. Calves/thighs must be held correctly: thumb on the flexor sides, fingers encircling the shank!

- Steep downwards traction is applied to both legs; the hands climb successively higher, alternating, until both hips have been delivered. Thumbs are parallel and next to the sacrum, the fingers encircle the thighs. In this hold, steep upwards traction, until the lower margin of the anterior shoulder blade emerges.

Afterwards classical arm extraction and delivery of the head (Smellie–Veit maneuver); see p. 253.

Complete breech, kneeling breech
Complete breech presentation. If the breech is mobile, it is pushed upwards; one foot is grasped and pulled downwards in order to perform the extraction.
- In a complete breech presentation, the anterior foot it pulled down and used for the extraction.
- In an incomplete breech presentation, the presenting foot is pulled down and used for the extraction.

The anterior foot is used in the complete breech for the same reason as in the frank breech. If it is not possible to push the breech up, the groin must be used for the extraction.

Kneeling breech. Both feet are used for the extraction in the kneeling breech, in the incomplete kneeling presentation the presenting knee is pulled down. A prerequisite is that the breech is mobile. If not, extraction is performed on the groin.

Frank breech
Three variations depending on the pelvic station of the breech:
1. Breech has not yet entered the PI (high, mobile breech). The frank breech is made into a single footling breech with the anterior foot presenting, so that it can be used to perform the manual extraction.

Note. The method of choice is pulling down the anterior foot. Prerequisite: termination of labor is necessary, conditions for breech extraction are fulfilled (p. 255).

No experienced person would think of attempting to perform an extraction on such a high breech. The breech does not offer good handholds for grasping and extracting: anterior hip. If possible, this feared maneuver is avoided. The anterior foot is pulled down, which relativizes the main difficulty of extraction.

Procedure (Fig. 8.101). The whole of the hand corresponding to the abdominal side of the baby is inserted. The fingers follow the breech along the anterior thigh to the foot. Index and middle finger take hold of the foot. The knee is bent and the foot drawn down until it appears in the vulva. Extraction as per the example on p. 255.

Practice tip. Only the anterior foot is drawn down!

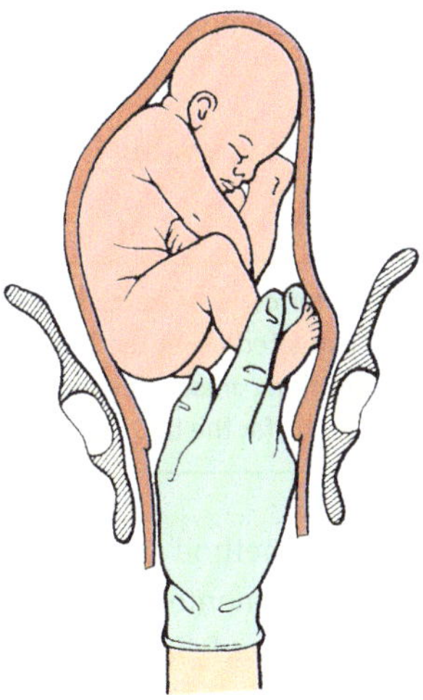

Fig. 8.101: Drawing down the anterior foot.

Reason. Only one foot, because drawing down a second foot would reduce the circumference of the presenting part, and because it is just as easy to take hold of and draw down one foot as two. The circumference of the breech, which paves the way for the largest part of the baby, the head, would be reduced by 1.5 to 2 cm if the second foot were drawn down. The anterior foot is used for the following reasons:

a) The back, which is anterior, remains anterior, which is crucial for the birth of the head.
b) In the rarer case that the back is posterior, drawing down the anterior foot would bring the posterior back towards the front.
c) If the posterior foot is extracted, the anterior hip can easily become trapped behind the symphysis pubis. In addition, the back can rotate posteriorly and the chin become trapped behind the symphysis pubis, which rarely happens if the procedure is performed skillfully.
d) The anterior foot is usually easier to reach and the extraction is more easily performed with it than with the posterior foot.
e) It corresponds to the birth mechanism that the anterior presenting part always takes the lead and is born first.

Difficulties extracting the foot. Extracting a foot is not simple: one comes into contact with the umbilical cord or it threatens to prolapse. If the cord is long, care must also be taken that it is not placed between the legs. It can also be difficult to get hold of the foot, especially if the anterior foot is particularly high in the fundus in front of the baby's face.

Pinard maneuver (Figs. 8.102, 8.103). In order to reach the foot more easily, the index finger is placed in the popliteal fossa of the anterior leg (Fig. 8.102), and the thigh is pressed firmly into the baby's abdomen: the leg flexes, the freed foot moves lower and can be grasped (Fig. 8.103).

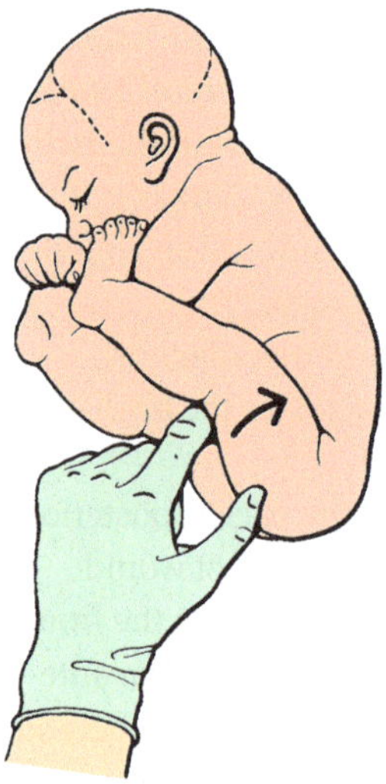

Fig. 8.102: Pinard maneuver to draw down the anterior foot. The index finger presses the thigh towards the abdomen in popliteal fossa.

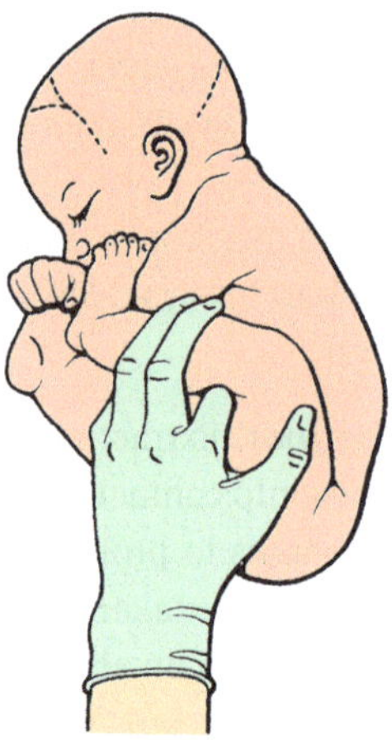

Fig. 8.103: Pinard maneuver to draw down the anterior foot. Middle and ring fingers bend the calf over the index finger in the popliteal fossa.

2. The breech is engaged (PI, midpelvis, PO)

Note. Extraction using the anterior foot is the method of choice in all 3 stations (PI, midpelvis, PO).

Anyone with experience would not attempt to perform an extraction using the breech at any of the 3 stations because it is not possible. The breech which is engaged in the pelvis does not offer good handholds for grasping and extracting.

The anterior foot is drawn down. This was easy when the breech was mobile above the PI.

In order to draw the foot of an engaged breech down – regardless of whether it is in PI, midpelvis or PO – the breech must be pushed right up out of the pelvis. It is only possible to perform the preparatory maneuver of drawing down the foot if the breech is above the brim!

Fracture of the femur results when an attempt is made to draw down the foot of a deeply engaged breech!

Pushing the breech out is easier the more mobile and the higher in the pelvis it is.

- It is easier to push the breech up out of the pelvis from the PI than from the pelvic floor.
- In the PI the breech is still mobile on palpation.
- On the pelvic floor it is engaged and immobile in the pelvis.

3. The breech is in the PO (it is visible in the vagina).

Note. Extraction using the anterior hip (groin) is the only possibility: the baby is extracted using the breech directly. A difficult, unusually tiring maneuver for the operator and extremely dangerous for the baby.

This convenient extraction method using the anterior foot cannot be implemented: the visible breech cannot be mobilized, it is so impacted in the soft tissue canal of the PO that the attempt to push it upwards is usually unsuccessful.

Procedure. A generous episiotomy is essential (conditio sine qua non). The soft tissue problems disappear in one move.

The index finger of the corresponding hand is inserted into the fold of the baby's anterior hip (gap between the trunk and the thigh which is extended against it). The index finger used is that with the same name as the anterior hip: in a right breech presentation (Fig. 8.104) the right index finger is inserted into the right (anterior) hip fold; in a left breech presentation the left index finger is inserted into the left (anterior) hip fold.
The other hand should support by encircling and holding the extracting hand above the wrist (Fig. 8.104).
An assistant should apply constant transfundal pressure from above using all their strength.

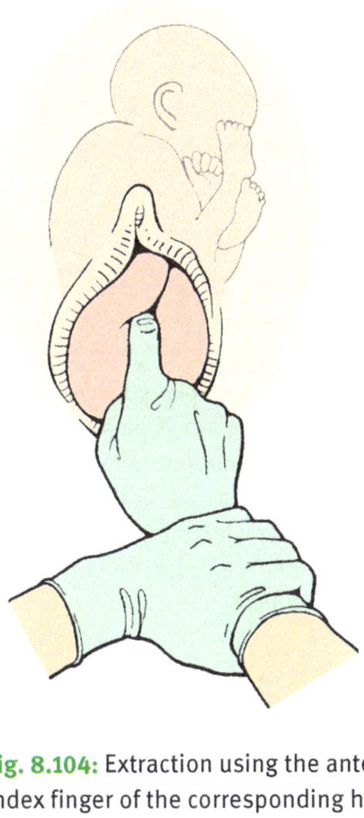

Fig. 8.104: Extraction using the anterior hip. The bent index finger of the corresponding hand is hooked into the anterior hip.

This is particularly important in this strenuous extraction in which the combined strength of both hands is transferred to the baby by only one finger.

In this position, the hands are drawn steeply downwards until the anterior hip appears below the symphysis pubis. The thumb of the drawing down hand is placed on the buttock of the hip which has just been born.
Traction is then applied steeply upwards until the posterior hip appears and is accessible. When this is the case, the index finger of the second hand is hooked into the hip fold and brings the second hip over the perineum. The thumb of the second hand is placed parallel to the other thumb on the posterior buttock. Constant downwards traction is applied and soon both legs slip out (if the second leg remains in the vagina, the trunk is simply bent slightly to the side and the leg slips out). Fingers 2–5 of both hands encircle the thighs; the thumbs remain on the buttocks. In this hold, steep downwards traction is applied in the same direction until the tip of the anterior shoulder blade is born.
Afterwards classical arm extraction and delivery of the head with the Smellie-Veit maneuver.

Note. Rules of breech extraction with epidural anesthesia or narcosis (summary).
Breech is above the pelvis. Anterior foot is drawn down and extraction performed using it, see p. 255.
Breech is engaged in the pelvis. Breech is mobile (PI) or no longer mobile (midpelvis, PO).
- Increase breech mobility.
- Push breech out of the true pelvis above the pelvic brim.
- Draw down the anterior foot and perform the extraction with it; see p. 260.
- Breech immobile in PO (visible deep in the vulva).
- Extraction with the finger on the anterior hip fold; see above.

Difficult extraction (arm, head extraction)

Difficult arm extraction

The baby is half born; one or both arms are extended or nuchal. The shoulders cannot be born because of this abnormal attitude.

Extended arms are an unpleasant complication because dealing with them lengthens the extraction procedure. Rapid resolution requires experience, skill, and the ability to act promptly and decisively.

Procedure (Fig. 8.105)

Note. Options are: extraction with the whole hand: simplest option, often successful; or Sellheim method: the arm is brought down by rotating the baby around its longitudinal axis.

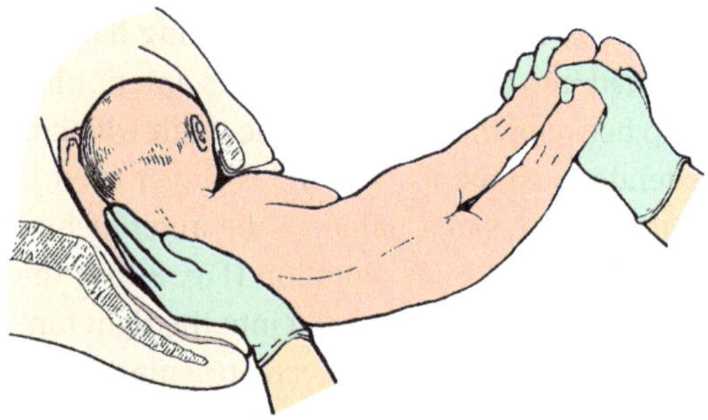

Fig. 8.105: Release of the extended arm using the whole hand (modified after Winter).

Release with the whole hand. If the baby is not too large, the goal is often reached. If the anterior arm is extended, it must be brought posteriorly into the sacral cavity using the plugging movement, as only here can it be released with the whole hand. The hand of the same name is inserted deep into the sacral cavity on the side of the baby's back and takes hold of the lower arm or upper and lower arm. The arm is moved past the side of the head and downwards (Fig. 8.105).

- Release of the arm is easier if the baby is elevated by the legs. This brings the posterior shoulder lower and the extended arm is easier to reach.

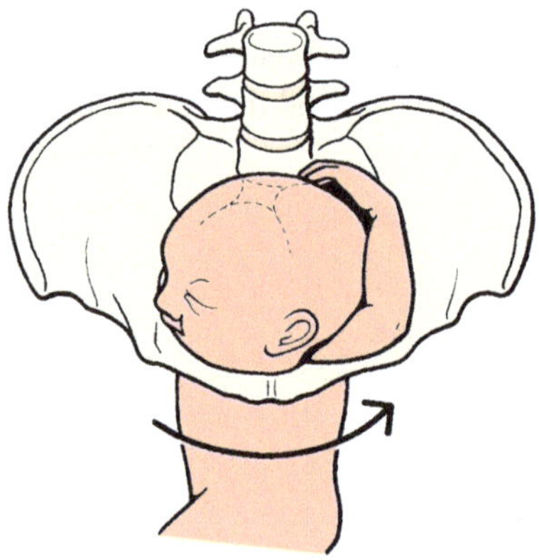

Fig. 8.106: Left breech presentation. Nuchal arm anterior (left). After release of the posterior arm the baby is rotated with a simultaneous plugging movement in the direction in which the arm is pointing (see arrow, clockwise; as seen by the operator, from below). The rotation occurs contrary to the rule, as the abdomen passes under the symphysis pubis. Rotation ends when the arm lies at the face. Extraction from the sacral cavity in the usual manner.

Sellheim method

Option 1. Anterior arm extended and lying in the nape of the neck (nuchal).

Procedure (Fig. 8.106, 8.107):

- First the posterior arm is released in the usual way.
- The baby is then rotated around its longitudinal axis with quick, plugging movements in the direction in which the extended arm points.

Option 2. Posterior arm extended and lying in the nape of the neck (nuchal).

Procedure. First the anterior arm is brought to the back and released in the usual way, and then the baby is rotated further in the same direction. The arm which was previously extended remains where it was until it eventually lies near the face. Extraction is then performed in the usual way.

Option 3. Both arms extended.

Rare! Most complicated scenario! Procedure: the anterior arm is first released by rotating posteriorly and extracting. Then the other arm

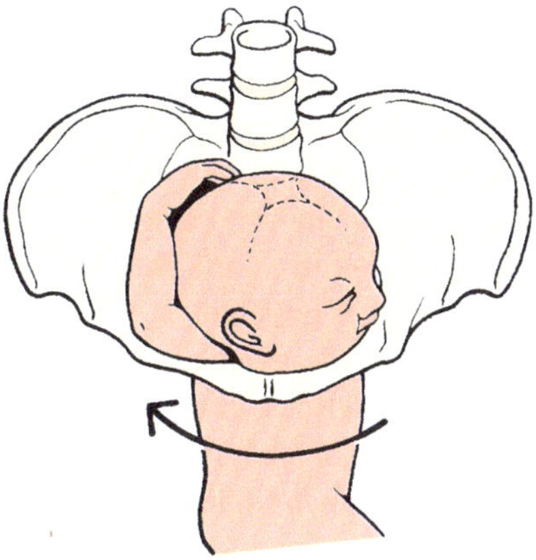

Fig. 8.107: Right breech presentation. Nuchal arm anterior (right). The posterior, not nuchal arm has already been released. The baby is rotated in the direction in which the extended arm is pointing (see arrow, counterclockwise). Here the abdomen also passes anteriorly under the symphysis pubis. Rotation ends when the arm lies at the face. Extraction from the sacral cavity.

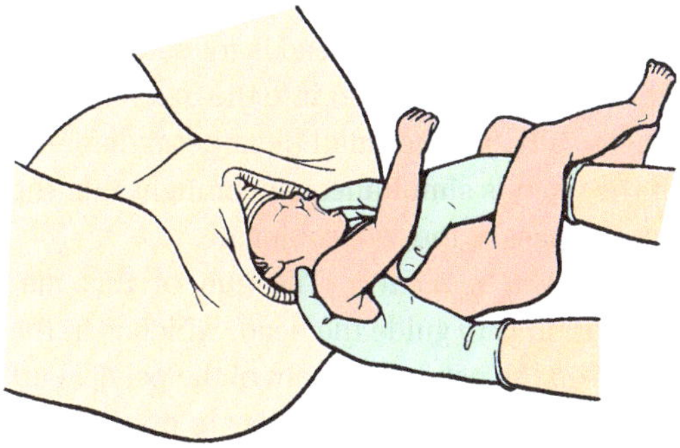

Fig. 8.108: Reverse–Smellie–Veit maneuver.

is brought to the face and extracted by rotating in the other direction.

Difficult head delivery

The baby is half born. The back is directly posterior, arms released, head in pelvis, baby's face is anterior, chin under the symphysis pubis.

Reverse Smellie–Veit maneuver (Fig. 8.108) is used:

- The external hand is placed under the baby's back and supports the neck in a fork-like hold with 2nd and 3rd fingers (Fig. 8.108). The baby rides backwards on the lower arm.
- The index finger of the internal hand is placed in the mouth, which is below the symphysis pubis, and brings the head into the APD and the chin to the chest. Downwards traction is applied until the brow hairline appears. Slow upwards traction (perineal laceration!) is then applied around the hypomochlion (brow hairline), allowing occiput and sinciput to be born.

The baby is half born; head does not enter the pelvis, back anterior or obliquely anterior.

The cause is usually unrecognized cephalopelvic disproportion.
In such cases, attempts and manipulations must on no account cause delays. The head is above, not yet in the pelvis. It has become entrapped above the PI.
A single maneuver confirms this assumption: The maternal abdomen is palpated above the symphysis pubis. (The abdomen must be covered with a sterile drape for every obstetrical operation). The head is palpated as a large firm object above the pelvic brim.
The Wigand-Martin-Winckel maneuver can often help.

Wigand–Martin–Winckel maneuver (Fig. 8.109).

As in the Smellie–Veit maneuver, the hand corresponding to the side the baby is facing is inserted into the vagina on the side of the abdomen/chest and along the front of the overstretched neck until it reaches the baby's mouth. The baby rests on the arm.

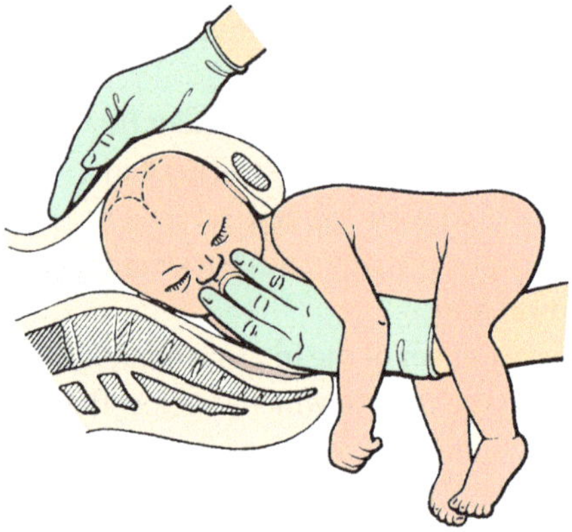

Fig. 8.109: Wigand–Martin–Winckel maneuver.

- The middle finger is inserted into the mouth; the second and fourth fingers are placed on the malar bones (taking care not to injure the eyes!).
- The thumb is placed under the lower jaw. In this hold, two maneuvers are performed:
  - The head is rotated into the transverse diameter so that the sagittal suture is in the transverse diameter, as is usual in the PI.
  - The head is extended, so that the smaller transverse head diameter, the bitemporal (8 cm) is brought into the narrow pass of the contracted true conjugate. If the head is flexed too far, so that the chin touches the breastbone, the larger transverse head diameter (biparietal, 9.5 cm) is brought into the pelvic APD.

This procedure can be used for a flat, contracted pelvis, or normal pelvis and too-large head.
If the whole pelvis is contracted, the head must be maximally flexed. The decision as to the extent of flexion of the head in order to get it to enter the pelvis is made by feel on implementation of the Wigand–Martin–Winckel maneuver.

Practice tip. The head which has been brought into the transverse diameter is not only drawn down into the pelvis, it is also simultaneously pressed into it from outside (from the maternal abdomen).

It is best for the interplay of traction and pressure when the external pressure is not applied by an assistant, but by the operator's free hand. Once the head has reached the pelvic floor, it is delivered using the Smellie-Veit maneuver: the external hand is placed in a fork-like hold on the shoulders as soon as possible.
The maneuver has two disadvantages:
- Time is lost; this is serious, as the baby can die during this stage of labor if the procedure takes longer than 4–5 min.
- Injury to the baby (and mother). Force must usually be applied to get the head into the pelvis. Death as a result of serious skull injury.

Smellie–Veit vs. Wigand–Martin–Winckel maneuver. Both maneuvers are similar externally. Differences:

Wigand–Martin–Winckel maneuver (see Fig. 8.109). The aim of the manipulation is to bring the high head (above the pelvic brim) into the pelvis. To this end, the head is rotated from the APD or oblique diameter into the transverse diameter (PI) and the small bitemporal diameter of the head is simultaneously brought into the narrow pass of the true conjugate
Smellie–Veit maneuver. The aim of this manipulation is to guide the head, which is in the pelvis on the pelvic floor, out of the pelvis. Part of manual assistance. In order to do this, the head, which is usually in an oblique diameter, is rotated into the APD and flexed (corresponding to the normal birth mechanism!).

8.3 Transverse lie/shoulder presentation

Definition. Fetal position in which the fetal and maternal axes are perpendicular or at an acute angle to one another (oblique lie). The smallest degree of an oblique lie is when the head deviates from the PI.

Classification. The following main shoulder presentations are classified according to the position of the scapula:
Dorsoanterior:
- Right scapula anterior (RSA): scapula anterior, right.
- Left scapula anterior (LSA): scapula anterior, left.

Scapula (dorso-)anterior presentations are the most common
Dorsoposterior:
- Right scapula posterior (RSP): scapula posterior, right.
- Left scapula posterior (LSP): scapula posterior, left.

Dorsosuperior and dorsoinferior transverse lies also occur.

Note. Transitory lies are more common than main lies!

Incidence. Transverse lies make up 1 % of all births, 75 % of those are multiparae, 25 % primiparae.

Etiology. Transverse lies occur in:
1. (Abnormally) large freedom of fetal movement. Multi and grand multiparae (lax uterus wall and abdominal musculature, yielding; 40 % of all causes), preterm deliveries (small fetus and relatively large AF volume), hydramnios, dead baby, second twin.
2. Normal lie obstructed in PI:
   a) Contracted pelvis (consider especially in primiparae!).
   b) Placenta previa.
   c) Multifetal gestation.
   d) Abnormal uterine anatomy (arcuate uterus, fibroids).

Prognosis. Birth is not possible from a transverse lie! SVD without assistance is possible in two exceptional cases: spontaneous rectification, spontaneous evolution (Evolutio spontanea) spontaneous expulsion.

Practice tip. Both exceptions are rare, so cannot be expected. The statement remains valid: Birth is not possible from a transverse lie.

Three types of spontaneous delivery. Prerequisite: extremely small babies (twins, preterm delivery), macerated fetus, strong contractions, broad pelvis.
- *Douglas method* (1819). The head remains above the symphysis pubis, the neck (hypomochlion) is behind it and the first shoulder is forced under it by the contractions (Fig. 8.110). Trunk and both legs are driven from the sacral cavity past the shoulder, behind the symphysis pubis and out of the pelvis, followed by shoulders and head. It is characteristic that the body folds in the upper spine.
- *Denman method* (1785). One shoulder is pressed laterally into the iliac wing, behind the symphysis pubis. The head is higher, laterally. The main difference to the Douglas method is that whereas in that method the body is folded in the upper spine, here it is the lower spine, usually the lumbar spine. The shoulders rise higher and the breech

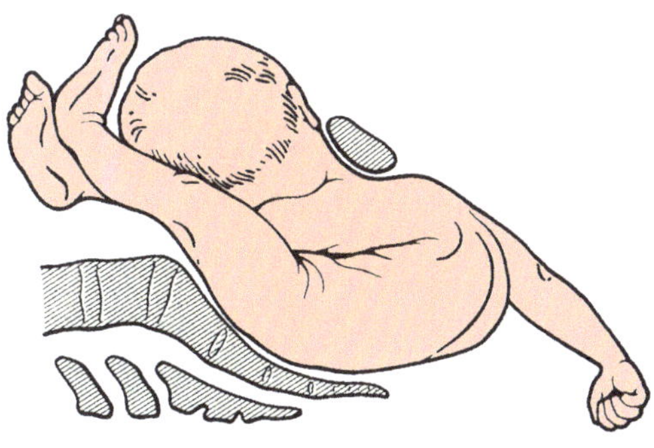

Fig. 8.110: Duncan method of spontaneous delivery.

and legs are expelled below the upper half of the trunk.

- *Conduplicato corpore, birth with doubled-up body* (Roederer, 1756). The fetus is doubled up on itself like a pocketknife and is expelled in this position (closed pocketknife). The body is folded in the thoracic spine. The head is forced deeply into the abdomen (Fig. 8.111).

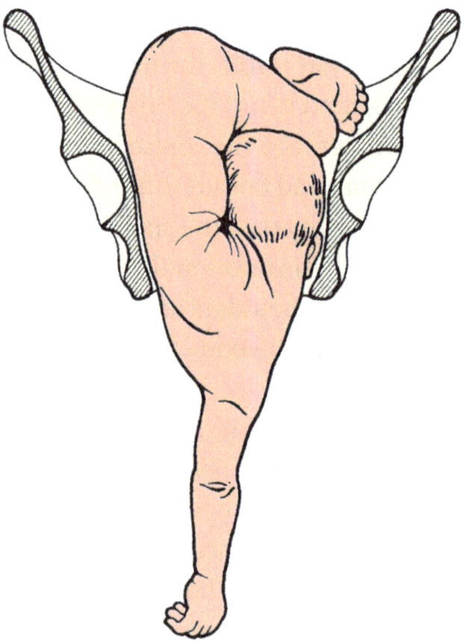

Fig. 8.111: Conduplicato corpore birth (after Stoeckel).

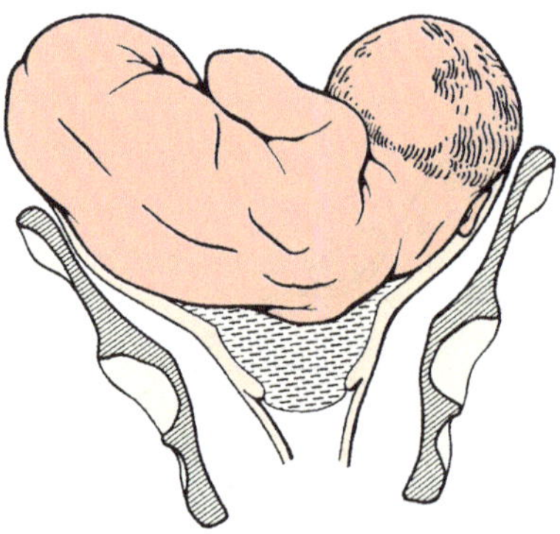

Fig. 8.112: Left scapula anterior (LSA; dorsoanterior) transverse lie with intact membranes (after Bumm).

8.3.1 Course of labor in transverse lie

There are three phases of the transverse lie birth, relating to the dangers for mother and baby in each labor phase:

Note. Phase 1 (→ phase of intact membranes). Baby at risk, mother not.
Phase 2 (→ begins with membrane rupture). Both mother and baby at risk.
Phase 3 (→ begins when cervix is fully dilated). Catastrophe for mother and baby.

Phase 1. Phase of intact membranes
As long as the membranes are intact, the baby floats above the pelvic inlet (Fig. 8.112); there is no danger!
The mother is not at risk because the shoulders do not begin to impact until the membranes have ruptured. The shoulders as leading part can descend lower into the pelvis, reflexively stimulate stronger contractions and become so firmly impacted that they can no longer be pushed back and out. This is known as an impacted shoulder presentation, and can cause a medical emergency at any moment: rupture of the uterine wall.

Note. Preventing the entry of the shoulders to the pelvis means avoiding the main danger of transverse lie: rupture of the uterus.

Babies in transverse lie are in danger! It appears that the transverse strain on the uterus and the resultant unfavorable placental hemodynamics are enough to pose a significant risk to the baby.
Monitoring the endangered baby: see p. 167.
Caution: avoid anything that may cause the membranes to rupture, in particular on examination.
Examination. Leading symptom of transverse lie is the empty pelvis!

- Leopold maneuver. This is enough, in many cases, to recognize a transverse lie.
- Sonography. Confirms the diagnosis and gives exact orientation: head! Back!

Phase 2. Dangerous phase

Note. Rupture of membranes (ROM; Fig. 8.113) means that both mother and baby are endangered.

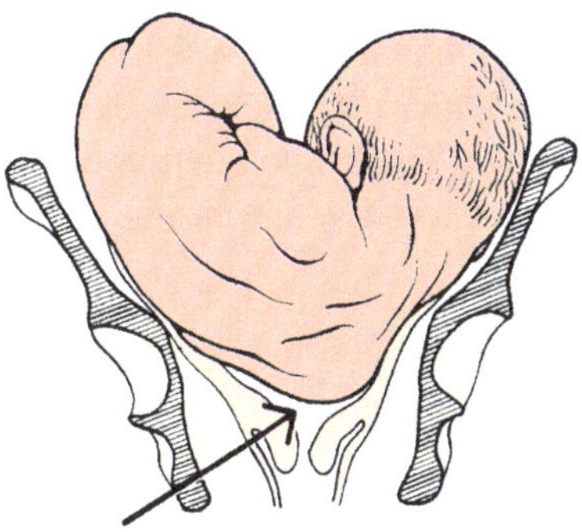

Fig. 8.113: Left scapula anterior shoulder presentation (LSA). Membranes have prematurely ruptured. Danger: one shoulder descends into the true pelvis.

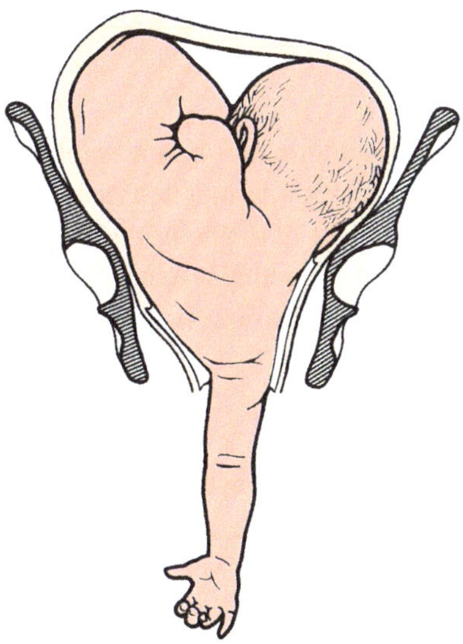

Fig. 8.114: Arm prolapse in LSA.

Main danger is impacted shoulder/s. The tip of the shoulder blade which was floating above the pelvis (Fig. 8.113) is forced towards and into the pelvic brim with the flow of AF (see Fig. 8.113, arrow): wedged-in shoulder, impacted transverse lie.

Pathological CTG, death of the baby. The placental circulation is impaired due to the transverse strain on the uterus and the loss of AF. This explains the not uncommon death of babies in a transverse lie.

Prolapsed arm (Fig. 8.114). The anterior-lying arm often (20–30 %) descends into the cervical canal or vagina. This is dangerous for two reasons:
- Impacted shoulders can result sooner, whereby the arm becomes axially centered in the birth canal more quickly.
- Cord prolapse. In addition, the cord can prolapse.

Cord prolapse. Cord prolapse alone is as common as arm prolapse: 10–20 %. It is not as alarming as in cephalic presentations as it does not become compressed.
Cord and arm prolapse or cord prolapse and shoulder descending towards the PI cause cord compression, which is life-threatening for the baby.

Complications of version
Ascending infection, which accompanies every premature and early ROM in prolonged labors, is mentioned last because in transverse lies mechanical dangers are in the forefront.

Examination
Vaginal. To be noted are:
- Cervical dilatation.
- Threatened prolapse of arm, foot, cord (cord palpable?).
- Cause of transverse lie?

Sonography. Position of head and back.

Phase 3. Catastrophic phase

Note. Begins when the cervix is fully dilated.

Wedged-in shoulders and impaction occur in the second phase of labor once the cervix has fully dilated.

Practice tip. Impaction can occur within minutes once the cervix is completely dilated! It can also take a number of hours if the expulsive contractions have not yet begun.

Neglected shoulder presentation (Fig. 8.115). The uterus contracts closer and tighter around the baby with every impacting contraction. The musculature retracts, thickening the fundal wall (arrow 1), and thinning that of the lower uterine segment (arrow 2). The baby, which is positioned largely in this increasingly overdistended section (arrow 2), is held in this unfavorable position not only because every contraction forces head and breech more firmly against the iliac wings, but also because each contraction forces it to fold further in on itself, usually folding in its most flexible section, the cervical spine. The descent of the shoulders results reflexively in stronger, more intense contractions, increasing to almost ceaseless tonic contractions and culminating in Tetanus uteri (continuous, extremely intense contractile state). These tonic contractions wedge the leading shoulder so deeply into the true pelvis that it cannot be removed by any means.

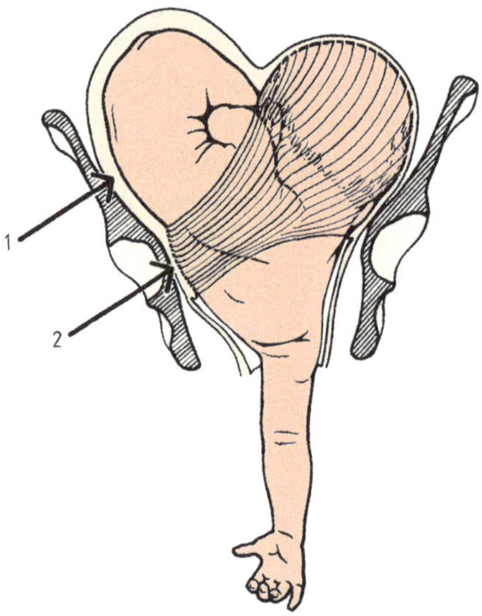

Fig. 8.115: Neglected LSA with prolapse of the right arm. The lower uterine segment is extremely distended both longitudinally and cylindrically (2) and is about to rupture. The hollow muscle of the uterine body is maximally contracted (1) and has retracted high above the body of the baby.

The end state of every untreated or incorrectly managed transverse lie has thus been reached, neglected shoulder presentation.

Note. Neglected shoulder presentation is the life-threatening end state of a untreated or incorrectly managed transverse lie, in which the baby is clamped so tightly in the extremely overdistended (both longitudinally and transversely) uterus that the slightest movement of the baby by the doctor's hand must lead to rupture of the uterus.

Examination

Vaginal. The shoulders are barely mobile, wedged onto the PI; they cannot be forced upwards (→ characteristic of the neglected shoulder presentation). If the umbilical cord is palpable, whether it is still pulsating is noted (babies are often damaged or dead).

8.3.2 Management of transverse lie

Note. Transverse lies are managed in hospital due to the high maternal and fetal mortality rates. Admission 2–3 weeks before EDD!

The danger to the fetus is explained by chronic placental insufficiency. This is caused by the impaired hemodynamics due to the unfavorable situation of placenta and fetus. The inadequate placental exchange can deteriorate acutely in particular once the uterine contractions set in, but also after the premature or early ROM so common in transverse lies, leading to intrauterine fetal death.

Hospital management
Before onset of labor, fetal monitoring (2–3 weeks before EDD).
- Daily CTG (see p. 36).
- Attempted external version with tocolysis (3 weeks before EDD; see p. 244).

Note. Once labor has begun: if external version is unsuccessful there are two methods to choose from: cesarean section or vaginal delivery (version, extraction). Which method is chosen depends on findings and course of labor.

Cesarean section. Fetal and maternal mortality can be reduced to a minimum (exceptions see below) if CS is performed, it is therefore the method of choice!

Indications for vaginal delivery:
- Stillbirth.
- Preterm delivery with estimated weight of < 500g.
- Second twin.
- No additional indication for CS (placenta previa, course of labor).

Management of vaginal delivery
Phase 1, intact membranes. ROM is delayed by any means possible until the cervix is fully dilated. Intact membranes prevent descent of the shoulders and are most favorable for version (see below).

Practice tip. Expectant management: Intervention is not performed in shoulder presentation as long as the membranes are intact and the cervix not fully dilated!

Prevention of ROM:
- Bed rest with elevated pelvis.
- Lateral supine position if contractions are strong, pelvis remains elevated.
- No uterotonics!

As there is no leading part, the full force of the contractions acts directly on the lower pole of the membranes (forebag). Contractions of moderate strength can therefore easily lead to ROM long before the cervix has completely dilated.
Amniotomy, version, extraction. The aim is that the cervix reaches full dilation before the membranes rupture. Once the cervix is fully dilated or (in multiparae) almost fully dilated, the membranes are ruptured and version (p. 340) and extraction (p. 246) immediately performed.
Placental separation. Immediately following this, the placenta is manually detached because after version and extraction the uterine cavity, in particular the lower uterine segment, must be examined in case rupture has occurred.

Phase 2, ruptured membranes. Immediate vaginal examination
- if the cervix is only slightly dilated CS is indicated;
- if the cervix is fully dilated, version and – after a pause – extraction.

Phase 3 Impacted shoulder presentation. Immediate and careful delivery under general anesthetic, high-dose tocolysis with beta$_2$ sympathomimetics (Fenoterol) until operation:
- Narcosis, if not already done before examination.
- CS if baby is living and undamaged.
- Decapitation or embryotomy if baby is dead or damaged.

Practice tip. Attempted version when shoulders are impacted is malpractice! After every procedure the uterus is manually examined!

8.4 Multifetal gestations

Definition. Babies which have simultaneously developed and are born in brief succession.

Incidence. Large geographical variations. Earlier the Hellin-rule was valid:
Twins 1 : 85/1 : 85.
Triplets 1 : 85^2/1 : 7,225.
Quadruplets 1 : 85^3/1 : 614,125.
Quintuplets 1 : 85^4/1 : 52,200,625.

Multifetal pregnancies are more common in **early pregnancy.**
Course of 325 twin pregnancies (Boklage 1990).
Rate of conception: 1 multiple to 1 singleton pregnancy.
Twin births: 19 %.
Singleton births: 39 %.
No living births: 43 %.

Twins. The rate of twin pregnancies decreased in most European countries in the 1960s from 12 to 9.5 in 1,000 pregnancies, and then returned to 12 from the early 1980s, and to 13–14/1,000 around 1990. A twin rate of 3.2 % of all live births was reported for the USA in 2006.

While the course of the 1960s and 1970s was caused by changes in age of/at parity (initially an increase of young parous women, later an increase of over 35 year olds), the increase from 1990 is due to reproductive medicine.

Higher order multifetal gestations. Dramatic increase since the late eighties: the rate of triplets in Germany increased by 170 % from 1975–1990, in the Netherlands by 300 %. Causes are ovulation stimulation and IVF.

Zygosity. Degree of relationship of multiples referring to the number of fertilized ova (zygotes), e.g., monozygotic (uniovular) and dizygotic (binovular).

Monozygotic (MZ) twins result from the division of a single embryo. Incidence 4/1,000 births.
- Embryofetal mortality. Higher than for dizygotic twins and singletons.
- Rate of malformation. Major malformations 2.3 % (1 % in singletons), minor malformations 4.1 % (2.5 % in singletons).

Monochorionic, monoamniotic twins have worse statistical results; if they are both girls the results are better.
Four types:
1. Dichorionic diamniotic (DCDA; 30 %), when the embryo splits before the 3rd day p.c.
2. Monochorionic diamniotic (MCDA; 65 %), when the embryo splits 4–8 days p.c.
3. Monochorionic monoamniotic (MCMA; 5 %), when the embryo splits 8–12 days p.c.
4. Conjoined twins develop when division occurs after day 13, incidence (Europe): 1/33, 000 births.

Dizygotic (DZ) twins result from the fertilization of two ova from two follicles.
The DZ incidence appears to correlate with the FSH level, which is influenced by light and dark periods; this would appear to be the reason that the rate of dizygotic twin conception is higher in Scandinavia in July than in January.
The incidence of dizygosity is influenced by the following factors:
- Assisted reproductive technology (ART), in particular hormonal stimulation of ovulation.
- Geographical differences (Africa 1/30 births, Asia 1/100, Europe 1/80).
- Maternal age. The prevalence of DZ increases with increasing maternal age.
- Parity. The probability of a DZ birth increases with increasing parity.

- Maternal weight and height; overweight and tall women have an increased risk of DZ.
- Family history.

Note. Multifetal gestations in the maternal family are more relevant than in the paternal family for the incidence of DZ twins. 2 % of dizygotic twin women, give birth to twins in contrast to 1 % if the fathers are DZ twins.

Superfecundation, superfetation. The simultaneous fertilization of two ova by two fathers in the same cycle (superfecundation) has not been demonstrated in humans. Equally inadequately proven is the ovulation of two follicles at different times in the same cycle, or from different cycles with fertilization (superfetation) and corresponding age difference of the fetuses.

Higher order multifetal gestations can develop from the fertilization of one, two, or more oocyte/s, or from division of one or more fertilized oocyte/s, so that a mixture of di- and monozygotic twins results.

Zygosity diagnosis postpartum. After delivery of the placenta macroscopic examination of the septum gives clues regarding zygosity.

Vanishing twin. The disappearance of an embryo or early fetus from a multifetal gestation is explained by resorption. An empty sac remains, or a Fetus papyraceus. Sometimes bleeding ex utero is clinically manifest.

Since refined sonographic diagnosis, numerous findings are available, including clinical, pathological and chemical.

Conjoined twins

Conjoined twins, pagus. Incomplete division on day 15–17 p.c. leads to development of conjoined twins (pagus). They are divided into completely symmetrical, incompletely symmetrical and asymmetrical pagus and classified according to the point of fusion.

- Thoracopagus: thorax–thorax fusion (Fig. 8.116).
- Craniopagus: head–head fusion.
- Ischiopagus: hip–hip fusion (Fig. 8.117).

Conjoined twins have the same sex; girls are more commonly affected (1.6 : 1), and 50 % have further malformations.

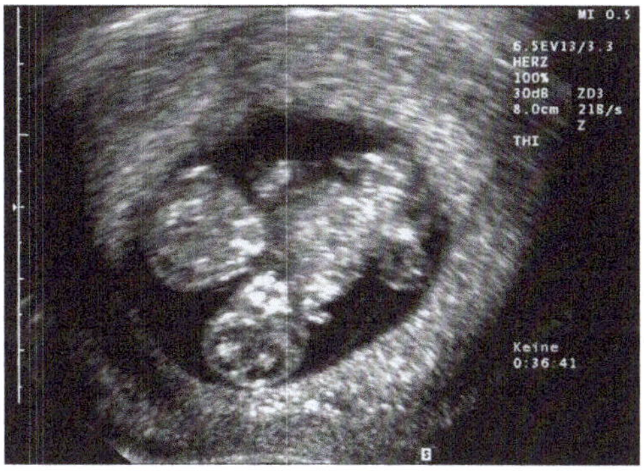

Fig. 8.116: Sonography of conjoined twins in week 10.

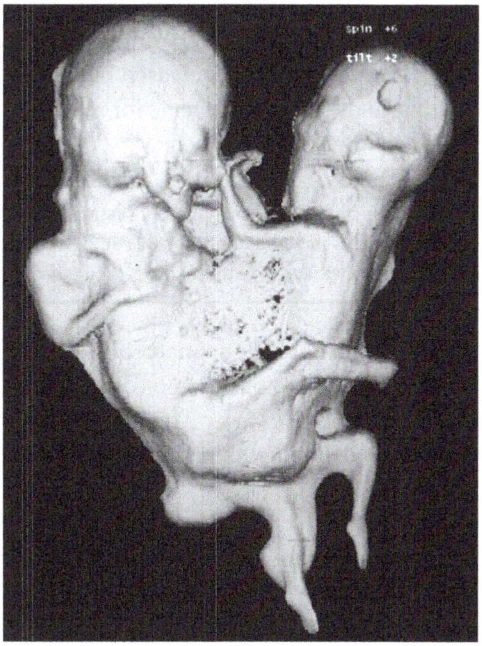

Fig. 8.117: Conjoined twins, week 14; postpartum surface reconstruction using computerized tomography.

The symmetrical double malformation is not always complete:
- Duplicitas. Body parts are doubled, e.g., two heads in dicephaly.
- Arcadiacus is a special malformation in monozygotic twins: one twin has no heart (acardiac twin) and is connected to the healthy twin‘s (pump twin) circulatory system via vascular anastomoses in the chorion.

Antenatal care involves: 1) sonographic diagnosis, 2) elimination of further malformations, 3) estimation of prognosis, 4) setting time and location of delivery, 5) neonatal care if necessary, 6) psychological support for the parents.

Maternal adaptation
The adaptation is more marked in multifetal pregnancy.
- *Cardiac output* (CO). In singleton pregnancies the CO is 25–30 % higher in week 32–36 (maximum level), in twin pregnancies 50–60 %; an additional 500 ml of blood is circulating.
- *Pregnancy anemia.* The increased blood volume and fetal requirements for iron and folic acid predispose to anemia.

Practice tip. The strain on the circulatory system in multifetal pregnancies is highest in week 32–36. (Caution: pregnant women with cardiac disease!)

- *Organ disfunction.* The spatial requirements of multifetal gestations promote mechanical disturbances in visceral organ function; the elevated diaphragm restricts breathing.

8.4.1 Antenatal care

Antenatal checkups
- Early diagnosis of multifetal gestation.
- Diagnosis of malformations.
- Prevention of preterm delivery.
- Recognition of intrauterine hypotrophy.

The antenatal checkups are to be performed fortnightly till 28 weeks, later weekly.

Indications for hospitalization
- Threatened preterm delivery.
- PIH.
- Maternal exhaustion, in particular in higher order gestations.
- Diabetes mellitus and gestational diabetes.
- Urinary tract infections.

Multifetal pregnancies are shorter:
- Twins. Rate of preterm delivery (< 37 + 0 weeks) 44.5 %, as opposed to 9.4 % of singletons (USA 1987). Duration of pregnancy 36 + 1 weeks in comparison to 39 + 2 in singleton pregnancies.
- Triplets. Gestational age on delivery 32 weeks.
- Quadruplets. Gestational age on delivery 30 weeks.

Causes. Overdistension of the uterus, mechanical stress on the cervix, reduced uterine perfusion and placental function.

Sonographic diagnosis. Sonographic assessment has led to prenatal diagnosis of multifetal gestations. This is beneficial for: management of the pregnancy, monitoring of mother and babies, intrapartal procedure and parental preparation. Perinatal mortality has decreased as a result of the high diagnosis rate of multifetal pregnancies.

Outcomes of sonography are:
- Diagnosis of multifetal pregnancy.
- Determination of gestational age.
- Monitoring of fetal growth. Head diameter and femur length growth curves correspond to those of singleton gestations.
- Nuchal translucency measurement, differentiated examination for malformations

- Cervical sonography.
- Diagnosis of chorionicity and placentation. In dichorionic pregnancies, a lambda-shaped membrane structure at the placental septum can be depicted in week 10–15.
- Separate placentae or one (fused) placenta.
- Chorionic septum (between the amniotic cavities). In monozygotic twins thin, in dizygotic thick.

Around 25 % of **monochorionic twins** suffer intrauterine growth restriction (IUGR), twin-twin or feto-fetal transfusion syndrome (FFTS or TTTS) or intrauterine fetal death. Perinatal death is 7 times as high in monochorionic as in dichorionic twins. The incidence of congenital anomalies is also markedly higher for monochorionic than for dichorionic twins. These facts illustrate that monochorionic twins represent a high-risk situation and require special antenatal counseling.

The diagnosis of twins must therefore always include diagnosis of chorionicity (monochorionic or dichorionic twins)!

Fortnightly sonographic assessment is to be performed from week 16 onwards in monochorionic twins for early diagnosis of IUGR or TTTS.
TTTS is recognized sonographically when there is discrepancy of AF volume between the twins: polyhydramnios of the receiver, oligohydramnios of the donor. Volume can be reduced to such an extent that the donor as smaller twin is pressed against the membranes (stuck twin).

Note. Monitoring fetal wellbeing: 1) AF volume, 2) non-stress test, 3) respiratory movement, 4) movement, 5) accoustic stimulation, 6) doppler velocimetry is indicated if risk factors exist: weight discrepancy, TTTS, pathological CTG.

Prenatal genetic diagnosis. Indication:
- Women > 35 years old.
- Prior pregnancy with chromosomal abnormalities.
- Parents with chromosome alterations.
- Psychological stress situation.

Methods. Amniocentesis in second trimester, chorionic villi sampling (CVS), early amniocentesis.
We recommend indigo-carmine in order to identify the amniotic cavity for amniocentesis.
Complication. The complication rate of amniocentesis is 5 times as high as in singleton pregnancy.

Selective feticide. Targeted reduction of higher order gestations to twin pregnancy via hysterotomy, heart puncture, injection of air, injection of cardiotoxic substances in order to reduce risks to mother and surviving fetuses. Selective feticide is ethically controversial. It would be preferable to introduce measures in reproductive technology to avoid multifetal gestation!

Method. Experienced groups recommend the transabdominal intrathoracic injection of potassium chloride. In the opinion of many authors the benefits for the surviving multiples justify the procedure.
Complication. In monochorionic twins there is the risk that the cardiotoxic substances will pass over to the other twin. Complete loss of pregnancy is to be expected in 10 %.

Main complications of multiple gestations:
- Shorter pregnancy length.
- Increased maternal risk.

Triplets:
- 20 % preeclampsia.
- 30 % anemia.
- 35 % PPH.

Quadruplets:
- 32 % preeclampsia.
- 25 % anemia.
- 21 % PPH.

Twin-twin transfusion syndrome (TTTS). Monozygotic monochorionic twins have interfetal vascular connections in the placenta:
- Arteriovenous, arterial, venovenous anastomosen on the chorionic plate.
- Arteriovenous shunts in the cotyledons.

They are the basis for a redistribution of blood, the causes of which have not yet been conclusively clarified. Consequences (Figs. 8.118, 8.119):
- Receiver. One twin is larger, polycythemic and develops hydramnios.
- Donor. The other is growth-retarded, develops anemia and oligohydramnios.

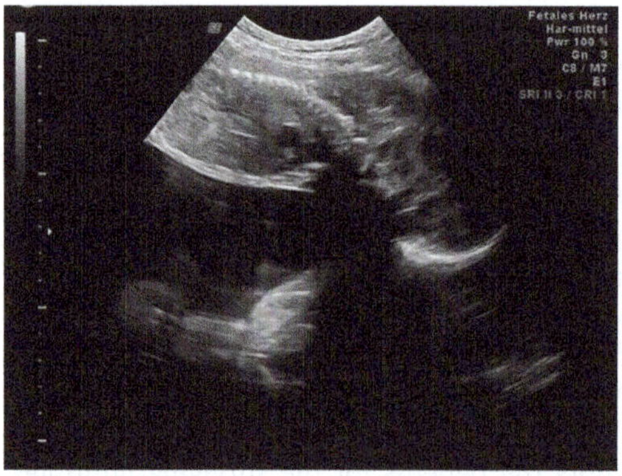

Fig. 8.118: Twin-twin transfusion syndrome (TTTS) with stuck twin as donor in week 25 + 3.

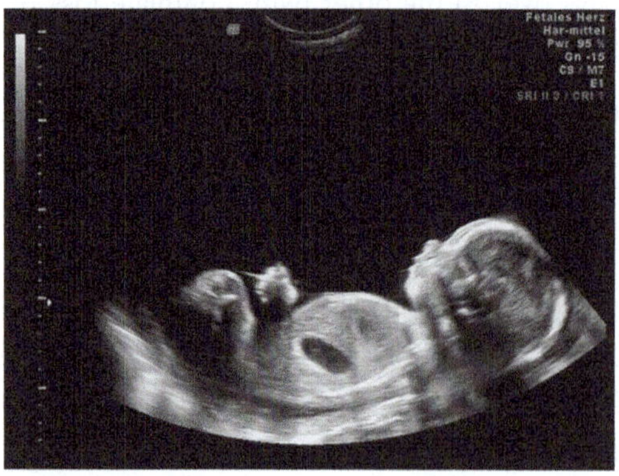

Fig. 8.119: Twin-twin transfusion syndrome with receiver in week 25 + 3.

Mortality rates are high (56–100 %). Intrauterine death occurs in 3–5 %, which results in twin-embolization syndrome in up to 14 %: thromboplastic material endangers the surviving fetus via disseminated intravascular coagulation (DIC) and infarctions with severe neurological disturbances.
Using ultrasound results, Quintero and colleagues have proposed a schematic staging of TTTS which correlates to the fate of the fetus:

Stage 1. Largest vertical pocket of AF: donor < 2 cm, receiver > 8 cm.

Stage 2. Bladder not visible for 60min (donor).

Stage 3. Abnormal Doppler results (zero flow or reverse flow in the umbilical artery pulsatile flow in the umbilical vein; reverse flow in ductus venosus).

Stage 4. Hydrops of one twin.

Stage 5. Death of one twin.

Therapy after early sonographic diagnosis:
- Selective laser coagulation of the chorionic vascular connections.
- Repeated amniocentesis and draining of amniotic fluid.

Intrauterine death. The intrauterine death of one or more multiples is common (1–5 % of all multifetal pregnancies). In addition to the parental state, particular attention is to be paid to the condition of the surviving fetus/es. The surviving fetus/es of monochorionic multiples often have neurological damage, thought to be caused by twin-embolization syndrome.

After death of a twin the surviving twin is at risk for the following:
- Fetal death (in monochorionic twins 12 %, in dichorionic 4 %).

- Neurological impairment (in monochorionic twins 18 %, in dichorionic 1 %).
- Preterm delivery (in monochorionic twins 68 %, in dichorionic 57 %).

The clinical consequences after the intrauterine death of a twin are disputed, as generally recognized prospective studies are not available. It appears reasonable to adopt expectant management alongside monitoring of mother and fetus after the death of a dichorionic twin. The pregnancy should be brought to an end in cases of monochorionic twins and the threatened death of the twin near term, because the surviving twin is endangered by the hypotension at the time of death of the co-twin. In cases where pulmonary immaturity is to be expected, the delivery should be delayed if possible until fetal lung maturity has been accelerated.

Reduction of the risk of preterm delivery. Multiples have higher perinatal risks.

Causes. High rate of preterm delivery, IUGR more common.
Rate of preterm delivery in twins. 30 %. 3–5 times higher than for singleton pregnancies.
- Early diagnosis of multifetal gestation.
- Regular sonography, cervical sonography.
- Cessation of work (from week 20), physical rest.

Obsolete: hospitalization if no further risk factors exist, preventative cerclage, prophylactic tocolysis.

Intrauterine growth restriction (IUGR). Incidence in multifetal gestations 60 %. *Causes:*
- Poor maternal nutritional status, reduced uterine perfusion.
- Umbilical cord anomaly.
- Transport capacity of the placenta, localization of the placenta.
- Unequal distribution of the total placental mass of the multiples, TTTS.

The elevated level of erythropoietin in cord blood, which indicates chronic hypoxia of the fetuses is of diagnostic value.

Concluding the pregnancy. Ending the pregnancy after 37 completed weeks is recommended to avoid intrauterine death.

Management of vaginal birth using prostaglandins to promote cervical ripeness, or IV oxytocin if cervix is mature.
Indications for primary CS:
- Triplets, higher order multiples.
- Monoamniotic twins.
- Twins with a sonographically estimated weight of < 1,800 g.
- Weight discrepancy between the twins, > 20 % in favor of the second twin.
- Leading twin in breech or transverse presentation.

8.4.2 Birth complications, mode

Birth complications

Malpresentations, malpositions, errors of attitude, extreme uterine distension are factors which predispose to complications:
1. Premature ROM, possibly before 36 completed weeks.
2. Abnormality, impediment to descent and entry into the pelvis.
3. Cord prolapse due to PROM and incomplete fit of leading part.
4. Locked twins due to collision of the heads.
5. Primary uterine hypotonia.
6. Long labor, protracted labor, secondary uterine hypotonia, maternal exhaustion.
7. Abruption of the second twin's placenta after birth of the first twin (hypoxemia of the second twin).
8. Atonic uterus in third stage.

Birth mode, management

A standardized birth mode for multifetal gestations is not generally accepted. The birth mode of twins differs from that of higher order multiples.

Triplets, higher order multiples

While in America CS is preferred, South Africa has a CS rate of 14 %. The majority were first detected in labor, so that no conclusions can be drawn from these numbers for Europe.

Vaginal delivery. Triplets born vaginally have worse postnatal status: lower Apgar scores, respiratory difficulties.

Complications alongside malpresentations and malpositions: placental abruption, asphyxia, cord prolapse, vaginal bleeding.

Note. Abdominal operative delivery. Triplets and higher order multiples are delivered via cesarean section.

The elective operation avoids some of the above-named complications and allows scheduling of obstetrician and neonatologist.
The organization of neonatal care and the availability of neonatal intensive beds is not to be underestimated as a problem. A further obstetrician is required, with experience in diagnosis of malpresentations and malpositions and their operative consequences. A third obstetrician follows the movements of the multiples sonographically during second stage.
Prerequisites for operating. The obstetricians are experienced in the operative delivery of multiples from malpresentations and malpositions, and with subsequent hysterectomy if necessary in cases of unstoppable PPH. The anesthetist is capable of treating shock.
Oxytocin is administered prophylactically after delivery of the babies to prevent uterine atony.

Twins

Lies and presentations must be known in order to decide on mode of delivery (Fig. 8.120).

Note. Monoamniotic and conjoined twins are delivered via CS, regardless of lie and presentation!

Monoamniotic twins. Two threatened complications on vaginal delivery:
- Head collision (rare). 1 : 1,000 twin births.
- The collisions are more common in monochorionic and monoamniotic twins than in dichorionic or diamniotic. They are accompanied by oligohydramnios.

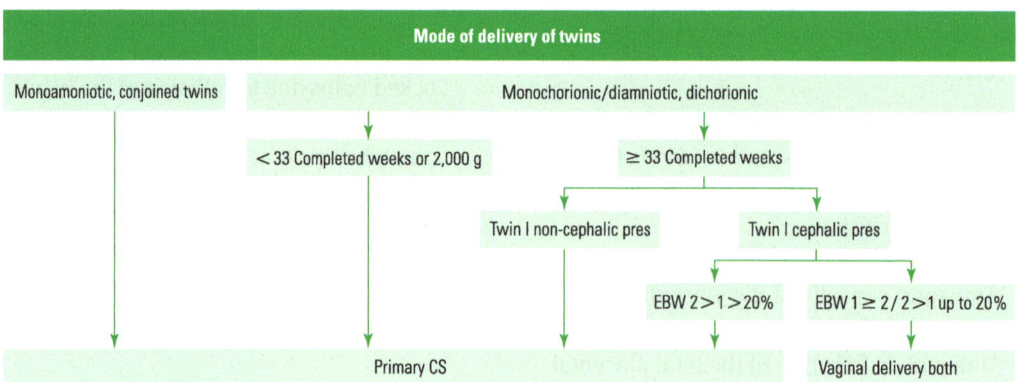

Fig. 8.120: Mode of delivery of twins (EBW = estimated birth weight, CS = cesarean section).

– Occluded cord with threatened intrauterine death occurs on descent of a twin in an acute phase.

Conjoined twins. Elective abdominal operative delivery raises the twins' chances of survival and avoids dystocia.

Diamniotic twins

Both in cephalic presentation. Can usually be delivered vaginally; no complications in 3/4 of all twins.

Indications for CS:
- Preterm labor and sonographically estimated birth weight < 1,800 g.
- Weight discrepancy between the twins, > 20 % in favor of the second twin.

Management of vaginal delivery of twins
- Simultaneous cardiotocography of both twins! If asphyxia of the first twin is suspected on the basis of the CTG, acid-base household is checked via FBS; if asphyxia of the second twin is suspected it is to be delivered operatively.
- Contractions are to be monitored; uterotonics are often required.

Birth management after delivery of the first twin

Second twins have a higher morbidity rate. Risk reduction:
- Diagnosis of lie and presentation (external examination, ultrasound).
- Oxytocin infusion to shorten the (brief) contraction-free interval after delivery of the first twin.
- Continuous cardiotocographic monitoring.
- Vaginal examination: Are the membranes intact? Which fetal part is presenting? Is it descending?
- Sonographic confirmation of lie and presentation.
- ARM on resumption of contractions and descent of the presenting part.
- Alternative: expectant management if CTG is normal (no signs of hypoxia).
- Operative delivery if CTG pathological.

Interval between first and second twin. Decision depends on heart rate pattern of the second twin:
- Prompt delivery of twins with pathological heart rates, often operative.
- Expectant management if heart rate pattern normal after birth of the first twin. However, longer intervals, which might allow the cervix to close, should not be allowed.

The interval length has been a topic of discussion for decades. While the attitude towards a set time limit was relaxed in Europe in the 1960s, Anglo-Saxon countries had a set interval of < 30 min to avoid asphyxia, placental abruption, cord prolapse and closure of the cervix. There is a correlation between the difference between umbilical cord artery values (twin 1 minus twin 2) of all twins and the length of this interval.
This relationship must be reconsidered in modern obstetrics in light of the heart rate pattern. If its heart rate is good, the second twin should be born within 30–60min.

Cephalic and noncephalic presentation. Birth management in cephalic–breech presentation or cephalic presentation – transverse lie is the subject of debate in America and Europe.
- USA: CS. This view is not shared in Europe.
- Europe: if the second twin is malpositioned or malpresenting the following options are considered: 1) external version, 2) combined version and extraction, 3) vaginal breech delivery.

External version. Reports on version of the second twin are conflicting. While some are successful, others are critical (threatened cord prolapse, loss of time).

Extraction of the second twin in breech presentation is a moderately stressful procedure (birth weight >1,800 g). Combined version (from transverse into breech presentation) and extraction is also successful if the operator is experienced.
Cesarean section. Combined version can be difficult in cases of oligohydramnios, dorsoinferior transverse presentation and macrosomia. In these cases CS is preferential to the difficult vaginal operative delivery.

Noncephalic presentation – cephalic or noncephalic presentation. CS is standard. Collision of the fetal heads is a lethal complication, if vaginally delivered and the first twin is in breech presentation.

No valid study data on the safety of vaginal delivery is available.

Third stage

Complications

Complications are to be expected with multiples. Causes are extreme distension and hypotonic uterine contractions.

- Impaired placental separation is more common.
- Separation is delayed.
- Incomplete placentae are more common.
- PPH after delivery of the complete placenta is more common. Atony is to be expected, particularly after operative deliveries, lasting a number of hours after delivery of the complete placenta.

Prevention of complications

- Rapid oxytocin infusion after delivery of the second twin!
- Monitoring of the uterus in the hours postpartum!

8.5 Pathological contractions, uterine dystocia

Definition. Abnormal contractions (see p. 147). Types: 1) hypotonic contractions (too weak, too seldom), 2) hyperactive contractions (too strong, too frequent), 3) hypertonic contractions (uterine baseline tone too high), 4) uncoordinated contractions.

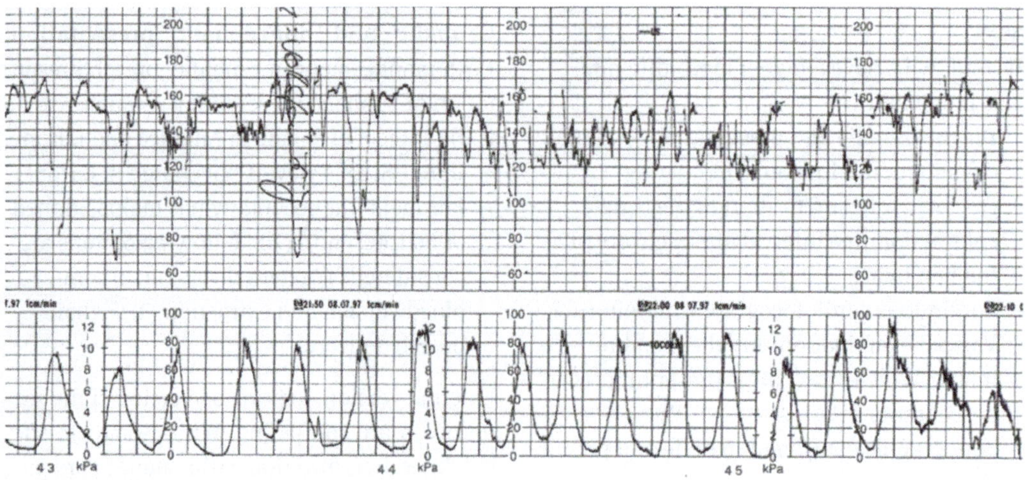

Fig. 8.121: Trace showing tachysystole (8 contractions in 10 min); 26-year-old para 2, week 37 + 3; SVD, boy, 3,390 g, 51 cm, Apgar 8/9/10, umbilical artery pH 7.30, umbilical vein pH 7.36.

Normal contractions are outlined on p. 147.
First stage contractions (IUP 40–50mmHg):
- Begin: regular contractions every 10–15 min.
- Later: every 3–5 min.

Contractions in second stage (IUP 60mmHg): every 3–4 min.

Hypotonic contractions. Anomaly of the driving forces; type of uterine dystocia; contractions too weak, too short, too infrequent to effect labor progress.

The intraamniotic pressure (or IUP) is 25–30 mmHg, or reduced contraction frequency of < 3/10 min is registered.
Not every abatement is due to hypotonic contractions. A brief physiological contraction-free interval occurs after ROM; the relationship to the amniotic sac is crucial.

Practice tip. As long as the membranes are still intact, hypotonic contractions are of secondary importance! Check if bladder is full, as a full bladder inhibits contractions reflexively!

Primary hypotonic contractions. The contractions are inadequate from labor onset. From the beginning the contractions are too seldom, too weak and too infrequent. Labor does not really get underway.

Causes. Obesity, overdistended uterus.

Secondary hypotonic contractions. The contractions are effective for a time, but begin to abate in the course of labor; they become shorter and weaker, the intervals between them become longer.

The main cause is tiring of the uterus and abdominal musculature, due to the strenuous work of labor, therefore secondary hypotonic contractions; ineffective labor due to exhaustion. It can be functional or due to an obstruction:
- CPD due to contracted pelvis, malposition or malpresentation (see p. 233).
- Rigid soft tissues, scarring and stenosis of the cervix, acute pubic arch angle, prominent tailbone or iliac spines.

These are the obstructions which exhaust the force of labor.

Hyperactive contractions. Differentiated into contractions which are too strong (IUP > 80–90 mmHg, hypertonic contractions), and contractions which are too frequent (≥ 4/10 min in first stage, tachysystole, Fig. 8.121).

Hypertonic contractions. Contractions with elevated uterine baseline tone. Uterine wall tension (baseline tone) or IUP between contractions > 12 mmHg.

Causes. Passive overdistension (e.g., hydramnios, multifetal pregnancy), muscular uterine hypertension or secondary hypertension due to tachysystole.
The strongest types of hypertonic contractions are tonic contractions or Tetanus uteri.
Uncoordinated contractions occur in cases of multifocal impulse development (e.g., left or right half of the fundus, other uterine segments); characterized by double contractions.
Differentiation of the types of contractions is no longer clinically relevant. Uterine dystocia, that is, inefficient labor, is in the foreground.

Treatment
Uterotonics for hypotonic contractions. At the onset of labor, physical measures are to be implemented: empty bladder and bowels! Warm bath or shower!

Practice tip. An enema is often the most effective uterotonic!

If the contractions do not improve, uterotonics are administered.

Uterotonics

Note.
Definition. Medications which stimulate contraction of the myometrium. Classification: uterotonics which stimulate the rhythmical contraction of the uterus and increase the frequency (oxytocin, prostaglandins [PGE_2]; see p. 278); uterotonics which cause prolonged contraction of the uterus: ergoline alkaloids.

Indication

Hypotonic contractions.
If uterotonics are unsuccessful, labor management should be reassessed and an end to labor be considered. Hypotonic contractions are often the result of a mechanical impediment to birth.

Prerequisite:
External and internal vaginal examination, cardiotocogram.

Contraindications

- Hypertonic or hyperactive contractions.

Tocolysis indicated (see below)! The disturbance in the progress of labor if the baseline tone of the uterus is already increased in between contractions cannot be favorably influenced by increasing the strength of the contractions.
- Extreme CPD.

Uterotonics are extremely dangerous if the disproportion between head and pelvis is extreme (contracted pelvis, hydrocephalus) or in malpresentations which preclude spontaneous delivery (transverse or oblique lie, mentoposterior face presentation).
- Pelvic floor resistance.

Extremely prominent tailbone, persistent occipitotransverse presentation which does not respond to position changes.
- Pathological heart rate pattern signifying imminent risk to the fetus (see p. 167).

Fetal condition must first be assessed by means of FBS.

Spasmolytics (muscle spasm suppressants). In contrast to uterotonics, spasmolytics have an antispasmodic effect on the cervix. Main effect is enabling cervical dilatation.

Indication. If cervix dilatation is markedly slow in first stage (rigid cervix), despite good contractions, some obstetricians prescribe pethidine.
These days a rigid cervix is seen as an indication for an epidural anesthesia.

Hyperactive and hypertonic contractions
Treatment, tocolysis. Suppression of contractions to reduce overactive contractility in labor.

Intravenous administration of Fenoterol to regulate contractions. Dosage: 2 mg Fenoterol in 500 ml electrolyte solution. Infusion speed about 10 ml/h.

Tip. In some cases of hypertonic contractions, uterotonics such as oxytocin can be given to stimulate contractions parallel to tocolysis infusion.
Side effects. Slight trembling, transitory palpitations, and tachycardia in addition in high doses, headache, muscle cramps, hypokalemia, hyperglycemia among others.

8.6 Arrested labor

Definition. Interruption of the normal course of labor in the pelvic inlet (PI), midpelvis or pelvic outlet (PO).

In many parts of the world, birth is managed according to normative regulations regarding the length of first and second stage. Factors such as the quality of the contractions, administration of uterotonics or conduction analgesics are often not considered. It is important to note that these normative regulations are not the result of prospective, randomized studies. The management of labor should therefore be more individualized, based on maternal and fetal wellbeing, rather than on empirically determined norms. These should serve as guides to rethinking labor management rather than indication for operative measures.

Arrested labor above or in the pelvic inlet. If contractions are good the cause is obstruction of some kind:

- Malpresentations and malpositions which preclude spontaneous delivery: transverse lie, oblique lie, high anteroposterior head, occipitoposterior presentation, mentoposterior face presentation, nasoposterior brow presentation.
- CPD. If the relationship between the fetal size and the maternal pelvis does not indicate difficulties, a possible cause is long pelvis with a high occipitoposterior presentation.
- Hydrocephalus.
- Rare obstructions: arm prolapse, pelvic tumors (Figs. 8.122, 8.123), extremely narrow soft tissue passage (scars, rigid cervix as a result of cervical cancer, and adhesion of the external os (Conglutination orificii externi).

Prognosis. Uterus rupture or septicemia, death of mother and baby.

Treatment. As outlined in the treatment guidelines of each of the abnormal and pathological situations.

Arrested labor in midpelvis occurs when contractions are hypotonic or the pelvis is generally contracted pelvis (p. 303).

Arrested labor on the pelvic floor. In addition to hypotonic contractions, can be caused by malpresentations and malpositions (deep transverse arrest); soft tissue or bony resistance.

The hypotonic contractions are due to the irregularities, which may also be present without hypotonic contractions. The laboring woman must not then be allowed to bear down for hours!

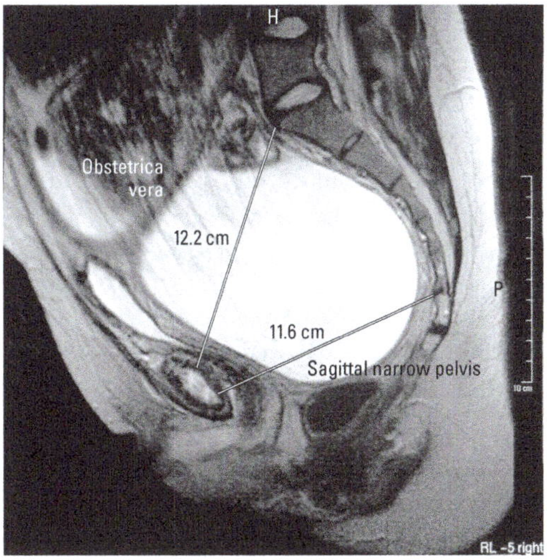

Fig. 8.122: longitudinal MRI showing pelvic dermoid cyst as birth obstruction.

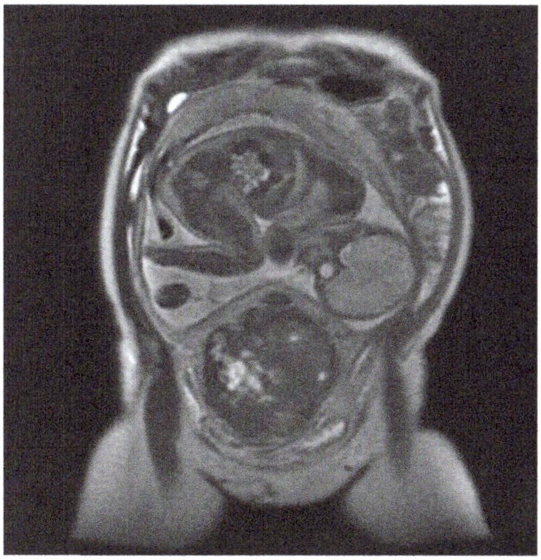

Fig. 8.123: MRI in week 36 showing large uterine fibroid as birth obstruction.

Note. Causes of arrested labor in second stage:
1. Hypotonic contractions: secondary hypotonic contractions, ineffective labor due to exhaustion.
2. Malposition or malpresentation. The most common are: deep transverse arrest, occipitoposterior and over-extended presentations (most commonly brow and face presentations).
3. Soft tissue resistance (perineum too high, too muscular or too rigid, extremely taut ligamentous attachment).
4. Bony resistance (prominent tailbone, contracted pelvic outlet, acute pubic arch angle).

Prolonged second stage increases maternal risk significantly. Chorioamnionitis, endometritis, injuries to the birth passage and uterine atony are significantly more common (ODDs ratio 4–9!). The risks to the baby are equally increased; the number of transfers to neonatal intensive care is considerably higher. Continuous cardiotocographic monitoring and – if necessary – FBS are to be performed.

Practice tip. The vaginal birth is to be ended operatively if the head has been on the pelvic floor longer than one hour and has failed to descend despite strong contractions, or if contractions are hypotonic and uterotonics are contraindicated.

8.7 Cervical priming and induction of labor

Definition. Pharmacological cervical ripening (= priming); induction of labor (IOL) before the onset of contractions by artificially rupturing the membranes (AROM, amniotomy: rupturing the membranes vaginally using ball forceps or amnioscope) or oxytocin infusion.

Indications. Mother and baby are at risk before the onset of labor in cases of:
- Prolonged pregnancy (p. 108).
- PIH, preeclampsia (see p. 74).
- Nonreassuring monitoring results (CTG, see p. 36, Doppler sonography, see p. 53, IUGR, see p. 107).
- Manifest maternal diabetes (p. 87), at term.
- PROM at term (see p. 105).

Contraindications:
- Placenta previa, vasa previa.
- Transverse lie.
- Higher order multiples.
- Twins with first twin in breech.
- Cord presentation, prolapse.
- Prior nonisthmic uterotomy.
- CPD.
- Chorioamnionitis.
- If administration of prostaglandins is planned: maternal asthma!.

Prerequisites
- Adequate personnel and equipment to monitor mother and fetus must be available.
- Immediate performance of a CS must be possible.
- Tocolysis must be available.

Planned delivery. In the absence of maternal or fetal risk signs and if the cervix is ripe, planned delivery in the form of IOL at term has become widespread. Whilst advocates cite organizational and medical advantages (planned admission for delivery, organization of family and professional affairs, avoidance of prolonged pregnancy), critics point out that it is an intervention in a natural process without medical indication.

Pharmacological IOL using:
- Intravenous oxytocin infusion.
- Intracervical prostaglandin gel.
- Intravaginal prostaglandin tablet.
- Intravaginal prostaglandin gel.
- Oral prostaglandin tablet.

1. Intravenous oxytocin infusion. This method has persisted. An intravenous drip is safer, more effective and can be better controlled than IM application, in particular for IOL. Contractions can be controlled within a few minutes by adjusting the number of drops/min.

Dosage. 6 IU oxytocin in 500 ml electrolyte solution.
Infusion speed. Begin with 1 drop/min; increase by 1 drop/min every 5 min.
Maximum dose. 30 drops/min should not be exceeded due to the risks for mother and baby if hyperstimulation occurs.
Overdose causes uterine hypertonus and tonic contractions of the uterus with the following three dangers: uterine rupture, intrauterine hypoxia, PPH in third stage.

2. Intracervical prostaglandin gel. 0.5 ml PGE_2 in 3 ml gel is applied intracervically to promote cervical ripening (softening or priming) → method of choice if cervix is unripe! Repeat if necessary after 6h. Vaginal delivery can be expected within 24 h in 80 % of cases.

Because prostaglandins are released and absorbed rapidly, CTG monitoring should be performed immediately after application for at least 2 h.

3. Intravaginal prostaglandin tablet. In particular for IOL in cases of ripe cervix, 3 mg PGE_2 tablets are available: 3 mg PGE_2 is placed in the posterior fornix of the vagina. Softening and dilatation of the cervix and effective contractions are achieved after 3–4 h, sometimes after 12 h.

CTG monitoring should be performed for 2 h after application because of the latent period, then as required, depending on contractions.

4. Intravaginal prostaglandin gel. A PGE_2 vaginal gel is available for IOL in cases of partially ripe cervix. Best induction results have been achieved by applying the gel twice 6 h apart. Contractions begin 20 min after application. Begin monitoring directly after administration.

5. Oral prostaglandin tablet. Oral administration of misoprostol (PG E_1 analogue) is prohibited in many countries. However, many positive experiences have been made worldwide using misoprostol for induction of a term baby, such that off-label use (after information and consent of the pregnant woman) is indicated from a medical-scientific standpoint.

Prior uterine operations are an absolute contraindication!
The initial oral dose consists of 25 µg misoprostol; increase is possible over 50 µg to 100 µg.
Vaginal **amniotomy** is an obstetrical operation. It is a general rule that the membranes are never digitally ruptured, but instead with an instrument such as ball forceps, a long Kocher clamp or special AROM instrument.

Method using sterile ball forceps (Fig. 8.124). Index and middle finger of the left hand are inserted into the vagina and search for the place at which the membranes are exposed. Transfundal pressure is applied to press the uterus downwards. The closed forceps are inserted with the right hand and guided along the fingers of the left hand to the membranes, which are clasped and torn, best during the contraction. Forceps are removed. Transfundal pres-

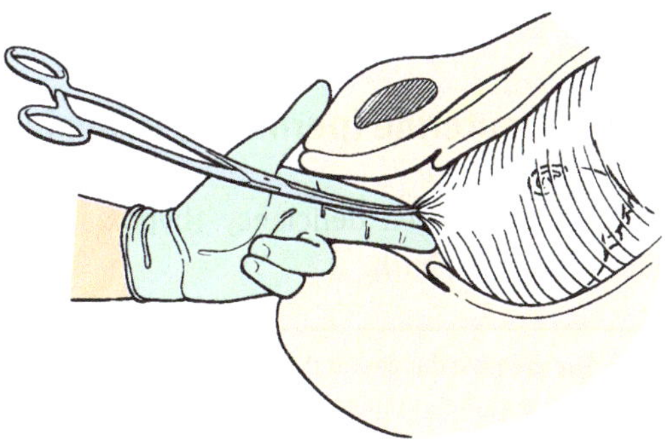

Fig. 8.124: AROM.

sure is applied to press the head into the pelvis. The fingers remain in the vagina to check whether the head descends and that prolapse of cord or small parts has not occurred. Uterotonics, if contractions moderate.

Practice tip. Tear a small hole so that AF flow is as slow as possible!

Prolapse of the umbilical cord or an arm occurs often more quickly than expected. Sometimes the prolapse only begins after AROM and goes unnoticed until, on internal examination sometime after repositioning, the prolapsed cord or arm are felt.

Method using amnioscope. Gentlest, safest and simplest method! A cannula (size irrelevant) is clamped in a ring forceps and inserted through the amnioscope. The membranes are punctured in direct view and the AF flows out. The size of the opening is selected as required. A small opening which allows slow flowing out of AF over 10–15 min is possible; this avoids cord prolapse if the head is high.

Continuous FHR monitoring is necessary during induction!
Management of birth after IOL must be based on the indication for IOL (maternal or fetal risk), labor progress and signs of fetal or maternal compromise (CTG, FBS, maternal temperature).

8.8 Intrauterine (perinatal) hypoxia

Definition. Oxygen deficiency (hypoxia) before and during birth.

Note. The greatest danger for the baby in labor is oxygen deficiency and the intrauterine acidosis it causes, with the possible consequences of organic brain damage to the baby. In addition to the significant problems for those affected, relatives, the high cost to society must be considered, which underlines the importance of diagnosis and prophylaxis.

Incidence. Severe intrauterine hypoxia resulting in sequelae can be expected in about 1 of every 500 births.

Etiology. Hypoxia in utero or during labor is the most common cause. Further causes: infection, cerebral hemorrhage, trauma, kernicterus, fetopathy.

10 % of infantile cerebral palsy cases (see clinical manifestation) are the result of intrapartal hypoxia.
Maternal causes:
- Inadequate oxygen supply: anemia, pulmonary disease, heart defect.
- Inadequate oxygen transport to placenta: arterial hypertension, hypertonic uterus, uterine tachysystole.

Placental causes:
- Insufficient gas exchange as a result of placental circulatory disturbance: PIH, prolonged pregnancy, placental abruption, placenta previa.

Fetal causes:
- Cord complication: entanglement, knot, prolapse.
- Anemia: post-hemorrhagic shock.

These maternal, placental or fetal causes of perinatal brain damage bring about neuronal cell death, especially in the parasagittal region of the cerebral cortex and the basal ganglia. The initial energy loss in the nerve cells and subsequent inflow of calcium, the post-ischemic inhibition of protein biosynthesis and the release of excitatory neurotransmitters and oxygen radicals all appear to be of great importance hereby. While these mechanisms have an effect in particular on the mature baby, in an immature fetus and ascending infection the post-ischemic inflammatory reaction with elevated tissue concentrations of cytokines plays a significant role.

The following criteria have been stated by the American College of Obstetricians and Gynecologists (ACOG; 1996), for cases of intrauterine hypoxia which could cause neurological damage:

- Umbilical artery pH < 7.00.
- Apgar > 5 min 0–3.
- Cramping, coma or hypertension in the neonatal period.
- Multiple organ damage (lungs, kidneys, GI tract, and cardiovascular system).

The clarification of the causes of brain damage, possible medical errors or avoidable brain damage is often sought later, on occurrence or diagnosis of neurological injury, and is often contentious. If the definition of intrauterine hypoxia causing neurological damage above is used as a basis, the link is improbable in most cases. However, imaging processes of the baby's brain in the first days of life help exclude or confirm hypoxia as the cause of an intrauterine oxygen deficiency situation.

Pathogenesis, pathophysiology. Fetal oxygen deficiency and increase in hydrogen ion concentration occurs in two ways:

1) Metabolic acidosis via intracellular lactic acid production as a result of anaerobic glycolysis in fetal tissues.
2) Respiratory acidosis via pCO_2 increase in pre-, intra-, or post-placental disturbance of the fetomaternal gas exchange.

Definitions

- Hypoxemia. Reduced oxygen content in blood.
- Hypoxia. Reduction of the partial pressure of oxygen (pO_2) in arterial blood (paO_2).
- Hypercapnia. Increase in arterial pCO_2.

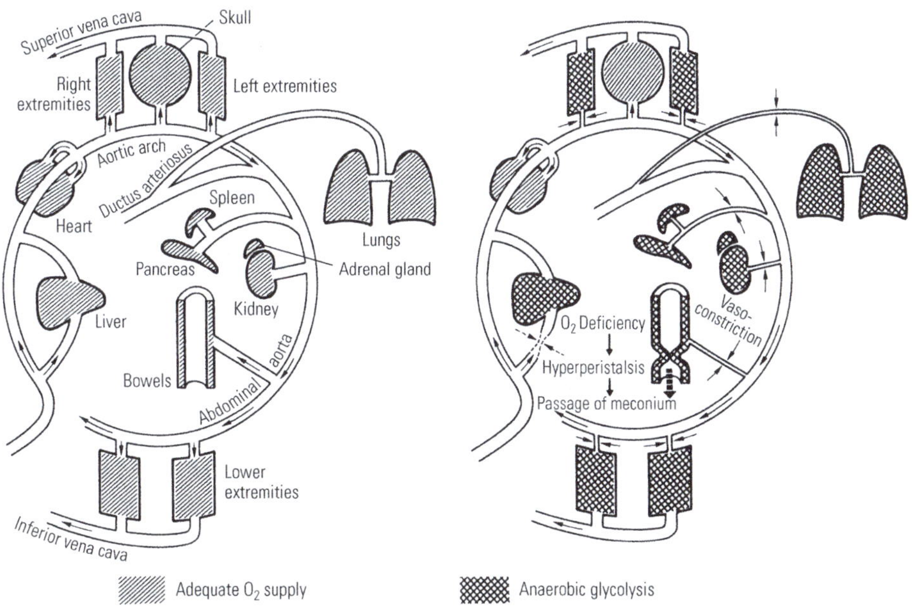

Fig. 8.125: Fetal circulatory system. Left normal (undisturbed) oxygen delivery, right decreased oxygen delivery: oxygen economization (after Saling).

Metabolic acidosis

Primary metabolic acidosis. FBS has shown that lactic acid overload often exists with or without mild hypoxia.

Oxygen economization (centralization) of the fetal circulatory system occurs when the oxygen supply slowly decreases (Saling). Vasoconstriction restricts or stops the blood flow to less important regions of the body (muscles, skin, intestines, lungs; Fig. 8.125). Oxygen benefits the vital organs: heart brain, placenta. The economization renormalizes the $paCO_2$.

Anaerobic glycolysis and lactic acid production (end-waste product of anaerobic glycolysis) occur in those tissues with reduced blood supply as a result of this economization. If the amount which enters the circulatory system is minimal, it may serve as an energy source for the organs before the acid concentration increases; lactic acid overload in normal or marginally reduced pO_2 levels. Metabolic acidosis occurs as a result of the overload of organic acids. Further breakdown, or rather the reconstruction of lactic acid, is only possible in the presence of oxygen.

Postnatal pH low. After birth and during the first 5–10 min, the pH reaches a low point (postnatal pH low), and then increases again: inflow of lactic acid from the "economized" tissues.

This effect is more marked in compromised neonates. If oxygen supply is adequate after delivery, circulation returns gradually to the "economized" regions of the body.

Note. The greater the intrauterine oxygen deficiency, the more extensive the "economization" is, and the greater the postpartum outflow of lactic acid. Consequences:

- *Intrauterine passage of meconium.* The local oxygen deficiency causes hyperperistalsis and passage of meconium.
- *Postterm pregnancy.* A longer-lasting oxygen deficiency of the skin, which has been only minimally supplied with blood, leads to signs of postterm pregnancy: cessation of sebum production, no vernix caseosa. Later occurrences: desquamation of the epidermal layer, redness of scrotum/labia, and flaky skin.

Respiratory acidosis

Metabolic acidosis, which occurs as a result of gradual oxygen deficiency, is to be compared with respiratory acidosis, caused by acute oxygen deficiency. The fetus is not acutely at risk over 1–2 min, as the tissues are relatively resistant to a short lack of oxygen. If such an intrauterine complication persists longer, however, over several minutes, the primary respiratory disturbance leads to metabolic reactions.

Secondary metabolic acidosis. Mixed acidosis occurs, and relatively quickly primarily metabolic acidosis: secondary metabolic acidosis.

Development of acidosis in complete oxygen deficiency. Animal experiments have shown that the pH value decreases by 0.1 pH units/min in the first 5 min after oxygen deficiency, after that every 3 min by 0.1 pH units/min (James).

Clinical manifestation (intrapartum). In addition to the acid-base household, the cardiovascular system has a balancing effect.

Mild oxygen deficiency mediates, via chemoreceptors (carotid sinus, aortic arch), an increase in cardiac output by increasing the heart rate (compensatory tachycardia).

Decreases in FHR coincident with contractions occur if oxygen deficiency persists.

Bradycardia with hypoxic damage to the myocardium and arrhythmias (disturbance of impulse stimulation and conduction) are the end results of hypoxemia and are extremely dangerous.

This emphasizes the importance of cardiotocographic and biochemical monitoring of the fetus (for cardiotocography see p. 167, FBS see p. 177).

Clinical manifestation (postpartum)

- Spastic paralysis as hemi-, di- or paraplegia.
- Reduced intelligence, speech development disorders, erethism, epilepsy.

Intrauterine diagnosis. Diagnosis of fetal well-being!

- FBS.
- Cardiotocography, electronic fetal monitoring.
- Blood gas analysis (Fig. 8.125, 8.126).

Practice tip. Blood gas analysis of O_2, CO_2 is unreliable: CO_2 production is reduced in anaerobic glycolysis, pCO_2 normalizes or remains elevated. CO_2 elimination is disturbed by the same intrauterine complication which caused the complication. The conclusions drawn from the pO_2 of fetal blood are even less reliable as the pO_2 normalizes after "economization" has occurred and therefore no conclusions can be drawn from it as to oxygen supply.

Prevention. Cardiotocography as screening method and FBS as method of diagnosis may be useful as early warning system of intrauterine asphyxia.

A prospective study (McDonald et al., 1985) which compared cardiotocography and auscultation has called the German concept of routine cardiotocographic monitoring as a screening method and FBS as a method of diagnosis in cases of suspected asphyxia into question. The discussion continues; conclusions have not been reached. It is only possible to suggest a concept of care which is acceptable for the mother which minimizes the number of compromised fetuses and with that the probability of – also forensically reproachable – brain damage as a result of hypoxia.

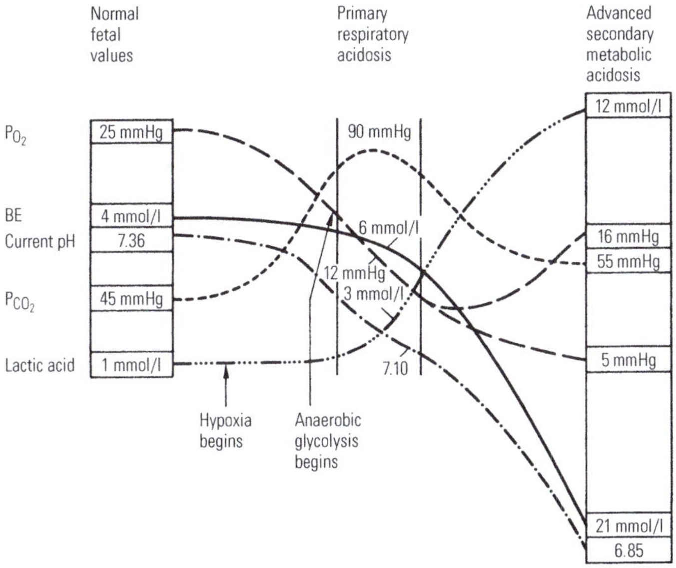

Fig. 8.126: Model of a brief intrauterine disturbance with hypoxemia, hypercapnia, acidosis (after Saling). To begin with, fetal oxygen deficiency (hypoxemia), followed by carbon dioxide overload (hypercapnia). If hypoxemia continues, anaerobic glycolysis occurs with rise in lactic acid: the respiratory acidosis becomes a metabolic acidosis. The current pH decreases, as a result of the rise in pCO_2; the base excess (BE) decreases as a result of the rise in lactic acid. Oxygen saturation rises again due to fetal O_2 economization as long as the compensatory mechanisms are not overextended.

8.9 Cord complications: presentation, prolapse

Definition. Complication in labor caused by the umbilical cord: the cord is presenting or prolapsed.

8.9.1 Cord presentation

Definition. Membranes are intact; the umbilical cord is felt in front of or near the fetal presenting part (Fig. 8.127).

Complication. Cord prolapse after rupture of membranes.

Note. Cord presentation, particularly in cephalic presentations, is the early stage of inevitable and dangerous cord prolapse.

Treatment

1. ROM is to be delayed until the cervix is fully dilated.
2. Retraction of the cord can be achieved by:
   a) elevation of the pelvis so that the presenting loop can slip back up. Even better: knee-chest position, followed by
   b) lateral supine position: the laboring woman is to lie on the opposite side to that on which the cord is presenting. If the cord is presenting on the left next to the head, which has deflected to the right, the woman is to lie on her right side with her pelvis elevated. The elevation of the pelvis allows the loop to slip back up, the right lateral supine position forces the head up against the left side of the pelvis and closes the gap: the head moves in the opposite direction to the breech!
3. Intravenous tocolysis supports steps 1 and 2.
4. Cardiotocogram. If the heart rate patterns become pathological the procedure for cord prolapse is to be followed (p. 167).
5. If the cervix is fully dilated, the membranes are artificially ruptured. Technique: p. 282. A birth assistant simultaneously applies transfundal pressure to press the head into the pelvis (see Fig. 8.131). If the cord loop is palpable on AROM, the head is pushed upwards and an attempt made to push the cord up and past it. If successful, expectant management.
   If the cord prolapses, however, the rules given below are followed.

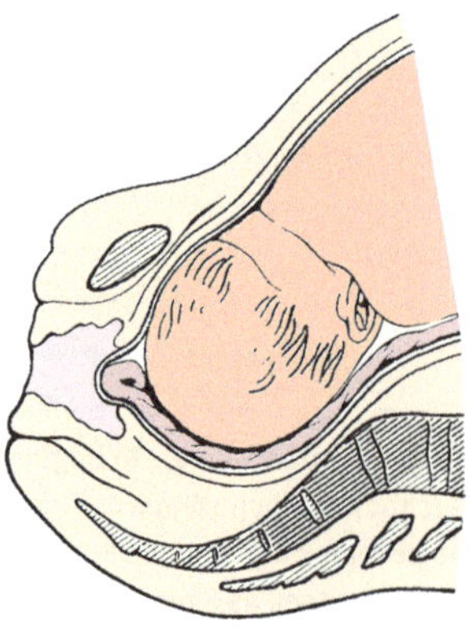

Fig. 8.127: Cord presentation.

8.9.2 Cord prolapse

Definition. Dangerous cord complication; one or more loops of the umbilical cord are felt in front of the presenting part after ROM, it is compressed (Fig. 8.128).

Etiology. Prolapse of the cord only occurs when there is a gap between the pelvis and the presenting part of the fetus. The larger the gap, the more easily prolapse can occur. Maternal causes: CPD. Fetal causes: transverse or

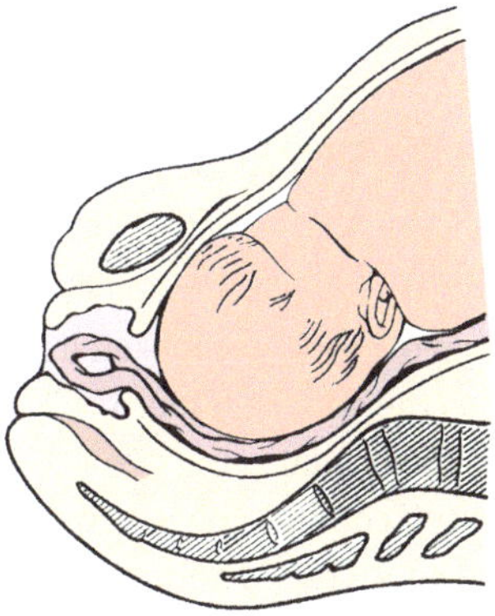

Fig. 8.128: Cord prolapsed.

oblique lie, breech presentation, preterm delivery, multiples, hydramnios, PROM, overlong cord, low-lying cord, placenta previa and low-lying placenta.

Incidence. 0.3–0.7 %, relatively seldom.

Pathophysiology. The cord is compressed between presenting part (e.g., head) and pelvic wall during contractions. Blood flow in the cord blood vessels is restricted. With descent of the presenting part permanent compression and occlusion occurs: the baby asphyxiates if decompression does not occur within minutes.

Note. *Occurrence.* Prolapse is 4–6 times more common in multiparous women, because the fit of the lower uterine segment is less tight at the beginning of labor than in primiparous women. Prolapse occurs most commonly in transverse lies, often in footling presentations, less often in breech and most rarely in cephalic presentations. It occurs in cephalic presentations if the head is laterally deflected, high or extended in first stage, and most commonly in cases of CPD.

Practice tip. The risk of cord compression depends on the presentation. It is highest in cephalic, less high in breech, in particular footling presentation, and relatively low in transverse lie.
In cephalic presentations the cord is immediately compressed in the narrow gap between the bony parts of the head and pelvis.
The cord can lie beside the soft breech in some cases for a long time before becoming fully occluded; this is even more valid for the footling presentation.
In transverse lie the prolapse is harmless as long as arm prolapse or descent of the shoulder and cord compression do not also occur (p. 266).

Timepoint. Cord presentation usually occurs before prolapse. On ROM the flow of AF flushes the cord down through the gap between presenting part and pelvic wall.

Clinical presentation, diagnosis
- Cardiotocogram. Pathological heart rate patterns directly after ROM or AROM.
- Immediate vaginal examination is the leading method of diagnosis. There is no possibility of error: a smooth cord as wide as a little finger is felt. Often only the tip of the cord is felt, sometimes one or more loops, or the cord is seen hanging out of the vagina. If pulsation is present it is clearly felt.
- Findings on cervical status, fetal presentation, station of presenting part, pelvic proportions.

Differential diagnosis. Bradycardia also occurs after ROM without cord prolapse. The loss of AF reduces the uterine space and intrauterine pressure and disturbs the hemodynamics of the uteroplacental vessels. This is rapidly compensated: the drop in FHR is transitory!

Treatment. Delivery must be expedited, IV tocolysis until operation begins!

Cord prolapse is one of the major, sudden occurrences in obstetrics. Its treatment requires prompt decision-making and unerring action.
If the cord has not pulsated for a long time and the baby is in a longitudinal lie, expectant management. Delivery of the dead baby is left to the forces of nature!
Duties of the midwife/birth assistant until arrival of the obstetrician:

- If the head is high, the woman is helped into the knee-chest position, or her pelvis steeply elevated. Bearing down is to be avoided.
- Cord prolapse is rare if the head is on the pelvic floor. The laboring woman is to bear down with all her strength to deliver the baby as quickly as possible.

Procedure according to presentation.
Cephalic presentation. The extent of cervical dilatation determines procedure:
- If the cervix is not completely dilated CS → method of choice (lowest fetal mortality!).
- Never attempt to reposition!
- Cervix fully dilated: consider vaginal delivery!

Low presenting head:
- VE or forceps.
- Never attempt to reposition!

High presenting head:
Cesarean section (gentlest form of delivery). In special cases (e.g., multiparous women) pressing the head into the pelvis, VE.
Condition. Cord pulsates; prompt action from decision to performance. During the preparation, which must only last a few minutes, the head is to be pushed upwards out of the vagina (sterile gloves) and held there until the beginning of the operation. Continuous FHR monitoring, i.v. tocolysis until operation.
Breech presentation. Although the risk of compression is lower, immediate action is recommended even if the CTG is normal.
Cesarean section is also the method of choice here, whether the cervix is fully dilated or not.
Transverse lie. Cord and arm prolapse make the cord prolapse equally dangerous as in cephalic presentation. Procedure: see below.

Prevention. Never rupture membranes if
- the pelvis is contracted and the head (breech)is high,
- the presenting part has not yet entered the pelvis,
- the cervix is not fully dilated in transverse lie.

Additionally:
- Never attempt to reposition a prolapsed arm in transverse lie, as the cord easily prolapses during this manipulation.
- Oblique lie (the breech oblique lie is to be particularly feared): the baby's abdomen lies above the pelvic inlet, whereby the cord presents above the cervix.

Prognosis. Unfavorable for the fetus. Fetal mortality 2%!

8.10 Arm complications: Compound presentation, arm presentation, prolapse

Definition. As in cord prolapse (p. 288), differentiated into compound presentation: abnormal lie of arm or hand beside or in front of the presenting part; membranes are intact. Arm prolapse: prolapse of an arm in labor after ROM.

Etiology, occurrence. In cephalic presentations with flat pelvis because the head is deflected laterally or high above the pelvic inlet, creating a gap between head and uterine wall through which an arm can slip (→ abnormal lie with or without CPD). In face presentations

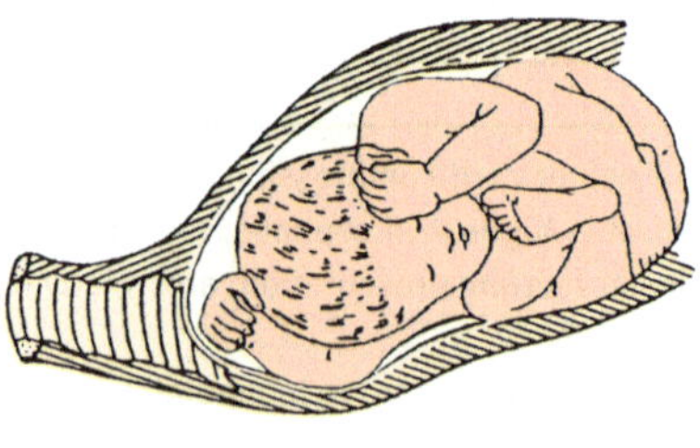

Fig. 8.129: Presentation of the right arm in ROA.

because the baby's chest lies close to the front, side wall of the uterus, which can force the arms down towards the PI. In transverse lies because the lack of a presenting part leaves the PI empty. In hydramnios because the baby always presents poorly and an arm can be flushed out in a gush of AF.

Clinical manifestation

Compound presentation (arm presenting in cephalic presentation) (Fig. 8.129). Arm prolapse is rare in such cases. It is not rare to feel a hand or arm lying beside the head when the membranes are intact. This does not interfere with the birth. The hand or arm usually retracts spontaneously as the head descends. Sometimes a hand is also born next to the head without disrupting the course of labor.

Nevertheless, the threatened arm prolapse is prevented by pelvic elevation and lateral supine positioning (→ on the opposite side to that on which the arm is presenting).
When the pelvis is elevated, the arm, which is wedged between the pelvic wall and the head, is freed and can be retracted towards the fundus. Supine positioning centers the head above the PI and closes the gap. If this is unsuccessful, positioning on the side on which the arm is presenting is attempted.

Compound presentation (prolapsed arm in cephalic presentation). There are two types (Fig. 8.130):

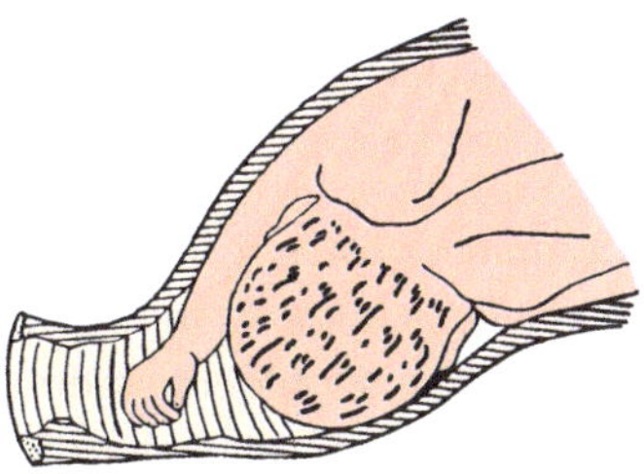

Fig. 8.130: Prolapse of the right arm in LOA.

- Incomplete arm prolapse, hand prolapse. Only the hand is felt beside the head; unimportant for birth (treatment as for arm presentation).
- Complete arm prolapse. The whole arm presents in front of the head. Dangerous for mother and baby, but rare.

Note. Spontaneous vaginal delivery. Birth can run its natural course under 3 conditions: 1) the arm is small (preterm delivery), 2) the arm is soft and can be compressed (stillbirth), 3) the arm (normal-sized) ends up lying in the hollow of the posterior pelvic wall near the sacral promontory.

Complications. Arrested labor and uterine rupture.

The prolapsed arm does not retract spontaneously and prevents the head from entering the PI; it remains above the pelvis or deflects onto the iliac wing on one side or the other (→ threatened cord prolapse!). This is particularly so in cases of CPD!
The prolapsed arm prevents the passage of the head through the pelvis. Labor is arrested when the head enters the pelvis next to (and with) the arm. The arm lies immobile next to or in front of the head, wedged in between head and the pelvic wall. It is trapped and can neither bend nor rotate. Rupture can also occur now.

Treatment. SVD is attempted.

Head has not yet entered the pelvis, is mobile above the PI. The prolapsed arm prevents entry of the head. The procedure is determined by the cervix.
Cervix fully dilated:
- Repositioning (see below), Hofmeier impression (Fig. 8.131), uterotonics are the method of choice.
- Cesarean section if the Hofmeier impression is unsuccessful.

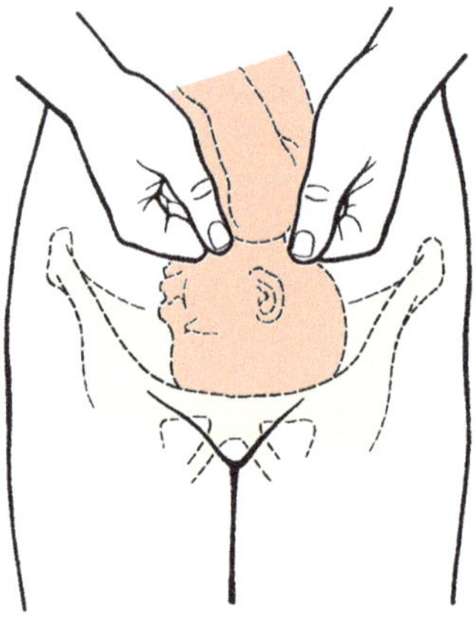

Fig. 8.131: Hofmeier impression.

Cervix incompletely dilated (cervix slightly dilated):
- Extremely unfavorable birth situation. Attempts at repositioning are unlikely to be successful.
- Cesarean section is the method of choice, in particular in cases of CPD.

Head has entered the pelvis. The prolapsed arm prevents passage of the head.
- Expectant management! Perform frequent vaginal exams to determine whether the head is spontaneously descending, then continue to wait, as VE is not at all simple.
- Uterotonics as soon as the contractions abate, titrated doses. The uterus is thoroughly examined: danger of uterine rupture! Intervene if labor is arrested.
- Repositioning and VE in general anesthetic.
- If repositioning is unsuccessful, the VE must be performed with the prolapsed arm.

Repositioning technique. If the laboring woman is cooperative, a repositioning without narcosis can be attempted in knee/chest position. The steep elevation of the pelvis (with a number of pillows) causes uterus and baby to sink towards the diaphragm to such an extent that everyone attempting to reposition small parts for the first time in this position is surprised at how mobile head and arm become as a result.

Practice tip. The repositioning of an arm in knee-chest position is successful more often than one expects.

The whole of the hand corresponding to the baby's abdomen is inserted into the uterus. The prolapsed arm is taken hold of and very slowly pushed back up and past the head and neck with four fingers. After repositioning, the arm is held in place (the obstetrician's hand remains in the uterus) and the woman is slowly helped back into her original position. An assistant presses the head back into the PI (→ Hofmeier impression; Fig. 8.131). As the arm can no longer prolapse, the obstetrician's hand is removed from the uterus. Uterotonics are administered and the VE applied if necessary.
Prolapsed arm in transverse lie see p. 266.

8.11 Shoulder dystocia

Definition. Arrested labor after birth of the head due to insufficient shoulder rotation.

Incidence. 0.2–3 % of vaginal deliveries, dependent on birth weight.

The incidence of shoulder dystocia is 2 % if the birth weight is 4,000 g, increases to 10 % in birth weights of 4,500 g, and reaches 40 % in weights of 5,000 g. On the other hand, more than half of shoulder dystocias occur in birth weights of < 4,000 g.

Classification. *High anteroposterior shoulders.* The bisacromial diameter is (almost) in the AP diameter above the PI. The shoulder rotation from the AP into the transverse diameter did not occur. *Deep transverse shoulders.* The bisacromial diameter remains in the transverse diameter in the pelvic cavity or almost on the pelvic floor. The shoulder rotation from the transverse into the AP diameter did not occur.

Etiology, risk factors
- Prior birth with shoulder dystocia.
- Macrosomia, in particular in cases of diabetes mellitus.
- Maternal obesity.
- Excessive weight gain in pregnancy.
- Postterm pregnancy, multiparity.
- Prolonged second stage.
- Vaginal-operative delivery from midpelvis.

Clinical manifestation, diagnosis
- Arrested labor after delivery of the head, absence of the external rotation of the head.
- When the shoulders are in the high AP position the head appears stuck to the vulva ("**turtle phenomenon**").

Complications. Fetal asphyxia, traumatic injury to the Plexus brachialis in 13 %, skeletal injuries, clavicle fractures in 5–7 %.

Treatment
High AP shoulders
- Performance or extension of an episiotomy (if possible!).
- Cessation of oxytocics, if applicable. Tocolysis!
- Change in position of the symphysis pubis (McRoberts maneuver).

McRoberts maneuver. The legs of the laboring woman are extended and bent dorsally along the longitudinal axis and then rapidly flexed in the hip joints. This lowers (→ away from the shoulders), then elevates the symphysis pubis (→ it may spring above the anterior shoulder. This is important for high AP shoulders!). The procedure is supported by **application of suprapubic pressure** with the fist; the mother's legs are flexed. In addition, when the legs are maximally flexed in the hip joint the pelvic outlet is enlarged (important in deep transverse shoulders).
- **Internal rotation of the shoulders.** 2 fingers of the hand corresponding to the baby's back are placed on the anterior shoulder blade. Pressure is applied to bring the shoulder into the transverse diameter (Fig. 8.132).
- Alternatively: two fingers of the hand corresponding to the baby's abdomen are placed on the posterior shoulder blade. Pressure is applied to the chest to bring the shoulder into the transverse diameter (Woods' maneuver).

Practice tip. Do not apply transfundal pressure (Kristeller maneuver) or traction to the head during this maneuver!

- **Delivery of the posterior arm.** The hand corresponding to the baby's abdomen is inserted and the posterior hand or lower arm of the baby is swept across the baby's abdomen. Flexion (Fig. 8.133) and extraction (Fig. 8.134).

Reduction of the bisacromial diameter frees the anterior shoulder so that it can be born. The anterior shoulder may need to be rotated by rotating the head posteriorly, and then this arm can also be delivered.
Overrotation of the head is no longer advisable.

Deep transverse shoulders:

Episiotomy. Position change of the symphysis pubis (as for high AP shoulders).

Internal rotation of the shoulders by an assistant: the shoulders are forced out of the transverse into the AP diameter with 2 fingers.

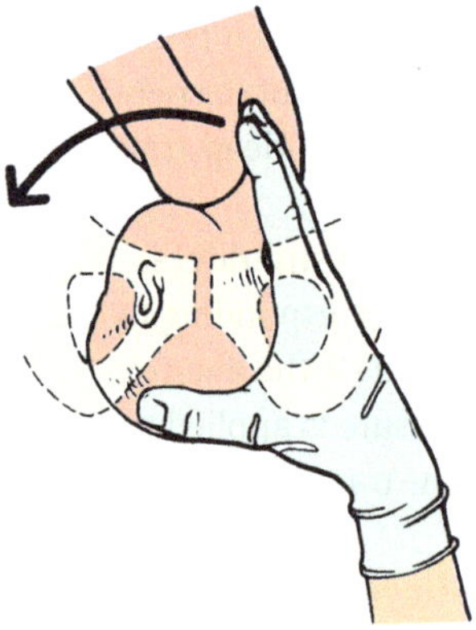

Fig. 8.132: Shoulder dystocia. Internal rotation of the high AP shoulders.

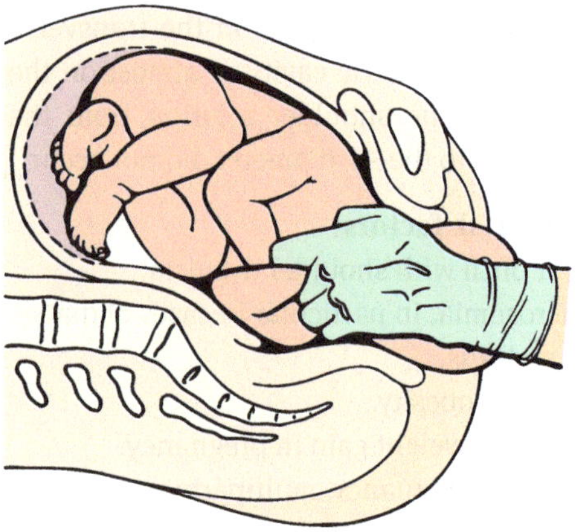

Fig. 8.134: Shoulder dystocia. Extraction of the posterior arm high AP shoulders.

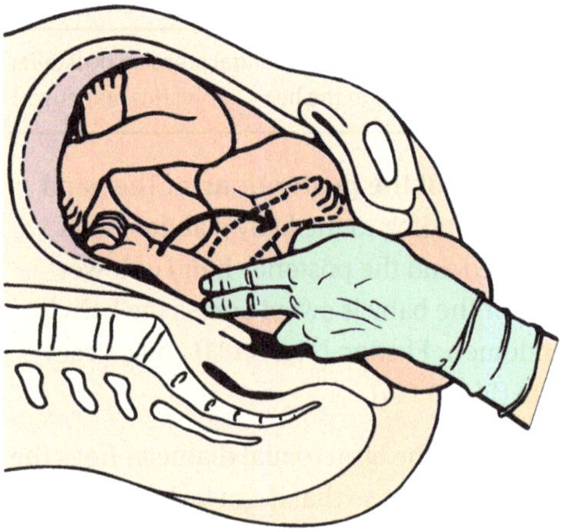

Fig. 8.133: Shoulder dystocia. Flexion of the posterior arm in high AP shoulders.

Prevention. The main risk factor is a history of shoulder dystocia, with a recurrence risk of 13.8 %! The indication for a primary CS should be made generously in such cases. (Lewis et al., 1995).

In order to prevent five cases of shoulder dystocia, if according to the prenatal sonographic EBW the birth weight will be greater than 4,500 g, 132 additional cesarean sections would be necessary (Gross et al., 1987).

8.12 Cephalopelvic disproportion (CPD)

Note. In the past, a common cause of complications in European obstetrics was the anatomically contracted pelvis. Problems with the mechanics of labor, types of pelvis, the mechanics of labor of these and obstetrical procedures were topics of broad discussion. The obstetrical situation has changed. The contracted pelvis has – for example due to the successful prevention of rickets as one of the important causes – become less important. Currently similar problems are clinically relevant, disproportion between fetal head and maternal pelvis. Diagnosis is divided into two types: anatomical and functional.

Etiology. Can be caused by a large head or a small, generally contracted pelvis, which is contracted evenly in all diameters of all planes, showing smaller measurements – miniature pelvis.

Anatomical diagnosis

- Vaginal and pelvic exams (p. 31) are standard.
- X-ray or MRI pelvimetry are reserved for individual cases.

Practice tip. Anatomical diagnosis involves determination of shape and degree of the bony pelvis: direct method of pelvimetry. In contrast to functional, it can be performed at any time, whether pregnant or not and during labor. These results must be compared with the results of sonographic fetometry.

Functional diagnosis comprises of history and observation of the course of labor.
Functional history:
- Course of prior births in multiparous women where CPD is suspected!
- Was CS necessary in prior births?
- Has the laboring woman had difficult births, perhaps stillbirths?

The prognosis depends on the answers to these questions in multiparous women.
Observation of the course of labor. In addition to the pelvis, head and contractions are decisive factors!
- Examination whether and how the head adapts to the pelvis.
- Will this head be able to enter this pelvis: head size, presentation, attitude, molding.
- Force of contractions.

Molding of the head. A small head, for example, can easily pass through an anatomically contracted pelvis; even a normal-sized head in some circumstances, if it adapts well under the force of the contractions, allows itself to be remodeled or configured.
It must be clarified that a normal-sized pelvis must be referred to as contracted in the case of a large, hard, nonadaptable head. It follows from this fact that a functionally contracted pelvis need not necessarily be an anatomically contracted pelvis.
The following two principles of functional diagnosis are different for primiparous and multiparous women:

1. *For primiparous women.* If the head is floating above the PI at the beginning of labor – and also in the last 2–3 weeks before labor – instead of in the PI, CPD should be suspected.
2. *For multiparous women.* If the head is still floating above the PI once the cervix is fully dilated and the membranes have ruptured, CPD should be suspected.

Three maneuvers are performed.

3. Fourth Leopold maneuver: no other external maneuver enables such an accurate determination of the level of the head in the pelvis and its passage of descent (p. 24).
4. Fifth Leopold or Zangemeister maneuver (Fig. 8.135) to determine whether the head protrudes anteriorly. Standing at the side of the supine woman, one hand is placed flat on the symphysis pubis (symphysis hand), the other (head hand) on the head above the symphysis pubis. There are three possibilities:
   a) Head hand is one finger-width lower than the symphysis pubis, no CPD (Fig. 8.136).
   b) Both hands are at the same level (Fig. 8.137), moderate CPD. SVD probable if contractions are good and head presentation favorable. Decision only possible after ROM. However, SVD

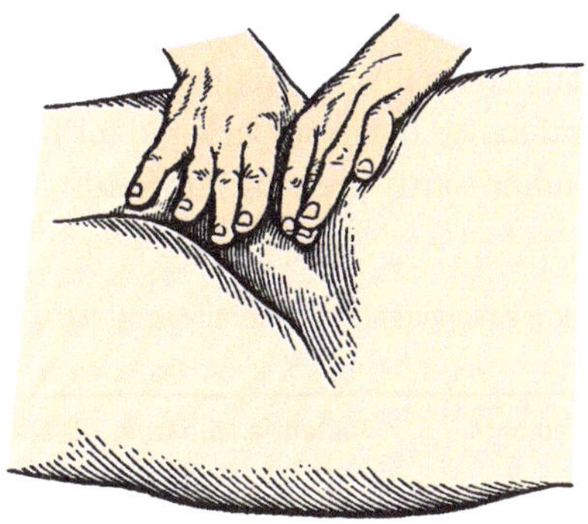

Fig. 8.135: Fifth Leopold or Zangemeister maneuver: both hands are at the same level, possible CPD.

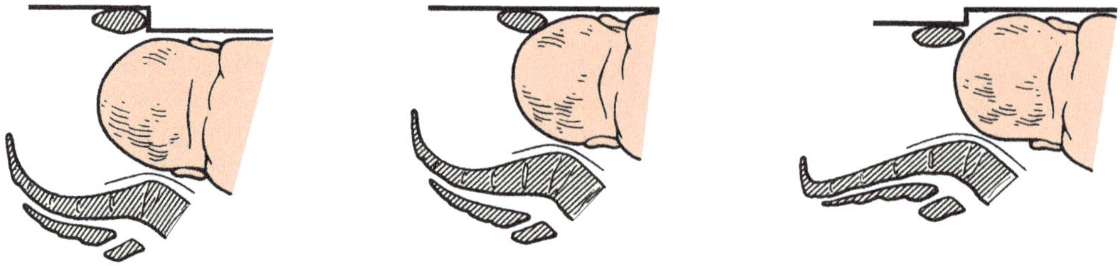

Fig. 8.136: Symphysis pubis is higher than the head engaged in the PI, the head fits the pelvis, no CPD.

Fig. 8.137: Head and symphysis pubis are at the same level, the head shears: moderate CPD. Good contractions and favorable presentation make SVD possible to likely.

Fig. 8.138: The head is higher than the symphysis pubis: significant to extreme CPD. Unfavorable prognosis.

is not to be expected if despite good contractions this finding does not alter after ROM.

c) Head hand is higher than symphysis hand; head is higher than the symphysis pubis. Significant to extreme CPD (Fig. 8.138). The head is not likely to enter the pelvis. This is also the case if the head is only slightly higher than the symphysis pubis.
d) The head is higher than the pelvis if the pelvis is contracted, the head too high, malpresenting or malpositioned or its entry is obstructed, e.g., due to hydrocephalus, prolapsed arm, pelvic, ovarian or uterine tumor.
e) Combined external-vaginal maneuver. The left index finger examines vaginally, the right hand goes to the head, externally. When the external hand moves the head back and forth, simultaneously pressing it towards the internal finger, a direct impression can be gained of the station of the head, its size, and whether it will fit into the pelvis.

8.12.1 Generally contracted pelvis

Definition. Pelvis with consistent shortening of all diameters in all planes (Tab. 8.4).

Diagnosis. Michaelis rhomboid: narrow, acute upper and lower angles, pointy rhomboid form.

Three characteristics are: consistent shortening of all diameters in all planes; pubic arch: acute angle, and Michaelis rhomboid: narrow, acute upper and lower angles.

Occurrence. Women with a generally contracted pelvis are usually small, delicate women. However, this form of narrow pelvis can also be observed in medium-sized women who are delicately built.

Tab. 8.4: Pelvic measurements in generally contracted pelvis.

Pelvic measurements (examples)	Distantia spinarum	Distantia cristarum	Distantia trochanterica	Distantia externa
Normal pelvis	26	29	32	20
Narrow (contracted) pelvis	23	26	29	19

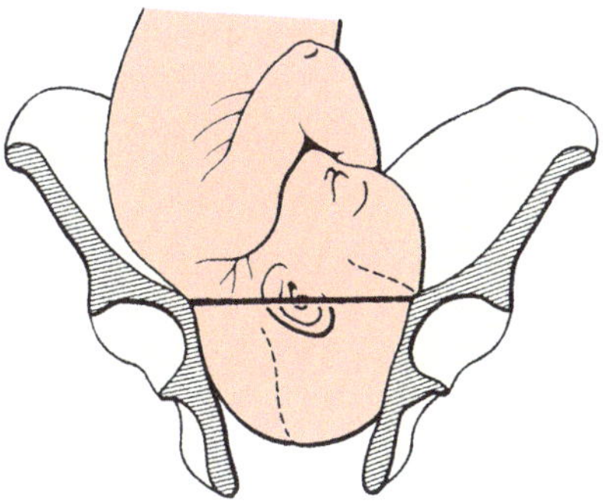

Fig. 8.139: Roederer attitude. Typical, favorable attitude of the head in a narrow pelvis: extreme flexion.

Mechanism of birth

Note. Adaptations in head presentation. Nature knows four methods of adaptation of the head to the limited space: 1) Roederer attitude, 2) lengthening of the head, 3) anterior and posterior asynclitism, 4) remodeling of the head.

1. Roederer attitude (Fig. 8.139). The head is maximally reduced in size due to its extreme flexion, so that the posterior fontanelle already becomes the leading part in the PI.

The posterior fontanelle is never felt laterally, but in favorable attitudes always, even in the PI, in the middle, centered in the axis of the birth canal.
It is the leading part in all levels of the birth canal, lowest point of the head. The sagittal suture is not in the transverse, but usually in one of the oblique diameters.
The posterior fontanelle is usually right or left lateral in the PI in a normal labor, and only begins leading when the head has entered the pelvic cavity.
Thus the longitudinally presenting head is slowly pushed through the resistances which are evenly distributed through all the pelvic planes with the occiput leading and deeply flexed. Only in this way can the head pass through all narrow pelvic planes with its smallest diameter. The adaptation of the head with the smallest possible and at the same time round cross-section is the best, because the internal pelvic dimensions are almost round in shape. Any attitude other than the Roederer is less favorable. Extended attitudes, for example, are extremely unfavorable.

2. Lengthening of the head. Typical molding. Only a head whose measurements have been correspondingly reduced can pass through a pelvis in which all dimensions are reduced. As the pelvis is shortened in equal measure in the anteroposterior, oblique and transverse diameters, a normal-sized head, which is to pass through this pelvis must also reduce its measurements in all diameters. It must be compressed in all diameters except in one, height.

The favorable form of adaptation through molding comprises of a shortening of all diameters at the cost of height, lengthening of the head, whereby the parietal bones are forced to overlap. The longitudinal axis is the only one which increases. The head adapts to the generally contracted pelvis by becoming longer.
This lengthening enables the entry to the pelvis and passage through to the pelvic floor. In contrast, the birth of the head in a curve around the symphysis pubis is made more difficult by this longitudinal extension.

3. Anterior and posterior asynclitism. In cases of extreme contraction, the sagittal suture is not felt in the birth axis on examination, but rather the concave surface of one of the parietal bones. The transverse sagittal suture is usually near the sacrum, sometimes also the symphysis pubis. The sagittal suture is therefore not synclitic (→ aligned with the axis of the birth canal), but asynclitic (→ unaligned with the birth axis). The anterior or posterior parietal bone has become the leading part:

a) Anterior asynclitism (Fig. 8.140; → severe anterior asynclitism, severe Naegele's obliquity).
b) In normal labor the sagittal suture often presents angled slightly towards the sacrum, asynclitically, for a brief period. This is known as physiological anterior asynclitism or Naegele's obliquity.
c) After ROM and lengthier labor a large caput is to be felt on the anterior parietal bone, on the posterior parietal bone a spoon-shaped impression or groove.
d) Posterior asynclitism (Fig. 8.141; severe posterior asynclitism, severe Litzmann's obliquity). Rare! The sagittal suture runs transversely and is felt angled towards the symphysis pubis. It has become the leading part.
e) Mild posterior asynclitism also occurs as a physiological presentation during pregnancy and at onset of labor, in particular in primiparae: physiological posterior asynclitism or Litzmann's obliquity.

Note. Buttonhole mechanism (Fig. 8.142) describes the asynclitic head presentation as adaptation to the pelvic form.

4. Remodeling of the head. The parietal bones are not only canted and pressed up against one another, but at the same time the higher parietal bone is forced some distance onto the internal surface of the lower one. This reduces the transverse diameter of the head significantly, the more moldable the head and the stronger the contractions the greater the reduction.

Anterior asynclitism (Fig. 8.143, 144). Common! The posterior parietal bone, which is always higher, is forced onto the internal surface of the lower anterior parietal bone. The difference in levels can often be felt as a step. With some practice, it is possible to feel whether the parietal bones are likely to overlap at all.

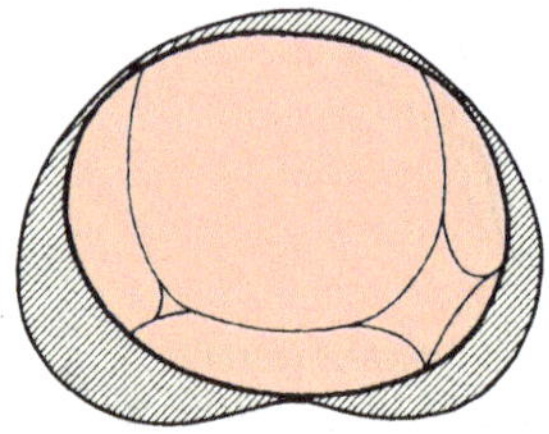

Fig. 8.140: Anterior asynclitism (severe anterior asynclitism, severe Naegele's obliquity).

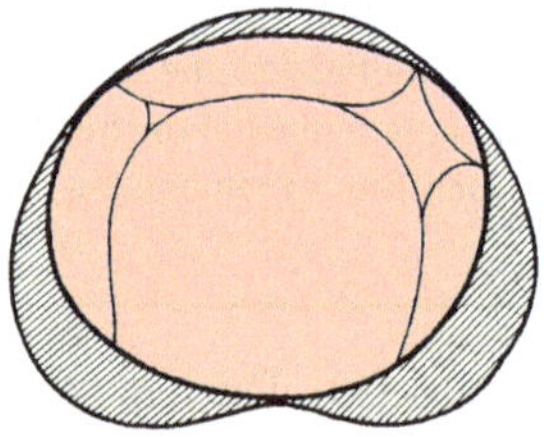

Fig. 8.141: Posterior asynclitism (severe posterior asynclitism, severe Litzmann's obliquity).

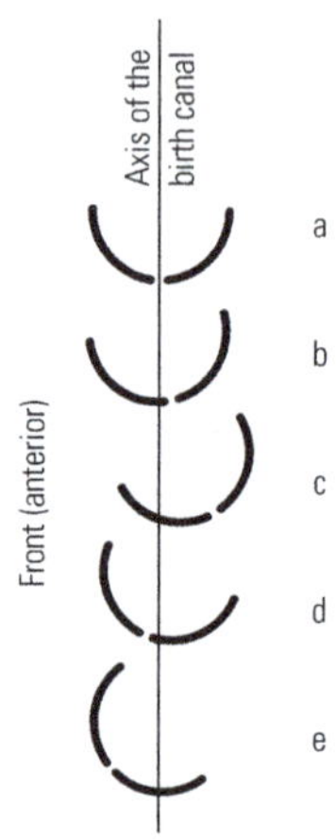

Fig. 8.142: Buttonhole mechanism. The head does not pass through the PI with its complete circumference in one go, but rather in two halves. One after the other the halves of the head pass through the contracted PI.

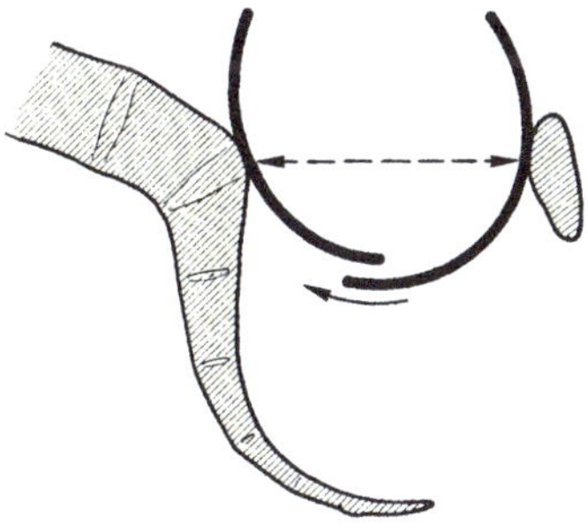

Fig. 8.143: Adaptation of the head through anterior asynclitism and overlapping of the parietal bones. Result is a reduced transverse diameter of the head.

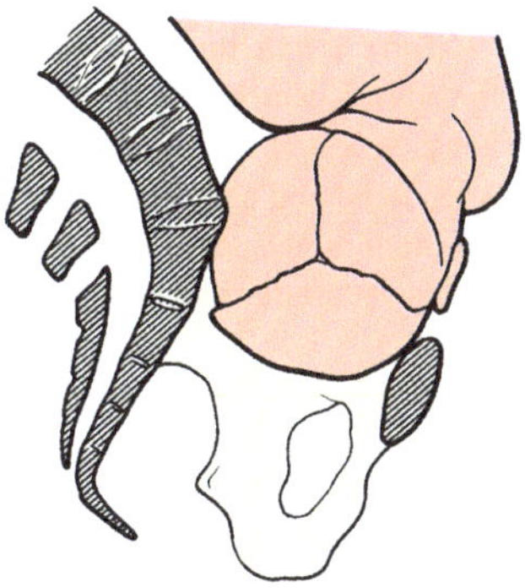

Fig. 8.144: Anterior asynclitism.

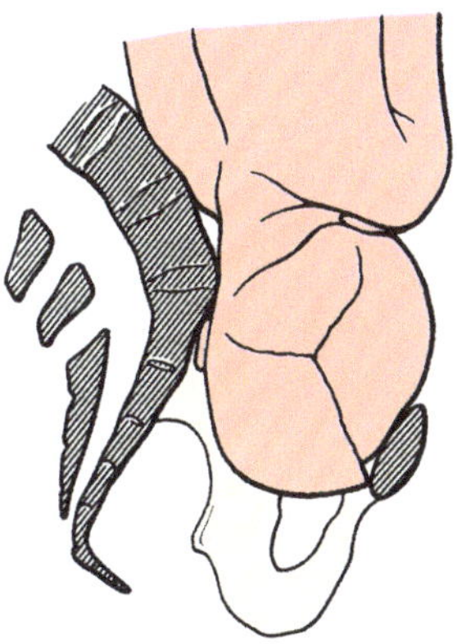

Fig. 8.145: Arrested labor in posterior asynclitism.

Note. Overlapping of the parietal bones reduces the transverse diameter of the head!

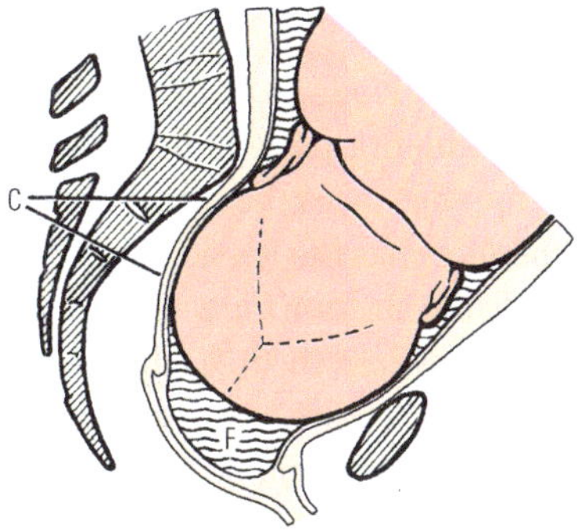

Fig. 8.146: Valve effect of the head in normal pelvis (after Bumm). The forewaters (F) are not connected to the AF; C = cervix.

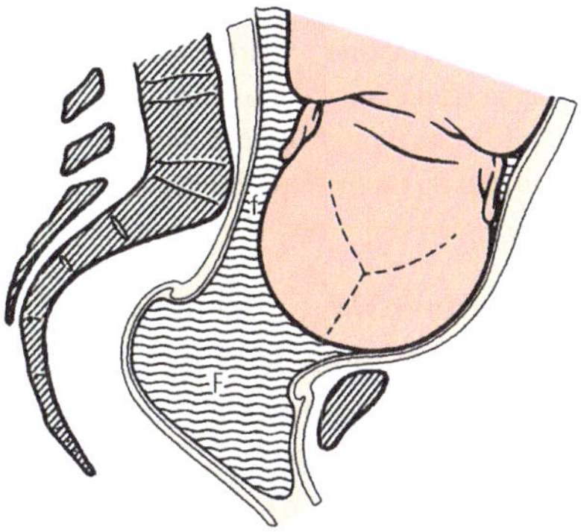

Fig. 8.147: In CPD, the forewaters (F) are freely connected to the AF in the uterine cavity. The head is above the pelvis and leaves free space (f) for the fluids to combine.

The degree of overlapping gives a palpable indication of the extent of the molding. The greater the amount of overlap, and the closer the transverse sagittal suture therefore becomes to the sacral promontory, the smaller the transverse diameter of the head and the greater the chance that the head will overcome the contraction by adaptation.

SVD is not possible in posterior asynclitism (Fig. 8.145)!

Posterior asynclitism is a further attempt by nature to adapt the relatively large head to the contracted PI, an attempt which is, however, always ineffective and leads to arrested labor. Reason: when the anterior parietal bone leads (Fig. 8.144), its free edge faces the sacral cavity, posteriorly; it therefore has the freedom to move lower and towards the back on descent. In posterior asynclitism, however, the free edge of the parietal bone comes up against the rear wall of the symphysis pubis and the pubic bones (Fig. 8.145), whereby all movement becomes impossible. In addition, the baby's posterior shoulder wedges upon the sacral promontory and becomes impacted. The head deflects anteriorly and protrudes above the symphysis pubis.

Note. Complications. Premature or early ROM, cord prolapse, arm prolapse, hypotonic contractions, prolonged labor. The two most dangerous complications are: ascending infection and threatened uterine rupture.

Premature or early ROM. In the normal relationship between head and pelvis the head seals the pelvis closed like a ball valve (Fig. 8.146). In CPD the head does not act as a seal, a dangerous free space is created. The forewaters (in the forebag in front of the head), which are normally separated from the main volume of AF by the head, are freely connected. With every new contraction a larger volume of AF is forced past the head into the amniotic sac. As the pressure of the contractions acts directly on the forewaters and the amniotic sac, this bulges tautly and becomes distended to such an extent that premature or early rupture of membranes occurs.

Cord prolapse. A dreaded moment is the rupture of membranes. The loop of cord which was already presenting is flushed out through the gap with the flow of AF into the vagina and outside: it falls out and lies in the vagina or in front of the vulva as a loop.

Practice tip. Cord prolapse is a threat in CPD as long as the head is not engaged (treatment see p. 288).

Arm prolapse. This event, which is characteristic in CPD, also usually occurs when AF flows; see p. 290.

Hypotonic contractions occur because the leading part descends very slowly or not at all in CPD, and as a result pressure on the cervical ganglia is missing.

Prolonged labor with threatened injuries to mother and baby (see below).

Threatened uterine rupture (p. 306).

Maternal injuries

Note. In CPD the head – if the contractions are sufficient – is pushed with considerable force onto and later into the pelvis over a long period of time (prolonged labor). Soft tissues between head and pelvis must bear this pressure: anterior (or more rarely, posterior) cervical lip, neck of the bladder, lower uterine segment (uterus rupture!).

Anterior and **posterior cervical lip.** Results of long-term congestion, obstruction of the venous outflow are:

- Edema of the anterior (Fig. 8.148) more rarely the posterior rim of the cervix, which looks like a fat, blue-red tumor.

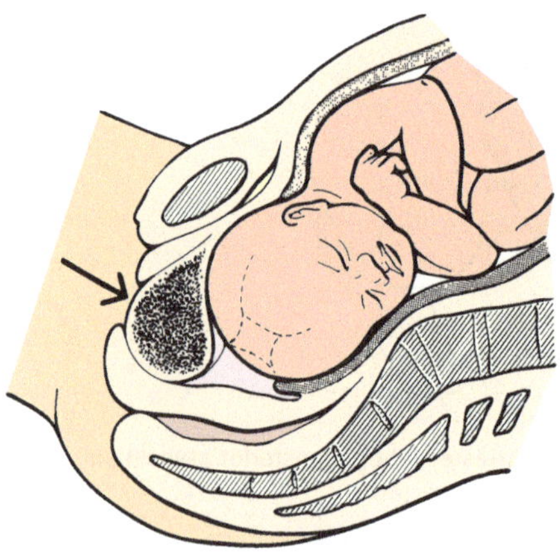

Fig. 8.148: Edema of the anterior cervical rim (arrow). The head compresses the bladder.

– Pressure necrosis of the rim of the cervix with extrusion of the necrotic tissue.

Urinary bladder and bladder neck. Strong pressure of the head presses the neck of the bladder against the anterior pelvic girdle. In this way, damage is caused to the tissue of the bladder (bloody urine!).

Consequences

Spontaneous urination not possible. Insertion of a catheter is often difficult, sometimes impossible. Nevertheless, it should be attempted. If this does not work, a finger is inserted into the vagina after preparation to push the head higher. The other hand attempts to insert the catheter with minimal force, which now always succeeds.

Hypotonic contractions. The hypotonic contractions which are almost always present worsen as a result of the full bladder, which appears as a large, full sack lying above the symphysis pubis: full bladder inhibits contractions!

Vesicovaginal fistula (VVF). The overfilling of the bladder causes at least an unpleasant paralysis of the bladder in the puerperium, sometimes (as a result of pressure necrosis) vesicovaginal or vesicocervical fistula.

Management of labor in CPD:

The first question in management of labor: is the disproportion so severe that cesarean section must be performed without delay or does this case belong to the group of CPDs in which expectant management must be followed? The comparison of the true conjugate (normal length 12 cm) and the BPD answers the question (Tab. 8.5).

Note. In moderate CPD expectant management is followed (restrictions see below). In extreme disproportion cesarean section is performed immediately on commencement of labor, or on a contraction-free uterus (→ elective CS). CS is also performed in the following indications (exceptions to the rule!): large, hard, poorly moldable head; abnormal presentations: breech, transverse lie, high AP head, posterior asynclitism; abnormal attitudes: brow, face presentation.

Expectant management

Rule in moderate CPD is expectant management (→ vaginal delivery). This strategy requires knowledge, experience and patience of the obstetrician.

Indications. Maternal and fetal wellbeing. Favorable presentation and attitude of the head: Roederer attitude, anterior asynclitism (p. 155 and 296).

If the head presents unfavorably expectant management is concluded.

No maternal tissue damage which force immediate operation:

- Urinary retention due to pressure trauma to the neck of the bladder.
- Bloody urine as a result of pressure trauma to the bladder.
- Edema or pressure trauma of the (anterior) rim of the cervix.
- Overextension of the lower uterine segment → rising retraction ring, especially when

Tab. 8.5: Management of labor results from the difference between the true conjugate and the biparietal diameter.

	Difference (true conjugate–BPD)	Management of labor
Moderate CPD	1 cm	Expectant management
Extreme CPD	0 cm and less	Cesarean section

it rises rapidly to or above the level of the navel → threatened uterine rupture.

Goal. Support of the entry and passage of the head through the narrow strait of a pelvis which is contracted completely or in one diameter.

Method

Positioning on the side of the posterior fontanelle. Goal is extreme flexion resulting in presentation of the occiput (p. 296): the pressure of the contractions must only act on the occiput in order to bring about entry and descent of the head.

Uterotonics. Contractions commonly play a decisive role in the course of labor in moderate CPD.

If after examination it can be assumed that the head will fit into the pelvis the contractions induce spontaneous entry into the pelvis.

Strong contractions. It may seem obvious to compensate for this deficiency by administering uterotonics. In particular if uterotonics are administered too early or in excessive doses however, the head, which is forced into the relatively narrow pelvis, would clamp the not-yet dilated and effaced soft tissues against the pelvic wall, would hold them there firmly in the rapid succession of strong contractions, so that they would not be able to efface. The cervix would be unable or only with difficulty to dilate.

If contractions are moderate, however, the soft tissues can retract over the head.

Moldability of the head. Positioning and regulation of contractions have the purpose of giving the head a favorable attitude and presentation for the available pelvic form, in order that it may be pushed into and through the pelvis. The moldability plays an important role hereby.

Note. Favorable assessment:
- Skull is small, narrow and soft.
- Sagittal suture is felt as a marked gap because the parietal bones lie movable next to one another.

Unfavorable assessment:
- Skull is large, broad and hard
- Sagittal suture is barely palpable because the parietal bones lie too closely together, so that they cannot overlap, or only minimally.

Final assessment. The definitive assessment as to whether or not the head will fit into the pelvis is not possible until the membranes have ruptured: the head cannot be remodeled as long as the membranes are intact.

Waiting period. One of the most difficult questions in treatment of CPD is how long should expectant management be followed when the head does not enter the pelvis despite conservative measures?

Practice tip. If after ROM, complete cervical dilatation and regular contractions the head has not entered the pelvis after 2–3 hours, expectant management is given up and a cesarean section is performed.

8.12.2 Funnel-shaped pelvis

Definition. The pelvic outlet is contracted; transverse diameter of the PO is greatly reduced (similar to a masculine pelvis); disproportion between baby's head and maternal PO.

Etiology. Congenital funnel-shaped pelvis in women with masculine habitus; acquired e.g., as kyphotic pelvis.

Incidence. High-grade funnel-shaped pelves are very rare; low-grade are commonly observed.

The **course of labor** corresponds to the situation of spatial contraction: easy entry and rapid passage of the head through the pelvis.

Abnormalities. The difficulties begin when the head has reached the pelvic floor. One of the three abnormalities usually occurs here:
- Rotation of the occiput does not occur.
- Development of a sinciput presentation.
- Development of deep transverse arrest.

8.12.3 Long pelvis

Definition. Cephalopelvic disproportion in labor with normal pelvic measurements and Michaelis rhomboid, in particular in cases of posterior asynclitism or high AP head.

Classification. Group 1: transitional pelvis. Group 2: assimilation pelvis. Group 3: assimilation-canal pelvis with 6 sacral vertebrae and missing sacral cavity, canal pelvis.

Etiology. There are two causes of the long pelvis: infantile pelvis, transitional vertebrae (assimilation pelvis).

Infantile pelvis. Pelvic development ceased at a stage of newborn development. The newborn pelvis is a long pelvis: missing sacral cavity, high sacral promontory, steep PI. The development to a true gynecoid (feminine) pelvis in puberty when the sacral promontory descends and the sacral cavity develops does not occur.
Transitional vertebra. The long pelvis is a normal pelvis plus transitional vertebra.
A transitional vertebra is the result of assimilation, the anatomical and functional adaptation to the neighboring spinal section. Obstetrically relevant transitional vertebrae are those on the lumbosacral junction.
The bony birth canal is lengthened by 2–3 cm (depending on the position of the vertebra) by the addition of a sixth (transitional) sacral vertebra, which results in a long pelvis: assimilation pelvis.

Transitional pelvis (Group 1; Fig. 8.149)

Definition. Normal pelvis plus lumbosacral transitional vertebra (4), which is not incorporated in the sacrum (as in group 2), but at the lumbosacral junction.

High sacral promontory. A functional lengthening of the bony birth canal accompanied by a high sacral promontory only occurs when the axis of the transitional vertebra is aligned with that of S1. High sacral promontory: spinal prominence at the lumbosacral junction which protrudes ventrally into the pelvis; caused by marked angling of the lumbar spine to the sacrum: Angulus lumbosacralis.
Double promontory. The transitional vertebra is often found bent backwards, which creates 2 promontories (Fig. 8.148): promontory I (1) is created by the upper edge of the transitional vertebra and promontory II (2) by the upper edge of the first sacral vertebra → double promontory.
Promontory I is as high as normal, which increases the angle of inclination of the PI (3). The axis of the transitional vertebra in Fig. 8.149 is almost in alignment with that of the sacral vertebra. The transitional vertebra is, however not yet fully sacralized, or it would have become the first sacral vertebra and its upper, ventral edge would have created the only promontory. The sacral vertebra, which is actually the first and has been relegated to second would not create a second promontory, but would only be involved in the creation of the sacral cavity.

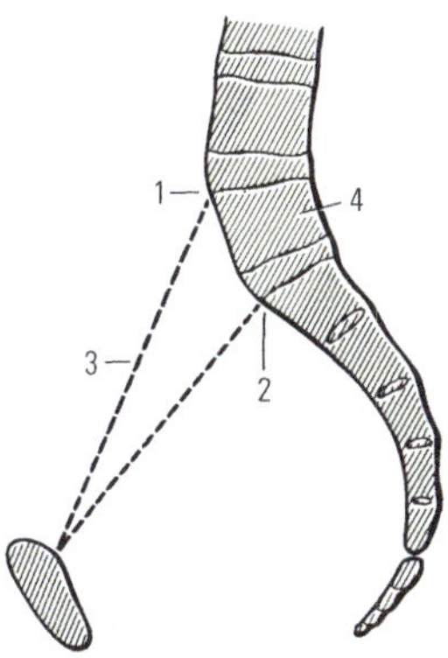

Fig. 8.149: Transitional pelvis. 1) Sacral promontory I, upper edge of the transitional vertebra; 2) sacral promontory II, upper edge of S1; 3) steep angle of inclination of the PI, 4. Transitional vertebra (after Kirchhoff).

Characteristics (Fig. 8.149). Lengthening of the bony birth canal with high sacral promontory and extremely steep angle of inclination of the pelvic inlet; double promontory is common.

Only the PI is abnormal, markedly deformed. The remainder of the birth canal is normal. The closer the longitudinal axis of the transitional vertebra is to that of the first sacral vertebra, the more this vertebra belongs anatomically and functionally to the sacrum, the more similar the group 1 pelvis is to that of group 2.

Assimilation pelvis with retained sacral form (Group 2; Fig. 8.150)

Definition. Normal pelvis plus lumbosacral transitional vertebra incorporated into the sacrum.

Characteristics (Fig. 8.150). Only anomaly: the transitional vertebra is completely incorporated into the sacrum; the first sacral vertebra becomes the second.

The pelvis shape is normal, as is the sacral cavity. It is, however, abnormally long, which creates a high sacral promontory and steep angle of inclination of the PI.
Fusion and inclusion of the transitional vertebra into the sacrum means that there is only one sacral promontory in this case, which with the symphysis pubis creates the narrowest section of the pelvis.

Note. An unusually steep angle of inclination of the PI is the cause of numerous obstetric complications.

Canal pelvis: Assimilation pelvis with absent sacral cavity (Group 3; Fig. 8.151)

Definition. Infantile pelvis plus assimilation of one lumbar vertebra into the sacrum; the sacrum has no concavity and is almost completely elongated. Sacral cavity and curve of Carus are absent. The bony birth canal has become a strait of equal width from PI to pelvic floor, therefore assimilation pelvis, or canal pelvis.

Characteristics (Fig. 8.151)
- The transitional vertebra is also completely incorporated into the sacrum in this case.
- The sacral cavity is missing. The whole of the birth canal is a straight tube of even width.

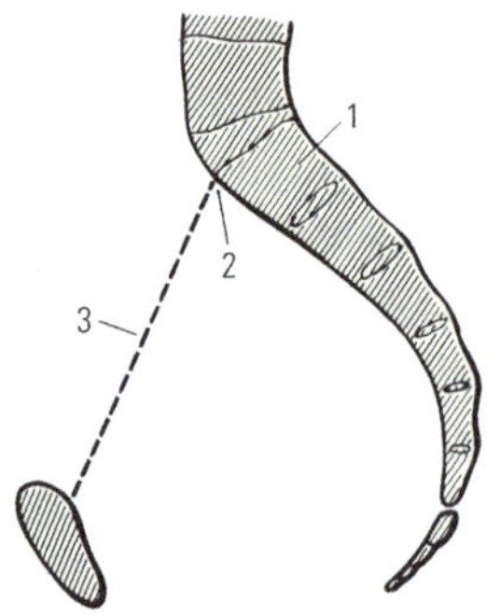

Fig. 8.150: Assimilation pelvis with retained sacral form. 1) Transitional vertebra incorporated into the sacrum; 2) high sacral promontory; 3) Steep angle of inclination of the PI (after Kirchhoff).

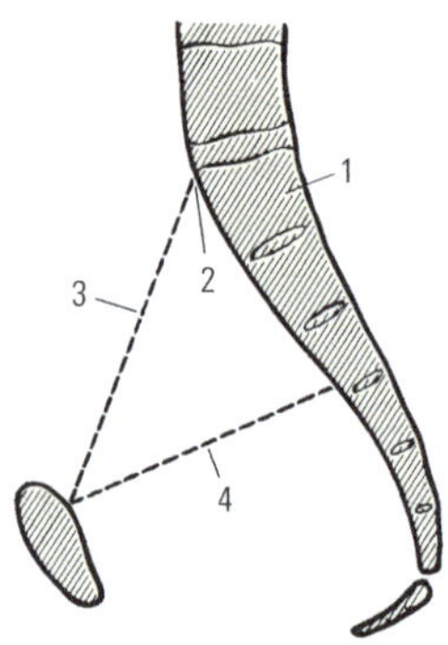

Fig. 8.151: Canal pelvis. 1) Transitional vertebra incorporated into the sacrum; 2) high sacral promontory; 3) steep angle of inclination of the PI; 4) connecting line between symphysis pubis and S2-S3 (true conjugate II).

- The sacral promontory is high, angle of inclination of the PI is steep, external conjugate is lengthened and the PI is often of longitudinal-oval shape (see below).
- The narrowest point is the connecting line between the symphysis pubis and the fusion of S2–S3 (true conjugate II), which lies far below the sacral promontory. It is often narrower than the normal PI: a reduced AP diameter often accompanies the above-mentioned anomalies!

Clinical manifestations of the long pelvis
- Despite good contractions the head remains floating above the PI (external pelvimetry, Michaelis rhomboid normal).
- Leopold maneuver: head usually overrides the symphysis pubis (normal pelvic measurements).
- Posterior asynclitism, head wedged on the symphysis pubis.
- Vaginal examination: sagittal suture felt very near the symphysis pubis.

Practice tip. Memory rule, long pelvis: normal pelvic measurements; head overrides the symphysis pubis. Internal examination: posterior asynclitism or high AP head. 40 % of all cases of CPD are caused by long pelves. SVD is only to be expected in 50 % of cases.

Diagnosis. X-ray imaging and MRI lead the diagnosis. This clarification should be sought after labors which suggest a long pelvis with regard to further births.

For the lateral image, the woman lies directly on her side on the x-ray table with extended legs. In order to measure the true conjugate a measuring instrument (e.g., after Büchner) is fixed at the level of the PI. The dimensions of the sacrum can also be assessed.

Mechanism of labor
Three moments disrupt the course of labor and explain the abnormalities:

First disruption. The bony birth canal is extended by one vertebra, the promontory is therefore higher.

This disruption affects only the PI, in which birth complications most commonly occur with a long pelvis.
In the normal pelvis a special mechanism traps the head in the pelvis: the head pushes up against the sacral promontory with one parietal bone and is held back on one side as a result. The cervical spine is slightly laterally flexed and convex in the direction of the abdomen, which aligns the axis of the skull vertically with the pelvic inlet.
This mechanism cannot work in a long pelvis: the sacral promontory is so high that the head cannot use it as a buffer in order to tip itself into the pelvis (Fig. 8.152).
The main mass of the head is already forced against the symphysis pubis below the sacral promontory at the onset of the first contractions. It is the buffer; here the head is slowed down for the first time and rides upon the symphysis pubis in the classical posterior asynclitic presentation (→ arrested labor).

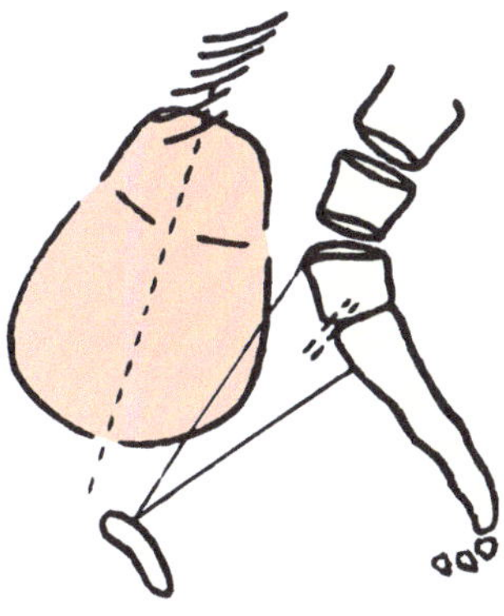

Fig. 8.152: First and second disruptions. The head does not find the trapping mechanism and the narrowest passage is below the true conjugate.

Note. On external examination an impression of CPD is gained without external indications of a contracted pelvis! A lateral x-ray confirms the diagnosis.

If the head does manage to enter the PI despite the PI deformity (1st disruption), the 2nd disruption threatens.

Second disruption. The narrowest section is created below the true conjugate, often recognizable as double promontory (cause: assimilated vertebra which presents in a transitional position and is often too prominent). The potential difficulty is shown in Fig. 8.153.

The sacral cavity is necessary so that the head can perform its second rotation, from the transverse over the oblique into the anteroposterior diameter in midpelvis, and from there its third rotation in a curve around the symphysis pubis. If the sacral cavity is missing, the second rotation cannot be performed because there is no space:

- Space for rotation, the space necessary for rotation in midpelvis is missing.
- The head passes through the whole birth canal from PI to pelvic floor with the sagittal suture in the transverse diameter (Fig. 8.153).

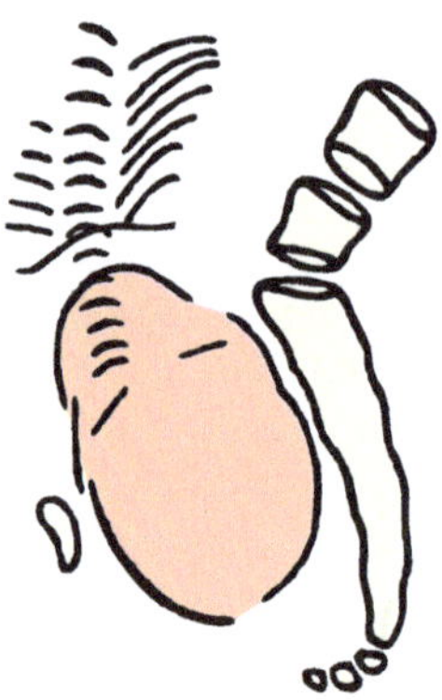

Fig. 8.153: Third disruption. The canal pelvis must be passed through with the baby's head (sagittal suture) in the transverse diameter until it reaches the pelvic floor

Note. Usually the head is already held up in midpelvis with the result that rotation from the transverse diameter over the oblique does not occur in midpelvis and mid-pelvic transverse arrest is found.

If the head descends to the pelvic floor with the sagittal suture in the transverse diameter, a further disadvantage follows in persistent occipitotransverse position: the lack of sacral cavity. The birth of the head, the movement around the symphysis pubis (→ third rotation), is a movement of extension only. Its execution requires the head to be in the correct starting position, with the sagittal suture in the APD.
The head is in the occipitotransverse position. The spontaneous delivery of the head around the symphysis pubis is therefore impossible (apart from exceptions). Therefore not only the space required for rotation is malformed by the missing sacral cavity, but also the space required for extension, the curve of Carus.

Anthropoid pelvis. As a result of the abovementioned developmental disturbance (→ infantile pelvis) the combination with an anthropoid (longitudinal-oval) pelvis is often found. It can only be confirmed by sitting x-ray images of the PI!). Further complications often result, malpresentations, malpositions, abnormal attitudes: occipitoanterior presentation, high AP head.

8.13 Uterine rupture

Definition. Uterine tear, rupture. Types: 1) complete rupture of the uterus with tearing of uterus and peritoneum; 2) incomplete rupture: the peritoneum remains intact; 3) Silent rupture: gradual, asymptomatic uterine rupture; 4) spontaneous rupture without the use of external force; 5) traumatic rupture caused by obstetrical operation. Classification also according to preferred sites and causes (see below).

Incidence. One rupture in 1,500 births, scar ruptures are most common.

Note. Classification

According to the site of laceration (Fig. 8.154):
- Tearing of Corpus uteri, lower uterine segment, cervix. Colporrhexis. Tearing of the cervix from the vagina (→ vaginal separation is classified as uterine rupture).
- The classical rupture is that of the lower uterine segment, the thinnest and most distended part of the uterus.

According to the cause:
- Rupture primarily due to overdistension: overdistension, scar rupture.
- Rupture primarily due to damage to the wall (after endomyometritis of a septic miscarriage).
- According to the rupturing forces: spontaneous, traumatic.
- According to peritoneal involvement: complete and incomplete rupture.
- According to the symptoms: with/without warning sign(s).

Etiology

Overdistension rupture. Tear of the uterine wall primarily due to overdistension. Causes:

1. Birth obstruction. All birth obstructions can provoke a rupture:
   a) CPD.
   b) Malpresentations and malpositions from which spontaneous birth is impossible: 1) transverse lie, 2) posterior asynclitism, 3) mentoposterior face presentation, 4) nasoposterior brow presentation, 5) high AP head.
   c) Fetal deformity, most commonly hydrocephalus.
   d) Mechanical displacement of the birth canal: ovarian or pelvic tumor.
   e) Rigid soft tissues (rare): cervical carcinoma, conglutinatio orificii externi (adhesion of the amniotic membranes to the cervical wall).

Practice tip. Overdistension rupture affects multiparae in 94 % of cases, in particular: 1) in CPD: overdistension → tissue trauma → scarring after first birth, rupture during a later birth; 2) if the baby is large; 3) if the births are in rapid succession (→ exhaustion factor). 6 % occur in primiparae.

---

2. Traumatic rupture (see below).
3. Uterotonics as infusion as long as the baby is still in utero.

Pathogenesis. The exertion of the Corpus uteri has a single goal in labor: expulsion of the baby from the uterine cavity, regardless of whether the resistances in the birth canal are normal, increased or – and this is the key issue here – insurmountable.

The greater the resistance, the greater the exertion and thus the force of contractions. Strength and number of contractions increase with increased resistance. If the resistance is insurmountable (→ hydrocephalus, impacted shoulder presentation), expulsion of the baby is impossible.

Tetanus uteri, hypercontractile state. If the resistance is insurmountable the force of the contractions becomes even stronger, the intervals

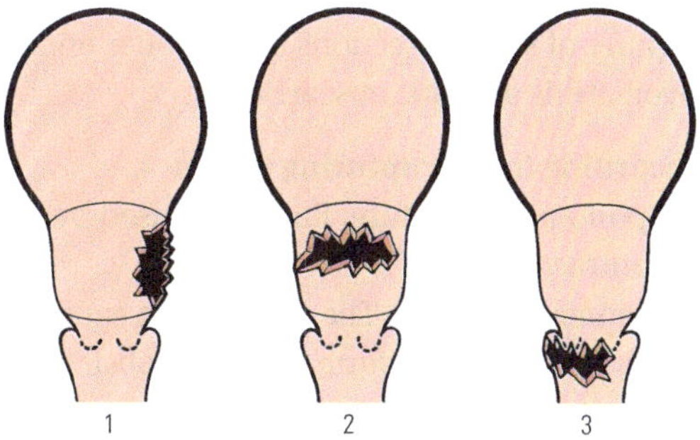

Fig. 8.154: Rupture of the uterus. Laceration of lower uterine segment as 1) longitudinal, 2) transverse, 3) colporrhexis (vaginal separation).

between them even shorter. The baby is forced into the lower uterine segment as a result. This is stretched more and more, overdistended. The thin wall becomes thinner with every new contraction. Result: hypercontractile state, continuous hypertonic contractions. Tetanus uteri describes extremely intense hypercontractility without pause. Rupture of the uterus in the lower uterine segment.

Note. Insurmountable birth obstruction plus hypertonic contractions = rupture of the uterus!

Scar rupture. Most common type of rupture! Laceration of the uterus in a scarred area (→connective tissue which is high in fiber and low in blood-vessels and cells) as a result of prior injury (history!) to the wall (e.g., CS), also due to normal tension of uterine muscles in pregnancy, but usually due to distension in labor. Cause:

Rupture of scars, particularly after:
- Cesarean section. The longitudinal section which used to be standard has been replaced by the transverse section of the lower uterine segment, which has led to a marked reduction in the rate of scar ruptures.
- Perforating injuries of the uterine wall (abortion, curettage after miscarriage), after transmural myomectomy, corrective uterine surgery.

Rupture of scarred sections of wall after endomyometritis of septic miscarriage.

According to the rupturing forces
- Spontaneous rupture. Rupture caused by contractions.
- Traumatic rupture. The obstetrician causes the tear during performance of an obstetrical operation (iatrogenic cause).

According to peritoneal involvement

Incomplete rupture (Fig. 8.155). Incomplete laceration of the uterus. Laceration of the uterus wall without tearing of the peritoneum: tear on one side of the lower uterine segment into the parametrium, sometimes also into the paracolpium without opening the abdominal cavity.

The leading symptom is a subperitoneal hematoma. As long as the peritoneum doesn't tear space is required (→ subperitoneal hematoma), into which the volume of blood oozes, raising the broad ligament and causing it to unfold.

Complete rupture (Fig. 8.156). Complete laceration of the uterus. Laceration of all layers of the overdistended section, including peritoneum with opening of the abdominal cavity. Gaping tear between the uterine cavity and the abdominal cavity. The following enter the abdominal cavity:
- Blood from the uterine arteries.
- Infected AF → infection.
- Possibly the baby.
- Placenta.

Practice tip. The laceration is generally lateral with injury to the uterine artery.

Clinical manifestation

Asymptomatic rupture (→ silent rupture). Scar ruptures are often asymptomatic, almost without warning signs, as are ruptures in hydrocephalus, overdose of uterotonics, traumatic uterine rupture (laboring woman in narcosis!).

Incomplete scar rupture
- Contractions slowly abate.
- No apparent bleeding.
- Shock symptoms (hemorrhage!) in late stage: haggard appearance, weak, fast pulse, hypotension.

Complete scar rupture (course not as dramatic as ruptures as a result of obstructed expulsion)
- Pain: spontaneous, on pressure.
- Abdominal guarding (defense musculaire).
- Shock.

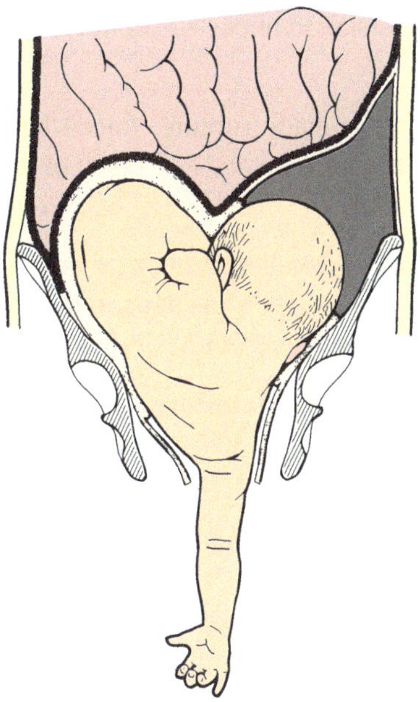

Fig. 8.155: Incomplete rupture.

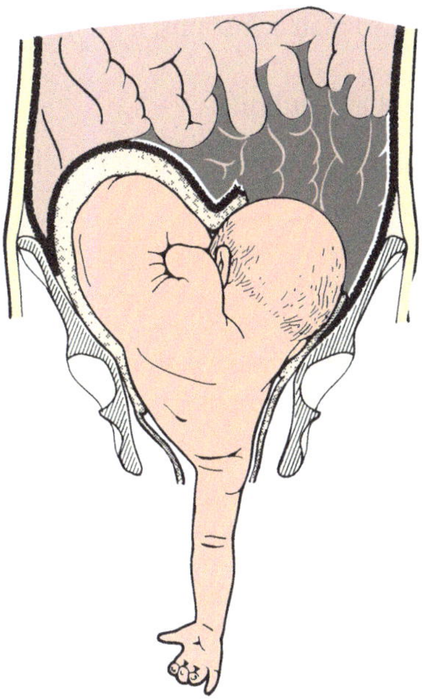

Fig. 8.156: Complete rupture.

- Fetal parts may be palpable through the abdominal wall.

Symptomatic rupture. Overdistension ruptures (insurmountable obstructions to expulsion, exception: rupture due to hydrocephalus, see above) announce themselves hours beforehand with warning signs:

1. Increased contractility to hypercontractility.
- One contraction after another without pause, so that the uterus is permanently contracted:
- – Hypercontractile state, highest degree of contractility.
- – Hypertonic contractions (→ danger for the baby) are continuous (→ Tetanus uteri) or single contractions in extremely rapid succession (→ Clonus uteri).
- The body of the uterus is maximally retracted. Consequences: points 2–6.

2. The retraction ring (Bandl's ring: upper border of the lower uterine segment) becomes apparent and rises to the level of the navel and higher.
- Distension of the lower uterine segment causes the retraction ring to rise, usually as a crooked groove. Rupture is imminent when the groove rises to the level of the navel or higher in a short time.
- Primiparae are less at risk than multiparae.

3. Unbearably painful contractions as though something inside were to tear. Sensitivity to pressure and tension between navel and symphysis.
- Overdistension of the lower uterine segment during contractions, and later in between contractions.
- Pain is unresponsive to epidural anesthesia

4. The round ligament of the uterus (ligamentum teres uteri) is stretched taut like a wire on one or both sides due to overdistension.

5. Facial expression: tortured, from anxious to mortal fear.

- The laboring woman complains, is restless and pale
- Pulse: fast, often fluttering.

6. Vaginal examination (in narcosis if not otherwise possible).
- The presenting part (head, shoulder) is floating above the PI.
- Head with large caput
- If the cervix is not completely dilated, rims are palpable due to entrapment and edema as bulging pillows.

Practice tip. Rupture of the uterus in presenting hydrocephalus is the exception. Its course is usually asymptomatic: the lower uterine segment is already overdistended in pregnancy. Rupture already threatens at the onset of mild contractions, in particular in cases of prior CS.

Symptoms of ruptured uterus

The surest sign is abrupt cessation of contractions after hypertonic contractions (see above). Rupture pain. The woman screams. She feels as though something in her abdomen has torn. Shock, anemia due to internal bleeding: weak, frequent pulse, hypotension, pale, extremely haggard appearance, cold sweat on the forehead, restlessness, dyspnea.
In cases of complete rupture the baby may enter the abdominal cavity, so that parts of the baby are palpable directly below the abdominal wall. There is usually bleeding from the vagina.
Vaginal examination. The presenting part (head, shoulder), which was previously fixed or impacted in the PI is now mobile and floating, sometimes no longer even reachable.

Contraindications. Never attempt vaginal delivery!

Examples of malpractice:
- Attempted forceps if entry of the head is impossible, in particular in hydrocephalus.
- Attempted version if entry of the head is impossible.
- Attempted version in impacted shoulder presentation.

Consequences: traumatic rupture, forced laceration of the uterus upon and as a result of an obstetric operation.

Complications. Hypovolemic shock (→ immediate danger), peritonitis (→ late danger) due to infected AF in complete rupture.

Procedure in threatened rupture

- Intravenous tocolysis with Fenoterol against hypertonic contractions.
- Operation, gentle delivery in general anesthetic.

Care must be taken of the extremely taut, paper-thin lower uterine segment in surgery; the lie of the baby must not be altered! No daring attempts at delivery.

Operative technique for dead fetus

- Cephalic presentations. Craniotomy (p. 343): perforation of the head and extraction with the cranioclast.
- Transverse lies. Decapitation: Severing of the head. Embryotomy: Severance of the trunk.
- Manual exploration of the uterus (see below), to prevent traumatic rupture of the uterus (see p. 306).

Operative technique for live baby

Cesarean section is the method of choice (possible exception in: hydrocephalus, severe birth defects), in some cases of stillbirth also (avoidance of interventional dismemberment, better uterine control).
Manual uterine exploration after every large obstetrical procedure, in particular after every version (combined, podalic).

Practice tip. The danger of rupture is greatest on version. Version is therefore the most dangerous operation for the mother!

- Forceps, decapitation, embryotomy.
- Manual extraction.
- Difficult assisted delivery, particularly if the head was above the pelvic brim.
- Perforation, if the head was not engaged (particularly in hydrocephalus!).
- The cervix must be inspected using of ring forceps postoperatively.

Procedure if rupture has occurred

Immediate laparotomy, even in seemingly hopeless cases!

We recommend a long, median incision of the lower abdomen: everything must happen very quickly! Removal of baby and placenta. Then assure a clear view! Effective hemostasis!

- The situation of the baby, whether it is alive or dead, whether it is still in the uterus or already in the abdominal cavity is completely irrelevant.
- Uterine extirpation is the method of choice (depending on location of the rupture) in complete rupture.
- Suturing may be sufficient in cases of incomplete rupture; it can become complete, however, so that here also hysterectomy by laparotomy is recommended.
- Ligation of the internal iliac artery for hemostasis, or suturing of the uterine arteries.

8.14 Management of birth after prior cesarean section

The risk of uterine rupture on vaginal delivery after transverse isthmus incision is less than 1 %. Rupture of the uterus here includes asymptomatic scar dehiscence as well as complete rupture with entry of the baby and placenta into the peritoneal space. After a number of cesarean sections the risk of rupture is approximately 3 %. If the cesarean section was performed by fundal incision or the classical vertical incision, or if the incision technique is unknown, scar problems are more common. Risk of rupture is 6 %, for example, after longitudinal uterine incision.

While earlier this risk was accepted in hospital managed births in Europe, and approximately 70 % of VBAC (vaginal birth after cesarean) attempts were successful as a rule, today the pregnant woman often elects to have a repeat cesarean section.

Absolute indications for repeat CS:

- Continuation of the indication for CS (e.g., pelvic deformity or nonobstetric indication).
- Nonisthmic incisions of the uterus.
- Prior uterine rupture.

Relative indications for repeat CS:

- Suspected macrosomia.
- Twins.
- Breech presentation.

The results of a study by Lydon–Rochelle and colleagues are important for management of VBAC. It was found that the risk of rupture for women with repeat CS and no contractions was 1.6 ‰, for women with spontaneous onset of labor 5.2 ‰, for women with induced labor without prostaglandins 7.7 ‰, and for women with labor induction using prostaglandins was 24.5 ‰. In this collective, induction of labor with prostaglandins carried the highest risk of rupture.

In management of VBAC labor, immediate operation must be possible! Pathological heart rate pattern, lack of or extremely delayed progress in labor, also after administration of oxytocics for uterine stimulation and conduction analgesia, claims of scar pain in the intervals between contractions or bleeding are clinical signs which should lead to an end of the trial of labor.

Routine uterine exploration after VBAC is no longer recommended. The earlier results of exploration are unreliable.

8.15 Amniotic fluid embolism (AFE)

Definition. Entry of AF into the opened uterine venous system of the mother (veins from the site of placental attachment, margin of the placenta, myometrium, cervix) on AROM, operation (CS, intrauterine procedures), traumas (placental abruption, rupture of the uterus, placenta previa, cervical laceration, hypertonic contractions in oxytocin overdose, Tetanus uteri) in labor or postnatally with shock.

Incidence. As fulminant event, AFE is rare: 1 in 30,000 to 50,000 births, maternal mortality 20–60 %; estimations as to the incidence of smaller AFE are not available, also due to the difficulties of diagnosis. Fetal mortality in AFE is given as 20–40 %.

Pathophysiology. It is not clear how AF enters the maternal circulation. Strong contractions, particularly after ROM and operative opening of maternal veins on uterotomy for operative delivery apparently promote the transfer of AF and its – also corpuscular – contents to maternal circulation. As a result, pulmonary microcirculation is displaced, pulmonary hypotension with resulting right-sided heart failure as well as left-sided heart failure and arterial hypotension occur, in addition to coagulopathy caused by the procoagulatory activity of AF.

Clinical manifestation

- Shock.
- Acute respiratory insufficiency.
- Coagulation disorders → afibrinogenemia with increased fibrinolytic activity, reduced platelet count in peripheral blood (30–40 %).
- Consumptive coagulopathy (DIC), caused by the thromboplastin content of AF (Hugo and colleagues, 1990).

Diagnosis. On the basis of the clinical symptoms only the suspected diagnosis can be made in hospital. Detection of corpuscular contents of AF in maternal central-venous blood (centrifuged blood sample) is recommended, but is not recognized as a sufficiently sensitive method, however. Histological evidence of AF material in pulmonary circulation confirms the diagnosis post mortem.

Differential diagnosis. Pulmonary embolism (no pulmonary pain in AFE, however!), pneumothorax, eclampsia, uterus rupture and left cardiac insufficiency.

Treatment. Intensive medical action (possibly intensive care ward!) for oxygenation, possibly intubation, and artificial respiration. Treatment with corticosteroids, volume substitution and infusion of fresh frozen plasma. Delivery via CS after stabilization of the mother!

References

American College of Obstetricians and Gynecologists. Operative vaginal delivery: ACOG practice bulletin no. 17. Washington, DC 2000

American College of Obstetricians and Gynecologists: Vaginal birth after previous Cesarean delivery. Practice Bulletin no. 115. Obstet Gynecol 2010; 116:450–463

American College of Obstetricians and Gynecologists. Committee Opinion No 369. Multifetal pregnancy reduction. Obstet Gynecol 2007; 109:1511

American College of Obstetricians nnd Gynecologists: Induction of labor. Practice Bulletin No 107. Obstet Gynecol 2009; 114:386–97

Barrett JFR, Hannah ME, Hutton EK, et al.: A randomized trial of planned Cesarean or vaginal delivery for twin pregnancy. NEJM 2013;369:1295–305

Boama V, Arulkumaran S: Safer childbirth: a rights-based approach. Int J Gynecol Obstet 2009; 106:125–7

Caughey A: Is there an upper time limit for the management of the second stage of labor? Am J Obstet Gynecol 2009; 201:337–338

Chauhan SP, JA Scardo, Hayes E, Abuhamad AZ, Berghella V: Twins: prevalence, problems, and preterm births. Am J Obstet Gynecol 2010; 203:305–15

Fitzpatrick M, McQuillan K, O'Herlihy C: Influence of persistent occiput posterior position on delivery outcome. Obstet Gynecol 2001; 98:1027

Gherman RB, Chauhan S, Ouzounian JG, et al.: Shoulder dystocia: The unpreventable obstetric emergency with empiric management guiclelines. Am J Obstet Gynecol 2006; 195:657

Gross T, Sokol R, \\/illiams T, Thompson K: Shoulder dystocia: A fetalphysician risk. Am J Obstet Gynecol 1987; 156:1408

Hannah MB, Nannah WJ, Hewson SA, et al.: Planned cesarean section versus planned vaginal birth for breech presentation at term: a randomised multicentre trial. Lancet 2000; 356:1375

Hannah ME, Term Breech Trial Collaborative Group: Outcomes at three month after planned caesarean vs. planned vaginal delivery for breech presentation at term. JAMAS 2002; 287:1822

Howarth GR, Botha DJ: Arniotomy plus intravenous oxytocin for incluction of labour. Cochrane Database Syst Rev 2001; 3:CD003250

Hutton EK, Hannah ME, Ross SJ, Delisle M-F, et al.: The early external cephalic version (ECV) 2 Trial: an international multicentre randomised controlled trial of timing of ECV for breech pregnancies. BJOG 2011; DOI: 10.1111/j.1471-0528.2010.02837.x.

Kelly AJ , Tan BP: Intravenous oxytocin alone for induction of labour. Cochrane Database Syst Rev 2001; 3:CD003246

Lydon-Rochelle M, Holt VL, Easterling TR, Martin DP: Risk of uterine rupture cluring labor among women with a prior cesarean delivery, N Engl J Med 2001; 345:3

Quintero RA, Kontopoulos EV, Chmait R, et al.: Management of twin-twin transfusion syndrome in pregnancies with iatrogenic detachment of membranes following therapeutic amniocentesis and the role of interim amniopatch.. Ultrasound Obstet Gynecol 2005; 26:628–33

Roberts D, Neilson JP, Kilby M, et al.: Interventions for the treatment of twin-twin transfusion syndrome. Cochrane Database Syst Rev 2008: CD002073

Rouse DJ, Owen J, Savage KG, Hauth JC: Active phase labor arrest: Revisiting the 2-hour minimum. Obstet Gynecol 2001; 98:550

Rouse DJ, Weiner SJ, Bloom SL, et al.: Second-stage labor duration in nulliparous women: relationship to maternal and perinatal outcomes. Am J Obstet Gynecol 2009; 201:357–360

Royal College of Obstetricians and Gynaccologists: Management of monochorionic twin pregnancy. Royal College of Obstetricians and Gynaecologists 2008; 51:1–13

Royal College of Obstetricians and Gynecologists: Shoulder dystocia. Green-top Guideline No. 42, March 2012

Stamilio DM, Fraser WD, Moore TR: Twin-twin transfusion syndrome: an ethic-based and evidence-based. argument for clinical research. Am J Obstet Gynecol 2019; 203:3–16

Surbek DV, Bösinger H, Hösli I, et al.: A double-blind comparison of the safety and efficacy of intravaginal Misoprostol and Prostaglandin E2 to induce labor : Am J Obstet Gynecol 1997; 177:1018

Whyte H, Hannah ME: Term breech trial collaborative group: Outcomes of children at 2 years after planned caesarean birth vs vaginal birth for breech presentation at term: The international randomised term breech trial. Amer J Obstet Gynecol 2004; 191:864

9 Obstetrical operations

9.1 Indication

Note. The indication provides the reason and the decision for operative delivery, the condition, prerequisite for the procedure, determines the type of operation.

Indication. Reason for the performance of a medical procedure (e.g., obstetrical operation), under consideration of risk-benefit and contraindications, whereby there is an obligation to inform the patient. Differentiated into absolute indication, compelling reason (→ immediate termination of labor, e.g., in severe fetal acidosis, life-threatening: vital indication) and relative indications. A conditional risk is present here; acute intervention is not necessary, however, from experience further waiting leads to worsening of the situation.

Prerequisite. In, for example eclampsia, labor progress and the current findings determine the relevant procedure for the indication. In the one case (head engaged and visible), labor can be terminated with an episiotomy; in another (head on pelvic floor, cervix completely dilated), with VE or forceps; in a third (high head, primipara) CS would be appropriate.
- Eclampsia is an indication for the termination of labor.
- Prerequisites determine the concrete method.

Only two indications exist in obstetrics: risk for the mother, risk for the fetus!
The indication for an obstetrical procedure arises from complications during pregnancy, in labor or in third stage. The danger hereby is to:
- The fetus only (placental insufficiency, cord prolapse).
- Mother and fetus (PIH).
- The mother only (PPH).

Note. The decision to intervene depends on the answers to three questions: Must I operate? Am I allowed to operate? Can I operate?

- Does the complication necessitate intervention? A lot of knowledge is necessary in obstetrics in order to do little.
- If the intervention is really indicated, must it be performed immediately? If not, wait. The obstetrician's greatest virtue is patience. Patience must not be taken too far however; risks are not to be taken.
- Are the conditions for the operation fulfilled? Have the four birth factors been considered and assessed: fetus, pelvis, contractions and cervical status? Has the laboring woman's general condition been assessed?
- Does the operator have practice and experience to perform the intervention?

Note. The worst mistake an operator can make is to attempt operations for which s/he is not adequately trained, alongside ignoring asepsis, antisepsis.

Obstetrical indication groups

Group 1: Maternal risks
- Heavy bleeding. Commonest causes:
  - Heavy bleeding in third stage (p. 380).
  - Placenta previa (p. 369).
  - Placental abruption (of a normally located placenta; p. 374).
  - Rupture of the uterus (p. 306).
- Maternal illness
  - PIH (p. 74), heart valve defect (mitral valve stenosis!), diabetes mellitus, pyelonephritis, nephrosis, infectious disease (pneumonia, febrile influenza, TB).
- Infection. Characteristics: temperature >38.5 °C, tachycardia.

- CPD.
- Excessively long labor.

Group 2: Fetal risks
- Fetal acidosis (p. 284).
- Acute bradycardia with head on the pelvic floor.
- Pathological CTG with closed cervix.
- Excessive length of labor (p. 208).
- Bleeding from velamentous insertion.

9.2 Preparation for the operation

Infection prophylaxis. The most important preparation is the behavior of the obstetrician, the observation of the principles of noninfection. Never touch the following without gloves:
- Wounds healing by secondary intention.
- Wound exudate.
- Infected dressings.
- Infected instruments.
- The smallest boil.

The operator removes rings, bracelets and the like before disinfection.
The following are to be observed with regards to the laboring woman:
Positioning. She can remain in a supine position for vaginal examination and episiotomy. Lithotomy position is required for all other procedures.
The buttocks must protrude over the edge of the bed.
Pain medication. Regional or pudendal analgesia (p. 184) is adequate for smaller obstetrical procedures (episiotomy, low forceps). Epidural anesthesia is advisable for VE or difficult forceps extractions. General anesthetic is rarely (internal podalic version and extraction of the second twin) necessary.
Disinfection of the external genitalia
- Pubic hair: prior to the operation the pubic hair in the posterior section of the vulva should at least be shortened, if not shaved. Always shave from front to back, never in the other direction.
- Cleansing with an antiseptic solution.

9.3 Episiotomy, perineotomy

Definition. Most common operation to enlarge the soft tissue birth canal. Usually performed preventatively, to prevent laceration and overdistension of perineum, vagina, muscles and fascia of the pelvic floor. Further, to ease operative delivery and terminate labor when the head is in the pelvic outlet.

Indication. The aim is avoidance of overdistension and laceration of the deep pelvic floor muscles, in particular the shanks of the levator ani.

For operations (→ before or during the operation): Forceps extraction, VE, complete extraction, manual assistance, in particular in primiparae.

Note. Not every vaginal-operative delivery necessitates an episiotomy!

In spontaneous deliveries (→ when the head is crowning or being born, always at the peak of a contraction).
- Rigid soft tissues (sportswomen, older primiparae).
- Unfavorable attitude (extended attitudes) of the head.
- Acute angle of pubic arch (unfavorable fit of the head, birth movement).
- Large head. The threatened perineal laceration announces itself by paling of the taut perineum.
- To expedite delivery. If head is crowning or being born and the FHR is indicative of hypoxia.

4–10 % of women complain of anal incontinence after delivery, 13–20 % suffer from flatus incontinence. Anal incontinence affects 30–60 % of women after sphincter damage (third or fourth degree laceration), the majority has flatus incontinence.

Restrictive use of episiotomy has demonstrated a reduction in traumatic injury to the area of the posterior peritoneum, less need for suturing and less faulty wound healing. Injuries to the anterior perineum are more common. No difference is shown between restrictive and routine episiotomy with regard to serious perineal and vaginal injuries, dyspareunia, urinary incontinence and various pain sensations.

Practice tip. Episiotomy has few advantages. The negative effects described predominate, so that it should only be indicated restrictively (large baby, shoulder dystocia, imminent fetal hypoxia among others).

Types. Lateral, median, mediolateral.

Lateral episiotomy. Incision with large, straight scissors 1 cm from the midline of the fourchette; incision direction towards the ischial tuberosity.

Mediolateral episiotomy. Healing is better when the scissors are placed directly at the posterior commissure (fourchette), mediolaterally, and the incision is made so that the ischial tuberosity lies above the extension of the imagined line of the incision. If standing on the right side (perineal protection), the incision is made towards the left, if standing between the legs (operative intervention) or on the left side, the incision is made to the right.

- Incision length. The requirement determines the length. Cuts less than 3–4 cm are pointless; they tear further or laceration occurs elsewhere. If the first incision is not adequate it is extended.
- Scissor hold. The flat sides of the blades are held at right angles to the tissue (Fig. 9.1). Otherwise the tissue is cut at an angle, which is not ideal for suturing and healing.
- Direction of incision: towards the ischial tuberosity.
- Transverse incision of the M. bulbospongiosus.

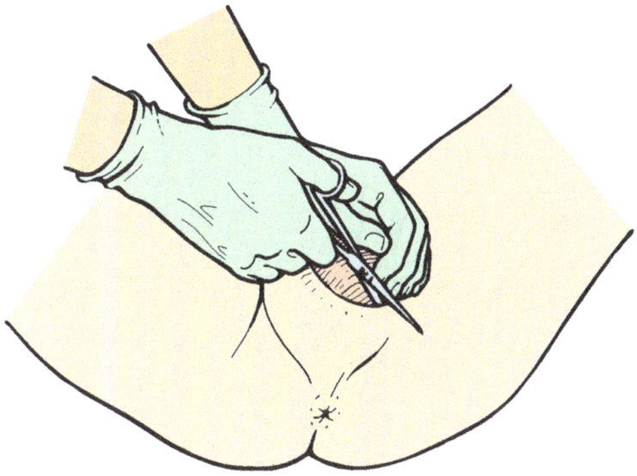

Fig. 9.1: Mediolateral episiotomy.

Median or midline episiotomy. The incision is made from the posterior commissure in the midline towards the anus.

- Direction of incision: incision of the M. bulbocavernosus along the course of the muscle fibers in the direction of the perineal body.
- The incision must not be closer than 1.5 cm to the anus (Fig. 9.2).

Advantages. Easier repair, better healing, less postpartum complaints.

Disadvantage. Danger of third and fourth degree extensions.

In choosing the type of episiotomy, it should be borne in mind that midline episiotomy is a risk factor for the development of fecal incontinence and is not suitable for avoidance of sphincter injury, regardless of maternal age, birth weight of the baby, length of second stage, contractions and method of instrumental delivery. However, in comparison with spontaneous perineal laceration, midline episiotomy shows a threefold higher risk for fecal incontinence

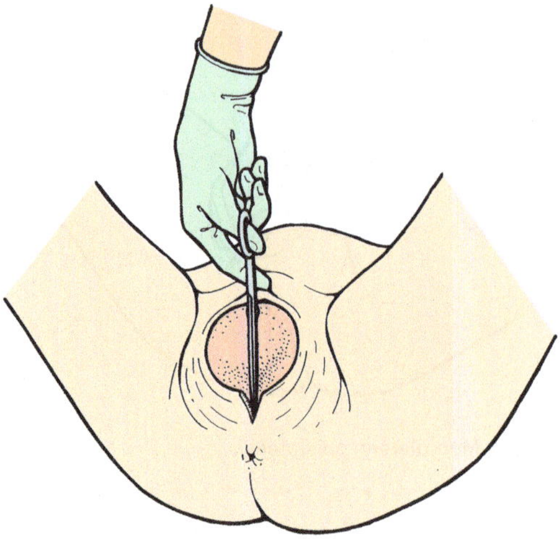

Fig. 9.2: Median or midline episiotomy.

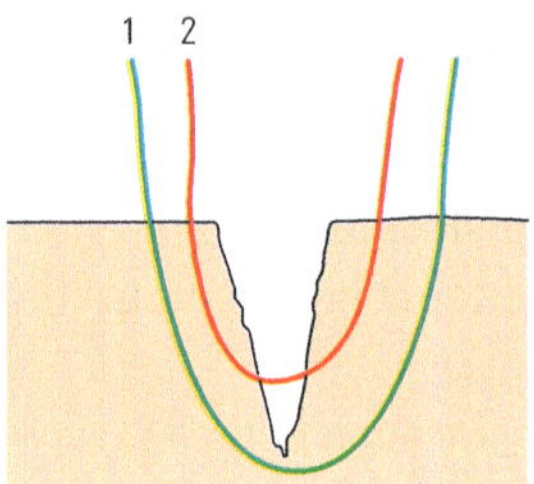

Fig. 9.3: Suturing technique: 1 correct, 2 false.

and double the risk of flatus incontinence after 3 or 6 months.

Episiotomy repair. The wound is a rhombus shape (Fig. 9.4) because of the gaping wound edges. Suturing is performed immediately after delivery of the placenta in epidural, pudendal or infiltration analgesia. Asepsis! Cleansing of the perineum with an antiseptic solution.

Anus is draped. Using 2 drape clamps, a sterile drape is hung from left to right so that the anus is draped. Suture material must not come in contact with the anus or the perianal region (→ infections!).

Wound area should be easily accessible. A clear view is most important! It is best to insert a sterile tampon (e.g., in the form of a tightly bound bag containing swabs) high into the vagina (spreads open the vagina, also soaks up blood flow from the uterus).

The inner- and uppermost corner (apex) of the wound is sought.

Ruptured blood vessels (rare!) must be clamped fast and stitched.

- Good healing if the wound surfaces are free of blood.
- Episiotomy wounds bleed sometimes, perineal lacerations seldom.

The first suture is placed in the apex (innermost corner) of the wound.

Suture material
- A Mayo–Hegar needle holder is used for suturing with a round needle (apart from the skin).
- Vaginal and buried perineal suturing with Vicryl® 3–0 .
- Skin sutures with Vicryl® 3–0 or for subcuticular continuous suturing Vicryl® 4–0.

Suturing technique. Wound pockets must be avoided! Suturing must encompass the complete depth of the wound (see Fig. 9.3). If the needle is guided as in Fig. 9.3 (2), a wound pocket of varying size is created, in which blood and wound exudate collect, later lochia. The drawn through suture causes infection!

Suturing sequence (interrupted suturing)

Vaginal suturing (Fig. 9.4). Stitches as in the diagram. The wound apex in the vagina is sought. The first stitch is placed here. Further single stitches are placed 1–2 cm apart to the frenulum. The wound surfaces to be brought together are swabbed frequently so that they are dry.

Needle holder is held parallel to the vaginal surface, horizontally.

Deep perineal suturing (Fig. 9.5). 2–4 deep (buried) stitches through the musculature. On beginning the suture, the left wound margin is raised with tweezers and a medium-sized needle is inserted directly below it and pushed deeply through to the other side, where the wound margin is also raised. The needle should come out as close as possible to the wound margin; the closer it comes out the better the alignment (approximation) of the wound surfaces.

The wound margins or skin must never be included in buried sutures!

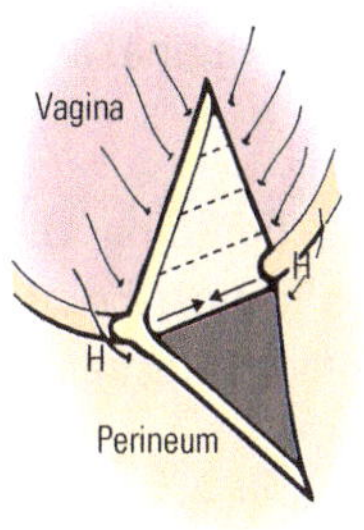

Fig. 9.4: Episiotomy repair. Vaginal suture, H = hymenal ring.

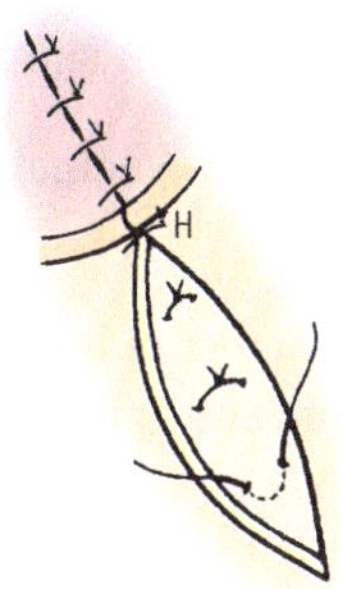

Fig. 9.5: Episiotomy repair. Deep perineal suture.

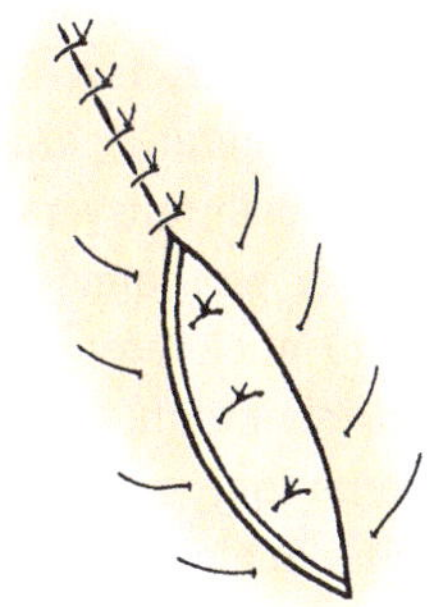

Fig. 9.6: Episiotomy repair. Skin suture with interrupted sutures.

Sutures here are also placed so that no pockets are created. The needle passes below the deepest part of the wound. The rectum must never be included!

Needle holder is held perpendicularly!

The buried sutures are knotted surgically. A further knot is added so that the thread may be cut short, which promotes healing of deep sutures.

Practice tip. If there is a danger of piercing the rectum (in particular in deep perineal suturing), the following trick is recommended: 2–3 needles are prepared and the well-moistened left index finger is inserted into the rectum. 1–2–3 stitches are made over the index finger of the left hand with the needle holder in the right until out of the danger zone. Gloves are changed and the knot is tied.

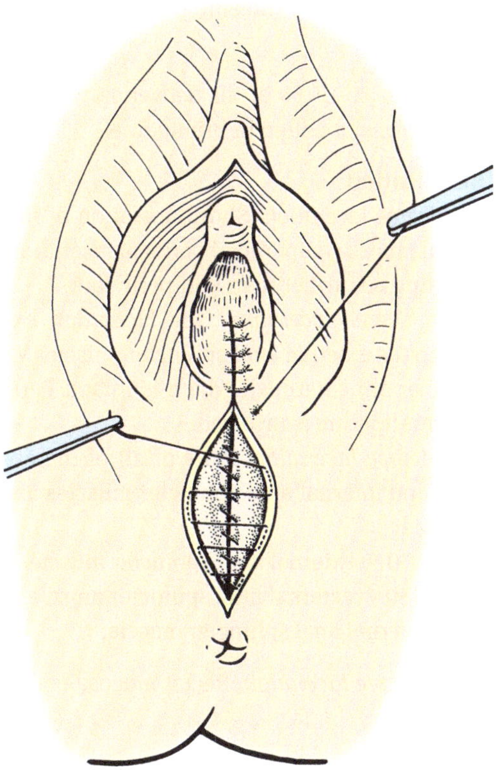

Fig. 9.7: Double-layered continuous perineal suture with subcuticular running suture.

Skin suture. Interrupted sutures (Fig. 9.6) from anterior to posterior. Needle holder is held perpendicularly! We recommend double-layered continuous perineal suturing with subcuticular running suture (Fig. 9.7).

Do not forget to remove the tampon from the vagina!

9.4 Laceration of the vagina, perineum, clitoris, labia

Laceration of the vagina, perineum

Definition. Soft tissue injury in labor involving laceration of vagina, perineal skin and perineal and pelvic floor musculature. Classification see below. Laceration of the birth canal is the correct term, as not only the perineum is affected, but also the vagina (bleeding from laceration p. 380).

Incidence. 20–30 % of all deliveries without episiotomy, more often in primiparae.

Classification

First degree laceration. Short laceration of the vaginal mucosa, superficial perineal laceration extending no further than mid-perineum.

Second degree laceration. The laceration extends to the external anal sphincter muscle (M. sphincter ani externus), which is intact. Perineal musculature is involved.

Third degree laceration. Parts or all of the external and internal anal sphincter muscles are lacerated:

- IIIa < 50 % external anal sphincter muscle.
- IIIb > 50 % external anal sphincter muscle.
- IIIc internal anal sphincter muscle.

Fourth degree laceration. Rectal mucosa is lacerated.

Repair of birth canal lacerations. Principle: approximate lacerated sections to their original position with sutures.

Timing:

- Wait until the placenta has been delivered in spontaneous delivery.
- Immediate suturing if the woman is under anesthesia (prior intervention).
- Suturing should occur within the first 30min.

Pain relief. Always carry out under local, conduction, or general anesthesia.
Drape the anus.
Ensure good accessibility to the wounded area (p. 318). A clear view is the most important thing.

First degree perineal laceration. Vaginal and perineal suture.

Vaginal suture (p. 316). If the Columna rugarum is severed on both sides it must be reattached with a row of interrupted suturing on each side.

Perineal suture. 2–4 skin sutures. The needle is inserted a few millimeters from the wound margin, passes deeply through the tissue and emerges at the corresponding place on the skin.

Second degree perineal laceration. Vaginal, deep perineal and skin sutures.

Superficial perineal suture. A number of interrupted sutures to close the wound and approximate the skin.

Anatomy. The longitudinal muscle fibers visible in second degree laceration originate from the thick Bulbocavernosus muscle. The transverse fibers below it from the deep transverse perineal muscle (see Fig. 7.16). Lateral lacerations involve the delicate superficial transverse perineal muscle. Lacerations or severance of the anterior levator sections are much rarer (occurrence: occipitoposterior presentation, sinciput presentation, face presentation, generally contracted pelvis due to acute angle of pubic arch).

Third and fourth degree perineal lacerations

Note. Procedure: 1) The sphincter ends are found. 2) The rectum is sutured: gloves and instruments are changed! 3) The sphincter is sutured. 4) The pelvic floor musculature is sutured. 5) Vaginal and perineal suturing as for second degree laceration.

1. Finding the sphincter ends. The sphincter ends are to be found directly subcutaneously where the radially folded skin of the anal region reaches the wound margins. The ends of the lacerated sphincter are deeply retracted. Finding them again is not easy for the beginner. Care must be taken not to sew something together similar to a sphincter. If one memorizes where the sphincter ends are to be found, the beginner must also find them (see Figs. 9.8 and 9.9).
   Each end is grasped with a Péan or Allis clamp and retrieved.
2. Repair of the rectum. If the rectum is injured it must be sutured first. Traction on the clamps, that is the sphincter ends, draws the wound margins of the rectum together and the wound becomes a slit. Closure of the rectum with Vicryl® 3–0 interrupted sutures is now easy. Sutures are placed 1 cm apart.
   Under no circumstances must the mucosa be involved (creation of fistulae!). This is achieved by sewing the perirectal connective tissue back-to-back (see Figs. 9.8 and 9.9).
3. Suturing of the sphincter: Gloves and instruments are changed!
   The anus is draped, both sphincter ends are retrieved with the clamps and reapproximated with several 3–0 PDS II interrupted sutures.
   Alongside the standard end-to-end approximation of the external anal sphincter muscle, overlapping approximation has been suggested. Initial prospective studies of both operation methods (end-to-end vs. overlapping) demonstrate advantages to the overlapping suturing technique (fecal incontinence, urge symptoms and perineal pain more seldom after 12 months).
4. Suturing of the pelvic floor. A row of interrupted sutures is placed above the row of rectal sutures through the pelvic floor musculature, in order to make a second degree laceration out of a third degree.
5. Suturing of vagina and perineum as for second degree laceration.

Postrepair treatment. Special postrepair treatment is not necessary. Whether the wounds heal well depends on the perineal suturing (suturing

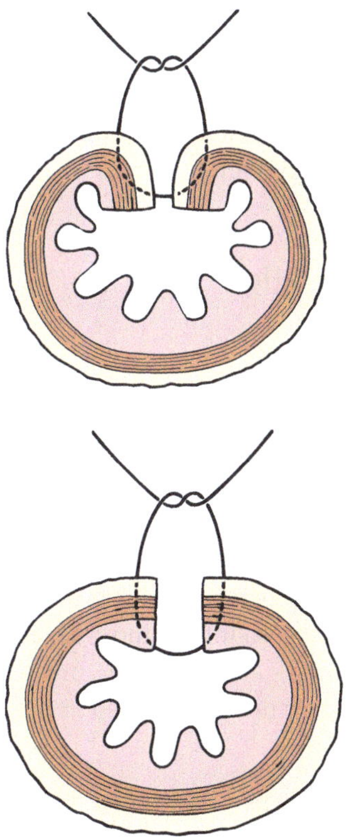

Figs. 9.8 and 9.9: Rectal suturing (after Martius). Involvement of mucosa is prohibited.

technique) and the lochia. Lochial congestion is to be avoided.
- Irrigation of the sutures after voiding (e.g., bidet) and careful drying are recommended.
- After repair of third and fourth degree lacerations laxatives bring relief, e.g., Lactulose syrup, 10ml twice a day (to avoid straining at stool); antimicrobial therapy for 5 days.
- Small steps when walking!

Note. Plastic surgery is possible 3–4 months after secondary intention healing.

Laceration of clitoris, labia

Clitoral lacerations bleed profusely (rupture of Crus clitordis) and the bleeding never stops on its own:
- Grasp with a clamp.
- Care: urethra! Deep suturing above and below the clamp.

Labial lacerations are abrasions and of no great importance. They are repaired with single interrupted sutures (Vicryl® 4-0).

9.5 Forceps operation

Obstetrical forceps.

Obstetrical traction instrument for forceps extraction made of two articulated blades (Figs. 9.10–9.13): Naegele, Kielland, Bamberger, Shute, Laufe forceps.

Naegele forceps (Figs. 9.14–9.18). The choice of forceps depends on personal experience of the operator. In some countries the Naegele forceps are preferred, and as such, unless otherwise stated, their use is described in this textbook.

Function of the forceps. The forceps is for traction. A certain amount of pressure to the head is unavoidable, however, and sometimes leads to injury of the baby.

Practice tip. Compression of the unmolded skull above the PI with the forceps to pull it into the pelvis is forbidden (→ malpractice!).

Indications, conditions. 2 questions must be answered before the forceps operation:

Indication. Is the use of forceps necessary (see indications for operative delivery, p. 315)?
Conditions: is the use of forceps possible?
6 conditions can/must be fulfilled in second stage for a live birth:
Three maternal:
1. Cervix must be fully dilated.
2. PO must not be too narrow.

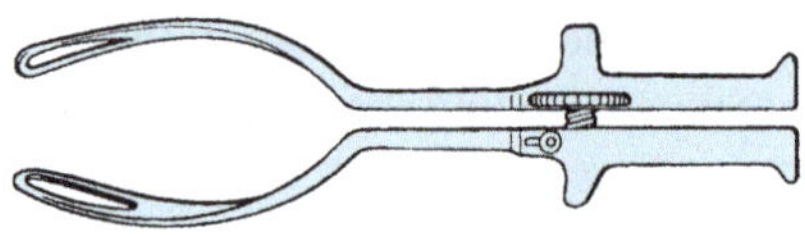

Fig. 9.10: Shute parallel forceps.

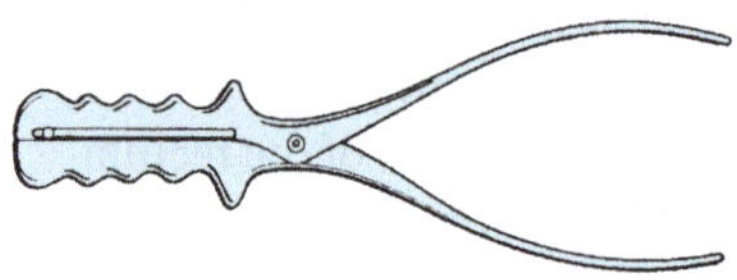

Fig. 9.11: Bamberger divergent forceps after Sipli–Krone.

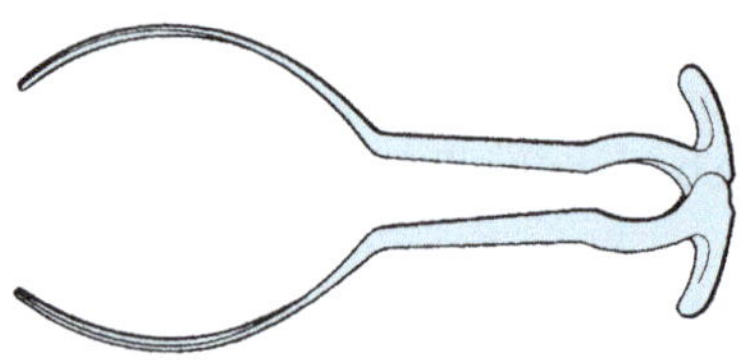

Fig. 9.12: Laufe divergent forceps.

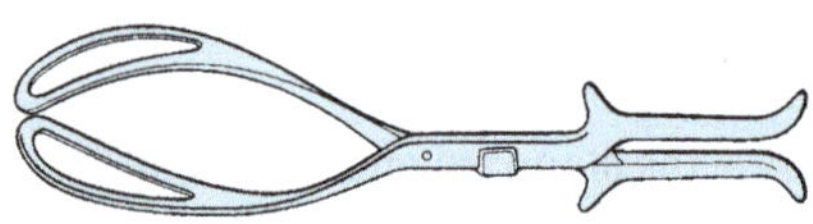

Fig. 9.13: Kielland forceps with crossed blades.

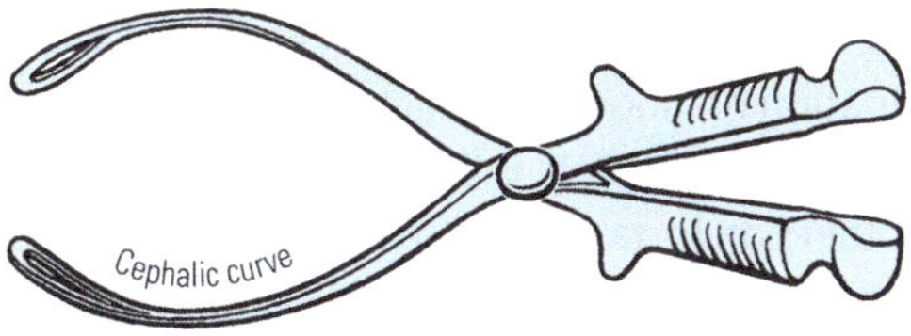

Fig. 9.14: Naegele forceps (from above).

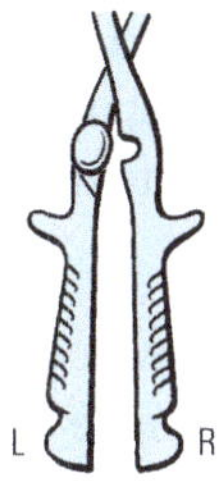

Fig. 9.17: Naegele forceps. The lock consists of pin and head on the left blade and notch on the right blade.

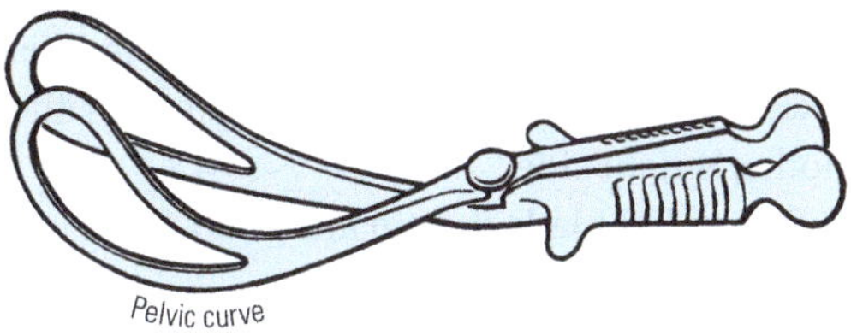

Fig. 9.15: Naegele forceps (from the side).

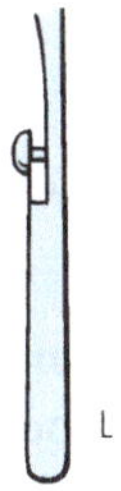

Fig. 9.18: Naegele forceps. Lock section of the left blade.

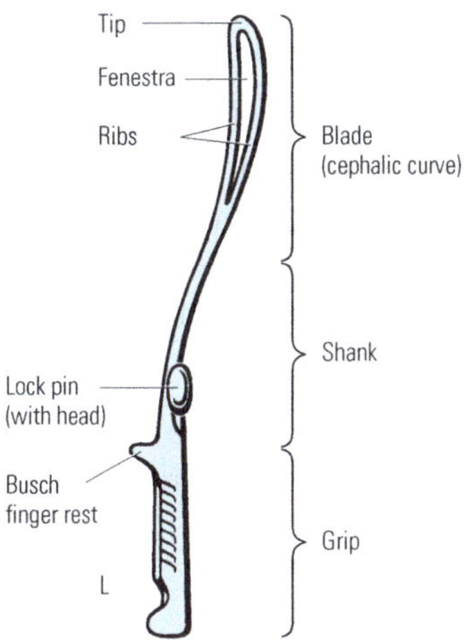

Fig. 9.16: Naegele forceps. Left blade and its parts.

3. Membranes must have ruptured or been ruptured.

Three fetal:
1. Head must be favorably positioned.
2. Head must not be too large or too small.
3. Baby must be alive.

Fully dilated cervix (→ most important condition!). If the intervention is urgent, the dilating cervix can be enlarged with incisions if necessary. If only a small lip is felt it is often possible to gently push this back over the head with the hand.

Forceps must not be used if the cervix is not completely dilated!
Only a completely inexperienced or unprincipled operator would attempt to insert the forceps through an incompletely dilated cervix and carelessly apply traction. Results are deep cervical lacerations with life-threatening hemorrhaging, laceration of the parametrium, rupture of uterine blood vessels. If the cervix is not completely dilated, one waits until it is, or performs an incision.
Pelvic outlet must not be too narrow as in generally contracted pelvis (→ acute angle of pubic arch) and funnel-shaped pelvis.

Membranes must no longer be intact. If they have not ruptured, AROM is performed with ball forceps when the bulging forebag presents.

If the membranes are intact when the forceps extraction is performed there is a danger that mechanical abruption of the placenta will occur (hemorrhage!).

Head must be favorably positioned, at least in midpelvis. On determining the fetal station the caput must be subtracted. It suggests that the level of the head is lower than it is.

The job of the forceps is to assist in delivery of a head which is in the pelvis; never draw a head from above the pelvis into it!
High forceps. The head must have entered the true pelvis with its largest circumference. It is engaged. Forceps extraction on this head is called high forceps and is no longer performed. Head must not be too large or too small.

Forceps are technically not applicable on a too large head (hydrocephalus) or a too small head (preterm delivery, anencephaly).

Whoever is in the situation of having to apply forceps in a very early preterm delivery will be surprised that the forceps slip off the too-small head because the cephalic curve is built for a normal head. Even more impressive is the experience in anencephaly: the skull is hereby so small that it cannot be fixed at all in the closed forceps. Forceps can also not be applied to a too-large head.

Baby must be alive. All forceps deliveries also involve more or less danger for the mother (see p. 332). If the baby is no longer alive and termination of labor is indicated, VE is performed (see p. 332), which is less dangerous for the mother; or in rare cases perforation followed by cranioclasm.

Application of the Naegele forceps
Rule 1: Holding and guiding the blades. The left blade is taken in the left hand and inserted on the mother's left side. The right blade is taken in the right hand and inserted on the mother's right side.
- On the left blade the pin and head of the lock are found (Fig. 9.16).
- On the right blade the notch of the lock is found (Fig. 9.17).

Rule 2: The left blade is inserted first. The right blade is inserted second and above the left, otherwise the forceps cannot be locked.

Rule 3: Application of the forceps to the head. The forceps are applied transversely to the head (Fig. 9.19, 9.20): the (transverse) diameter of the blades of the forceps (Figs. 9.21 and 9.22) is perpendicular to the longitudinal diameter of the head (Fig. 9.22; sagittal suture).

The longitudinal diameter must be known. In OP and sinciput presentations it is represented

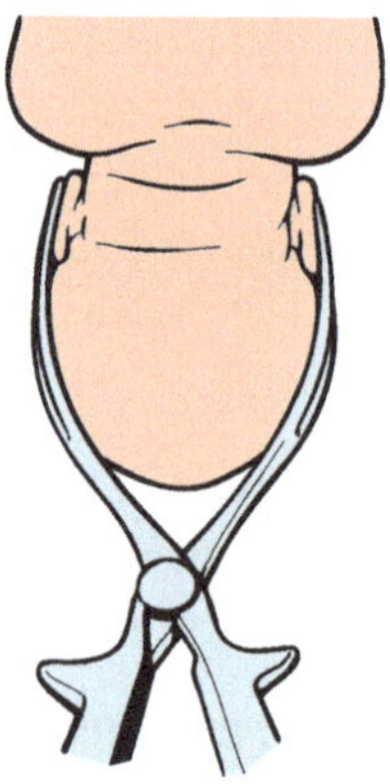

Fig. 9.19: Forceps are applied transversely to the sides of the head (Exception see p. 213).

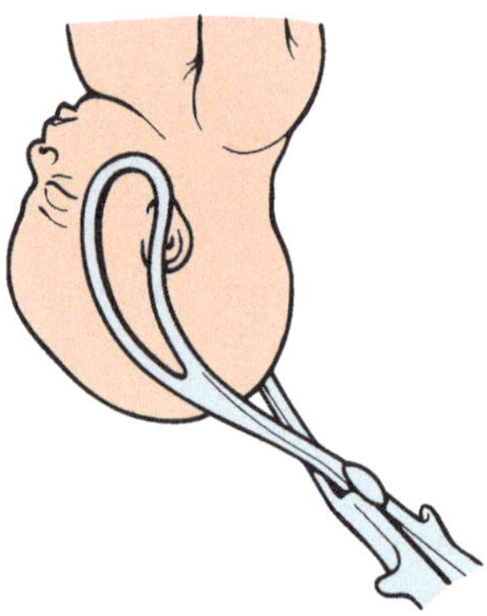

Fig. 9.20: Transversely applied forceps seen from the side.

by the sagittal suture, in face presentations by the facial axis.
The (transverse) forceps are inserted as follows:

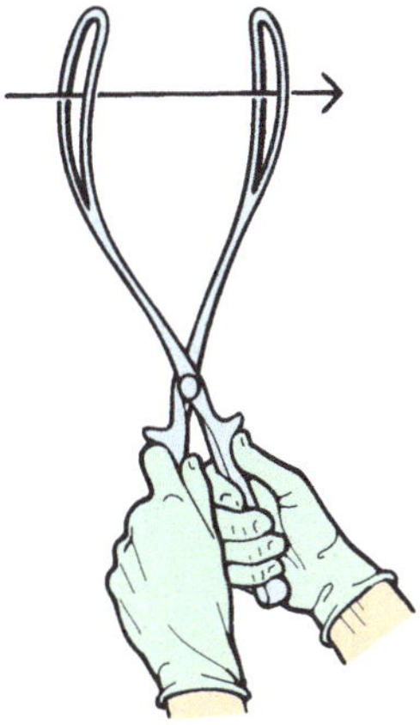

Fig. 9.21: Transverse diameter (arrow) of the forceps.

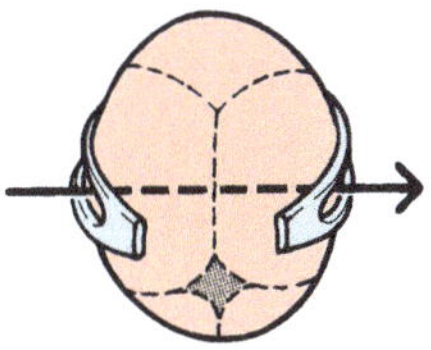

Fig. 9.22: (Transverse) diameter of the forceps (*dashed arrow*) is perpendicular to the longitudinal diameter of the head (sagittal suture).

- OA presentation – perpendicular to the sagittal suture.
- OP presentation – perpendicular to the sagittal suture.
- Sinciput presentation – perpendicular to the sagittal suture.
- Face presentation – perpendicular to the facial axis.

Practice tip. There is one exception to the rule that the forceps are applied transversely to the head: in deep occipitotransverse presentation (see p. 213) they are applied obliquely to the head.

Rule 4: Preparatory holding of the forceps (Fig. 9.23). Before the forceps are applied, they are held closed in front of the positioned woman (Fig. 9.23) in the way that they are later to be applied to the head. The left hand holds the left handle hereby, the right hand the right handle.

The tips of the forceps point toward the leading part:
- Posterior fontanelle in OA presentation.
- Posterior fontanelle to brow in OP presentation.
- Anterior fontanelle in sinciput presentation.
- Chin in face presentation.

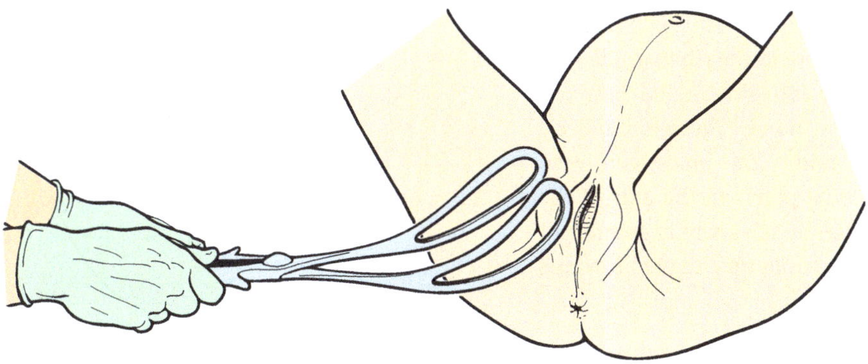

Fig. 9.23: Preparatory holding of the forceps.

The pelvic curve of the forceps is held so that it corresponds to the curve of the pelvic axis, with the concavity upwards (Fig. 9.23).
The correct preparatory holding of the forceps before application is extremely valuable. The advantage of the demand that the left hand hold the left and the right hand hold the right handle becomes obvious when the head is at an oblique angle.
There are no exceptions to this rule.

Rule 5: Protection of soft tissues. Before the forceps are introduced, at least two fingers, better four (fingers 2–4, half hand) are inserted into the vagina. The fingers are pushed deep between head and vagina. The thumb remains outside and is abducted at right angles (Fig. 9.24).

On introduction of the left blade, the fingers of the right hand; on introduction of the right blade, the fingers of the left hand are inserted to protect the vagina. The protecting hand must not be removed as long as the blade is being inserted! It is removed when the blade is finally in place.

Rule 6: Introduction of the first, left blade (Fig. 9.24). The left blade is held between thumb and index finger of the left hand at the far end of the handle as if it was to be dropped, and then held vertically in front of the vulva. The abducted thumb of the right hand is placed on the posterior rib of the blade (Fig. 9.24) and simply applies pressure to the rib to guide it so that it slides gently into the vagina between head and protective hand. The left hand on the handle only guides the blade gently so that it slides into the pelvis in the axis of the birth canal: the handle is slowly lowered (not pushed!) and at the same time moved towards the mother's right thigh.

No force is to be exerted on introduction of the blade. It must be introduced as gently as a probe! Never push the blade into the vagina: it will slide in by itself.

Rule 7: Introduction of the second, right blade (Fig. 9.26). The right blade is correspondingly introduced above the left blade. The handle is lowered and moved towards the left thigh of the mother.

Rule 8: Locking of the forceps and manual check (Fig. 9.27 and 9.28). The two crossed blades lie on top of each other and have been lowered to the perineum. They are locked with light pushing movements.

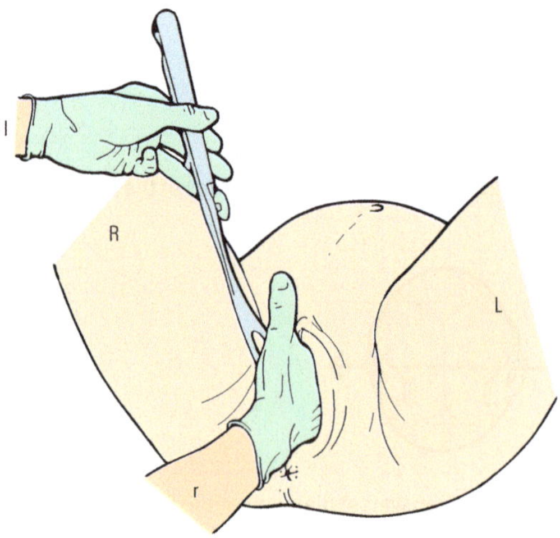

Fig. 9.24: Introduction of the first, left blade.

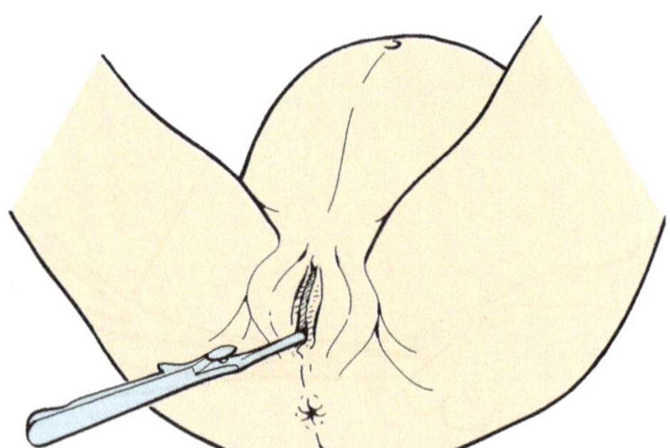

Fig. 9.25: Correctly applied left blade.

The Naegele forceps can only be locked if the right blade is above the left blade.

Difficult closure of the forceps
- The blades are crooked, not aligned on one plane but at oblique angles to each other. Remedy: the hands grasp the handles and tilt the blades in opposite directions.

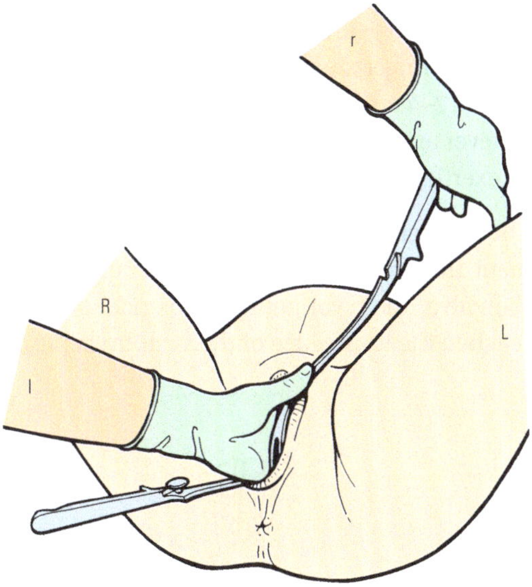

Fig. 9.26: Introduction of the second, right blade.

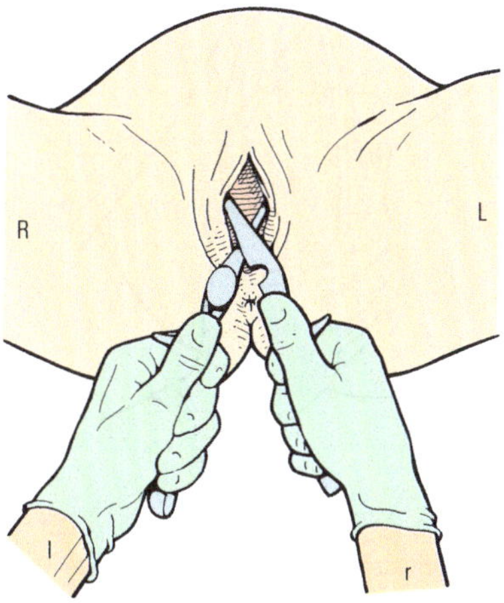

Fig. 9.27: Locking the forceps.

- The pin cannot be brought into the notch because one blade is higher than the other.
- Remedy: After a protective hand has been inserted in the vagina, the blade which is too low is carefully raised. If this is unsuccessful, removal and reintroduction of one or both blades will be.
- The forceps cannot be closed because the right blade was inserted first.
- Remedy: Removal and reinsertion of the right blade above the left blade.

Manual check. After locking the forceps a manual check is immediately performed! One hand holds the forceps; the other is inserted into the vagina and ensures that:
- Both blades are correctly applied to the head.
- No soft tissues have been trapped by the forceps: cervix, parts of the vagina, external genitalia.

Extraction
Rule 1: Holding the forceps (Fig. 9.29). The left hand holds both handles from above; the 2nd and 3rd fingers of the right hand are placed in the Busch finger rests.

The left index finger is inserted into the gap between both forceps handles to avoid overcompression of the head.

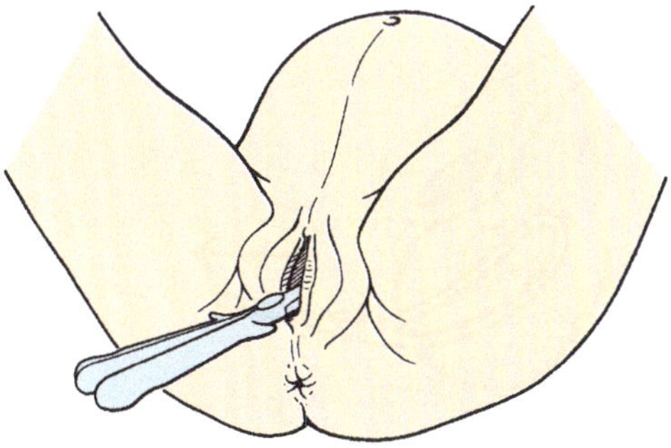

Fig. 9.28: Correctly applied, locked forceps. Handles point in the direction of traction.

The positioning of the hands is different for a face presentation (see p. 230).

Rule 2: Direction of traction. The natural birth mechanism is simulated with forceps.

Prerequisite for the use of forceps is knowledge of birth mechanics and familiarity with the mechanics of expulsion in vertex presentations.

Traction in the direction of the handles (Fig. 9.30). Horizontal traction is applied until the leading part is visible in the vulva:
- Posterior fontanelle in OA presentations.
- Posterior fontanelle to brow in OP presentations.
- Anterior fontanelle in sinciput presentations.
- Chin appears in the vulva in face presentations.

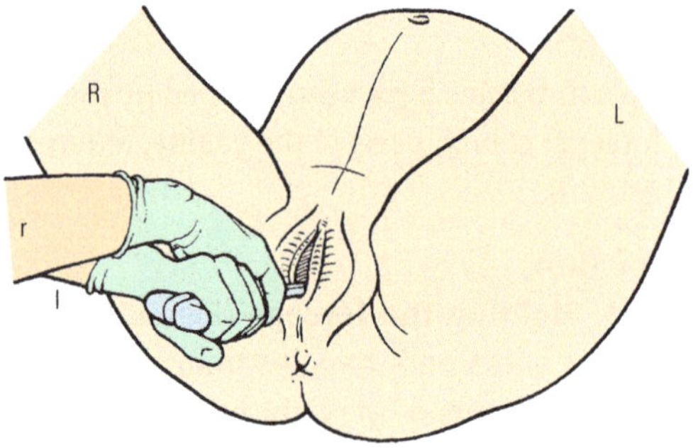

Fig. 9.29: Holding the forceps. Left hand encircles the handles from above; right hand is placed over the left, second and third fingers over the Busch finger rests. (Warning: this operator has forgotten to place the index finger between the handles!).

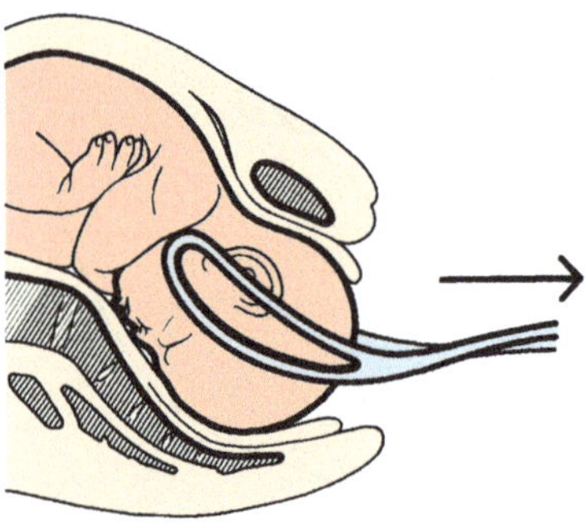

Fig. 9.30: Horizontal traction in the direction of the handles.

Position and hand change
- Position change to the left side (Fig. 9.31).
- Hand change. The right hand alone takes over the forceps; the left needs to be free to guard the perineum. The right hand is now placed across the handles (Fig. 9.31), so that index finger and thumb are above and fingers 2–4 are below the finger rests. Reason: lever arm is smaller for the desired reduced exertion of force.

The hand change is necessary, because the moment the leading part (see above) appears in the vulva, the pivot point (hypomochlion) has reached the lower edge of the symphysis pubis

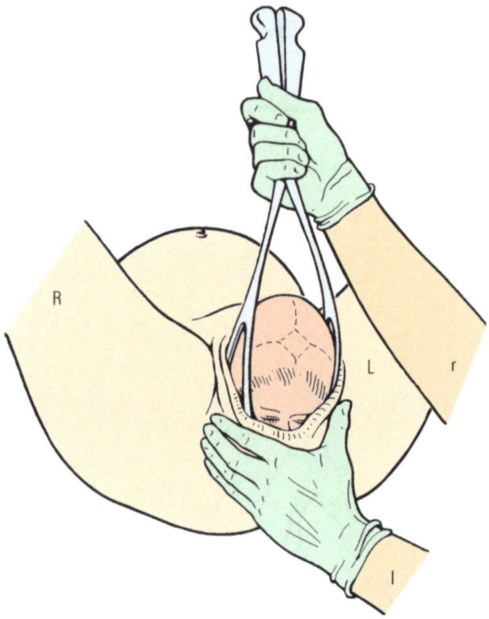

Fig. 9.31: Position (move to the left side) and hand change (right hand remains alone on the forceps, left on the perineum). Handles are raised, traction discontinued.

and rotation around the symphysis pubis and perineal protection must begin.

Pivot points are:
- Neck hairline in OA presentations.
- Anterior fontanelle, brow hairline in OP presentations.
- Brow hairline (and below) in sinciput presentations.
- Hyoid bone in face presentations.

Traction is discontinued after position and hand change, only elevation is performed:
- The right hand raises the handles of the forceps (Fig. 9.32) and moves them slowly and carefully (→ greatest perineal distension) in an arc till they are vertical, and further in the direction of the mother's abdomen (Fig. 9.33). The head is hereby guided in a curve around the symphysis pubis; the curve of Carus is negotiated.

Note. Main movements of the forceps operation: horizontal traction (in the direction of the handles), until the pivot point has reached the lower edge of the symphysis pubis. Characteristic: leading part is visible in the vulva. Elevation of the handles, to allow the head to rotate around the symphysis pubis.

Once the head has been completely born, the forceps are removed. The delivery of the baby follows as for spontaneous delivery (p. 197).

Forceps on oblique presenting head

The head is found in an oblique diameter in midpelvis or (not infrequently) on the pelvic floor. The head is in the left oblique diameter (LOD; sagittal suture from left anterior to right posterior; Fig. 9.34) or in ROD (sagittal suture from right anterior to left posterior; Fig. 9.36). As always (exceptions see below) the forceps are placed on the sides of the head. The blades (their transverse diameter) are thereby brought into an oblique pelvic diameter, in the oblique diameter perpendicular to that of the sagittal suture. One of the blades is brought laterally to the front, the other into the sacral cavity opposite. The left blade is introduced first.

Example 1. Sagittal suture in LOD, posterior fontanelle left, anterior (Fig. 9.34).

Preparatory holding of the forceps:
- The tips must point towards the posterior fontanelle, left anterior. When the forceps are held in the position that they are to be applied to the head, one sees that one blade needs to be left posterior, the other right anterior.

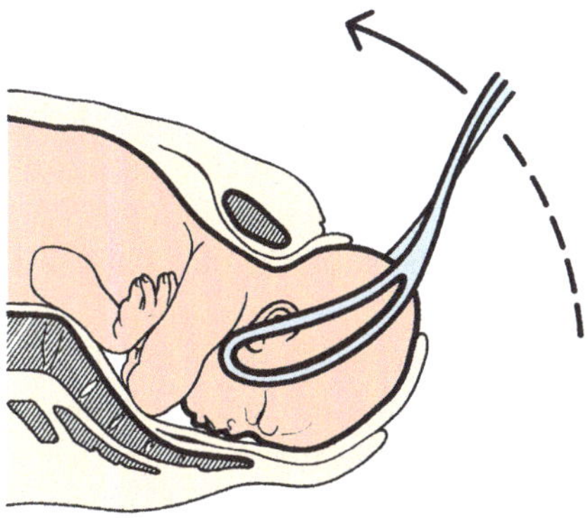

Fig. 9.32: Raising the handles of the forceps to guide the head in a curve around the symphysis pubis.

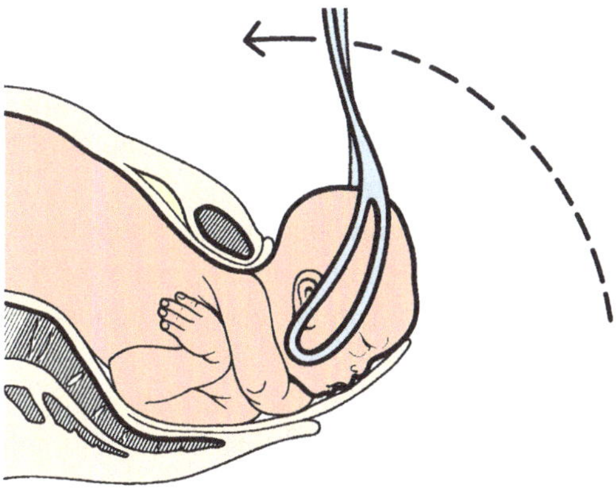

Fig. 9.33: The handles are elevated in the direction of the mother's abdomen to a vertical position.

Which blade belongs where is apparent when the forceps are correctly (p. 325) held:

- The blade which will be placed left posterior is held in the left hand, is therefore the left blade. Correspondingly, the blade which ends right anterior is the right one. This reflection is of practical value! Even experienced operators don't hesitate to make it.

The blade which needs to be posterior (in this case, the left blade), which belongs left, posterior, is introduced into the vagina without difficulty in the usual manner.
Introduction of the anterior blade (in this case, the right blade), which needs to be right, anterior (Fig. 9.34). The blade, which needs to be oblique and anterior, cannot be introduced anteriorly due to lack of space on the right. The descending pubic bone blocks direct anterior insertion.

- The blade is migrated. The blade which needs to be anterior is introduced into the vagina posteriorly, towards the sacral cavity and then moved towards the front.

Note. The blade which migrates is always that which comes to the front!

In this case it is the right blade which moves. First it is introduced right posteriorly into the sacral cavity as usual. As soon as it is correctly applied to the head in the soft tissue canal, the hold on the forceps (until now, as if holding a fountain pen) is altered:
The handle is firmly held in the whole hand like a racquet from now on. Movement of the blade now begins, in which both hands are equally involved.

- The outer hand (here the right) lowers the handle and at the same time moves the blade in such a way that it moves on the head directly from right posterior to right anterior (Fig. 9.35).
- The inner hand (here the left) is permanently active: it not only continues to cover the blade as usual (prevention of soft tissue injuries), but must also actively take hold of the blade from inside and help bring it in an arc around the head towards the front, hereby supporting the outer hand.

If the inner hand does not actively assist, movement of the blade is unnecessarily difficult. Once the anterior blade is in place the forceps are locked. A manual check is made that the forceps are correctly applied and extraction is begun.

- Traction is applied in the direction of the handles!
- When the head is in an oblique diameter traction and rotation are applied –simultaneously!

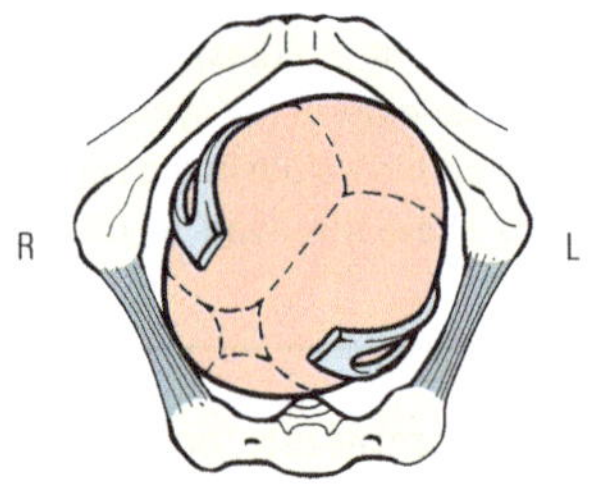

Fig. 9.34: Sagittal suture in LOD, forceps are applied in ROD.

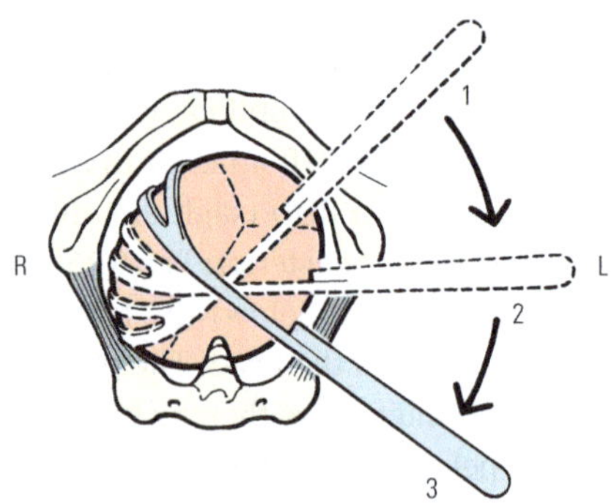

Fig. 9.35: Migration of the right blade.

Note. A rotational movement of the forceps is never to be performed without simultaneous traction!

Rotation is performed so that the lateral-lying posterior fontanelle is brought towards anterior, in this case (Fig. 9.32), anti-clockwise. Continue in the usual manner.
A third main movement is added to those already learnt, traction in the direction of the handles and elevation of the handles: traction with simultaneous rotation.

Example 2. Sagittal suture in ROD, posterior fontanelle right anterior (Fig. 9.36).

Naegele forceps are applied in LOD (Fig. 9.36)
- Left blade must end up left anterior, right blade must be placed right posterior.

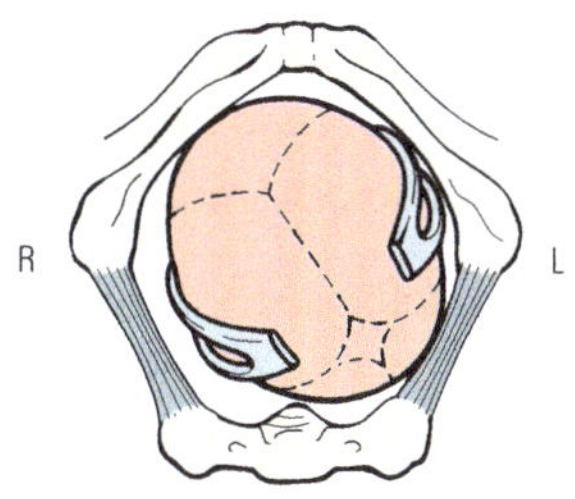

Fig. 9.36: Sagittal suture in ROD, forceps are applied in LOD.

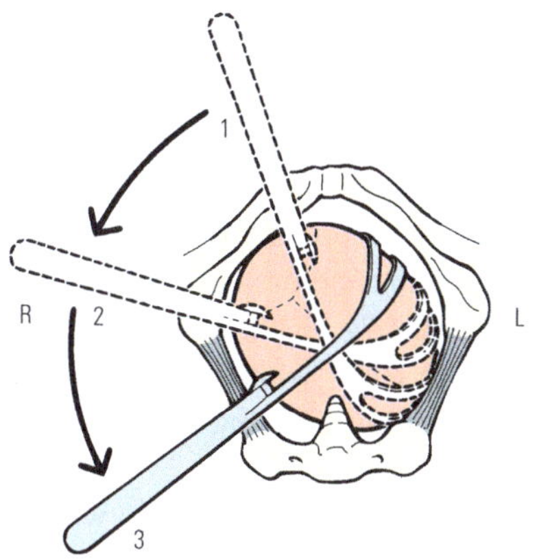

Fig. 9.37: Migration of the left blade.

- The left blade must therefore migrate (Fig. 9.37).
- As always, the left blade is introduced first.
- While traction is applied, clockwise rotation is simultaneously performed.

The technical rules of the art of forceps have thus been discussed. Several hours on a model suffice to practice their use. Forceps operations are different in practice (see below).

Risks, prognosis. Even the experienced operator cannot avoid injuries; this lies in the nature of the method! Forceps are simply not as gentle as nature in the normal course of labor!

Prognosis. The operator's experience, skill and technique are crucial, alongside the quality of diagnosis:
- Station of the head.
- Attitude and presentation of the head.
- Cervical status.
- Soft tissue status.
- Condition of mother and baby.

Head. Station, attitude, presentation. To use forceps is to imitate the natural birth mechanism. Clear findings of what is presenting (OA, OP, sinciput or something else) are necessary.
A command of vertex presentations is necessary. Anyone unfamiliar with the mechanism of birth (at least the movement of expulsion) of all cephalic presentations must not attempt a forceps extraction.
Someone attempting to treat a sinciput presentation as an OA presentation, for example, would cause great damage.
Controlled pressure. The mistake is often made of pressing the left hand, which holds the handles of the forceps closed, too tightly together during traction. This can lead to serious head injury. Pressure is unavoidable, or the head would not follow and the forceps would slip off. It must, however, be as minimal as possible.

- Overcompression is life-threatening: laceration of the tentorium, intracranial hemorrhage, skull fracture.
- After closure of the forceps a gap remains between the handles, which must be held open during application of traction by placing a cloth or finger in it.

Traction is applied horizontally, or in the direction of the handles (see above). Over and above that, it is a matter of feeling to find the direction of least resistance into which the handles must be brought.

Practice tip. The extent of trauma to maternal soft tissues is determined by the type of traction. Each application of traction must be slow and calm! Apply traction intermittently during contractions. Pause after each application.

Intermittent traction. As long as there is no need for great haste, traction is applied intermittently, coincident with the expulsive contractions! Pauses aid distension of the soft tissues and reduce the pressure of the forceps on the skull. The blades are slightly loosened in the lock during the breaks.
Guide the head. The head must be particularly slowly and carefully guided around the symphysis pubis on crowning and birth. Birth over the perineum should take several minutes. This makes protection of the perineum easier.
Main dangers to mother and baby are injuries.

Maternal injuries. Common: perineal laceration, longitudinal vaginal laceration (particularly when the head has been rotated), clitoral lacerations, cervical lacerations (usually extending from the free lip of the cervix), tearing or severance of one of the levator shanks (even when the walls of the vagina are uninjured). Therefore:

Note. After every forceps extraction inspection for lacerations is carried out: of the vagina using large specula and of the entire cervix using clamps.

Rare are: vesicovaginal and rectovaginal fistulae.

Injuries to the baby. Common are: laceration of the tentorium with ruptured veins (particularly V. cerebri) or Sinus transversus, sinus petrosus superior and consecutive hemorrhaging in the posterior cranial cavity: death as a result of compression of the medulla oblongata. Further: skin abrasions, contusions, hematoma, nerve paralysis (particularly N. facialis, good prognosis), skull fracture, which is often accompanied by rupture of the venous sinus.

9.6 Vacuum extraction, ventouse extraction (VE)

Definition. Form of operative assistance for delivery of the baby's head using vacuum cup, which is placed on the scalp and firmly applied to it by means of negative pressure; creates a caput succedaneum (known as "chignon").

Instruments. The flat, metallic suction cup is the main part. It comes in 3 sizes: 60, 50, and 40 mm diameter. The suction cup is placed on the scalp. With the aid of a tube system, a vacuum bottle and a pump the air is slowly pumped out of the cup, which is firmly applied to the head after 2–3 min as a result. The negative pressure is displayed on the pressure gauge and regulated. The vacuum creates a caput succedaneum, the size of which corresponds to the cup size.

As an alternative silicon extractor cups are used. They create no chignon, but adapt to the shape of the head (Fig. 9.38). Reduced force of extraction is possible with them; they are therefore most useful in assisting delivery from the PO or pelvic floor.
In recent years extraction instruments with a hand pump for creating negative pressure have been developed: Kiwi® Fig. 9.38, and estab-

lished themselves – also for transabdominal delivery of the head in CS.
On extraction of the head the hand holds the tube which leads to the cup, traction is not applied to the tube but to a traction chain which runs through it, and is attached by means of a plate inside the cup.
Once the head has been delivered the vacuum is released by opening a valve and the cup removed. Cup, tube and chain can be sterilized.

Indication, conditions. As for forceps extraction, before a VE is performed 2 questions must be answered: indication: is the VE necessary (see indications for operative delivery, p. 315)? Conditions: is the VE possible?

There are **five conditions** for the VE.

Three maternal:
- Cervix must be fully dilated.
- PI and PO must not be too narrow.
- Membranes must no longer be intact.

Two fetal:
- Head must be in a favorable position for VE.
- It must be possible to attach a cup to the presenting part.

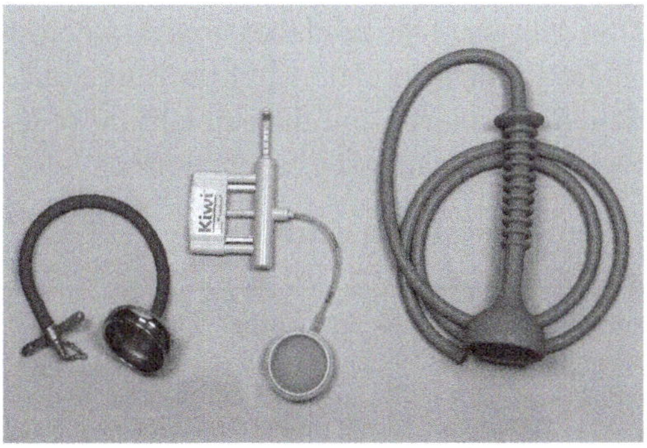

Fig. 9.38: Vacuum extraction cups. Left metal cup, right silicon cup, both to be attached to an air pump; in the center a cup with hand pump to create negative pressure.

Cervix must be fully dilated. A VE is only performed on an almost completely dilated cervix in exceptional cases. It will be easily possible to push the narrow lip back during the attempt.

PI and PO must not be too narrow. CPD must not be present, in particular in VE from the PI.

The operator recognizes when the head does not respond to traction, discontinues the VE and performs a CS.
If the PO is contracted, the special type of PO contraction known as funnel-shaped pelvis and the acute pubic arch angle are to be considered.

Membranes must no longer be intact. Otherwise AROM is performed (p. 282) before the VE.

Head must be in a favorable position for VE. Determine station of the head (see diagnosis of level of descent p. 162). In contrast to forceps, VE from PI (high VE?) is allowed, in particular in arrested labor.
Contraindication of pelvic inlet VE is intrauterine acidosis.

It must be possible to attach a cup to the presenting part. Attachment is impossible in anencephaly and face presentation.

Technique. The laboring woman is in the lithotomy position in bed or operating chair. The obstetrician sits in front of her. Outlet or pelvic floor VE may be possible without analgesia. Conduction anesthesia (epidural anesthesia) is recommended for more difficult VE, also from mid-pelvis.

The metal cup is placed on the leading part of the baby's head so that the small metal thorn on it corresponds to the leading part. The cup is lightly pressed onto the head, whereby neither cervical lip nor vaginal tissue is trapped. The pump is switched on and an artificial caput slowly created. This should completely fill the cup as a prerequisite for the firm attachment of the cup to the head. A vacuum of 0.3kg/cm^2 is created. After a 2–3 min pause and a check that no cervical or vaginal tissue has been trapped it is increased to a maximum of 0.9 kg/cm^2.

Traction coincident with contractions. Traction is only applied during contractions with increasing and abating force.

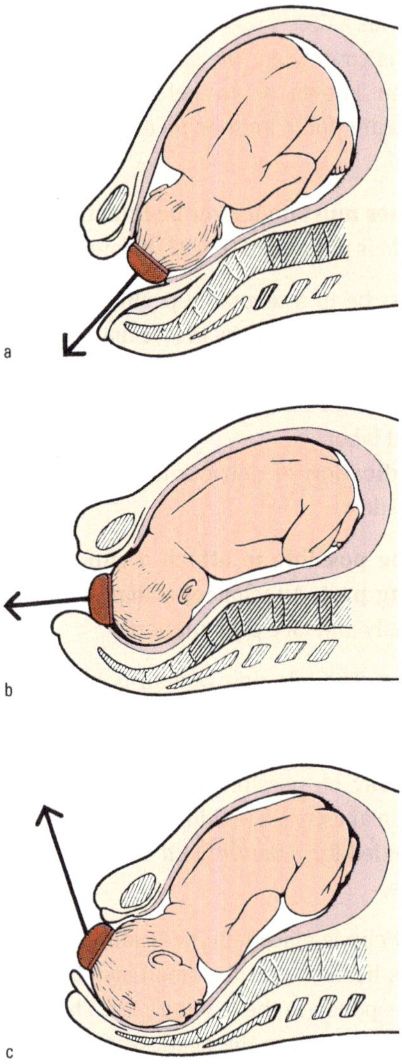

Fig. 9.39a, b, c: Vacuum extraction. Application and direction of traction (arrow) for different stations of the head.

Direction of traction. Traction is applied in the direction of the pelvic axis (Fig. 9.39). In the interval between contractions the instrument is released. The contractions become stronger or return due to pressure on the cervical ganglia and reflex.

Controlled traction. The maximum exertion must be felt on practice and the head delivered very slowly. If cup detachment is felt, traction must be discontinued. The cup reattaches.

Cup detachment. The cup detaches when traction is applied in the wrong direction. It is reapplied without difficulty; however, there is a risk of intracranial pressure variations and scalp abrasions, particularly if the VE is prolonged or continuous traction is applied.

Caput succedaneum. This method potentially causes a substantial caput, which may look frightening, but resolves completely (Restitutio ad integrum) within 12–24 h.

Rotation of the head. Rotating the cup can bring about the desired head rotation. It is usually more successful if the cup is applied eccentrically and the head is rotated in the direction in which rotation is desired. The descending, or rather extracted head often only follows the rotation when it has reached the pelvic floor.

After delivery of the head the pump is switched off. During delivery of the trunk pressure equalization is achieved and the cup falls off of its own accord or can easily be removed.

Forceps vs. vacuum extraction

Note. The preference for one or other of the two vaginal operative methods depends rather on the obstetrical school, and with which method more personal experience exists, as prospective studies are not available.

Forceps extraction. Risk for the mother: soft tissue injury.

Risks for the baby. Soft tissue injury, forceps mark, intracranial hemorrhage, skull fracture.

Vacuum extraction. Risk for the mother: none.

Risks for the baby: cephalhematoma, intracranial pressure variations, retinal hemorrhage, intracranial hemorrhage, skull fracture.
VE is not performed in:
- Preterm deliveries < 32 weeks.
- Sonographically estimated birth weight of ≤ 1,600 g.

Vaginal operative delivery is a predisposing factor for the development of fecal incontinence. VEs cause significantly less injuries to maternal perineum and vagina. Anal ultrasound detected occult sphincter defects in 82 % of women after forceps extractions and 48 % after VE.
Current practice is summarized in Tab. 9.1.
Delivery from pelvic floor. Forceps and VE are equivalent, in particular when the sagittal suture is in the AP diameter. Crucial here is the urgency and personal experience.
Delivery from mid-pelvis. VE is superior to forceps. The head is not forced to rotate, but rather autorotates when space permits. The additional space requirements for forceps do not apply.

Tab. 9.1: Preferred method of vaginal-operative delivery method (VE, forceps) dependent on findings.

Diagnosis	Forceps preferred	VE preferred
Head on pelvic floor, sagittal suture AP	+	
Head on pelvic floor, fetal indication	+	
SGA	+	
Head on pelvic floor, sagittal suture oblique or transverse		+
Head above pelvic floor		+

9.7 Cesarean section

Definition. Cesarean section (CS). Operative termination of pregnancy or labor under surgical opening of the abdominal wall and uterus and delivery of the baby (→ Sectio caesarea intraperitonealis supracervicalis). Performed under general anesthetic or epidural anesthesia in supine position with a slight left tilt (prophylaxis against supine hypotensive syndrome).

Indications. Indications for CS are undergoing a change: they are dependent on the risk that the CS itself poses for the mother and potential complications and sequelae. CS has been recognized and implemented as an emergency measure for the rescue of the mother for about 100 years, and as an emergency measure for the rescue of the baby (initially only term fetuses, later, in the last 30 years also for the rescue of preterm fetuses) for about 50 years. Saving the life of the baby then played the main role, while today the prevention of damage to the fetus is in the forefront (change in indication to damage prevention). Advances in obstetrics and neonatology are clearly measurable in the collective of women with life-threatening abnormalities and their prevention by CS from the improved figures of maternal mortality and morbidity, and the drastically increased chance of survival and damage-free survival of even extremely small preterm babies. The low rates of maternal mortality and morbidity achieved make it easier for the obstetrician to establish an indication.

In addition, there has been a development over the last 15 years towards increased requests for CS in the absence of any medical indication (known as Cesarean delivery on maternal request, or CDMR).
Increase in rate of CS. The change in obstetrics described and other factors have led to a worldwide increase in the rate of CS (central Europe

1960 3 %, USA 2007 32 %). The following reasons exist: older parous women, for the first and following births, increasing newborn weight, early recognition of imminent hypoxia, the use of cardiotocography without FBS, avoidance of difficult vaginal-operative delivery methods, avoidance of or insufficient experience with vaginal-operative maneuvers in breech delivery, the desire of the parents and the obstetrical team for scheduling, the low stress tolerance of the laboring woman and her partner in labor, fear of pelvic floor damage resulting in prolapsed genitals, urinary and anal incontinence, reduced stress for the – potentially compromised, possibly immature – fetus, fear of the pain of contractions, avoidance of litigation conflicts.

Types of indication in relation to onset of labor. Two types:
- **Primary** (= primary indicated, elective) CS before onset of contractions or before ROM.
- **Secondary or emergency** (= secondary indicated) after onset of labor or ROM.

Some secondary cesarean deliveries are emergency interventions in which labor should be terminated as rapidly as possible. The time from decision for CS to delivery (so-called **decision to delivery time**) is particularly important in this group and should not be longer than 20min.

Absolute indications. If there is a compelling reason for the termination of pregnancy or labor, this is an absolute indication for CS, for example in the case of abnormalities endangering mother and baby, such as in the life-threatening bleeding from the uterus, fetal hypoxia, cord prolapse or uterine rupture. This group makes up about 10 % of all cesareans.

The absolute indications for rescuing the mother without consideration for the baby in the forefront shaped the classical obstetrics of our fathers and grandfathers. Maternal injuries from vaginal-operative deliveries performed to avoid the mortality and morbidity associated with CS were also accepted. In obstetrics today, every chance is consciously taken for the baby if absolute indications are maternal indications for the termination of the pregnancy.

Relative indications. If a conditional risk exists, abnormalities or risk factors are present which suggest that the capacities of mother and baby will be exceeded during labor; the relative indication for a CS is established. For example in cases of prepathological cardiotocogram and increased blood flow resistance in the umbilical artery, in IUGR, prolonged labor in cases of mild maternal cardiac disease or arrested labor in mid-pelvis in a brow presentation. This group makes up about 80 % of all cesareans.

The consideration of benefits for mother and baby as a result of the shortened or avoided labor and the risks of the operation for mother and baby is at the center of the relative indications. The improvement in operational and anesthesia methods, the availability of blood and blood substitutes, thrombosis prophylaxis, and antimicrobial therapy have reduced maternal morbidity and mortality, and as a result the chances for the unborn child, even in cases of extreme immaturity, are significantly higher.
The changed conditions in obstetric practice, the introduction of obstetrical quality controls, and the altered goal of ensuring not just survival, but damage-free survival have led to the increased rate of CS in the last 30 years. It is not possible to provide lists of schematic indications, in particular for relative indications. In such cases establishment of indication is dependent on numerous hospital conditions, the findings of the pregnant and laboring women, the organizational level of the hospital and many more. It is not schematization of the decision that is required in relative indications, but

individualization and generous preventative establishment of indications. Dependent on the organizational level of the hospital, questions such as lack of experience in vaginal breech deliveries or inexperience in performing vaginal operative delivery techniques will be incorporated in the establishment of indications.

It is clear that, particularly in the area of relative indications the advent of preventative thinking which has increased the rate of CS, has also undoubtedly improved the chances of the babies. For example an LGA or macrosomic baby after prior shoulder dystocia, a 13 % probability of recurrence is given. If Erb's palsy resulted from shoulder dystocia in a prior birth, generous, preventative indication from the mother's perspective, and from the responsible obstetrician's perspective is understandable, particularly if a macrosomic baby is expected.

The preventative attitude in obstetrics was thus formulated by Huch in 2000: "Weighing up of the benefits between cesarean mortality on the one hand and fetal and maternal morbidity risk in vaginal-operative delivery on the other determines the decision for absolute and relative indications for CS today." And Max Hirsch as early as 1927: "Abdominal delivery therefore takes the place of artificial preterm delivery, high forceps, version and extraction and dismemberment of the fetus". Max Hirsch's expulsion from Germany, the emphasis of natural forces have unfortunately suppressed these thoughts for decades.

Cesarean delivery on maternal request (CDMR). Approximately one in ten CSs – this is the estimated number – is performed today in the absence of medical indication. Possible reasons for a desire for CS are fear of labor and the unavoidable pain, reduction of risks for the baby, fear of pelvic floor injury with the dangers of urinary and anal incontinence and genital prolapse.

The possibility of planning is often seen as an advantage of CS near term, for example for a multipara. If additional risk factors happen to exist, for example White D – diabetes mellitus or a prior liver transplant establishing an indication is easier.

The short- and long-term advantages and disadvantages of elective cesarean must be brought up in the informed consent discussion and on establishing an indication: increased risk of infection, increased rate of postoperative anesthesiological problems (after epidural or spinal anesthesia), delayed breast feeding begin, increased incidence of placenta previa and faulty implantation in following pregnancies, increased risk of uterine rupture in a subsequent vaginal delivery, higher incidence of respiratory morbidity of the baby (Boyer and colleagues), including incidence of RDS, decreased rate of PPH and operative complications, decreased incidence of urinary stress incontinence and of intracranial hemorrhage, neonatal asphyxia and encephalopathy, neonatal infections as well as birth injuries to the baby.

A feared complication in a subsequent pregnancy is faulty placentation such as placenta increta or percreta in placenta previa on the uterine wall in the region of the old CS scar. If this has not been diagnosed in pregnancy, severe intraoperative hemorrhaging with dramatic consequences can be expected. Antenatal diagnosis allows for a differentiated operation and treatment plan (Henrich and colleagues).

The placentation risks described increase with repeated cesarean sections. According to Silver and colleagues, Placenta accreta occurred in 0.24 % of first, 0.31 of second, 0.57 of third, 2.13 % of fourth, 2.33 % of fifth and in 6.74 % of sixth and all further CS deliveries. Placenta accreta was found in 67 % of cases of placenta previa in the fifth or upwards CS deliveries. Hysterectomies were necessary in 9 % from 6 CS and above.

Primary and secondary indicated cesarean section. The most important indications for CS today are:
- Prior CS (p. 311).
- Breech presentation.
- Arrested labor.
- Hypoxia.

Breech presentation. Management of birth of singleton breech presentation has been controversially discussed since the seventies. The discovery that breech babies were more frequently affected by acidosis and more often compromised after vaginal birth than after CS (Kubli) resulted in the recommendation that all breech babies be delivered per CS. In spite of comprehensive studies on this topic (Hannah), a clear recommendation for pregnant women at term is difficult. Although the original recommendation was confirmed in the multicenter study quoted, doubts have been raised as to the methodology of the study. Therefore, after individual risk assessment, vaginal delivery continues to be a reasonably safe and gentle birth mode for term babies in a breech presentation.

The following indications for primary CS in singleton breech presentations are recognized (guideline): IUGR (< 10 percentile), sonographically estimated weight ≥ 3,800 g, fetal disproportion (head circumference >> abdominal circumference), footling presentation, pelvic anomaly. The indications for secondary CS are made according to the standard obstetrical principles.

Arrested labor. If progress is arrested in first or at the beginning of second stage despite good contractions, mother and baby are at risk for birth injuries or septicemia as a result of ascending infection. In such cases termination of the birth via CS is indicated.

In spite of the commonly used definition of arrested labor (no progress for over 2 hours despite good contractions), it is not possible to standardize indications because many subjective influences are involved (assessment of the contractions, variability of findings among other things). Maternal fever and/or tachycardia are clinical parameters, however, which should lead to a reevaluation of birth management. Establishment of an indication for CS as opposed to vaginal operative delivery in second stage has changed. Whereas earlier, high forceps and vacuum extractions were regularly practiced, in obstetrics today, difficult vaginal operative deliveries are avoided in favor of CS because of the risk of injury to mother and baby which these interventions pose.

Threat of hypoxia. Although fetal hypoxia in labor can be sufficiently accurately diagnosed using fetal blood sampling (FBS), the diagnoses "imminent hypoxia" and "fetal distress" are often given in routine clinical practice as imprecise descriptions of fetal condition. Only lectronical fetal monitoring solely can be mentioned in this context. It is generally to be used as a screening method. In certain FHR patterns indicative of hypoxia, the diagnosis of "fetal hypoxia" can then be made using FBS, with the consequence of termination of labor by CS as response. If electronical fetal monitoring alone is used, an increased number of operations to terminate labor can be expected.

Operating technique. Transperitoneal delivery of the baby through the opened lower uterine segment (Sectio caesarea intraperitonealis supracervicalis) is almost exclusively practiced.

The pregnant or laboring woman is positioned in a supine position at a 15° lateral tilt on the operating table. Opening of the peritoneal cavity is performed via the suprapubic Pfannenstiel incision. After incision and division of the bladder peritoneum and separation of the bladder, a 2-cm-long incision is made in the midline of the lower uterine segment (Fig. 9.40). The uterotomy is extended bluntly to the

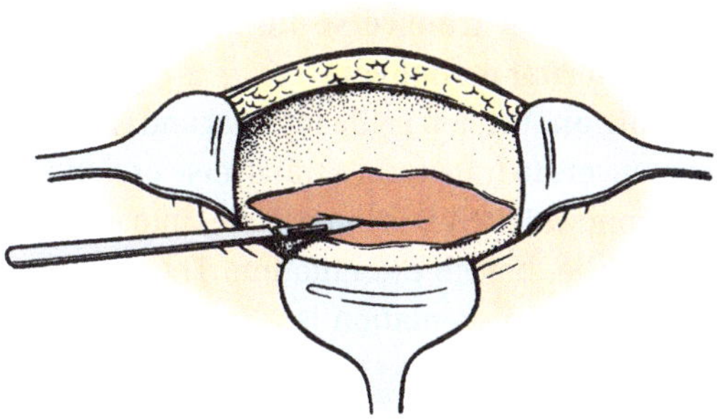

Fig. 9.40: Incision of the lower uterine segment in the midline after separation of the bladder.

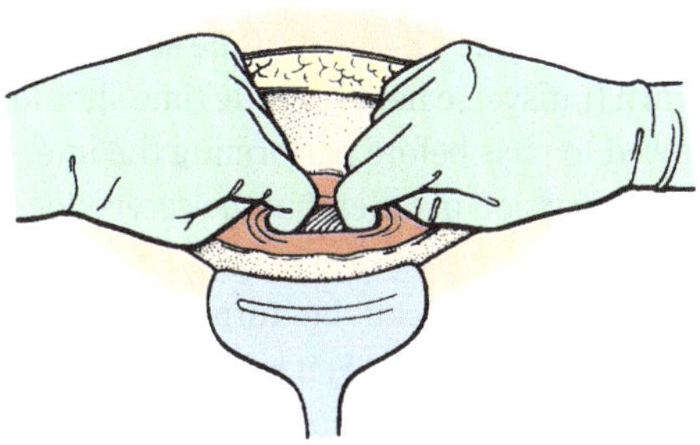

Fig. 9.41: Lateral digital extension of the incision in the lower uterine segment; rupture of membranes is to be avoided if possible.

left and right with the fingers (Fig. 9.41). After delivery of the baby, complete placenta, and amniotic membranes, the uterotomy is usually closed in one layer with interrupted or running sutures. A Canadian multicenter study (Bujold and colleagues, 2010) found significantly lower rates of uterine rupture for closure of the uterotomy in two layers.

Alternative methods of operation. Variations from this procedure are to be considered in some cases. Some obstetricians prefer, for example, the isthmo-cervical longitudinal incision for babies in breech presentation and < 1,500g.

Misgav-Ladach CS method (so-called gentle CS). The skin incision is made 3 cm below the connecting line of the anterior superior iliac spines (ASIS; spinae iliacae anteriores superiors), significantly higher than the Pfannenstiel transverse incision. Subcutaneous tissue and fascia are opened 2–3 cm in the midline, and then the fascia below the subcutaneous tissue is opened with half-open scissors. The rectus muscles are manually separated by pushing to either side, the peritoneum is opened bluntly by stretching with the finger and the hole in the peritoneum manually extended. The uterotomy is performed above the peritoneal flap without separating the bladder. After the placenta has been manually removed, closure of the uterotomy is performed with a continuous locking stitch from the operator to the assistant. The peritoneum is not closed, the fascia suture is continuous, the subcutis remains open, and skin closure is made with three back-and-forth sutures and the use of four Ellis clamps for 5 min.

Various studies have demonstrated shorter operating times, reduced blood loss, reduced requirements for pain relief, and shorter hospital stays of this modified technique in comparison to the classical Pfannenstiel technique. Studies on the question of whether leaving the visceral and parietal peritoneum open has consequences have found no disadvantage in peritoneal nonclosure.
Since cesarean delivery has become a routine procedure, many modifications to the technique and to postoperative management have been developed, whereby not all steps have been separately evaluated with adequate study methods. Today the following validated methods are implemented: single-dose antimicrobial prophylaxis, nonclosure of visceral and parietal peritoneum, not suturing the subcutaneous layer if < 2 cm, thrombosis prophylaxis with low-molecule heparins, early mobilization, early intake of fluids and solids instead of elaborate IV fluid administration and special postoperative diet.

Intraoperative complications
- Injury to the urinary bladder.
- Injury to the ureter.
- Hemorrhage, coagulation disorder < 0.5 %.
- Amniotic fluid embolism.
- Anesthesia incident.

Maternal morbidity in the puerperium
- Endometritis up to 10 %.
- UTI up to 10 %.
- Faulty wound healing or infection up to 10 %.
- Anemia ≤ 0.5 %.
- Pneumonia ≤ 0.5 %.
- Thrombosis, embolism ≤ 0.5 %.
- Subileus, ileus ≤ 0.5 %.
- Septicemia ≤ 0.5 %.

Maternal mortality. 1 death in 59,000 cesarean sections.

9.8 Combined version

Definition. Artificial alteration of the fetal lie (rotation in the uterus), to make delivery possible or easier. Most dangerous intervention for the mother in labor. Today only used for the second twin

Classification. Version can be from transverse lie, breech or cephalic presentation.

9.8.1 Version from transverse lie

Two possibilities: external version and combined or internal podalic version from transverse lie (version using internal and external maneuvers).

External version from transverse lie. Only external maneuvers are used (procedure as for external cephalic version from breech presentation, p. 244).

Version from transverse lie using internal and external maneuvers
Definition. Version using internal and external maneuvers to transform a transverse or oblique lie (from which SVD is impossible) into a longitudinal lie, breech presentation. The thus created breech presentation is a footling breech, presenting with one or both feet.

Indication. Transverse lie of the second twin (→ internal podalic version).

Timely version is that performed when the cervix is fully dilated, as with the second twin. After delivery of the first twin, if the second remains in a transverse lie, very little time should be allowed to pass before performing the internal podalic version in order that the cervix does not close again.
How well the baby can be turned depends mainly on the volume of AF; it is largest if membranes are intact, less the more time has passed since ROM occurred.
A dead baby in transverse lie can be delivered via internal podalic version and extraction. The cervix must be completely dilated in order that extraction may then be performed.

Method of internal podalic version
Conduction or general anesthesia is obligatory! Without analgesia the woman would bear down, contractions would begin, and version would be impossible. In addition, an arm or the umbilical cord could prolapse.

External examination, if necessary sonographic diagnosis. The side on which the breech is lying must be known to ensure that the correct hand is used.

Positioning of the woman in labor. Version is begun in a supine position. If, during the operation it becomes clear that the feet are not reachable when the mother is supine she is to be assisted on to her side, the side on which the breech is lying. The birth assistant helps repo-

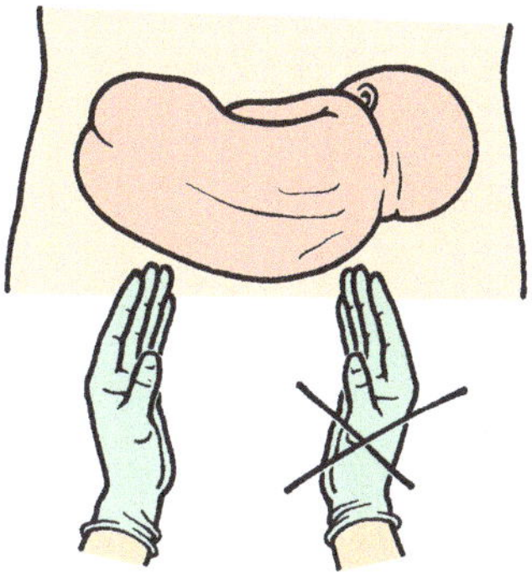

Fig. 9.42: Left transverse lie, left hand is inserted.

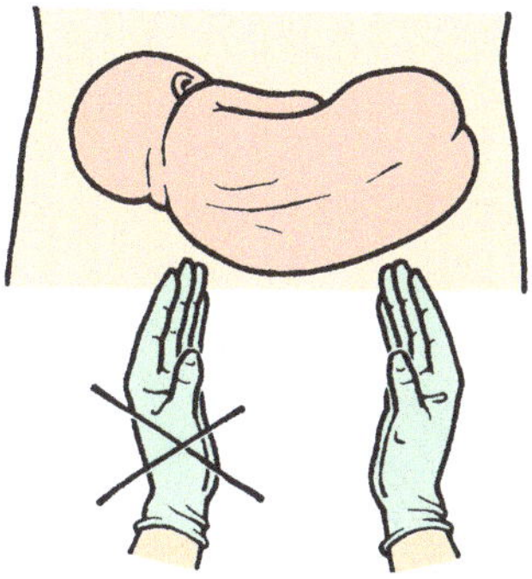

Fig. 9.43: Right transverse lie, right hand is inserted.

sition the woman, the hand of the operator remains in the uterus. The birth assistant lifts the one leg over the head of the operator.

Sterile external hand. A sterile drape must be placed on the woman's abdomen. The external hand must remain sterile; it may be necessary that the hand working externally become the internal hand. This is impossible, however, if it has previously been placed on the unsterile abdomen.

Selection of the internal hand (Figs. 9.42 and 9.43). The hand which corresponds to the breech (feet) is introduced into the vagina:
- Left hand (Fig. 9.42) in left transverse lie (head left, breech right).
- Right hand (Fig. 9.43) in right transverse lie (head right, breech left).

Selection of the foot. In dorsoanterior transverse lie the lower foot is used, in dorsoposterior both feet.

Steps. Version is to be performed with slow, smooth movements! The internal wall of the uterus is to be touched as little as possible as contractions may be stimulated, or an internal contraction ring created, which would restrict the mobility of the baby.

Three steps (Tab. 9.2).

Tab. 9.2: Three steps of internal podalic version from transverse lie.

Step I	Step II	Step III
Hands at the head (Fig. 9.45)	Hands at the breech (Fig. 9.46)	External hand at head, internal hand at foot (Fig. 9.47)

Step I. Both hands at the head. Head and shoulder are pushed up (Fig. 9.45)

Aim. To free the pelvic inlet, that is, push the presenting part, the shoulder, out of the PI so that the hand can be introduced into the uterine cavity.
- The external hand pushes the head away from the iliac wings towards the fundus.
- The fingers of the internal hand are pressed together in a conical form (Fig. 9.44) and inserted into the uterus via rotational movements. It pushes the shoulder upwards in the same direction in which the head is being pushed externally. The shoulder is presenting in the PI and blocks the entry, and thus access to the uterine cavity.
- If the shoulder cannot be pushed upwards, elevating the pelvis helps.

Step II. Both hands on the breech. Grasping the foot (Fig. 9.46).

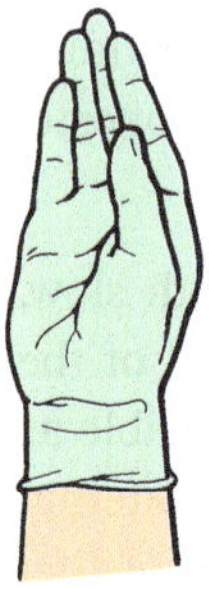

Fig. 9.44: Conical form of the fingers of the internal hand on insertion.

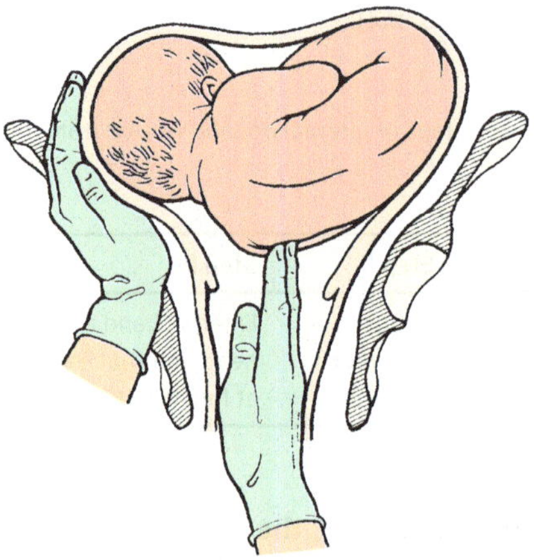

Fig. 9.45: Internal podalic version from transverse lie: Step I: hands at head.

Proceeding slowly, cautiously, and calmly is the quickest way to achieve the goal of finding the foot.

- The external hand pushes the breech firmly into the pelvis towards the internal hand.
- The internal hand feels from the shoulder along the side of the baby to the breech, which is pushed towards it by the external hand. The hand feels along the breech to the thigh, from the thigh to the foot/feet. Foot/feet is/are grasped without exertion of traction!

Identifying the foot. Recognizing the foot is not easy, when it has to be found by the hand amongst four extremities which are pressed together in an enclosed space. The foot lies

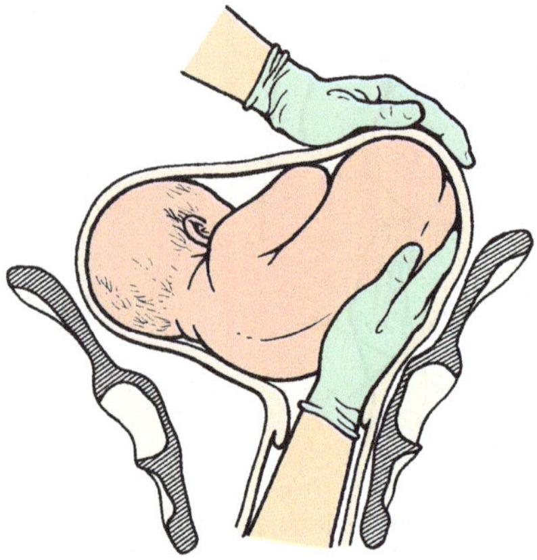

Fig. 9.46: Internal podalic version from transverse lie: Step II: hands at breech.

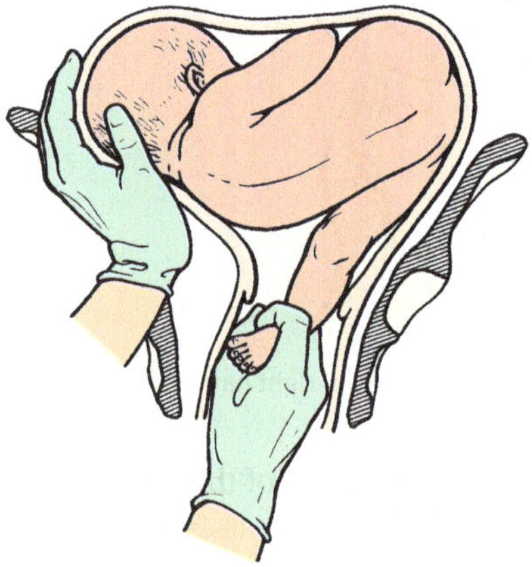

Fig. 9.47: Internal podalic version from transverse lie: Step III: external hand at head again, internal hand at foot.

- usually posteriorly in dorsoanterior transverse lie,
- usually anteriorly in dorsoposterior transverse lie, crossed in front of the abdomen,
- near the head if the legs are extended.

Practice tip. Differential diagnosis: hand vs. foot. Don't grasp the hand! Feel carefully whether hand or foot was grasped! Rule: follow along the side of the baby with the internal hand, over breech, thigh and calf to the foot, in this way, no hand will be grasped.

The external hand is just as important as the internal in the version. Each act begins with the external hand. The success of the procedure depends on both hands working together.

Step III. External hand at the head again, internal hand on the foot (Fig. 9.47). Beginning the version:
- the external hand goes back to the head at the side and pushes it upwards, towards the fundus;
- when the head follows the upwards pressure, the foot (or feet) held by the internal hand are slowly pulled down and guided out.

Practice tip. The version will not be successful if the foot is removed before the head is pushed upwards!

The version is completed when the head is felt in the fundus and the knee is visible and remains in the vulva.
2–3 min pause between version and extraction. The extracted foot is released, the operator washes in the antiseptic solution and waits, observing the cardiotocogram. Advantages:
- The arms and head, which have been moved from their positions by the version, have time to reassume their normal positions. If the extraction is continued directly after the version the arms extend and delivery of arms and head will be difficult.
- The baby needs time to recover after the version.

Only the inexperienced continue immediately with the extraction without letting go of the foot.

9.8.2 Version from cephalic presentation

Definition. Rotation of the baby (today only performed on the second twin) from a cephalic into a breech presentation using combined maneuvers. Procedure similar to that of internal podalic version.

9.9 Dismembering operations: perforation, cranioclasm

Perforation

Definition. Dismembering operation on living or dead fetus. The intrauterine perforation of the fetal head allows brain matter to escape and reduces the size of the skull, making passage through the birth canal possible or easier.

Indication. Hydrocephalus (see p. 136) of live fetus.

Perforation was seldom performed on a live baby. The only indication was hydrocephalus.

Conditions. Cervix must be 3–4 cm dilated. An incompletely dilated cervix is not a contraindication for perforation!

For cranioclasm the cervix must be further dilated.

Procedure in four steps

Step 1. The head is fixed in place from outside. It is a mistake not to let the head be pushed firmly into the pelvis from outside. The birth assistant holds the head firmly in place from above so that it can safely be perforated from below.

Fixation prevents the head from retreating when the perforator is pushed into it and the perforator from slipping and perforating the bladder for example.

Practice tip. Fixation of the head is so important that it is only somewhat exaggerated to say: it is not the operator who perforates the skull by inserting a sharp instrument into it from below, but the person who firmly presses the head into the pelvis from above until perforation is complete.

Step 2. Introduction of the left hand to find the perforation site. If the head is high it is difficult to reach. The left hand must penetrate deeply in order to reach the head. Sagittal suture and fontanelles are felt. Perforation should be performed in a suture or fontanelle. If possible, the operation is performed with good visibility using large specula.

Step 3. Perforation of the head. The Smellie perforator (blades inside; Fig. 9.48) and the Naegele perforator (blades outside) are available.

The perforator is held firmly in the right hand, while the left is held around the instrument to protect tissues. The perforator is introduced carefully and slowly into the vagina, protected by the left hand, with lowered handles. The tip of the instrument is placed on the scalp over the perforation site. The axis of the perforator must be perpendicular (Fig. 9.49). From this point on, energetic fixation of the skull from above, outside, is crucial. The tip of the perforator is sunk carefully and very slowly into the scalp. A certain amount of pressure is required with minimal force. Once this has happened, it will feel as if the tip of the perforator is stuck in the galea. It can now no longer slip towards the bladder or rectum. Only now, when this feeling is present, can the instrument perforate the chosen site on the fetal skull with firm, increasing pressure and simultaneous brief rotation of the instrument. Care must hereby be taken that the instrument is held perpendicular to the skull until it is deeply embedded in the skull and can no longer slip out. The left hand is then removed from the vagina, the handles are taken in both hands, opened and closed (Fig. 9.50). The perforator is rotated 90°, again opened and closed. Perforation is complete. The instrument is closed and removed.

Step 4. Expulsion of brain matter is assisted with dressing forceps, irrigation. Once the

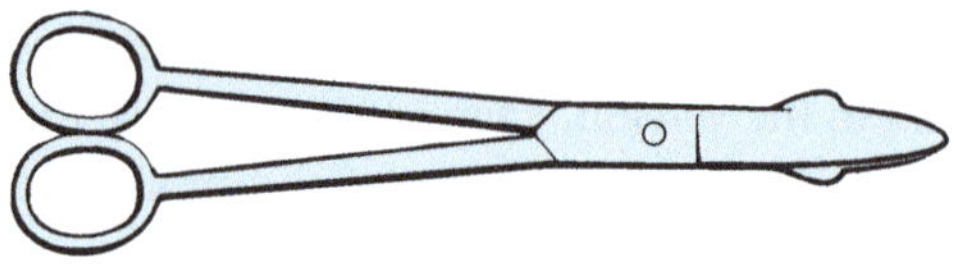

Fig. 9.48: Smellie perforator (blades inside).

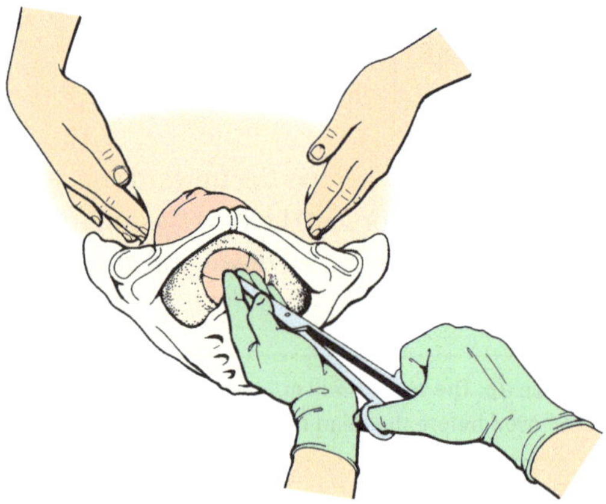

Fig. 9.49: Perforation of the head (I; Stoeckel).

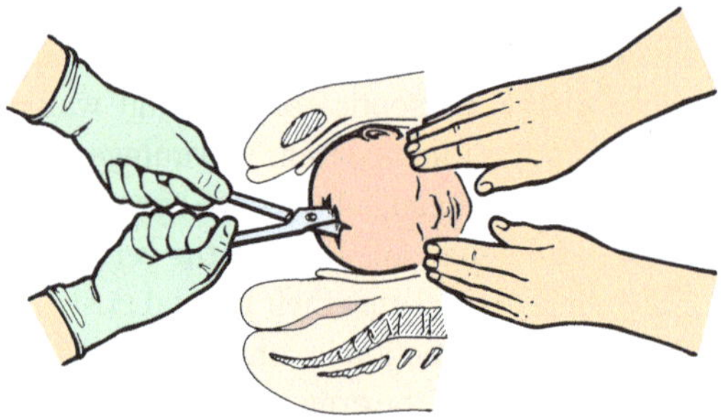

Fig. 9.50: Perforation of the head (II).

skull has been perforated and brain matter has escaped, the operation is complete; the threat to the mother's life has been diverted.

Cranioclasm is not always necessary after perforation, especially as it is a much more difficult procedure.
It is now possible to wait for spontaneous delivery. If contractions are good the empty, compressed skull will soon be born.

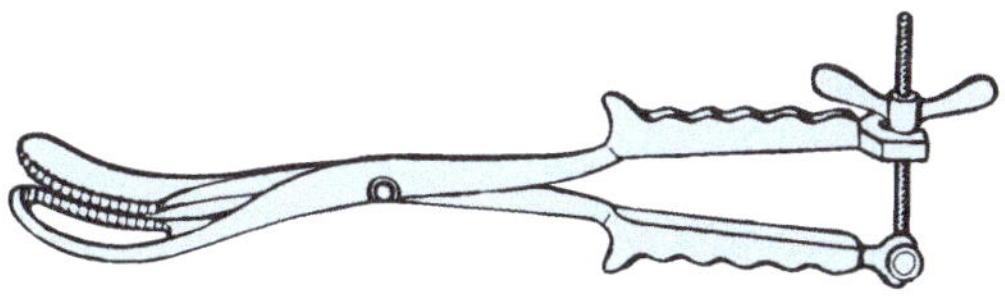

Fig. 9.51: Braun's cranioclast.

Note. Repeated for less experienced doctors: it is the perforation, not the cranioclasm which removes the mother from danger!

Cranioclasm

Definition. Compression of the perforated skull with the cranioclast and extraction of the fetus by the perforated head.

Conditions

- Cervix ≥ 6–7 cm.
- True conjugate ≥ 6 cm.

Method. Braun's cranioclast (Fig. 9.51). We recommend Braun's cranioclast, which has two parts:

- Inner blade: solid with rough, ribbed surface.
- Outer blade: smooth, fenestrated.

Before the instrument is inserted it should be understood how the ends of the blades fit together (Fig. 9.51). Then orientation should be gained as to which side the face/occiput is on.

Practice tip. The cranioclast is prevented from losing its hold when the blades grasp the face or the occipital plate.

The parietal bones should be avoided, as they are easily detached. It is best to position the blades over the face. The face bones resist detachment; they loosen, but are not easily detached. The occipital plate is softer.

Six steps

Step 1. Insertion of the inner blade. The inner, solid blade is inserted first (Fig. 9.52) and pushed as deeply as possible into the head through the perforated opening in the direction of the part of the skull to be grasped.

Most important is fixation of the head from above, as for the perforation.

Step 2. Insertion of the outer, fenestrated blade (Fig. 9.53).The hands steadying the head from outside must release it for this step; otherwise it is not possible to insert the second blade correctly or high enough. The blade must cover as much of the face as possible. The second (internal) hand covers the blade and guides its tip to the face.

An assistant must hold the inner blade or it will fall out.

Step 3. Articulation of the blades in the lock. The blades are now brought together loosely in the lock, the wing nut attached and lightly tightened. The further apart the handles are, the more is grasped, the better the cranioclasm sits. Articulation of the blades in the lock is not equivalent to closure of the instrument as in forceps. The instrument is not closed until it is tightly screwed (Step 5).

Step 4. Manual check. Check whether the inner blade penetrates the skull as deeply as possible and the outer blade has not trapped a portion of cervix or vagina.

Step 5. Closure, screwing together. The cranioclast is screwed together as tightly as possible with the screw and wing nut (Fig. 9.54) so that it cannot slip off. After screwing together another manual check is performed just in case.

Step 6. Traction (Fig. 9.55). Traction is slowly applied in the direction of the pelvic axis:

- First steep downwards traction.
- Then more horizontally.
- Then increasingly upwards.
- Finally steeply vertical.

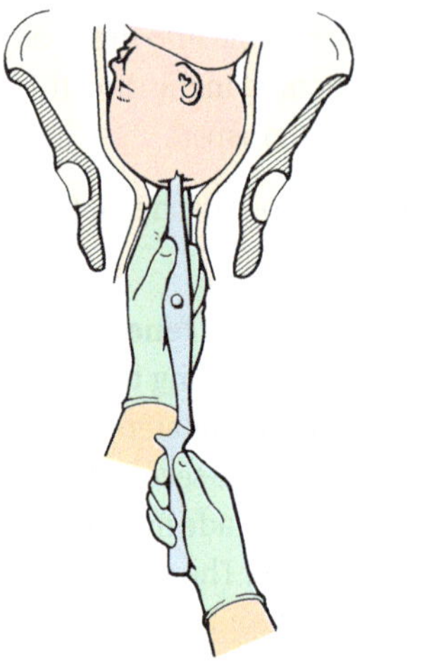

Fig. 9.52: Cranioclasm (Step 1). Insertion of the inner, solid blade as deeply as possible, head is firmly fixed from above.

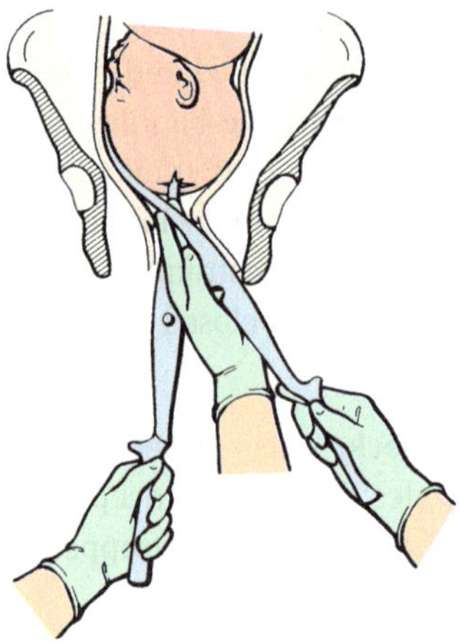

Fig. 9.53: Cranioclasm (Step 2). Insertion of the outer blade. Cover as much of the face as possible. Head released.

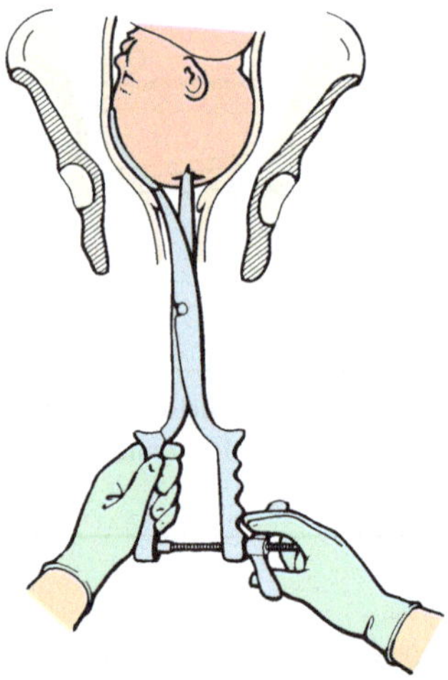

Fig. 9.54: Cranioclasm (Step 5). Blades are tightly (!) screwed together.

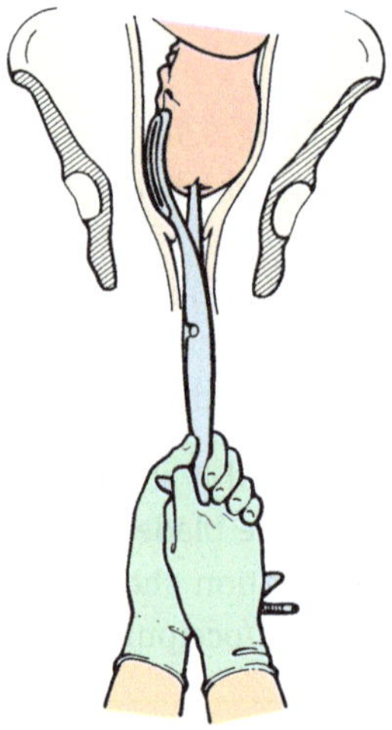

Fig. 9.55: Cranioclasm (Step 6). Manual check, slow traction. Direction of traction is the direction of the handles.

Practice tip. Always apply traction in the direction in which the handles are pointing (direction of traction is the direction of the handles!) The smaller the cervix opening, the slower the traction.

After each application of traction one hand is inserted into the vagina to check. If the rim of the cervix is too taut traction is discontinued. A pause is made with the head in position before the extraction is continued. Care must be taken of sharp bone edges or splinters, which are covered with the fingers or removed with Boer's bone forceps (Fig. 9.56).

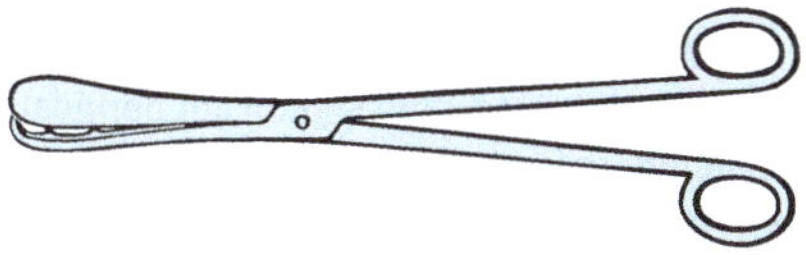

Fig. 9.56: Boer's bone forceps.

If the fetus is macerated, it is often not possible to apply the cranioclast, or the bones detach. In such cases, 2–3 strong grasping clamps (best: Collin clamps) are used to grasp and extract the skull. Boer's bone forceps are also suitable for grasping and extracting.
After extraction the uterine cavity is manually explored and vagina, perineum and cervix are inspected (large specula, good lighting).

Perforation of the after-coming head. If the after-coming head remains stuck above the pelvic brim (contracted pelvis, hydrocephalus) in breech delivery the baby can only be saved with the Wigand–Martin–Winckel maneuver (p. 263).

If a head cannot enter the pelvis, perforation of the after-coming head is to be performed; a technically difficult maneuver due to the thick soft tissues of the neck.

Two methods

Occiput anterior, behind the symphysis pubis (Fig. 9.57). The fetus is pulled firmly downwards by the feet. The posterior edge of the sternocleidomastoid muscle is sought. The perforator is inserted from this edge and pushed through the soft tissues in an oblique angle towards the base of the skull. The perforator is withdrawn and the finger inserted in the soft tissue canal thus created. The finger is pushed up towards the place where the spine meets the base of the skull. The gap between atlas and the base of the skull is sought, and the perforator is inserted into it with minimal force. The posterior atlantooccipital membrane is hereby pierced. After a number of lever-

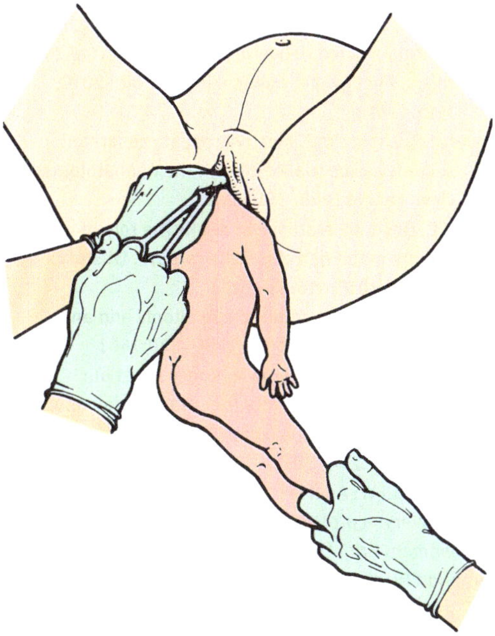

Fig. 9.57: Perforation of the after-coming head.

ing movements of the perforator the foramen magnum is open and brain matter can escape. Stirring movements can be made with dressing forceps in order to speed up the escape of brain matter. Extraction of the collapsed head by the trunk follows.

Occiput posterior, chin behind the symphysis pubis. The base of the skull is penetrated from the floor of the mouth. The perforator is inserted at the front of the neck and through the soft tissues between the branches of the lower jaw in the direction of the base of the mouth.

References

Bahl R, Patel R, Swingler R er al.: Neurodevelopmental outcome at 5 years after operative delivery in the seconcl stage of labor: a cohort study. Amer J Obstet Gynecol 2007; 197:147

Berghella V, Baxter JK, Chauhaın SP: Evidence based surgery for cesarean delivery. Amer J Obstet Gynecol 2005; 193:1607

Boucoiran I, Valerio L, Bafghi A, Delotte J, Bongain A: Spatula-assited deliveries: a large cohort of 1065 cases. Eur J Obstet Gynecol Reprod Biol 2010; 151:46–51
Boyers SP, Gilbert WM: Elective repeat caesarean section versus trial of labour: the neonatologist's view. Lancet 1998; 351:155
Bujold E, Goyer M, Marcoux S, et al.: The role of uterine closure in the risk of uterine rupture. Obstet Gynecol 2010; 116:43–50
Chaliha C, Sultan AH: Midline episiotomy and anal incontinence. Brit Med J 2000; 320:1601
Dahlke JA, Mendez-Figueroa H, Rouse DJ, et al.: Evidence-based surgery for cesarean delivery: an updated systematic review. Amer J Obstet Gynecol 2013; 207:294–306
Faridi A, Rath W: Anal incontinence after vaginal delivery: a prospective study in primiparous women. Brit J Obstet Gynaecol 1999; 106:1107
Fernando RJ, et al.: Repair techniques for obstetrical anal sphincter injuries: a randomized controlled trail. Obstet Gynaecol 2006; 107:1261
Gei AF, Pacheco LD: Forceps: Still an option? Current Women's Health Reviews 2008; 4:56
Hannah ME, Hannah WJ, Hewsorı SA et al: Planned caesarean section versus planned vaginal birth for breech presentation at term: a randomised multicentre trial. Lancet 2000; 356:1375
Holmgren G, Sjoholm L, Stark M: The Misgav Ladach method for cesarean section: method description. Acta Obstet Gynecol Scand 1999; 78:615
Kolas T, Saugstad OD, Daltveit AK, et al.: Planned cesarean versus planned vaginal delivery at term: Comparison of newbom infant outcomes. Am J Obstet Hynecol 2006; 195:1538
Lydon-Rochelle M, Holt VL, Easterling TR, Martin DP: Risk of uterine rupture during labor among women with a prior Cesarean delivery. N Eng J Med 2001; 345:3
Lyell DJ, Caughey AB, Hu E, Daniels K: Pertoneal closure at primary caesarean delivery and adhesions. Obstet Gynecol 2005; 106:275
National Institutes of Health: State-of-the-Science Conference Statement: Cesarean Delivery on Maternal Request. Obstet Gynec 2006; 107:1386
Richter R, Bergmann RL, Dudenhausen JW: Previous caesarean or vaginal delivery: Which mode is a greater risk of perinatal death at a second delivery. Eur J Obstet Gynecol Reprod Biol 2007; 129:51
Rieger N, Wattchow D: The effect of vaginal delivery on anal function. Aust N Z J Surg 1999; 69:172
Robinson JN, Norwitz ER, Cohen AP, et al.: Episiotomy operative vaginal delivery, and significant perineal trauma in nulliparous women. Obstet Gynecol 1999; 181:1180
Robson M, Hartigan L, Murphy M: Methods of achieving and maintaining an appropriate cesarean section rate. Best Practice & Research Clinical Obstetrics and Gynaecology 2012; http://dx.doi.org/10.1016/j.bpobgyn.2012.09.004
Royal College of Obstetricians and Gynaecologists: Operative vaginal delivery. Guideline No. 26. Revised October 2005
Royal College of Obstetricians and Gynecologists: Operative vaginal delivery. Guideline No. 26, January 2011
Samuelsson E, Ladfors L, Wennerholm UB et al: Anal sphincter tears: prospective study of obstetric risk factors. Brit J Obstet Gynaecol 2000; 107:926
Signorello LB, Harlow BL, Chekos AK, Repkr JT: Midline episiotomy and anal incontinence: retrospective cohort study. Brit Med J 2000; 320:86
Silver RM, Landon MB, Rouse DJ, et al.: Maternal Morbidity associated with multiple repeat Cesarean deliveries. Obstet Gynecol 2006; 107:1226
Smith GCS, Pell JP, Cameron AD, Dobbie R: Risk of perinatal death associated with labor after previous Cesarean delivery in uncomplicated term pregnancies. JAMA 2002; 287:2684
Stark M, Chavkin Y, Kupfersztain C, et al.: Evaluation of combinations of procedures in cesarean section. Int J Gynecol Obstet 1995; 48:273
Sultan AH, Stanton SL: Occult obstetric trauma and anal incontinence. Eur J Gastroenterol Heparol 1997; 9:423
Sultan Al, Johanson RB, Carter JF,: Occult anal sphincter trauma following randomized forceps and vacuum delivery. Int J Gynecol Obstet 1998; 61:113
Sultan AH, Monga AK, Kumar D, Stanton SL: Primary repair of obstetric anal sphincter rupture using the overlap technique. Brit J Obstet Gynaecol 1999; 106:318
Tempest N, Hart A, Walkinshaw S, Hapangama DK: A re-evaluation of the role of rotational forceps: retrospective comparison of maternal and perinatal outcomes following different methods of birth for malposition in the second stage of labour. BJOG 2013; DOI: 10.1111/1471-0528.12199
Tolcher MC, Johnson RL, El-Nashar S, Colin P: Decision-to-incision time and neonatal outcome:

A systematic review and meta-analysis. Obstet Gynecol 2014;123:536–48
Watson F, Owen P: Perineal trauma following vaginal delivery without episiotomy. Eur J Obstet Gynecol Reprod Biol 2010; 148:202–3
Zeitlin J, Di Lallo D, Blondel B et al: Variability in cesarean section rates for very preterm births at 28–31 weeks of gestation in 10 European regions: results of the MOSAIC project. Eur J Obstet Gynecol Reprod Biol 2010; 149:147–152

10 Antepartum and postpartum hemorrhage

Overview

Antepartum hemorrhage (APH)

- First half of pregnancy: Miscarriage. Molar pregnancy, p. 360. Trophoblastic tumor, p. 362. Ectopic pregnancy, p. 363. Cervical carcinoma.
- Second half of pregnancy: Placenta previa, p. 369. Placental abruption, p. 374. Varicose hemorrhage. Cervical carcinoma.

Intra- and postpartum hemorrhage (PPH)

- First stage: Placenta previa, p. 369. Low-lying placenta, p. 369. Placental abruption, p. 374. Marginal sinus bleeding. Rupture of the uterus. Uterus rupture is rare in first stage, can occur in hydrocephalus (p. 136), however.
- Second stage: Rupture of the uterus, p. 306. Bleeding from laceration, p. 388. Labial, clitoral laceration, p. 320. Velamentous insertion.
- Third stage: Atonic PPH, p. 380. Factor I deficiency hemorrhage, p. 377.

Fibrinogen (Factor I) deficiency hemorrhage (see p. 374) in:

- Abruption of a normally located placenta, p. 374.
- Retained products of conception, p. 109.
- Miscarriage (septic shock), p. 357.
- Amniotic fluid embolism (AFE; often fatal pulmonary embolism of a laboring woman due to AF material). Treatment of coagulation disorders in AFE, p. 312.
- Generally, in severe hemorrhage.

10.1 Miscarriage, spontaneous abortion

Definition. Premature termination of the pregnancy by expulsion of a dead embryo/fetus with a birth weight of ≤ 500 g.

Stillbirth. A fetus is classed as stillborn when it does not demonstrate any of the definitive signs of a live birth (heartbeat, natural breathing, pulsation of the umbilical cord) after separation from the mother's body.

Preterm delivery. If the fetus ≤ 500 g is alive (detection of heartbeat, natural breathing, pulsation of the umbilical cord), it is a preterm delivery and is registered as a live birth.

Incidence. 10–15 % in relation to the number of births (clinically accountable spontaneous abortions). Losses of early embryos, which usually run a subclinical course, are not considered (see Fig. 10.1).

Risk of recurrence. The risk of recurrence after a spontaneous abortion is 24 %, after two consecutive spontaneous abortions it rises to 26 %, after three (→ see recurrent spontaneous abortion, p. 357) to 32 %.

Etiology. Differentiated into induced and spontaneous abortions.

10.1.1 Induced abortion

Definition. Therapeutic abortion, termination of pregnancy. Induced termination (usually instrumental) of pregnancy.

Medical indications. Maternal: the life and health of the pregnant woman are endangered.

Note. If there is a medical indication, termination is possible at any time in the pregnancy.

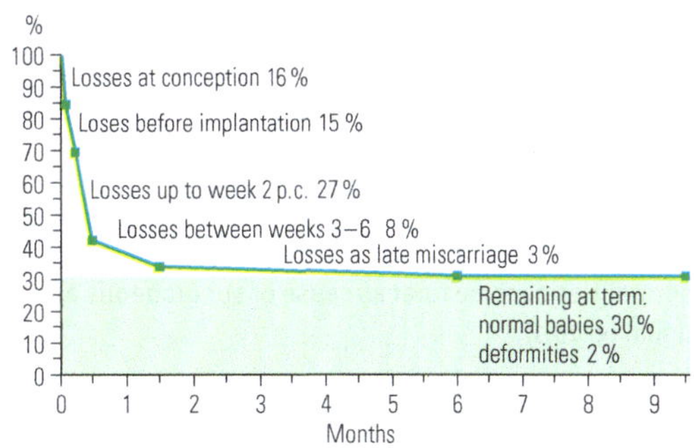

Fig. 10.1: Fate of fertilized ova (Witschi 1969).

10.1.2 Spontaneous abortion

Definition. Abortus spontaneus; miscarriage in the absence of external influences, nonintentional abortion; natural termination of pregnancy as a result of ovular or maternal causes.

Note. Types. 1) Nonfebrile, uncomplicated spontaneous abortion. Miscarriage in temperatures of <38 °C. 2) Febrile, uncomplicated spontaneous abortion. Endometritis without salpingitis, parametritis. 3) Febrile, complicated spontaneous abortion. Endometritis, salpingitis, parametritis.

Ovular causes of abortion. Nonviable products of conception are the most common cause: blighted ovum > 50 (–70) %, molar pregnancy.

Note. Every second spontaneous miscarriage is due to nonviable products of conception!

Chromosomal abnormalities are caused by faulty cell division during meiosis of the egg cell. Such cytogenetic causes are responsible for half of the blighted ova.
- Autosomal trisomies predominate, with 50 %.
- Polyploidies, primarily triploidies, account for 20 %.
- Monosomy X accounts for 25 %.
- Chromosomal structural aberrations 5 %.

While the aberration rate in live births is 0.5 % and early miscarriages 50–60 %, spontaneous abortions are nature's regulators. Aneuploidies increase with maternal age; the risk of recurrence is doubled.

Note. With increased gestational age, chromosomal abnormalities become rarer as cause of spontaneous abortion (Fig. 10.1).

Exogenous factors. Poisoning by mercury, organic solvents, radiation and medication.

Molar pregnancies
- Molar embryo. Embryonic material is deformed or atrophied.
- Blighted ovum. Gestational sac without embryo.
- Blood mole. After death of the products of conception in the embryonic phase, the chorionic cavity detaches from its site of attachment which leads to bleeding around and into the embryonic material.
- Fleshy mole. Blood mole after loss of hemoglobin and organization of contents.
- Breus' mole. Partial development of hematoma between chorion and decidua (subchorionic hematoma), which causes the amniotic cavity to bulge inwards.
- Hydatidiform mole; see p. 360.

Note. Half of all spontaneous abortions cannot be therapeutically influenced. Nonetheless, if children are desired and the pregnancy is intact, possible miscarriage must be treated.

Maternal causes of spontaneous abortion

Genital organs
- Retardation of uterine growth and lack of space. Hypoplastic uterus, malformation (bicornuate, subseptate uterus), intrauterine adhesions (IUA, Asherman's syndrome), uterine fibroids. Small subserosal fibroids do not disturb a pregnancy.
- Faulty protection of the lower pole of the ovum. Absent mechanical protection, e.g., in large cervical laceration and cervical incompetence (cervix as mechanical closure apparatus).

Luteal phase defect. The conceptus only requires progesterone from the ovary (corpus luteum graviditatis) in the first 4–6 weeks of gestation. The chorionic epithelium of the placenta produces relatively high amounts of progesterone from the second month of pregnancy.

- Progesterone is essential for the pregnancy, particularly in the first days (production of decidua, storage of glucosaccharides in the endometrium, implantation of the oocyte and development of the placenta). In contrast, its effect on uterus motility is controversial.
- Disturbed thyroid gland function and poorly controlled diabetes mellitus prior to conception or in early pregnancy are potential causes.

Infectious diseases

- Highly feverish infections cause miscarriages, in particular as a result of triggering contractions, which expel the conceptus.
- In addition viral infections (HSV, CMV) play an underestimated role.

Psychological factors

Psychological trauma, shock, agitation.

Immunological causes. Recent studies have shown that couples with high HLA (human leucocytic antigen) system similarities have an increased rate of miscarriage. The similarity inhibits the synthesis of antibodies which protect the conceptus.

Note. The course of the miscarriage is: immediate (→ early abortion, complete abortion) or in two stages (→ late abortion, incomplete abortion).

History. LMP, bleeding, subjective symptoms which indicate ectopic pregnancy: Sudden, colic-like pain, faintness, dizziness, threatened collapse.

Clinical manifestation

- Take temperature!
  - Temperatures > 37.9 °C indicate febrile miscarriage
  - Temperatures > 39 °C indicate septic miscarriage.
- Bimanual examination with sterile gloves whether:
  - The external os is closed or open (an open external os is normal in multiparae).
  - The cervical canal can be penetrated or even passed through.
  - Products of conception are felt in the cervical canal.
  - Adnexa: thickened cords, tumorous swelling, sensitive to touch.
  - Size, position (retroflexion!) attitude, and in particular consistency of the uterus are noted.
  - Parametria: free or infiltrated, particularly to the sides and back.
  - Recto-uterine pouch (Pouch of Douglas): doughy, soft (retrouterine hematoma, ectopic pregnancy) or tumorous masses (tumor in the Pouch of Douglas, tubal pregnancy).

Diagnosis. Transvaginal ultrasound (TVUS or TV sonography, TVS) is the leading method of diagnosis: intact pregnancy (live fetus)?

HCG detection is comparatively less important; normal serum hCG levels have a better prognosis than low levels.
The combination of transvaginal sonography and hCG measurement increases the diagnostic value:

Practice tip. Serum hCG levels of 2,000 mU/ml imply an intrauterine chorionic cavity of 4–7 mm diameter. If transvaginal ultrasound does not detect it, an ectopic pregnancy is likely.

Speculum examination. Intensity and frequency of bleeding.
Injury. Cervix, vagina, posterior fornix.
Blood count. RBC count, differential WBC count.

Complete abortion (Abortus completus), early abortion

Definition. Miscarriage in the first trimester (early abortion) with loss of the complete conceptus (Abortus completus, complete abortion; Fig. 10.2).

Pathogenesis. The conceptus is a complete mass, surrounded by villi, chorion villosum (powder puff shape, not yet differentiated into chorion frondosum and chorion laeve). If contractions occur, the villi, which at this time are not yet firmly anchored in the decidua, detach and the complete conceptus (embryo with amniotic sac, chorionic cavity) is expelled (Fig. 10.2).

Bleeding is the first symptom and continues until the contents of the uterus have been expelled.
Bleeding. The chorionic villi create intervillous spaces and there is no area around the conceptus which could detach without blood loss. The same is true for the lower pole, internal os, where detachment usually begins.

Clinical manifestation, diagnosis

- Bleeding and loss of conceptus.
- If the complete conceptus has been expelled, diagnosis is confirmed!
- Cervical canal is completely open, may have already begun to close up again.
- Bleeding ceases as the uterus rapidly becomes smaller.
- Uterus is smaller (not uncommon: normal size) than it should be for gestational age.

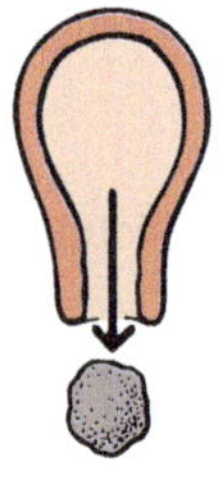

Fig. 10.2: Complete abortion.

Differential diagnosis. Incomplete abortion.

Treatment

- Curettage of the uterine cavity after every miscarriage (from week 6 to week 20).
- Blunt curettage if the placenta is incomplete. Remains which do not allow themselves to be detached from the wall must be (carefully!) removed with a sharp curette (exception).
- Suction curettage if cervix is not sufficiently open, as forced opening of the cervix can usually be avoided.
- Dilatation of the cervical canal up to weeks 8–9 to Hegar dilator 12, 13; after that no longer necessary.

Incomplete abortion (Abortus incompletus), late abortion

Definition. Incomplete, two-stage abortion, late abortion (after 12 weeks); more dangerous than complete abortion.

Occasionally the embryo is also expelled in weeks 1–12, alone or with part of the amnion and chorion, so that embryonic membranes are retained in the uterine cavity and later expelled (incomplete abortion). Bleeding continues until the remains have been expelled.
On completion of formation of the placenta between weeks 16–20 the fetus can be born.

Clinical manifestation

- Bleeding, contractions, loss of AF.

Practice tip. From week 12–13, the abortion (late abortion) tends to take place in two stages, like a birth: contractions, ROM, AF loss, first stage, second stage, birth of the fetus (pause) birth of the placenta (Fig. 10.3).

- Fetal loss, placenta in utero. Sections of the placenta or chorion may have been expelled.
- Cervical canal widened.

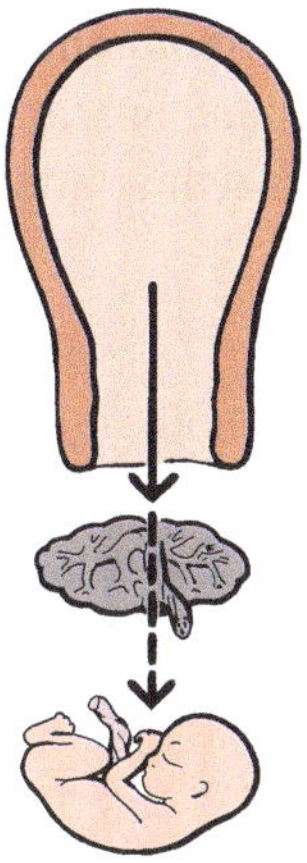

Fig. 10.3: Incomplete abortion.

Treatment

- From week 13 onwards instruments must not be inserted before the placenta or most of it has been expelled: danger of hemorrhage, perforation!
- Manual placenta removal. If the placenta is not expelled spontaneously it must be detached and removed manually. If the cervical canal is not dilated enough for the finger, dilatation with the Hegar dilator (18–22). Remains are removed with the large blunt curette.

Practice tip. The later the late abortion occurs, the less appropriate purely surgical evacuation is.

- Dilatation of the cervical canal is only necessary in the early weeks.
- Medical management poses a therapeutic alternative to surgical treatment of incomplete and complete abortion. Since the speed of the procedure is no longer top priority (as in the age of illegal abortions), controlled observation of physiological processes like the expulsion of uterine contents and medical support can be applied. In addition to surgical treatment, expectant and medical management (administration of mifepristone and/or misoprostol) are possible. According to Ballagh and colleagues, only 10 % of women require curettage.

There are different methods of **medical abortion**; as yet no one method has been definitively accepted:
Day 1: 800 µg misoprostol vaginally.
Day 3: Sonography: products of conception retained in utero?
If retained products detected: repeat vaginal dose of 800 µg misoprostol.
If the uterine cavity is empty, no further administration.
Day 8: Curettage, if products of conception are detected sonographically.

Inevitable miscarriage (Abortus incipiens), beginning miscarriage

Definition. Miscarriage has begun and is no longer stoppable. Contractions and heavy bleeding are present, cervical canal and internal os are more or less open.

Clinical manifestation

- Cervix effaced, internal os dilated.
- Lower embryonic pole has entered the cervical canal.

Diagnosis

- Morphological and histomorphological examination of the material obtained on curettage (chromosomal abnormality?).
- From a human genetics viewpoint, examination of the abort material is not performed. Karyotypic evaluation is carried out on parental blood samples after the third spontaneous abortion. On the other hand, evidence of aneuploidy can provide the parents with a rational basis for processing their experience.

Treatment

Inevitable abortion up until 13 completed weeks. Support of the process which has begun but is delayed.

To **soften the cervix** 1 mg Gemeprost is placed in the posterior fornix 3 h before surgery.
Alternatively: 200 µg misoprostol can be taken orally 10 h before the procedure.
Early abortions can only be surgically evacuated with curettage. Dilatation with Hegar dilator 12, 13 beforehand. The risk of perforation is very low as the uterine wall is relatively thick at this point.

- If products of conception are protruding from the cervix, they are removed with the use of specula and Winter abortion forceps.
- Curettage of the uterine cavity to remove villous remains and decidua.

Inevitable abortion between 13 and 23 completed weeks. Surgical evacuation only after expulsion of part or all of the products of conception; after the inevitable abortion has become a complete or incomplete abortion.

The further advanced the pregnancy is, the more difficult (fetal head detaches easily) and dangerous (heavy bleeding, soft, thin uterine wall) it is to remove the products of conception. The curette is lost in the large uterine cavity. Risk of perforation! If blood loss allows expectant management, treatment as follows:

- 200 µg misoprostol orally, 24 h before induction of labor, to prepare the cervix.
- To soften the cervix 1 mg Gemeprost vaginally, repeat every 4 h
- If treatment fails (no delivery within 48 h), continuous infusion of Sulproston, 500 µg in 500 ml, 2–8 ml/min, max 1,500 µg/24 h.

Contraindication: prior CS or other transmural operation!
Curettage is performed after expulsion, as in complete and incomplete abortion (see above). Life-threatening hemorrhage requires (rare) immediate curettage and abortion forceps (after dilatation with Hegar dilators).

Threatened miscarriage (Abortus imminens)

Definition. Threatened or imminent miscarriage with contractions or light bleeding and closed cervical canal.

Clinical manifestation

- Light bleeding or contractions or both, cervical canal closed.
- In early pregnancy contractions manifest as lower back or suprapubic pain.

Examination. Cautious and not more frequently than every 10–12 days.

Diagnosis. Sonography!

- Intact pregnancy detected from 6 weeks' gestation, existence of the fetus (cardiac action, movement of extremities).
- Measurement of conceptus.

Differential diagnosis (bleeding before 16 weeks). 1) Intact intrauterine pregnancy. 2) Molar embryo, blighted ovum. 3) Missed abortion. 4) Incomplete abortion. 5) Ectopic pregnancy. 6) Hydatidiform mole.

Prognosis. As there is a relationship between the extent of villous detachment and the intensity and duration of blood loss, the type of hemorrhage has prognostic character. On the other hand, a single, even heavier bleed is not necessarily critical. Unobserved bleeding cannot really be considered. For this reason alone, threatened miscarriage should be under clinical observation!

Treatment

- Physical and bed rest, if possible in hospital.
- Abstinence from sexual intercourse (prohibition!).
- No application of ice or heat (stimulation of uterine muscles).
- Regulation of bowel movements with gentle (no drastic) laxatives.

Corticosteroids or diazepam are not advisable.

Prognosis. Unfavorable if:
- Bleeding continues over >2–3 weeks.
- Contractions become more frequent or even regular.
- Growth of the embryonic sac is retarded.
- Embryonic movements and cardiac action are missing.
- Serum levels of hCG are too low.

Habitual abortion (Abortus habitualis), recurrent abortion

Definition. If three or more consecutive pregnancies end with spontaneous abortion, it is termed habitual abortion (also recurrent abortion, recurrent pregnancy loss or RPL). Types: habitual early abortion (up to 12 weeks), late abortion (from 12 weeks).

Etiology. Manifold causes. In addition to the causes of miscarriage already discussed, the following causes must be discussed in habitual abortion, although analysis of the cause is difficult and unsatisfying in individual cases.
- Cytogenetic causes in early abortions.
- Ascending infections.
- Endocrinological findings. Hyper- and hypothyreose, detection of thyroid peroxidase (TPO) antibodies, polycystic ovary syndrome (Metformin treatment of women with PCOS and insulin resistance reduces the rate of abortions), Luteal phase defect (serum progesterone levels! Consider progesterone replacement!), inadequately controlled diabetes mellitus, hyperprolactinemia.
- If TSH levels in the upper norm are found, indicating latent hypothyreose with normal levels of peripheral thyroid hormones, increased risk of miscarriage is expected. Treatment with L-Thyroxine is recommended.
- Uterine findings. Uterine malformations (arcuate, subseptate uterus), synechiae after curettages, isthmo-cervical incompetence, intramural or submucosal fibroids.
- Immunological causes. Maternal defense reaction to the genetically different embryonic tissue (treatment attempts with lymphocytes or immunoglobulins were unsuccessful).
- Thrombophiliac causes. Factor V Leiden mutation, prothrombin polymorphism (low-molecular weight heparin from week 8!), antiphospholipid syndrome (low-molecular weight heparin plus 100 mg Aspirin!)
- Environmental factors. Contact with heavy metals, organic solvents; incomplete knowledge of influences, risks difficult to calculate.
- Psychological causes. Clarification difficult, however it is a recognized fact that tender loving care (personal, frequent attention from a physician) can be successful.

Treatment. The factors listed occasionally permit the consideration of special therapeutic measures, the effects of which are controversially discussed. Study-based recommendations do not exist. It is also not possible to give a validated recommendation on active (autologous lymphocytes) or passive (IV immunoglobulins) immunization.

Missed abortion, silent miscarriage

Definition. Silent miscarriage; retention of dead, immature products of conception in the uterus over weeks or months; can lead to dead-fetus syndrome.

Clinical manifestation. Disproportion between date of LMP and size of uterus!

Diagnosis
- Sonography (from weeks 6–10) is the leading method of diagnosis: absence of movement of fetal extremities and cardiac action.

- Hormones. Increased urinary secretion of hCG and serum hCG or β-hCG levels are helpful in difficult cases.

Complications. Dead-fetus syndrome. Consumptive coagulopathy caused by retention of a dead fetus in utero (> 5 weeks). Treatment see p. 110.

Treatment. Medical. Prostaglandins induce an artificial abortion:

- 1mg Gemeprost vaginal suppository (optimum efficacy after 4–6 h)
- Infusion of 1,000 μg Sulproston in 1,000 ml fructose over 10 h.

Active treatment if medical fails. Suction curettage < 12 weeks.

Febrile abortion (Abortus febrilis), septic abortion

Definition. Febrile miscarriage; types: 1) uncomplicated febrile abortion (local infection of the endometrium); 2) complicated febrile abortion (with salpingitis); 3) septic abortion with pelveoperitonitis and threatened septic shock. Temperature > 37.9 °C indicates a febrile abortion, temperature > 39 °C a septic abortion.

Febrile abortion

Clinical manifestation

- Uncomplicated febrile abortion: local infection (endometrium) with temperatures between 38–39 °C. No salpingitis, peritonitis.
- Complicated febrile abortion: salpingitis (pain on pressure), local peritonitis (acute abdomen with abdominal guarding). Usually high fever, in some cases only slightly elevated temperatures.

Treatment. Antimicrobial therapy; curettage once high temperatures have ceased.

Septic abortion, septic shock

Septic abortion. Most severe form of febrile abortion with threatened septic shock.

Septic shock (bacterial shock, toxic shock syndrome or endotoxic shock). Usually caused by bacterial endotoxins of Gram-negative pathogens. Occurrence: most common in febrile abortion, rarer in PROM with fever (chorioamnionitis), septic ovarian thrombosis, pyelonephritis gravidarum.

Incidence. Febrile abortion is accompanied by arterial hypotension in 5 % of cases: first symptom of shock! Incidence of endotoxic shock appears to be rising. Mortality: >10 % in intensive care.

Etiology. Gram-negative pathogens: usually E. coli, Clostridium perfringens.

Pathogenesis. Endotoxins activate monocytes which release mediators (TNFa, interleukins). These cytokines have a procoagulatory effect on the endothelium and cause disseminated intravascular coagulation (DIC) in and displacement of the terminal vessels, ischemia of kidneys, lungs, CNS, muscles, later diffuse tissue necroses with multiple organ failure.

Kidneys. Acute renal failure (→ shock kidney), with oliguria, anuria, sometimes polyuria. On healing, chronic renal insufficiency.

Lungs. Interstitial pulmonary edema (→ shock lung, acute respiratory distress syndrome or ARDS), which may be followed by an intra-alveolar exudation. Edema leads to faulty gas diffusion and with that to respiratory insufficiency.

CNS. Cerebral edema, meningoencephalitis.

Musculature. Destruction of muscle tissue with increased consistency, spontaneous pain and pain in response to pressure.

Heart. Myocardial insufficiency with tachycardia, increase in central venous pressure and decrease in mean arterial pressure.

Consumptive coagulopathy in generalized intravascular coagulation. Consumption of plasma coagulation factors (fibrinogen, factors V, VII; p. 377). Pathological hemorrhaging is, however, rare, as excessive fibrinolytic activity rarely occurs.

Pathophysiology. In septic abortion, shock manifests initially as arterial hypotension; often, however, it begins with a hypercirculatory (hyperdynamic) initial phase with increased cardiac output, tachycardia, reduced peripheral vascular resistance; arterial blood pressure is initially normal, later reduced, hyperventilation, beginning respiratory insufficiency, followed by hypocirculatory late phase with reduced cardiac Output, high peripheral vascular resistance, hypotension, DIC, acute renal failure, ARDS.

Clinical manifestation. Generalized infection with:
- Fever following chills, temperature ≥ 38 °C, occasionally without rise in temperature!
- Genitals: putrid discharge, moderate tenderness of uterus and adnexa.

Leading symptoms of shock:
- CNS. Drowsiness, restlessness, stiff neck, meningitis, paralysis.
- Lungs. Tachypnea, compensatory hyperventilation, respiratory insufficiency.
- Kidneys. Acute renal failure with oliguria, anuria (shock kidney), in some cases primary polyuria.
- Circulatory system. Tachycardia and hypotension (reduced venous blood flow to the heart).
- Musculature. Spontaneous and pressure pain of the muscles of the extremities, raised consistency of muscles.
- Unclear abdominal pain in some cases.
- Hemorrhagic skin necroses on nose, forehead and cheeks.

Diagnosis
- Body temperature.
- Hourly urinary output (in-dwelling catheter and urometer), contents.
- BP and pulse half-hourly.
- Respiration: BGA.
- Peripheral circulation, CVP.
- Water-electrolyte balance.
- Acid-base household.

Pathological coagulation parameters. Thrombocytopenia, hypofibrinogenemia, clot observation test.

Treatment

Shock prophylaxis
- Intravenous line and volume administration, plasma substitute solution, CVP < 14 cm H_2O!
- Oxygen supplementation if necessary.
- Antimicrobial therapy after antibiogram. If pathogen unknown combination of Mezlocillin 3 x 2 g i.v. and Metronidazole 3 x 500 g i.v. daily.
- Uterine evacuation with prostaglandin: Sulproston, 1–8 mg/min.
- Monitoring of the parameters listed under diagnosis.

Shock treatment
- Volume administration, if necessary vasoactive substances. Dopamine (200–600 mg/min) or Norepinephrine (Noradrenaline; up to 100 mg/min).
- Antimicrobial therapy see above.
- Corticosteroids. Prednisone, prednisolone (5mg per kg body weight) every 4 h.
- Treat renal insufficiency .
- Treat pulmonary disfunction.

Eliminate the source of infection if shock does not respond to therapy within 6–8 h:

- Curettage if cervical canal is open.
- Abdominal hysterectomy if cervical canal is closed.

10.2 Gestational trophoblastic disease (GTD)

Classification. Gestational trophoblastic disease encompasses: benign GTD: molar tumor, hydatidiform mole, and malignant GTD: nonmolar tumor or trophoblastic tumor.

Hydatidiform mole

Definition. Hydatid mole, molar pregnancy, vesicular mole. Degeneration of the placental chorionic villi into vesicles up to the size of grapes filled with a light-colored fluid, simultaneous proliferation of cytotrophoblast and syncytiotrophoblast.

Etiology. Evidently an early developmental disorder of the products of conception. Cytogenetic examinations have shown that the chromosomal composition of hydatidiform moles is a diploid karyotype (46XX or – rarely 46XY). The genetic material of the cell nucleus is of paternal; the DNA of the mitochondria is of maternal origin. There are also tetraploid, triploid and aneuploid hydatidiform moles.

Incidence. There are marked geographical differences: Japan: 2 : 1,000, Europe 1 : 1,000.

Histopathology. Stroma and chorionic epithelium are affected. The stroma absorbs fluid and swells (hydropic swelling). It is transformed

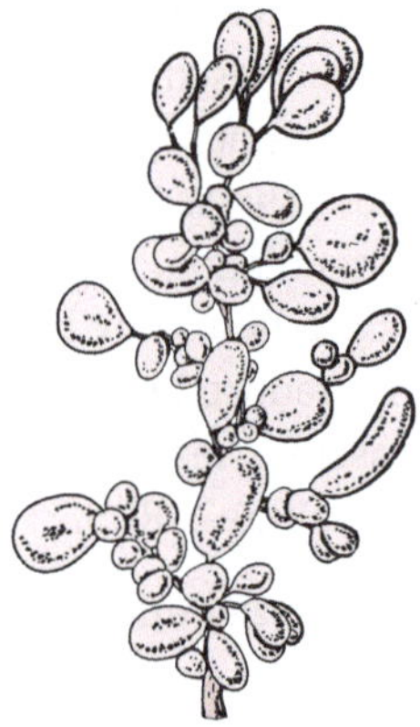

Fig. 10.4: Degenerated villi in hydatidiform mole.

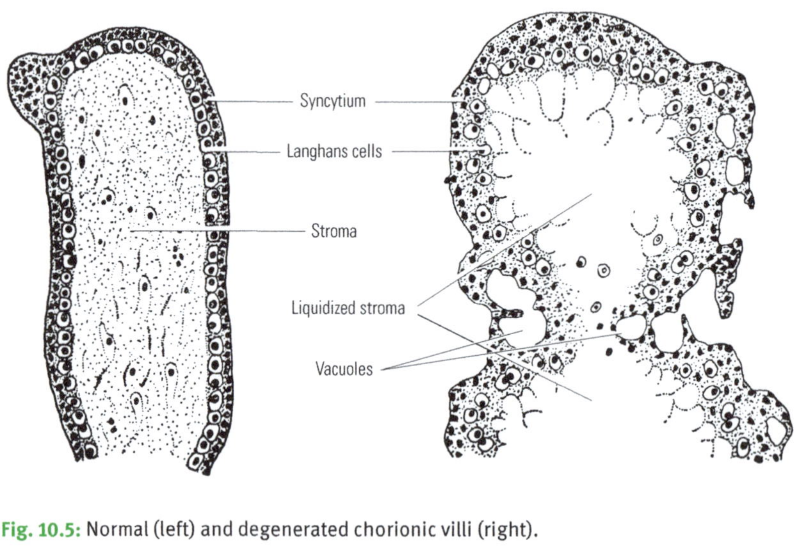

Fig. 10.5: Normal (left) and degenerated chorionic villi (right).

into a slushy, liquefied mass. Stromal cells are dissolved. Chorionic epithelium (syncytium, Langhans cells) is extremely proliferative, loss of order, altered shape: size and vacuole creation.

Pathogenesis. Villi are similar to trees with very fine, even, thin branches which are anchored with each other and with the decidua. The nature of the hydatidiform mole is that these fine villous branches are blown up like bubbles (vesicles) and thicken (Figs. 10.4, 10.5): from match head size to as large as peas or larger; rarely as large as grapes.

Usually all villi have degenerated to vesicles (complete mole); rarely only some (→ partial mole).

The complete uterus is filled due to swelling and proliferation of the mushy mass of fluid-filled vesicles.

The fetus has died, disintegrated and been reabsorbed.

Clinical manifestation

- The leading symptom is the conspicuously soft and large (fundal height) uterus, too large for gestational age (menstrual history).
- Absence of vital signs: no cardiac action, movement (chorionic epithelium is unfit for the exchange of substances, leading to fetal demise).
- Vaginal bleeding as a result of detachment of degenerated villi.

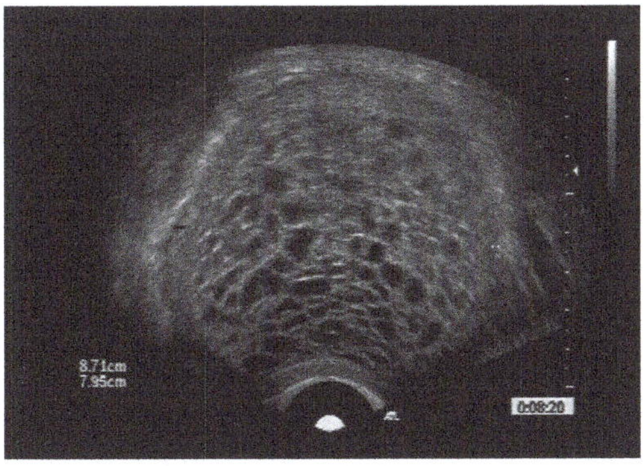

Fig. 10.6: Ultrasound image of a hydatidiform mole at the beginning of second trimester.

Diagnosis

- Ectopic proliferation of chorionic epithelium: pea- to cherry-sized blue-red knots in the vaginal wall.
- Detachment and passage of the vesicles (degenerated villi) from the cervical canal.
- Sonography. Cystic masses and clots in the uterus: "snowstorm" (Fig. 10.6).
- Repeated high levels of hCG (≥ 500,000–1 million units) are the leading diagnostic method. The proliferation of epithelium causes excessive hCG production.
- Theca-Lutein cysts: overproduction of hCG induces lutein cysts in the ovaries (in 10 %), bilateral ovarian cysts can grow to the size of a baby's head.

Theca-Lutein cysts are follicle cysts, lined with granulosa lutein cells which develop from an atretic cell after failed ovulation.

Usually resolve spontaneously after removal of the hydatidiform mole and cessation of hormone production. Operation if they have not disappeared within 3–4 months.

Complication. Trophoblastic tumor (see below).

Treatment. Hydatidiform mole is to be treated as an abortion. Some particularities apply:

Prostaglandins (i. v. Sulproston, dosage p. 356) support spontaneous expulsion and are the remedy of choice if bleeding is light and the complete mass of the hydatidiform mole is still in utero. Curettage is necessary afterwards.

Suction curettage if bleeding is heavy.

- If the cervical canal is not sufficiently dilated, careful dilatation with Hegar dilators. Alternative: 1mg Gemeprost vaginally 3–6 h preoperatively.

- Curettage must always be performed afterwards. Retention of chorionic tissue can cause bleeding and hormone release over weeks.
  - 1 ampoule (= 1 ml: 5 IE Oxytocin + 0.25 mg Methylergometrine) of Syntometrine i.v. reduces the size of the uterus and causes thickening of the walls, which reduces the risk of perforation.
  - Cautious and slow inspection with a large curette.

Note. Curettage in hydatidiform mole is a life-threatening procedure! Two dangers threaten: perforation of the soft, pulpy, in places extremely thin uterine wall; hemorrhage from the gaping vessels of the overdistended uterus.

Follow-up examination

- Weekly ultrasound, control of clinical findings, hCG levels (quantitative).
- Immunological hCG tests are negative 3 weeks after removal of the hydatidiform mole, serum β-hCG after 12 weeks.
- If serum β-hCG is positive after 12 weeks metastases must be sought: sonography of the upper abdomen, CT, MRI, if necessary brain and liver scintigraphy.

Trophoblastic tumor

Definition. Tumor which develops from cells of the syncytiotrophoblast or cytotrophoblast of the placenta (→ gestational trophoblastic disease, GTD) or from germ cells (endodermal sinus tumor, EST or yolk sac tumor).

Nonmetastasizing trophoblastic tumor. GTD in the uterus as persisting or invasive mole and choriocarcinoma.
Metastasizing trophoblastic tumor. GTD outside the uterus: no liver, brain metastases (low risk, good prognosis) or choriocarcinoma, high hCG excretion, liver or brain metastases (high risk, poor prognosis).

Incidence. 5–10 trophoblastic tumors in 100,000 live births.

Occurrence

In 50 % after a hydatidiform mole, seldom after partial mole.
In 25 % during or after normal pregnancy.
In 25 % after miscarriage or ectopic pregnancy.
Primiparae and older pregnant women are particularly at risk.

Pathogenesis. Trophoblastic neoplasia, which proliferates beyond the decidua, enters the bloodstream and spreads (metastasizes) to distant tissues: lungs, liver, brain, knots in the vagina.

Note. Metastases have the special characteristic of being capable of resolution: they heal via connective tissue organization and are termed benign metastases.

Clinical manifestation

Three leading symptoms are: bleeding, uterine enlargement, rise in hCG levels
Bleeding

- Bleeding continues after surgical evacuation (hydatidiform mole, miscarriage).
- Treatment-resistant bleeding in puerperium.
- Renewed bleeding.
- Placental polyps in puerperium, after abortion.

Uterus soft, large, minimal involution.
hCG (p. 60) remains positive or becomes positive again.
Further symptoms:

- Lung metastases (common). Shortness of breath and bloody sputum.
- Metastases in the vaginal wall (common).
- Brain metastases with cerebral symptoms.
- Liver metastases with icterus, uncharacteristic upper abdominal complaints.
- Vulva metastases as blue-red or blue-black knots which tend to bloody degeneration.

- Tumor perforates the uterine wall: hemorrhage into the abdominal cavity, possibly with shock.
- Ovarian tumor. Theca-lutein cysts due to excess hCG.

FIGO scoring system:
- I: Disease is confined exclusively to the uterus.
- II: Spread to other genital organs (vagina).
- III: Pulmonary metastases with or without involvement of uterus, vagina and true pelvis.
- IV: Advanced metastases in brain, liver, kidneys, GI tract.

Diagnosis
- Serum or urinary hCG levels.
- Ultrasound examination.
- CT, MRI, angiography of the pelvic arteries, scintigraphy.

Diagnostic curettage (abrasion) is no longer relevant due to fear of transferring tumor material and because histological diagnosis is not sought.

Treatment. Hysterectomy only in cases of heavy bleeding.

Methotrexate (cytostatic agent, folic acid antagonist) is the drug of choice against trophoblastic tissue. Dosage 15–25 mg/day oral, i. m. or i. v. over 5 days; total dose of a: 75–125 mg.

- Measurement of success is the drop in hCG
- Duration of treatment: 5–6 courses, then normal urinary hCG excretion.
- Interval between two courses should, depending on condition, be 7-15-20 days long

Side effects. Administration of methotrexate causes side effects:
- Leukopenia and thrombocytopenia.
- Mucosal ulcers in mouth and throat region (gingivitis, stomatitis).
- Vomiting, diarrhea, icterus.
- Blockage of tubular secretion in the kidneys.

Monitoring during therapy:
- Hemogram.
- Serum methotrexate concentration.

Leucovorin (active folic acid) is a methotrexate antidote and is administered in cases of toxic reactions (1 Ampoule = 1 ml or 3 mg)
- Dosage: begin with 1–2 ml daily (3–6 mg) i. m., depending on the severity of the reaction.

Metastasized tumor. Polychemotherapy with Methotrexate (dosage see above) and Actinomycin (0.5 mg/day over 5–7 days). Combination with other cytostatic agents as required, e.g., Etoposide.

Follow-up examination after chemotherapy has ended.
Weekly hCG level monitoring for the next 2 years!
An oral contraceptive is indicated for avoidance of a pregnancy after hydatidiform mole or trophoblastic tumor. Ultrasound and endocrinological diagnosis are advisable in a subsequent pregnancy on the one hand; however a normal pregnancy – also after chemotherapy against malignant GTD – can be expected.

10.3 Ectopic pregnancy

Definition. Pregnancy in the abdominal cavity or ectopic pregnancy; pregnancy outside the uterus: extrauterine pregnancy. Preferred sites: Fallopian tube, ovary, abdominal cavity. Life-threatening in cases of intraperitoneal hemorrhage.

Classification. Tubal pregnancy. The commonest ectopic site is in the Fallopian tube (99 %; Fig. 10.7).

Ovarian pregnancy. Fertilisation of the ovum, e.g., after ovulation, and implantation in the ovary, destroying the corpus luteum.
Abdominal pregnancy. Peritoneal pregnancy, primary (initial) implantation and development in the peritoneum (usually the Pouch of Douglas).
The following statements refer only to tubal pregnancy. Ovarian and abdominal pregnancies are rare (together 1 % of all ectopic pregnancies).

Incidence (Fig. 10.7). 1 ectopic pregnancy in 100 deliveries. Risk of recurrence after ectopic pregnancy 10 %, after repeated tubal pregnancy 50 %. Mortality 0.2 %

Etiology. The zygote implants as soon as it is able to on days 5–6 p.c.

Note. Causes are either obstructions in the oviduct (the fertilized ovum is obstructed on its path to the uterus) or impaired tubal motility.

Oviductal obstructions. Main cause is tubal inflammation (→ salpingitis) after gonorrhea, febrile abortion, puerperal inflammation.

Effects of salpingitis:
- Adhesion of the mucosal folds creates a net, in whose mesh the migrating fertilized ovum becomes trapped; particularly in the broad ampullary segment.
- Pockets penetrating deep into the musculature and small cavities in the tubal wall are created when abscesses heal, in particular in the narrow isthmic segment.

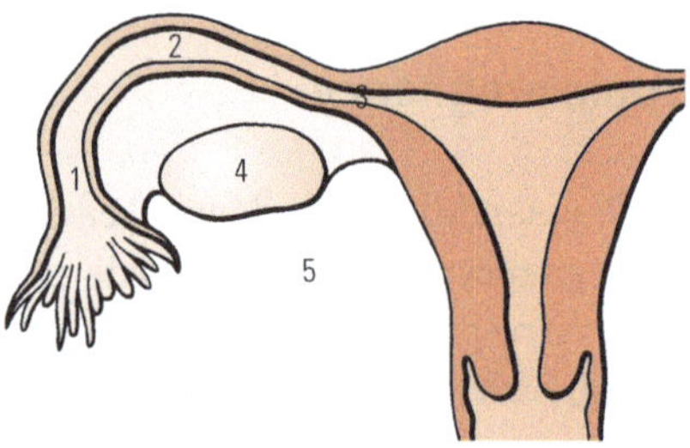

Fig. 10.7: 99 out of 100 ectopic pregnancies are sited in the tube, usually in the ampullary segment (1), more rarely in the isthmic (2), even more rarely in the interstitial segment (3). Ovarian (4) and abdominal (5) pregnancies are rare.

Endometriosis causes narrowing of the interstitial tubal segment and leads to a labyrinth of side passages.
Uterine operations (ventrofixation) can displace the tube by bending it.

Impaired tubal motility. Main cause is ovarian insufficiency with tubes which are long, narrow-lumened, and weak muscled (hypoplastic, infantile), with incomplete ciliation, which impairs transport of the ovum (tubal motility is a condition for the transport). Additionally, the hypoplastic tube is much more susceptible to ascending infection (salpingitis) than a normal, functional tube.

Transport of the ovum is also restricted in a tube which is stretched over an ovarian tumor (longer path, narrow lumen, motility impossible).
Intrauterine devices disrupt tubal motility and are also thought to cause tubal pregnancies.

Pathological anatomy. Tubal pregnancy causes: tubal abortion, tubal rupture or completion of the pregnancy (rare, here not discussed).

Practice tip. General rule. Implantation of the ovum in the Ampulla tubae (broad, ampullary segment) leads to tubal abortion (Fig. 10.8), in the isthmic segment (narrower) or (rarely) interstitial segment to tubal rupture (Fig. 10.9). Tubal abortion is 6–10 times more common than tubal rupture.

Tubal abortion (Fig. 10.8). The fertilized ovum adheres to the mucosal folds of the ampullary segment of the tube and implants in such a way that a portion sits in the muscle wall; the other

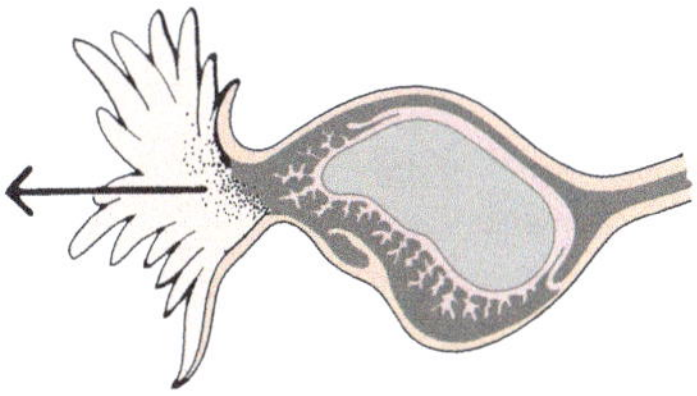

Fig. 10.8: Tubal abortion.

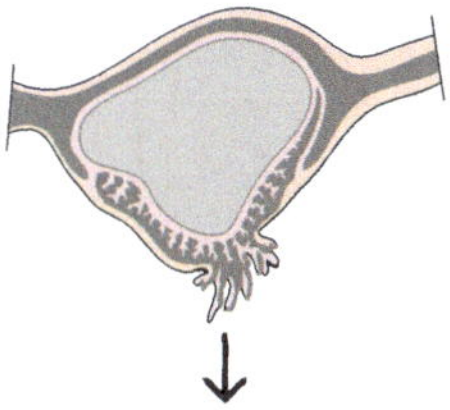

Fig. 10.9: Tubal rupture.

protrudes into the lumen. This site is unsuitable and degenerates.

After a number of weeks the thin mucosal capsule on the internal side of the tube ruptures (internal embryonic capsule rupture), with contraction of the tube and bleeding. The detached products of conception are moved back along the tube in the direction of the Ostium abdominale, the fimbriated end; it returns by the same path it entered the tube.

Tubal rupture (Fig. 10.9). The fertilized ovum adheres to the mucosal folds or in a blind passage in the wall of the isthmic segment (Isthmus tubae). Development of the embryo occurs within the wall (intramural).

Trophoblasts, or rather villi, invade the wall and erode it, whereby the wall of the embryonic capsule perforates into the abdominal cavity: external embryonic capsule rupture with tubal rupture hemorrhage.
Arterial hemorrhage. The ruptured vessels belong to the ovarian arteries. Result is heavy, sudden arterial hemorrhage into the abdominal cavity.
1–2 l of blood can be hemorrhaged intraabdominally within 20–40 min. Rupture hemorrhages are life-threatening!
Retrouterine hematocele. A portion of the blood lands and coagulates in the Pouch of Douglas (rectouterine cul-de-sac). As after tubal abortion, it is palpable as a soft, doughy tumor from the vagina, from where it can also be punctured.

Clinical manifestation. There are 3 defined stages: Stage 1: intact tubal pregnancy, asymptomatic. Stage 2: Embryonic material in the tube dying or dead, bleeding in the tube, few symptoms. Stage 3: Hemorrhaging from the tube, peritoneal shock.

Stage 1: asymptomatic

Definition. Embryo and tube are intact, one or (more rarely) two periods are missed, implying (uterine) pregnancy. Implantation and the first weeks of pregnancy are normal.

Pregnancy hormones effect enlargement and softening of the uterus (→ proliferation of decidua!).
The uterus is only rarely of normal size for gestational age. The mucosa is always transformed into normal decidua.

Diagnosis. Sonography. No intrauterine pregnancy, decidual transformation of the endometrium; the tubal implantation is often depicted, in some cases retrouterine fluid.

Stage 2: minimal symptoms

Definition. Hemorrhage within the tube, no bleeding outside the tube, 6–8 weeks since LMP.

Practice tip. Bleeding (usually spotting) in women of child-bearing age 6–8 weeks p.m. (period 2–4 weeks overdue) arouse suspicion of extrauterine pregnancy or abortion.

Three leading symptoms

1. Amenorrhea
2. Hormone-related uterine bleeding, continuous spotting, 6–8 weeks p.m. Caused by disintegration and expulsion of the decidua from the uterus. After 6–8 weeks the corpus luteum graviditatis disintegrates with decline and expulsion of the decidua: bleeding! This bleeding is not obligatory:
   a) Tubal rupture often occurs without bleeding because the rupture occurs before the embryo has died.
   b) Tubal abortion is normally accompanied by bleeding, sometimes only minimal and brief bleeding or bloody discharge.
3. Unilateral, often contraction-like pains, periodically returning once uterine bleeding begins. Cause: detachment, later contraction of the tubes when the embryo enlarges the lumen on its path to the ampulla.
   a) Tubal abortion. Episodic attacks of pain with pain-free intervals (→ slow course of tubal abortion over weeks). DD: salpingitis.
   b) Tubal rupture. Intense pain (→ rupture pain) in stage 3 from a state of complete health.

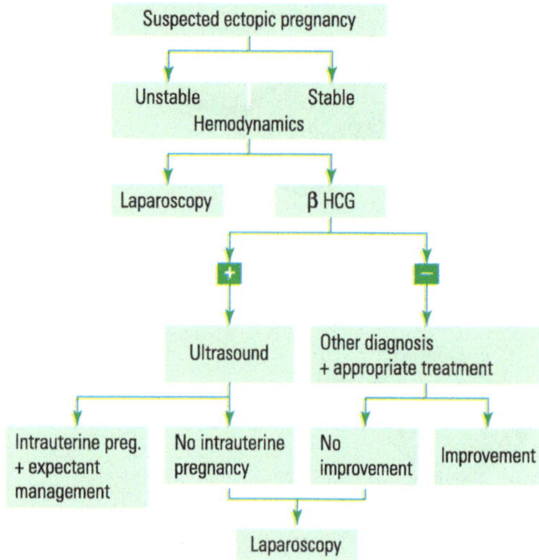

Fig. 10.10: Diagnostic procedure in extrauterine pregnancy (secondary amenorrhea, lower abdominal complaints, uterine bleeding, unclear vaginal exam findings).

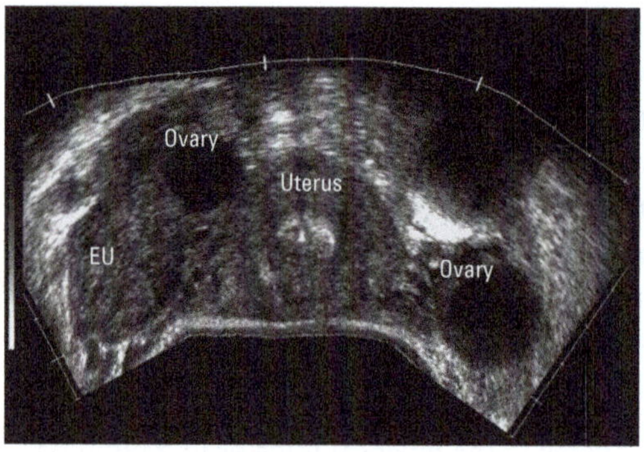

Fig. 10.11: Tubal pregnancy right, lateral to the ovary; transverse section of uterus and adnexa, panorama image.

Diagnosis (Fig. 10.10)

- Intrauterine pregnancy is often indicated by increased vaginal congestion, slightly enlarged and relaxed uterus. Minimal swelling in the tubal pregnancy.
- Cervix is tender to the touch. Ovarian pain when the uterus is moved.
- Palpable adnex tumor (hematosalpinx).
- Pregnancy can be detected in maternal serum a few days after implantation via β-hCG.
- Ultrasound diagnosis (Fig. 10.11). TVS (intraperitoneal) accumulation of blood in the Pouch of Douglas, extrauterine embryonic material is often detectable (Fig. 10.12).
- Laparoscopy. After creating a pneumoperitoneum with about 3L of CO_2, the tubes and ovaries are inspected using an introduced optical device and diagnosis confirmed.
- In unclear cases, diagnostic curettage (abrasion)! It is indicated when there is a

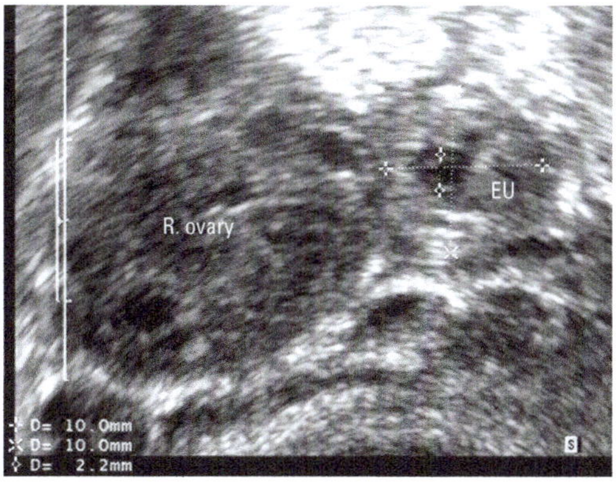

Fig. 10.12: Transvaginal sonographic oblique section in week 6: 1) ovary with follicles; 2) tubal pregnancy (1 cm). Trophoblastic tissue and chorionic cavity with a diameter of 2.2 mm.

suspicious history with continuing uterine bleeding (10–12–14 days), no findings on palpation of the adnexa and negative immunological pregnancy test.

Histology

- Fetal material and decidua confirm the abortion.
- Only decidua, no fetal material: abortion in which the complete embryo has been expelled, ectopic pregnancy.

Stage 3: Peritoneal shock

Definition. Bleeding from the tube into the abdominal cavity, stage of peritoneal shock, alarm signals.

Tubal abortion

Peritubal hematoma (Fig. 10.13). The blood trickling out of the tube does not reach the abdominal cavity, but collects earlier, and coagulates to a palpable hematoma surrounding the end of the tube; it can become as large as a fist or larger and sinks into the Pouch of Douglas due to the effect of gravity.

Retrouterine hematocele (Fig. 10.13). Smaller amounts of intraabdominal blood collect in the

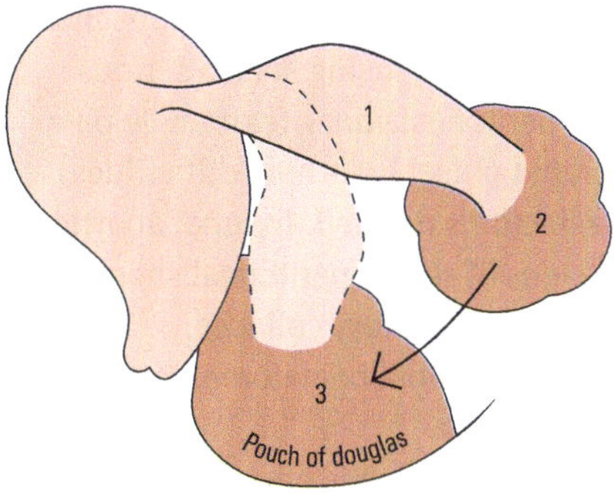

Fig. 10.13: Hematomas: 1) hematosalpinx; 2) peritubal hematoma; 3) retrouterine hematoma.

Pouch of Douglas behind the uterus. The blood coagulates and, together with the peritubal hematoma already there, creates a doughy hematoma (retrouterine hematocele) which can easily be palpated from the vagina.

Four leading symptoms

1. Unilateral adnexal pain, perianal pain, passage of wind is painful. Most contraction-like pains are caused by tubal contractions (p. 366) and peritubal hematoma. The retrouterine hematoma causes rectal complaints (see above), e.g., painful passage of wind.
2. Numerous peritoneal shocks over the course of weeks manifest as attacks of weakness: sudden feeling of weakness, pale face, pointy nose, cold sweaty forehead, tachycardia; occur as a result of contact of blood with the peritoneum.
3. Even a small amount of blood trickling into the abdominal cavity next to the peritubal hematoma can cause peritoneal shock, which need not be dramatic the first time: “As I was about to sit down at the table I had a sudden pain on my left lower side, felt dizzy, and fainted”. This may pass after a small bleed on the peritoneum, and repeat once or twice at hourly, daily or weekly intervals, until

one day a larger volume of blood reaches the peritoneum causing such a serious bout of peritoneal shock (extremely pale face, rapid pulse, breathing difficulties) that a doctor is notified. In tubal abortion these signs of severe peritoneal shock can increase to circulatory collapse.
4. Findings: peritubal hematoma, retrouterine hematocele.
5. On palpation, which is often difficult due to abdominal guarding, one of the 3 types of hematomas (Fig. 10.13) is felt. If first only a hematosalpinx (hematoma no. 1) is present, the somewhat thickened tube is felt next to the relaxed and enlarged uterus on one side. If a peritubal hematoma (hematoma no. 2) has developed, a soft, doughy, diffuse thickening is felt at the farthest end of the tube. It can become larger than a man's fist in a very short time. If a number of spills of blood have flowed into the abdominal space or if the peritubal hematoma has lowered itself into the Pouch of Douglas, the Pouch of Douglas is felt to be somewhat bulging and the retrouterine hematoma (hematoma no. 3) is felt.
6. Uterine bleeding as in stage 2.

Tubal rupture

Abrupt intraabdominal inundation of blood. Source of the bleeding is ruptured vessels in the tubal walls. Life-threatening, threatened exsanguination.

Three leading symptoms. In contrast to tubal abortion: single attack from a state of wellbeing!

1. Sudden lower abdominal pain.
2. The onset of pain can usually be given to the minute, something has torn in the abdomen, and the correct side is indicated. The pain is so extreme that breathing is difficult. Sometimes pain is experienced in the upper abdomen, below the ribs or in a shoulder or upper arm. This is caused by irritation of the phrenic nerve: when a large volume of blood reaches the diaphragm of a supine patient the phrenic symptom is triggered (pain in shoulder and upper arm).
3. Peritoneal shock: pallor, weak pulse, breathing difficulties.
4. Within one minute, the face loses its normal coloring and becomes extremely pale (→ pathognomonic for tubal rupture)! The rapid pulse can disappear very quickly. Breathing difficulties are always present.
5. Acute abdomen (internal hemorrhage). Abdomen is sensitive to touch and as hard as a board!
6. Within seconds of the rupture the abdomen is diffusely sensitive and so tense and painful that not even light touch is bearable anywhere: acute abdomen. Only immediate laparotomy can avert a catastrophe.

Diagnosis. According to the clinical manifestion (→ leading symptoms).

Differential diagnosis (Tab. 10.1). Characteristic of tubal abort: periodic, slow, trickling hemorrhage from intervillous spaces which results in three hematomas: hematosalpinx, peritubal hematoma, retrouterine hematocele (Fig. 10.13). Characteristic for tubal rupture: sudden, excessive intraabdominal arterial hemorrhage (p. 365).

Treatment

- Laparoscopic salpingotomy or salpingectomy are the methods of choice. Today the tube is usually retained; the ovary if possible.
- In the last 10 years **laparoscopic instillation procedures** have been introduced: Prostaglandins, glucose solutions,

Tab. 10.1: Differential diagnosis of ectopic pregnancy (tubal abortion, rupture) according to clinical manifestation (leading symptoms).

Clinical stage	Tubal abortion	Tubal rupture
Stage 1: Embryo and tube intact	Stage 1: Asymptomatic	Stage 1: Asymptomatic
Stage 2: Dead or dying embryo; Bleeding into the tube possible, hematosalpinx	Stage 2: Uterine bleeding 6–8 weeks after LMP. Unilateral, contraction-like pains in lower abdomen. Tube is usually not yet palpable, does not become palpable until development of a hematosalpinx.	Stage 2: Asymptomatic; There is usually no stage 2 in tubal rupture: no bleeding because the tube ruptures before demise of the embryo.
Stage 3: Bleeding from the tube into the abdominal cavity	Stage 3: A number of episodes of weakness over weeks (peritoneal shock). Findings: gradual development of peritubal hematoma, retrouterine hematocele.	Stage 3: A single, severe attack (peritoneal shock), which occurs suddenly in a state of complete wellbeing. In brief: acute abdomen with internal hemorrhage!

Methotrexate are instilled into the ectopic pregnancy. The tubal pregnancy is usually reabsorbed.
- Systemic Methotrexate treatment. Proliferation of trophoblastic tissue is inhibited, therefore the ectopic pregnancy can be successfully treated with Methotrexate, particularly if hCG levels are < 4, 000 mIU/ml, a 92 % success rate has been described. The success rate declines if hCG levels are higher.
- Dosage: single dose 50 mg per kg body surface.
- Monitoring of hCG and hemogram on day 4 and 7 after treatment begin, hCG levels weekly till no longer detectable. Around 20 % of patients require a second injection, a few also a third. Abdominal ultrasound to monitor free fluid in the abdomen, in particular if Hb falls.

10.4 Placenta previa

Definition. Atypical localization of the placenta; the inner wall of the lower uterine segment is covered by placenta; 4 types are defined, dependent on the amount of cervix covered (see classification), whereby the cervix by definition is 3 cm dilated.

Note. Classification in 4 types:
1. Placenta praevia totalis, total placenta previa: the internal os is completely covered by the placenta (Figs. 10.14, 10.17).
2. Placenta praevia partialis, partial placenta previa; the internal os is partially covered by the placenta (Figs. 10.15, 10.18).
3. Placenta praevia marginalis, marginal placenta previa: the lower edge of the placenta reaches the internal os or covers it with a small segment (Figs. 10.16, 10.19).
4. Low-lying placenta: the part of the placenta which is in the lower uterine segment does not reach the internal os with its lower edge (Fig. 10.20). The lower edge is ≤ 5 cm from the internal os.

In the age of **transvaginal sonography** this traditional classification can be replaced by a modern one, which includes clinical consequences:

Distance of the margin of the placenta from internal os:
- **> 20 mm:** vaginal delivery desirable, no indication for primary CS due to placental location

- **11–20 mm:** increased likelihood of antepartum hemorrhage and for CS indication as a result
- **0–10 mm:** Antepartum hemorrhage is highly likely and CS will most likely be necessary

Occurrence. In multi- and grand multiparae, older primiparae; particularly after pregnancies or curettages in close succession; after CS; less often in primiparae.

Incidence. 1 placenta previa in 200 births.

Etiology. Unclear. A large placenta in a multipara, endometrial lesions and primary isthmic implantation play the main roles.

Large placenta. The most important etiological indication is the enlarged placenta in multi- and grand multiparae, in whom mucosal lesions are frequently found (see below).
Endometrial lesions due to inflammation, endometritis corporis, abortions, curettages, atrophy after pregnancies in quick succession, scars after CS. Consequence: reduced perfusion and insufficient nutrients for the conceptus, which doesn't implant in the upper section of the uterine cavity as a result, but instead in the lower uterine segment.
Primary isthmic implantation. The primary site of implantation of the conceptus is the lower uterine segment instead of in the mucosa of the uterine body. Rare.
Pathogenesis. The further the cervix dilates, the more stretched the internal os and with it, the placenta, becomes. The degree of coverage increases from 1mm to 3 cm!
The placenta previa is implanted low in the uterus, it covers the inner wall of the lower uterine segment to varying degrees, the opening of the internal os is completely or partially covered (Figs. 10.17, 10.18) or not reached (Figs. 10.19, 10.20).
The placenta is so positioned that it lies closer to the vagina than the presenting part of the fetus: it precedes the baby (P. previa) and more or less covers the exit route.

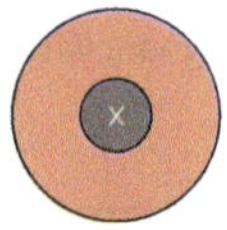

Fig. 10.14: Total placenta previa (cervix 3 cm dilated).

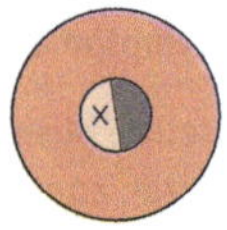

Fig. 10.15: Partial placenta previa (x = exposed membranes; cervix 3 cm dilated).

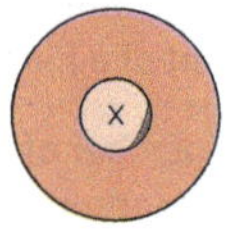

Fig. 10.16: Marginal placenta previa (cervix 3 cm dilated).

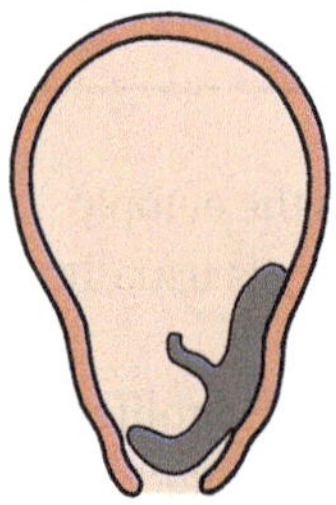

Fig. 10.17: Total placenta previa (fetus not depicted).

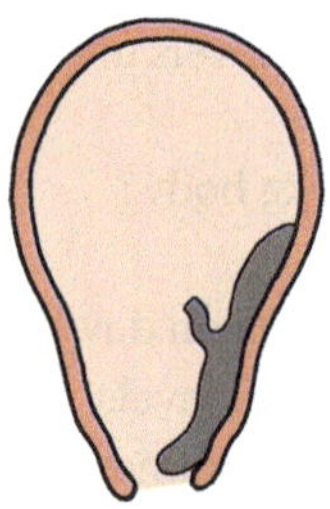

Fig. 10.18: Partial placenta previa (lateral; fetus not depicted).

Note. The greatest danger is that the placenta detaches and hemorrhages in the last weeks of pregnancy, at the latest in labor.

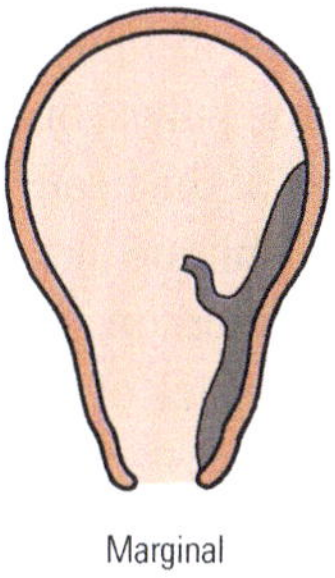

Fig. 10.19: Marginal placenta previa (fetus not depicted).

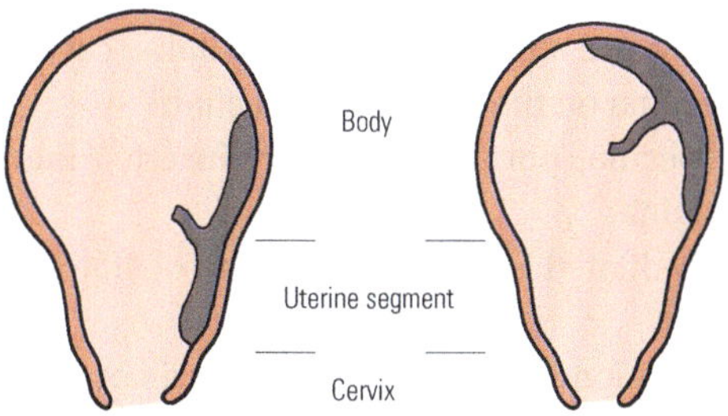

Fig. 10.20: Low-lying placenta (fetus not depicted).

Fig. 10.21: Normal site of placental attachment (high position; fetus not depicted).

If the placenta is positioned normally in the fundus (see Fig. 10.21), detachment usually does not occur until the baby has been born. The lower uterine segment is stretched from the onset of the first and weakest contractions. It effaces and thins – in contrast to the main body of the uterus, whose walls contract in every contraction! If the placenta is attached there, this results in:

- Maternal hemorrhage. As the section of the placenta which is attached to the lower uterine segment cannot stretch, its base is removed from under it once contractions begin, causing it to detach. This results in hemorrhage in the area of detachment, because the villi are removed from the decidua basalis and the intervillous spaces are ruptured.
- Fetal hemorrhage. Fetal villous vessels and larger placental vessels may rupture on placental separation: fetal Hb and RBC can be detected.
- Fetal hemorrhage is responsible for a number of fetal deaths due to placenta previa.
- Posthemorrhagic shock of the newborn (pallor, apnea, bradycardia) as a result of hemorrhage.

One of the most serious complications of birth! As the strength of the contractions increases, a growing section of placental surface is detached from the inner wall of the lower uterine segment: if the contractions increase in strength and cervical dilatation progresses, the previa hemorrhage becomes heavier, life-threatening!

Antenatal counseling. On the one hand, diagnosis of the location of the placenta as early as possible is important; on the other hand, it is also a known fact that the incidence of placental location on or near the internal os decreases with gestational age, particularly during the second trimester. As a result, women with the diagnosis of placenta previa **before week 20** often have a completely normal pregnancy outcome and birth. Early diagnosis of an abnormally located placenta therefore worries the pregnant woman needlessly and may also lead to unnecessary considerations regarding the mode of delivery.

A particularly interesting fact is that TVS diagnosis of abnormal placental location in **weeks 20–23** correlates to the pregnancy outcome, or rather to the mode of delivery:

- **Low-lying placenta.** High probability of normal course of labor.
- **Placenta covers the internal os by less than 25 mm.** High probability of spontaneous regression, further ultrasound examinations are indicated to monitor placental location.

– **Placenta covers the internal os by more than 25 mm.** High probability that placenta previa will persist and delivery will be by CS.

Practice tip. TVS to determine the placental attachment site between weeks 20–23 is sensible and allows a prognosis to be made regarding course of pregnancy and mode of delivery.

Clinical manifestation

Note. Leading symptoms are: 1) bleeding (→ cardinal symptom!); 2) malpresentation; 3) primary uterine inertia; 4) PPH.

1. **Bleeding** (→ cardinal symptom!) in pregnancy or labor.

Practice tip. Placenta previa bleeding occurs before ROM. Bleeding after ROM is not due to placenta previa!

Antenatal hemorrhage (→ after week 28). Warning bleeding. Bleeding due to placenta previa often occurs at rest, nights, and also during the day on movement. Occasionally mild contractions are present. The initial hemorrhage is never life-threatening, although it may make a threatening impression (warning bleed). Further hemorrhages occur at intervals of days or weeks. Their severity can never be predicted. A severe, life-threatening hemorrhage may follow a mild one.

Note. The severity of hemorrhaging increases successively, as does the anemia. Frequent, mild hemorrhages also cause anemia.

Hemorrhage at the onset of labor. The initial hemorrhage can occur with the first contractions in first stage.

Hemorrhage in labor from placenta previa is severe, often life-threatening for mother and baby!

2. **Malpresentation.** The placenta occupies a section of the entry to the true pelvis, obstructing normal presentation of the head. Malpositions, transverse lies, oblique lies and breech presentations are common.
3. **Primary uterine inertia** due to lack of pressure on the cervical ganglia.
4. **Postpartum hemorrhage**, see p. 380.

Diagnosis

Speculum examination in cases of acute hemorrhage. Never perform digital examination, but use sterile specula to examine cervix and vagina on the gynecological chair!
The specula, not the fingers are inserted into the vagina:
- How dilated is the cervix? Degree of effacement?
- Is the blood coming out of the cervix or from somewhere else?
- Is the hemorrhage very severe, severe, moderate, or slight?
- Cervix still closed, slightly open, 3–5 cm or more dilated?
- Membranes intact or ruptured?
- Exclude cervical carcinoma.

Sonography
- In acute hemorrhage. Placental location (already occurred in antenatal care), exclude retroplacental hematoma.
- Is placenta previa the cause of the hemorrhage (Fig. 10.22)?

Note. TVS has a diagnostic certainty of >99 % in placenta previa!

- Degree. Marginal, partial, total?
- Early diagnosis before warning bleed occurs (Fig. 10.22).

The possibility of placenta accreta must be excluded.

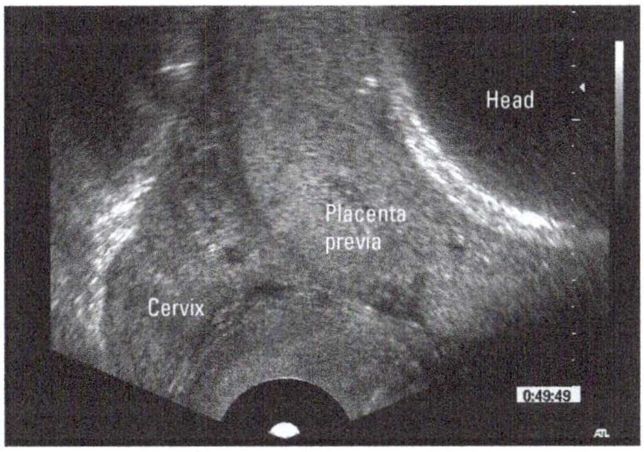

Fig. 10.22: Sonogram of a total placenta previa close to term.

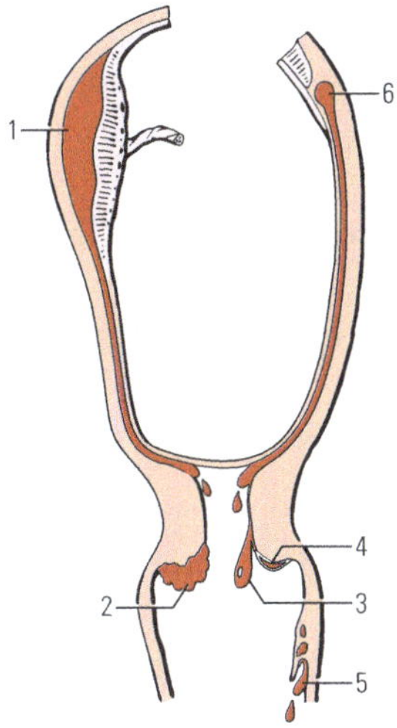

Fig. 10.23: Main hemorrhage sites in a term pregnancy (excluding placenta previa): 1) placental abruption) 2) cervical carcinoma; 3) cervical polyp; 4) cervical erosion; 5) varicose bleeding; 6) marginal sinus hemorrhage.

If placenta previa has been diagnosed the possibility of placenta accreta/increta/percreta must be considered, particularly after prior CS. Normally a hypoechogenic space is found between placental tissue and bladder, created by the myometrium and the retroplacental myometrial blood vessels. In cases of faulty placentation this space is absent; the placenta penetrates the wall of the bladder directly.

Differential diagnosis. 70–80 % of hemorrhages in the second half of pregnancy are due to placenta previa! In 20–30 % the bleeding has another source (Fig. 10.23):

1. Placental abruption (p. 374).
2. Cervical carcinoma. Excluded on speculum examination!
3. Cervical polyp. Speculum examination!
4. Cervical erosion. Speculum examination!
5. Arroded varicose veins of the vagina or clitoris bleed intensively are therefore impossible to overlook.
6. Marginal sinus bleeding (rupture of the Sinus circularis placentae), also in normally located placentae.

Complications. Risks for the mother: severe hemorrhage, exsanguination, infection, sepsis. Risks for the baby: hypoxia. The surface area of the site of placental attachment is reduced on detachment of the placenta from its base, which leads to a potentially considerably reduced oxygen supply. Posthemorrhage shock, exsanguination. The baby bleeds to death on detachment of the placenta as a result of rupture of villous or large placental blood vessels.

Treatment

Note. Whether delivery is vaginal or by cesarean section is decided by: volume of blood lost, intensity of the bleeding, degree of placenta previa, maternal and fetal conditions.

Procedure in mild hemorrhage

- Blood typing (already performed in antenatal care!).
- Ensure availability of compatible, cross-matched blood .
- Bed rest. Going to the toilet is allowed. Constipation is to be avoided!
- Bloody sanitary napkins are to be kept and shown so that bleeding intensity can be monitored.

- Observation.
- Hemogram. Hb < 9 g/100 ml means transfusion is necessary.
- CTG.
- Tocolysis suppresses contractions and thus new hemorrhages (see p. 102).
- Treatment to stimulate fetal lung maturation with 2 × 8 mg Betamethasone IM.
- Rh-negative women receive anti-D prophylaxis.

Procedure in cases of heavier hemorrhaging
CS or vaginal delivery?
- Same measures as for mild hemorrhage if urgency permits.
- Decision is based on results of speculum examination, TVS (see diagnosis).

Absolute indications for cesarean section
- Severe hemorrhage, cervix only slightly dilated, viable fetus.
- Hemorrhage which is life-threatening for the mother, minimally dilated cervix, nonviable or dead fetus.
- Total and partial placenta previa.

Cesarean section is the only procedure which can safely and quickly eliminate maternal and fetal risks.

Vaginal delivery
Indication. Membranes intact, hemorrhage mild or moderate, cephalic presentation, external os ≥ 5 cm, marginal placenta previa (forebag is felt in the cervix).

Procedure:
- 3 steps of management: 1) AROM. 2) Head is pressed from above into the pelvis. 3) Administration of uterotonics. AROM and entry of the head can stop the bleeding and begin the birth!
- The striking effect of AROM is brought about by the descent of the head on release of the forewaters. It compresses the detached section of the placenta against the inner wall of the lower uterine segment.
- If AROM is successful, vaginal hemostasis can be expected.
- If hemostasis does not occur, CS is performed.

Technique in three acts:
- AROM is performed with amnioscope. Risk of cord prolapse (placenta previa is the high presenting part). Never digitally rupture the membranes. The finger causes further placental detachment!
- Introduction of the head. During AROM a birth attendant presses the head firmly into the pelvis from above with both hands. In cases of obesity the Kristeller maneuver is more effective.
- Uterotonics are administered if contractions are absent or insufficient. Only now can the necessary force be created.

Third stage. In placenta previa, the birth of the baby is the beginning of a new danger period, third stage: severe hemorrhage is virtually a characteristic!

During vaginal delivery, hemorrhage is stopped by compression of the detached section of placenta. Postpartum this compression stops. The placenta detaches from its site of attachment and bleeds. In addition, the bleeding lower uterine segment contracts poorly. For this reason hemorrhage is still a threat after CS and complete removal of the placenta.

10.5 Placental abruption

Definition. Abruptio placentae; partial or complete detachment of the (normally located) placenta (in contrast to placenta previa) during the second half of pregnancy or in labor (Fig. 10.24) with maternal hemorrhage from the blood vessels of the site of attachment and retroplacental hematoma.

Placenta previa also detaches prematurely, its incorrect site is, however, the cause of detachment!

Incidence. Serious cases with classical symptoms are rare (0.2–0.5 %), mild and asymptomatic (see below): 1 %. Risk of recurrence in subsequent pregnancy 5–15 %, after two successive pregnancies with placental abruption 25 %!

Etiology. Unclear in 50–70 %. Causes in 30–50 % are: PIH, trauma, extreme uterine reaction after ROM, birth of second twin.

- PIH (see p. 74): Damage to capillary walls resulting in permeability and hemorrhage between uterine wall and site of placental attachment, which causes placental abruption: "The drama takes place in the capillaries" (Couvelaire).

Mechanical exogenous causes:

- Trauma (falling onto the abdomen, blow), in addition to a short cord (→ traction on the placenta).
- Extreme uterine reaction to a sudden drop in intrauterine pressure after: ROM in hydramnios, birth of the first twin.
- Result: rapid reduction of the size of the site of placental attachment, partial detachment, or detachment of the second twin's placenta.

Pathogenesis. Origin of the blood. Bleeding begins with detachment of the placenta from its site of attachment. It comes from small maternal blood vessels, rarely with fetal blood mixed in.

Practice tip. The more severe the hemorrhage, the larger the detached area.

Types of hemorrhage

Concealed hemorrhage (20–30 %). Blood collects in the space between the detached placenta and the inner wall of the uterus and creates a hematoma. If detachment occurs centrally (Fig. 10.25): retroplacental hematoma.

Mixed hemorrhage (concealed and revealed; 70–80 %). Not a major hemorrhage! Only possible if a marginal part of the placenta has detached. The blood makes its way between the membranes and inner uterine wall and flows through the cervical canal and vagina (Fig. 10.25).

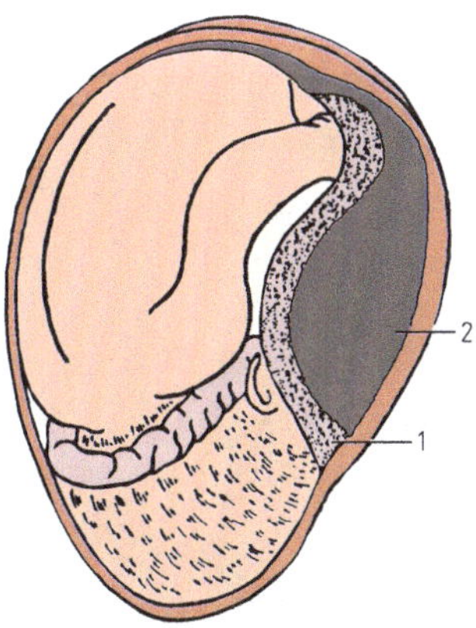

Fig. 10.24: Placental abruption: 1) completely detached placenta; 2) retroplacental hematoma.

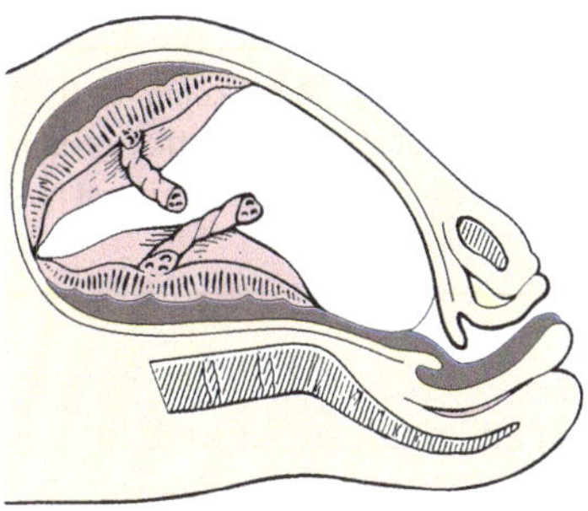

Fig. 10.25: Placental abruption. Top: centrally detached placenta with retroplacental hematoma. Bottom: placenta detached centrally and marginally with retroplacental hematoma and external bleeding.

Practice tip. Blood loss in placental abruption hemorrhage is mostly internal; the perceived vaginal bleeding is no indication of the extent of the hemorrhage!

Clinical manifestation

Note. In the majority of cases its occurrence is sudden, without warning; PIH is present in one third.

Subjective symptoms:
- Pain. Dominated by the sudden, intense pain in the lower abdomen, often described as piercing.
- General unwell feeling, combined with anxiousness, dizziness, fainting, shortness of breath, loss of consciousness. Sometimes a feeling of fullness and abdominal tension is described.
- Fetal movements are no longer felt.

Objective symptoms in severe cases:
- Mild vaginal bleeding is the most common symptom (70–80 %)! In 20–30 % the bleeding is internal (concealed).
- Shock. Pallor, colorless lips, hands, rapid, light pulse, hypotension.
- In particular the rapid loss of facial coloring indicates the severity.

Practice tip. The (mild) vaginal bleeding contrasts the extreme facial pallor, which is mainly caused by shock.

Note. Asymptomatic abruptions. More common than symptomatic are mild cases of abruption, with no symptoms or only mild ones in which the abruption is not recognized until delivery of the placenta.

Diagnosis
1. Uterus is taut and rigid, as if it were in a hypertonic state (even without contractions). The rigidity is a result of the hematoma.
2. Uterus is sensitive to touch, often so extremely that external examination is not possible. Cause: overdistension of the perimetrium (uterine serosa).
3. Points 1 and 2 make misdiagnosis of ruptured uterus possible.
4. Signs of hypoxia or missing cardiac action in CTG.
5. Ultrasound. Retroplacental hematoma (Fig. 10.26), in particular in anterior, not always in posterior placentae.
6. Fresh retroplacental hematomas have fewer echoes than the placenta.
7. Older retroplacental hematomas cause bulging of the placenta, no echogenicity.
8. Doppler sonography: no flow in the hematoma!
9. Placenta. Contains a bowl-like depression. Clots are adhered to its surface.

Differential diagnosis. Placenta previa (vaginal bleeding, no pain or uterine rigidity; p. 369), ruptured uterus, further hemorrhage causes (see DD placenta previa, p. 369).

Complication. Couvelaire syndrome, coagulopathy.

Couvelaire syndrome (uterine apoplexy; Apoplexia uteri)
Severe form of placental abruption with extravasation into the muscle wall (myometrial hem-

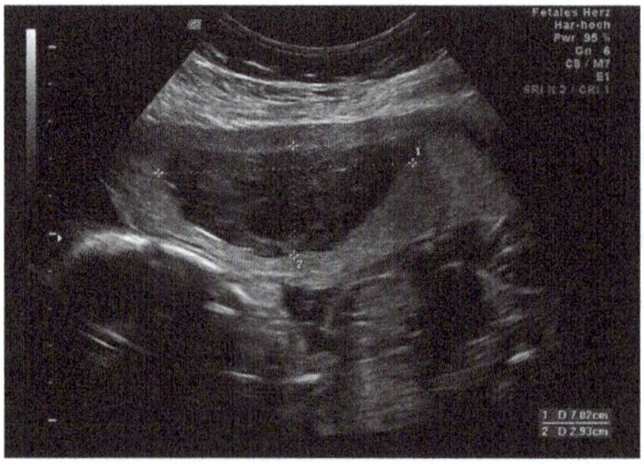

Fig. 10.26: Sonographic diagnosis of placental abruption with a retroplacental hematoma.

orrhage; no retroplacental hematoma) of the body of the uterus (→ uteroplacental apoplexy; Apoplexia uteroplacentaris). Muscle fibers are split and degenerate. The blood may pass through the serosa into the abdominal cavity (acute abdomen!)
Uterine serosa is a dark bluish-red to black, which Couvelaire compared to the appearance of an ovarian cystoma which has hemorrhagically infarcted after torsion.

Blood coagulation disorder (coagulopathy)
Etiology. Unclear. Activated coagulation factors (from thromboplastin) enter the maternal bloodstream from the retroplacental hematoma and the uteroplacental bed. In addition, fibrinolysis is excessively activated as a result of an inflow of tissue plasminogen activator (tPA) from the myometrium.

Pathogenesis, pathophysiology

Note. Coagulopathies after placental abruption and other complications of pregnancy and labor go through several phases: 1) phase of increased coagulation; 2) phase of coagulation and reactive fibrinolysis in the terminal vessels; 3) phase of manifest consumptive coagulopathy; 4) phase of profuse hemorrhages and pronounced organ failure.

Phase 1. Coagulation is activated without major changes to laboratory parameter being detectable.

Phase 2. Clots are formed in the terminal vessels (vascular pathway: arterioles → capillaries → venules) which activates fibrinolysis. With this, the consumption of coagulation factors and platelets begins.

Phase 3. If this process continues, coagulation and fibrinolysis also continue in the terminal vessels:
- Fibrinogen is broken down to fibrin, whereby the formed blood elements are enclosed in fibrin's fiber net → phase of increased coagulation, disseminated intravascular coagulation (DIC in the terminal vessels). Due to the consumption of fibrinogen (→ fibrin) and other coagulation factors this phase is termed consumptive coagulopathy (DIC).
- Microcirculatory disorder with damage to organs and tissues. Clots block the terminal vessels and reduce microcirculation. Hypoxia and metabolic acidosis cause tissue damage (kidney, liver, lungs, brain, spleen), later irreparable tissue necroses. In this phase of coagulation disorders such life-threatening tissue damage characterizes the disease.
- Acute renal failure (→ oliguria, anuria) with shock is in the foreground clinically.
- Fibrinolysis. The organism is capable of dissolving fibrin clots in the terminal vessels by fibrinolysis. Using proteolysis, plasmin breaks down fibrin and fibrinogen into degradation products. The blocked vascular pathway arterioles → capillaries → venules is reopened, microcirculation resumes. Tissue damage may be resolved.
- Hyperfibrinolysis with hypo- or afibrinogenemia. Fibrinolysis can be excessive, resulting in destruction of fibrin and fibrinogen. The fibrinogen level sinks: hypofibrinogenemia, fibrinolytic syndrome, defibrination syndrome.
- Fibrinogen deficiency hemorrhage from the wound surface of the uterus results, which initiates or intensifies shock. These hemorrhages are often life-threatening.

Note. Dangerous coagulation disorders manifest with a fibrinogen level of < 100 mg/100 ml (rare!). Normal level of plasma fibrinogen in pregnancy: 400–600 mg/ml.

Phase 4. Condition with life-threatening hemorrhage and severe organ failure.

Diagnosis. Coagulation status!
- Clot observation test. Screening test in afibrinogenemia or hyperfibrinolysis which measures the coagulation time of 1 ml of whole blood (reference value is 8–12 min at 22°); dissolution of the clot within 1 h suggests hyperfibrinolysis.
- Platelet count, fibrinogen level, platelet function, AT-III and thrombin time-
- Hemoglobin. Blood group and Rhesus factor should be known from antenatal care!
- Renal function. Urinary output (catheter!), creatinine, electrolyte (renal insufficiency).
- Acid-base status. BGA: picks up respiratory and metabolic disorders (pH, pCO_2, standard bicarbonate, base deviation: BE).

Treatment. Obstetric treatment. Shock and coagulopathy must be treated!

Obstetric management

Note. Goal. Rapid delivery: hemorrhage and hypofibrinogenemia increase; shock prophylaxis.

Abdominal operative delivery if the fetus has a chance of survival: EBW! Gestational age!

CS due to maternal indication can be avoided if vaginal birth progresses rapidly and coagulation remains stable (half-hourly monitoring). However, even if the fetus has died and coagulation status is normal a maternal indication for CS may still exist.

Vaginal delivery if fetus is dead or its chances of survival are very low:
- AROM is the most important measure, regardless of fetal station or cervical dilatation.
- Digital cervical dilatation, IV oxytocics.
- Intensive monitoring: BP, urinary output, coagulation, BGA.
- If necessary, treatment of shock and coagulopathy (see below).
- A universal time limit for the duration of labor is not possible; all obstetric measures are aimed at expediting delivery.
- Hysterectomy is only indicated in cases of severe PPH.
- If the uterus is atonic postpartum and treatment unsuccessful, it must be removed, whether delivery was vaginal or by cesarean.

Practice tip. Uterine discoloration in Couvelaire syndrome (p. 376) is not an indication for hysterectomy!

Treatment of shock. Coagulation disorder occurs and worsens if treatment for shock is not begun early and followed through:
- Cross-matching; infusion, central venous line.
- Volume replacement therapy: plasma replacement (hydroxyethyl starch; HES), plasma protein solution or fresh frozen plasma (FFP) until blood is available.
- Dosage based on effect: raised BP, lowered pulse, rosy periphery, warm face.
- Transfusion (whole blood or erythrocyte concentrate).
- Procedure in cases of renal insufficiency (in-dwelling catheter to monitor urinary output!), disruption of acid-base household and respiration.

Shock is controlled if urinary output is >30–40 ml/h.

Treat coagulation disorder (bleeding tendency)
- Obstetric treatment. Expedited delivery is the most important measure.
- No heparin while bleeding persists or there is increased risk of hemorrhage!
- Adequate volume substitution to ensure microcirculation continues. General rule: 1 ml blood loss is replaced by 3 ml crystalloid solution.
- Correction of metabolic acidosis, if present.

- FFP contains coagulation and fibrinolysis factors and is to be administered generously to compensate for consumption.
- Erythrocyte concentrate must be available. Begin infusion within 30 min if blood loss is around 1,500 ml.
- Platelet concentrate if platelet count < 50,000/µl.
- Antithrombin (AT III) replacement in AT III deficiency: 25 U/kg body weight.
- Fibrinogen concentrate 50 mg/kg body weight.
- Recombinant Factor VIIa after all other medical measures have been attempted: for example 100 µg/kg body weight as bolus injection.

Prognosis. The danger for the mother after placental abruption is high; in severe cases, if a third or more of the placenta is affected, it is unavoidable for the baby:
- Mother: Mortality 1 %, morbidity 20–30 %.
- Baby: usually dies in severe cases. Perinatal mortality: 20–50 % due to hypoxia (detachment of ¼ of the placenta kills the baby), exsanguination.

10.6 Velamentous insertion

Definition. Pathological insertion of the umbilical cord into the membranes. The 3 blood vessels (one Vena umbilicalis, 2 Aa umbilicales) run between amnion and chorion, branching apart before reaching the placenta.

Types. Central, lateral and marginal insertions are normal.
- Central insertion: attachment in the middle of the placenta.
- Lateral insertion: eccentric attachment.
- Marginal (or Battledore) insertion: at the edge of the placenta.
- Velamentous or membranous insertion: attachment into the membranes.

Incidence. About 1 %.

Clinical manifestation
Velamentous insertion is clinically relevant when the umbilical blood vessels, which run exposed and unprotected through the membranes, are in the vicinity of the cervix (vasa previa), or are compressed against the pelvic wall by the presenting fetal part. Only the fetus is at risk:
- Exsanguination (vaginal bleeding is fetal blood), if one of the larger vessels ruptures on ROM; the fetus dies quickly.
- Hypoxia, if unprotected vessel /s is/are compromised.

Diagnosis.

Before ROM:
- Palpation of pulsating blood vessels in the membranes in the cervix.
- CTG: variable decelerations on descent of the presenting part and compression of the blood vessels.
- Ultrasound and Doppler sonography: detection of vasa previa.

After ROM:
- Sudden hemorrhage on rupture of membranes.
- CTG: severe variable decelerations.

Differential diagnosis. 1) Placenta previa and low-lying placenta can be ruled out: bleeding before ROM, stops immediately on ROM. 2) Placental abruption can also be ruled out: placental abruption is accompanied by severe internal hemorrhage and poor general condition of the mother, which is unaffected by velamentous insertion despite heavy vaginal bleeding. 3) Marginal sinus bleeding in a normally located placenta.

Treatment. Goal of therapy is expedited delivery as the baby is in great danger.
- Vaginal delivery if the head is low, by forceps or VE.
- If, as seldom occurs, diagnosis has been made before ROM and the CTG is good, expectant management is possible. ROM must be delayed until the cervix is fully dilated.
- Abdominal operative delivery minutes after onset of hemorrhaging if the prerequisites for vaginal delivery are not fulfilled and the baby is alive and viable.

Antenatal diagnosis of vasa previa. The high risk of vasa previa can be reduced, in particular if the diagnosis is made antenatally. The pregnant woman is hospitalized from week 28 and delivery is by cesarean section at 35 weeks (see also recommendations of the **International Vasa Previa Foundation** – www.vasaprevia.org).

10.7 Postpartum hemorrhage (PPH)

Definition. Abnormal blood loss (normal = 200–300 ml) after birth or abortion, 2–4 h postpartum > 500 ml, after cesarean section > 1,000 ml.

Note. Classification. Cause 1. Hemorrhage from the site of placental attachment is the most common (gaping uteroplacental blood vessels) in cases of incomplete or after complete placental separation. Two types: PPH before placental separation (separation hemorrhage) and PPH after separation (atonic PPH). **Cause 2.** Laceration hemorrhage from soft tissue injury: usually cervix, more rarely clitoris and labial lacerations, even more rarely episiotomy wounds, isolated vaginal lacerations, very rarely perineal lacerations. **Cause 3.** Hemorrhage due to coagulation disorder (hypo- or afibrinogenemia). It is not rare for the bleeding to originate from the site of attachment as well as from a laceration!

10.7.1 Separation hemorrhage, atonic PPH

Definition. Excessive bleeding due to impaired placental detachment before (separation hemorrhage: early hemorrhage) or after expulsion of the placenta (atonic PPH).

Separation hemorrhage (before placental expulsion). Excessive bleeding from the site of attachment usually occurs when the placenta partially detaches.

Etiology. Functional and anatomical- pathological causes.

Functional causes:
- Atonic hemorrhage in cases of adherent placenta (Placenta adhaerens; Fig. 10.27). Main cause is restricted uterine contractility.
- Contractions after delivery have a limited effect on the placenta:
  - Location (tubal placenta). Placenta is in a corner near the tube and the postpartum contractions barely reach it.
  - Shape. Flat: Placenta membranacea or anularis (ring-shaped placenta; middle section of the placenta is atrophied).
  - Size. Abnormally small placenta.

Anatomical-pathological causes (impaired placental detachment):
- The placenta does not detach at all! Due to a partial or complete lack of decidua (prior deep curettage, cesarean section or removal of myomas) the chorion frondosum is attached directly to the myometrium. Depending on the degree of attachment, this is termed **Placenta accreta**, increta (Fig. 10.28) or percreta (into the serosa or neighboring organs).

Incidence. About 1 in 500–7,000 births, the incidence is increasing due to the increasing rate of cesarean sections; impaired separation is due to placenta previa in 20 % of cases.

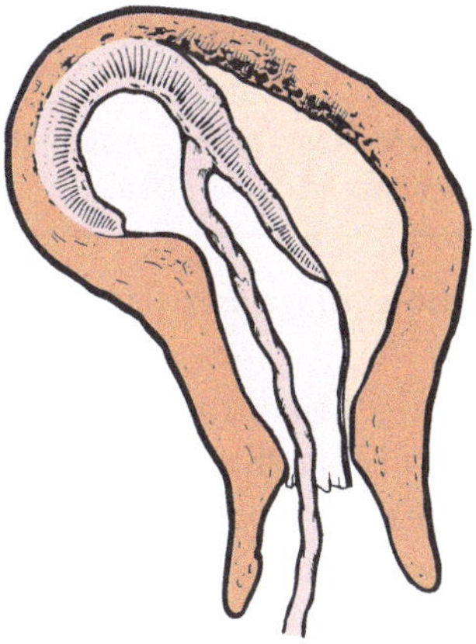

Fig. 10.27: Adherent placenta; common!

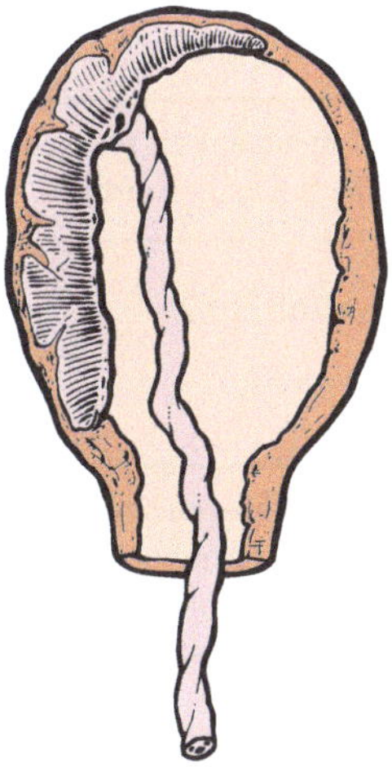

Fig. 10.28: Placenta accreta, or rather increta.

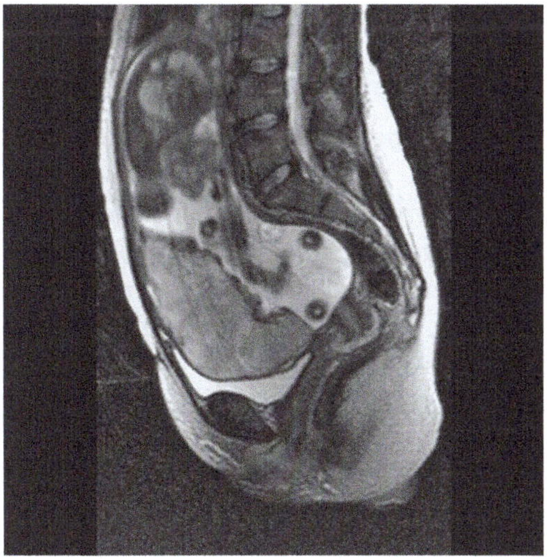

Fig. 10.29: Magnetic resonance imaging: anterior placenta with placenta percreta.

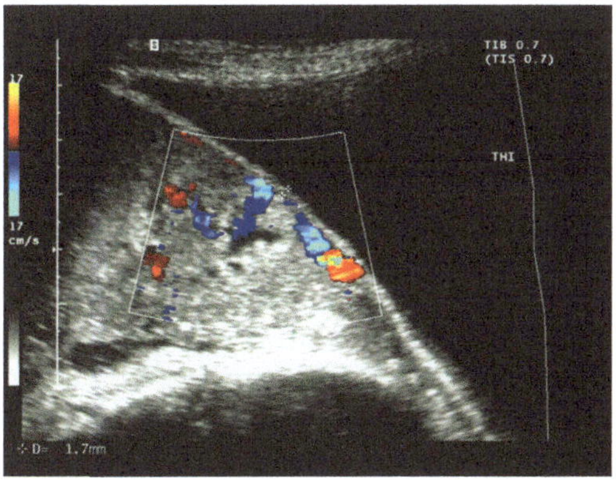

Fig. 10.30: Sonographic findings in low-lying placenta and placenta increta.

Antenatal diagnosis. The placental invasion of the myometrium is seen on ultrasound examination, and color Doppler sonography detects the increased vascularization of the bladder wall (Figs. 10.29, 10.30).

Treatment. Usually not suspected until the placenta does not separate and difficulties are encountered on manual separation with artificial layers of separation and the risk of perforation. In these, usually dramatic, cases treatment must be consistent with the treatment program for atonic PPH with IV prostaglandins and operative measures culminating in hysterectomy. When the above-named risk factors are present, diagnosis should be made antenatally if possible. As mode of delivery, cesarean hysterectomy can then be chosen or a decision made to either perform a focal incision of the uterine wall in cases of impaired placental separation with clearly demarcated abnormal attachment, or uterotomy and delivery of the baby, leaving the placenta in situ, with the possibility of postoperative administration of methotrexate.

Atonic PPH (hemorrhage after placental separation)

Atonic uterus with incomplete placenta. Hemorrhage results when part of the placenta or a succenturiate lobe is retained in the uterine cavity, because the uterine musculature cannot contract sufficiently.

Practice tip. A retained fragment of placenta (bean-sized is sufficient) is life-threatening! If placental tissue is missing, or ruptured blood vessels are found at the edge of the placenta or in the membranes, a manual exploration must be performed immediately!

Note. Causes of retained placental tissue:
- Hemorrhage immediately after expulsion of the incomplete placenta; rare.

More common are:
- Hemorrhage in the puerperium. Most common cause of puerperal hemorrhage (p. 412), which can be severe.
- Puerperal infection (septicemia; p. 406), originating from an infection of the placental polyp (dead tissue!).
- Transformation of the placental tissue into a trophoblastic tumor (see p. 362).

Succenturiate lobes. Ruptured blood vessels on the membranes and at the edge of the placenta are evidence of one or more succenturiate lobes.

Atonic uterus with complete placenta

Practice tip. Atonic PPH also occurs in the absence of risk factors in history, findings and course of labor.

Clinical manifestation, diagnosis (see Tab. 10.2)
- Source of hemorrhage: hemorrhage from the site of attachment, usually in cases of atonia and after placental separation, or from a laceration; inspection of the cervix.
- Coagulation parameters. Hypo- or afibrinogenemia (p. 376)?
- Placenta and membranes are inspected directly after delivery: defects? Succenturiate lobe?

Note. Inspection of placenta and membranes is the most important condition for the prevention of hemorrhage.

Differential diagnosis. See Tab. 10.2

Treatment

Note. Excessive blood loss before or after expulsion of the placenta is the most common cause of maternal death! Principle of treatment is pharmacological prophylaxis.

Pharmacological prophylaxis. Uterotonics are administered when the leading head crowns, the shoulders are born, or the after-coming head emerges in breech presentation. Results are: re-

Tab. 10.2: Differential diagnosis atonic hemorrhage (common!) and laceration hemorrhage (rare!).

Hemorrhage from the site of attachment	Laceration hemorrhage
– Uterus hypotonic, soft, often abnormally large and high. – Delayed vaginal hemorrhage (several minutes) after birth of the baby, because the uterine cavity fills up first. Intermittent episodes of profuse vaginal bleeding. – If the uterus is hypotonic it slowly becomes firmer after massage or uterotonics → atonic hemorrhage from the site of attachment (hemorrhage may also be occurring from a laceration!)	– Uterus is hard, firmly contracted, small. – Vaginal bleeding commences immediately after birth of the baby; continuous (not intermittent). Speculum examination, laceration must be found! – The uterus becomes firm after massage or uterotonics, bleeding continues.

duced blood loss, shorter third stage. General prophylaxis: uterotonics are administered after every birth. Targeted prophylaxis: uterotonics are administered if indicated.

Indications (targeted prophylaxis).
History:
- Prior PPH.
- Multipara.
- Rapid birth succession.
- Postterm delivery.
- Prior CS.
- Frequent abortions.

Note. Women with a history of severe PPH must deliver in a hospital!

According to findings and course of labor:
- Uterus has emptied too rapidly: after operative delivery (CS!), forceps and version with extractions; after VE.
- Overdistended uterus; in twins, hydramnion, in particular with large, heavy babies
- Uterine fatigue: after overcoming CPD, prolonged labor.
- Lax uterus: after long narcosis, overadministration of spasmolytics shortly before third stage.
- Hypotonic uterus: after primary or secondary uterine inertia, continuous IV oxytocin.
- Uterine tumor: fibromyomas, endometriosis.
- Malformed uterus: arcuate, subseptate uterus.

Uterotonics

3 units of oxytocin i.v.
Oxytocin infusion, as continuous IV infusion, possibly continuation of oxytocin infusion which was used in labor (see below).
- Increase dosage to 400 ml/h until third stage is completed (placenta has separated, been expelled and is complete)

Practice tip. Leave intravenous line in place! Atonic hemorrhage can suddenly occur after birth of the complete placenta and can be treated via the cannula. If the placenta is incomplete and manual exploration is necessary or an episiotomy needs suturing, intravenous access is available for administration of narcotics.

PPH before placental separation (separation hemorrhage)

Treatment plan in five steps

1. **i.v. uterotonics**
   a) 3 IU oxytocin i.v. (intravenous line) or
   b) Oxytocin infusion (6 IU in 500 ml electrolyte solution).
   c) Oxytocin is easily controlled (rapid acting, short duration of action). Placental separation is not made more difficult, and a placenta which has already separated will not be trapped.
   d) Plasma expanders: administration of 500–1,000 ml (e.g., crystalloid and colloid solutions) to prevent hypovolemic shock. The infusion rate can be increased in case of shock (rapid pulse, hypotension).
   e) FFP for volume replacement and prevention of a coagulation disorder.
   f) If more than 20 % of the total blood volume (calculation: 9 % of the woman's body weight) has been lost, erythrocyte concentrate must be given; if platelet count is < 50,000/µl, infusion of platelet concentrate!
2. **Empty bladder (catheter), uterine massage**
   a) If the woman is unable to urinate, catheterize. A full bladder inhibits contractions in first, second and third stage. A full bladder also causes a separated placenta to be retained in the uterine cavity.

   b) Light uterine massage, rubbing with the fingertips (midwife). Do not press firmly or squeeze!
   c) Icepack.
   d) If the placenta has separated, expel immediately with the Credé maneuver.
   e) If the placenta has not yet separated: preparation for manual removal (lithotomy position, disinfection), meanwhile
3. **Credé maneuver without anesthetic.** If unsuccessful:
4. **Credé maneuver under anesthetic (Fig. 10.31).** Final external attempt!

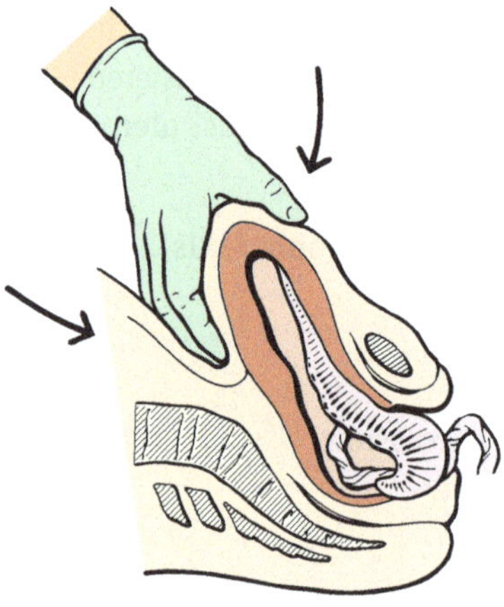

Fig. 10.31: Credé maneuver.

Method: the maneuver requires force, but not violent pressure or squashing! If uncontrolled force is used there are two dangers:
   a) Uterine inversion, if the uterus hasn't been made to contract strongly.
   b) Pressure and bruising of muscles and decidua mobilize thromboplastin (thrombokinase), which leads to coagulation disorder (see p. 376).

Practice tip. The Credé maneuver, particularly if performed under narcosis (relaxed abdomen!), is a valuable maneuver to separate the adherent placenta.

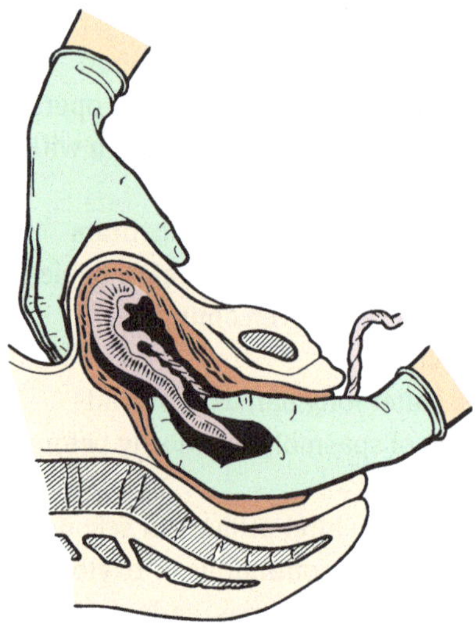

Fig. 10.32: Manual placenta removal.

If the Credé maneuver is also unsuccessful, manual removal must be performed.

5. **Manual removal of the placenta** (Fig. 10.32). Performance under the same narcosis after unsuccessful Credé maneuver. Method:
   a) It is recommended that right-handers insert the left hand and use the right hand externally. More strength is required from the external hand, which pushes and holds the uterus towards the internal hand.
   b) The external (right) hand always begins. It takes hold of the fundus from above and below and forces the uterus downwards into the pelvis until the external os is almost visible in the vulva.
   c) The internal (left) hand is now inserted directly into the external os without touching the vagina. This is achieved with the use of a large Bumm speculum, which bridges the short stretch: vulva → introitus → external os.

d) The external hand can release the uterus for a moment and give the umbilical cord, which is hanging out, a tug to tauten it, so that the internal hand can quickly follow the tight cord to the site of the placenta, where it then finds the separated edge of the placenta.
e) The internal hand is flattened and inserted between placenta and uterine wall. Pay attention to the layer! The external hand forcefully pushes the attached part of the placenta towards the internal hand. It can best be removed with the little finger side of the hand, in a slow and cautious (risk of uterine perforation!) sawing movement.
f) The force must be exerted by the external hand. The internal hand needs only to find the gap between the uterine wall and the placenta and to receive the placenta. Most failures are the result of ignoring this rule. Force must not be used to remove any parts of the placenta! After separation of the placenta, the internal hand remains in the uterus. The site of implantation is now inspected. First the external hand pulls firmly on the umbilical cord to remove the detached placenta from uterus and vagina. The internal hand, which has remained in the uterus, can move freely and explore the site of attachment once more to determine whether placental tissue has been retained.

Note. Difficulties of manual removal
- Entrapped placenta (placenta incarcerata: cramp of the internal os). A cramp of the internal os can narrow the entry so that it is not possible to enter the uterine cavity. The hand remains in the vagina under narcosis. Usually the cramp ceases after a few minutes. The separated placenta is often found in the cavity, it was incarcerated.
- Placenta accreta, increta, percreta, see p. 380.

PPH after placental expulsion (atonic PPH)

Atonic uterus with incomplete placenta. Manual exploration to extract retained placental tissue or succenturiate lobe/s:
- Method as for manual removal.
- If digital removal is difficult, curettage using the large Bumm curette is recommended.
- Manual exploration also if fever is present, if a bean-sized or larger fragment of placenta is missing.

Atonic uterus with complete placenta (see above: indications, targeted prophylaxis).

Treatment program in 7 steps
1. **Rapid oxytocin infusion i.v.**
   a) 20 IU oxytocin in 500 ml basic solution, infusion rate 500 ml/h.
2. **Fundal pressure, rub up a contraction, ice pack, empty bladder. Uterotonics are most effective when the bladder is empty!**
   a) Administration of uterotonics, Credé maneuver to remove intrauterine blood.
   b) Following these measures, a contraction is stimulated with gentle rubbing.
   c) Do not knead. Contractions cannot be stimulated by kneading.
3. **Fundal pressure and monitoring of the uterus.** A hand holds the well-contracted uterine fundus from above (Fig. 10.33): thumbs anterior, four fingers posterior, holding it firmly. It does not make sense to hold a uterus which is not well-contracted. The uterus is held in this way so that it cannot refill with blood and rise, and the state of contraction can be monitored.

   a) Tonization is supported by careful stroking and rubbing movements with the fingers.
   b) If the uterine tone decreases (uterus soft, relaxed) the hold changes and anterior and posterior walls are pressed firmly together and forcefully into the pelvis towards the vulva to prevent it from filling with blood again.
   c) Speculum examination! Cervical laceration?
   d) Coagulation disorder (p. 377).
   e) The focus is often on the uterus in PPH, and the fact that there may be other causes is often forgotten.
4. **Prostaglandins**
   a) Sulprostone: infusion. 500 µg in 500 ml electrolyte solution in 60–120 min (4–8 ml/min) or
   b) misoprostol suppository 800–1,000 mg.
5. **Removal of blood clots, manual exploration (silent rupture?)**
   a) Remove blood clots which prevent contraction of the uterus.
   b) Manual exploration, whether clots are adhered to the wall or placental tissue retained (although the placenta appeared to be complete). Clots adhering to the wall also reduce contractility of the uterus, are therefore a potential cause of hemorrhage.
   c) Manual exploration whether uterine rupture has occurred.

Manual removal method. After disinfecting the hand it is inserted in the uterine cavity and removes blood clots and membranes if necessary. Afterwards the cavity is explored to exclude the possibility of laceration.

Hamilton's maneuver to compress the uterus (Fig. 10.34): uterine walls are pressed together for a long time (in severe cases 1–2 h), so that hemorrhage into the uterine cavity does not resume.

– The external hand presses the uterus firmly against the internal hand. The internal hand is made into a fist and so positioned in the vagina that the knuckles are directed towards the anterior wall of the uterus. Firm pressure and counterpressure of the external and internal hand, pressing anterior and posterior walls of the uterus firmly together. In addition, both hands simulta-

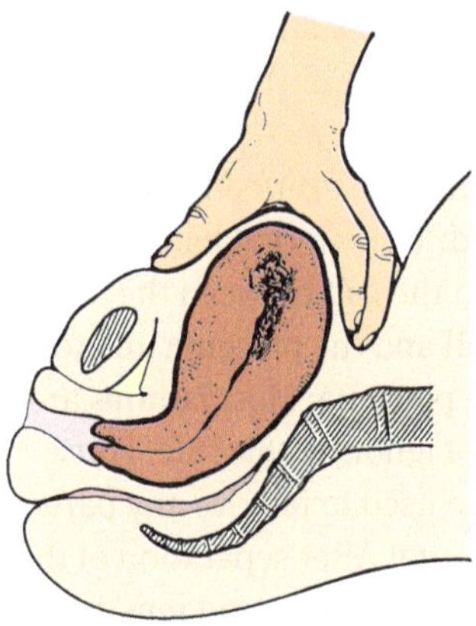

Fig. 10.33: Holding the uterus.

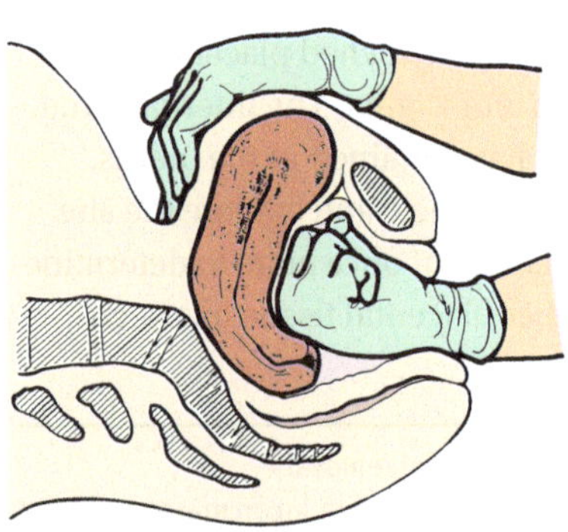

Fig. 10.34: Hamilton's maneuver (punching-ball maneuver) for the control of atonic PPH with internal and external hand.

neously massage the uterus lightly, without releasing the firm hold on the organ.
- External hand. The individual fingers lightly tap the posterior uterine wall.
- Internal hand. The fist is slowly rotated from side to side so that the knuckles lightly massage the anterior wall. In this way, regular contractions are stimulated.

Note. Aortal compression (Fig. 10.35). Last resort, although compression of the abdominal aorta is simple: The fist is used to press the aorta against the spine for 15–20 min. This causes hemostasis and further steps can be undertaken in peace.

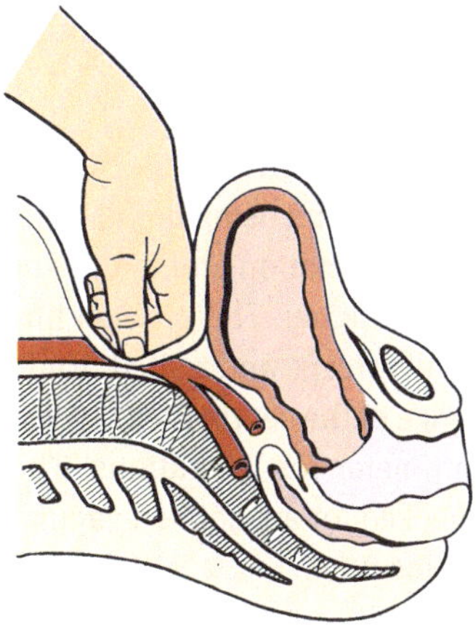

Fig. 10.35: Manual aortic compression.

6. **Operative measures.** If the measures listed above are unsuccessful (= hemostasis), operative measures to be considered include laparotomy with
   a) B-Lynch sutures (Fig. 10.36) with Vicryl® BT-3 (Ethicon) or Safil® HR 48 (Braun) or other uterus compression sutures,
   b) Ligation of the hypogastric artery (Aa iliacae internae; Fig. 10.37) or clipping of the uterine artery in addition to
   c) Total or supracervical hysterectomy.

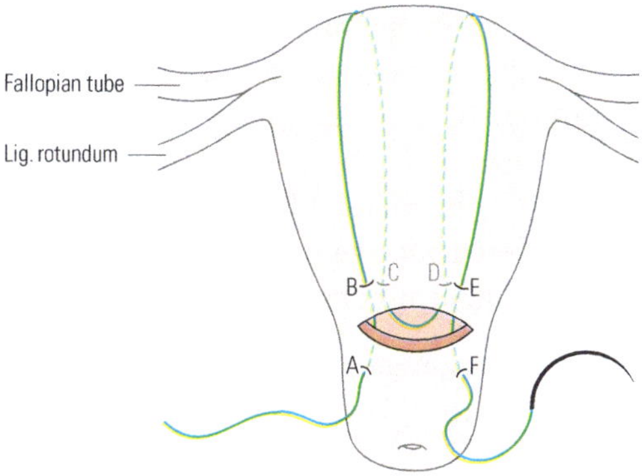

Fig. 10.36: B-Lynch uterine compression suture.

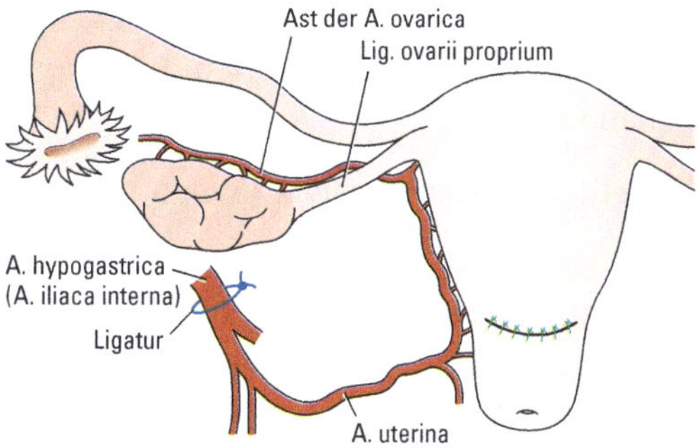

Fig. 10.37: Uterine arteries and ligation possibilities for atonic PPH.

The **Tamponade Balloon** (SOS Bakri Tamponade Balloon, Cook Ob/Gyn, USA) has been suggested for temporary reduction of atonic PPH. In appropriate cases (non-life-threatening blood loss, time and transport justifiable), and if a radiologist is available, **intravascular embolization** of the uterine arteries with gelatin and/or microparticles is a very suitable method.

Note. Do not leave consideration of and preparation for an operation or interventional treatment too late!

---

7. **Coagulation disorder** (→ acute hemorrhagic syndrome, coagulopathy; treatment see p. 377).

10.7.2 Hemorrhage from a laceration

Definition. Hemorrhage from soft tissue laceration wounds in the post-placental period (contrast: hemorrhage from the site of placental attachment, see p. 380); uterus is contracted, without afibrinogenemia.

Etiology. Laceration of cervix (see below), vagina, clitoris (p. 320) or perineum.

The cervix is the most frequent source of hemorrhage!

Cervical laceration

Definition. Laceration of the cervix, usually during delivery, e.g., if the cervix is not completely dilated or is widened too quickly via dilatation.

Emmet tear = scarred cervix (from a previous birth).

Etiology. High cervical tears occur if operative delivery is performed too early, incorrectly or badly and if the cervix is incompletely dilated after:
- Version and extraction.
- Forceps/VE delivery.

Preferred location is the lateral cervix, usually unilateral. The tear runs longitudinally upwards, begins at the external os and can extend to the internal os.
If the cervical branch of the uterine artery ruptures, heavy bleeding results. In addition, broad, deep opening of the parametrium often occurs.

Clinical manifestation

Early hemorrhage:
- Monosymptomatic. Severe PPH with well-contracted uterus, if the cervical branch of the uterine artery is ruptured.
- Sometimes bleeding may not occur even from a high extended tear (cervical tears are often overlooked).

Late hemorrhage:
- In the puerperium if hemostasis occurred and it was not sutured.
- In cases of ascending infection in the puerperium due to bacterial migration into the circulatory system, into the parametrium and paracolpium.

Note. The smallest cervical tears can cause parametrial infiltration and serve as the port of entry for fatal puerperal septicemia.

Diagnosis
- Clotting parameters (exclude afibrinogenemia).
- Inspect vagina and cervix with broad speculum and ball forceps (PPH often occurs coincidentally).

The cervix must be examined and inspected for laceration all the way around using broad specula after version with extraction and forceps or VE from mid-pelvis or higher. The cervical lips are grasped with ball forceps and pulled firmly downwards. The edge of the cervix is examined centimeter by centimeter for lacerations! The vagina must be checked for an isolated vaginal laceration at the same time.

Treatment. Laceration is sutured with 2 maneuvers:

- Firm fundal pressure is applied to push the uterus into the pelvis.
- Broad specula are inserted. The external os is immediately visible. It is grasped with Collin clamps and firmly pulled downwards (Fig. 10.38).

Suturing technique. No time is to be wasted with preparations!

After the tear has been located and the cervix positioned (Fig. 10.38a), needle, needle holder, suture, and tweezers are required. Suture is Vicryl® 3-0 and needle should be not too large.

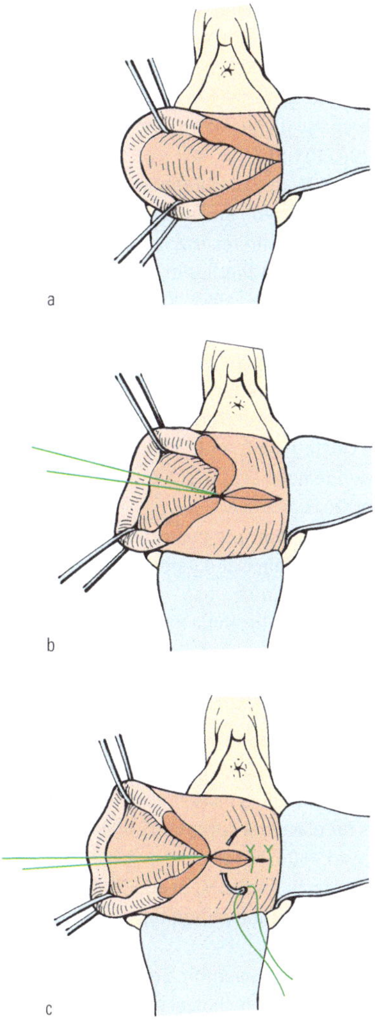

Fig. 10.38: Cervical laceration, examination and suturing: a) examination; b) first suture; c) identification and suturing of the apex of the cervical laceration.

Beginner's mistake. Trying to place the first suture at the apex of the laceration. This is not possible, at least not in longer tears. Lose no time with such experiments! The first suture is placed at the highest point of the laceration which can be comfortably reached. Include the complete cervix (Fig. 10.38b) and as much tissue as possible.

Knot and apply traction until the apex becomes visible (Fig. 10.38c). The ruptured artery is often found here, and is sutured. The tear is now sutured from the apex. Always use round, never sharp needles! Danger of damaging other blood vessels!
If the laceration extends beyond the internal os, laparotomy is performed.

Prophylaxis. Never apply forceps or perform a foot extraction until the cervix is definitely fully dilated! No extraction on the breech and no forceps or VE if cervix is not completely dilated! Do not allow bearing down if cervix is not fully dilated.

References

Ananth CV, Berkowitz GS, Savitz DA, Lapinski RH: Placental abruption and adverse perinatal outcomes. JAMA 1999; 282:1646

Ananth CV, Demissie K, Smulian JC, Vintzileos AM: Relationship among placenta previa, fetal growth restriction, and preterm delivery: a population-based study. Obstet Gynecol 2001; 98:299

Ananth CV, Savitz DA, Williams MA: Placental abruption and its association with hypertension and prolongecl rupture of membranes: a methodologic review and meta-analysis. Obstet Gynecol 1996; 88:309

Becker RH, Vonk R, Mende BC, et al.: The relevance of placental location at 20–23 gestational weeks for prediction of placenta previa at delivery: evaluation of 8650 cases. Ultrasound Obstet Gynecol 2001; 17:496

Bernirschke K, Kaufmann P: Pathology of the human placenta. New York, Springer 2000

Bodelon C, Bernabe-Opitz A, Schiff MA, Reed SD: Factors associated with peripartum hysterectomy. Obstet Gynecol 2009; 114:115–23

Condous GS, Arulkumaran S, Symonds I, et al.: The `tamponade test' in the management of massive postpartum hemorrhage. Obstet Gynecol 2003; 101:767

Dashe JS, McIntire DD, Ramus RM, et al.: Persistence of placenta previa according to gestational age at ultrasound detection. Obstet Gynecol 2002; 99:692

Delotte J, Novellas S, Koh C, Borıgain A, Chevallier P: Obstetrical prognosis and pregnancy outcome following pelvic arterial embolisation for post-partum hernorrhage. Eur J Obstet Gynecol Reprod Biol 2009; 145:129–32
Eckman MH, Erban JK, Singh SK, Kao GS: Screening for the risk for bleeding or thrombosis. Ann Intern Med 2003; 138:W15–24
Empson M, Lassere M, Craig J, Scott J: Prevention of recurrent rniscaırriage for women with antiphospholipic antibody or lupus anticoagulant. Cochrane Database Syst Rev 2005; 2:CD 2859
Goldstein DP, Berkowitz RS: Prophylactic chemotherapy of complete molar pregnancy. Semin Oncol 1995; 22:157
Gris JC, Mercier E, Quere I et al: Low-molecular weight heparin versus low-dose aspirin in women with one fetal loss and a constitutional thrombophilic discorder Blood 2004; 103:3695
Gülmezoglu M et al: WHO multicentre randomized trial of misoprostol in the management of the birth stage of labour. Lancet 2001; 358:689
Henrich W, Fuch I, Ehrenstein T et al: Antenatal diagnosis of placenta percreta with planned in situ retention and methotrexate therapy in a woman infected with HIV. Ultrasound Obstet Gynecol 2002; 20:90
Kulier R, Gulmezoglu, AM, Hofmeyr GJ et al: Medical methods for first trimester abortion. Cochrane Database Syst Rev 2004; 2:CD 002855
Laughon SK, Wolfe HM, Visco AG: Prior caesarean and the risk for placneta previa on second-trimester ultrasonography. Obstet Gynecol 2005; 128:105
Niiinimäki M, Jouppila P, Martikainen H, Talvensaari-Mattila A: A randomized study comparing efficacy and patient satisfaction in medical or surgical treatment of miscarriage. Fertility Sterility 2006; 86:367
Oppegard KS, Abdelarov M, Nesheim BI et al: The use of oral misoproston for pre-abortion cervical priming: a randomized tria of 400 versus 200 microg in first trimester pregnancies. Br J Obstet Gynaecol 2004; 111:154
Oppenheimer LW, Farine D: A new classification of placenta previa: Measuring progress in obstetrics. Am J Obstet Gynecol 2009; 201:227–9
Oyelese Y, Catanzarite V, Prefumo F: Vasa previa: The impact of prenatal diagnosis on outcomes. Obstet Gynecol 2004; 103:937
Rai R, Cohen H, Dave M, Regan L: Randomised controlled trial of aspirin and aspirin plus heparin in pregnant women with recurrent miscarriage with phospholipids antibodies or antiphospholipid antibodies. BMJ 1997; 314:253
Royal College of Obstetricians and Gynecologists: Placenta praevia, placenta praevis accreta and vasa praevia: diagnosis and management. Green-top Guideline No. 27, January 2011
Royal College of Obstetricians and Gynecologists: Antepartum haemorrhage. Green-top Guideline No. 63, Nov. 2011
Seifer DB: Persistent ectopic pregnancy: an argument for heightened vigilance and patient compliance. Fertil Steril 1997; 68:402
Sharma A, Suri V, Gupta I: Tocolytic therapy in conservative management of symptomatic placenta previa. Int J Gynaecol Obstet 2004; 84:109
Society of Maternal-Feta] Medicine: Placenta accreta. Am J Obstet Gynecol 2010; 203:430–439
Tikkanen M, Nuutila M, Hiilesma V, et al.: Prepregnancy risk factors for placental abruption. Acta Obstet Gynecol Scand 2006; 85:40
Toivonen S, Heinonen S, Anttila M, et al.: Obstetric prognosis after placental abruption. Feta Diagn Ther 2004; 19:336
World Health Organization Scientific Group: Gestational trophoblastic disease. Technical report series 692. WHO, Geneva 1983
Yao M, Tulandi T: Current status of surgical and nonsurgical management of ectopic pregnancy. Fertil Steril 1997; 67:421
Zhang J, Gilles JM, Barnhart K, et al.: A comparison of medical management with Misoprostol and surgical management of early pregnancy failure. N Engl J Med 2005; 353:761

11 Normal puerperium

Definition. Period of time after the birth (postpartum, p.p.) in which the changes to the woman's body brought about by pregnancy and childbirth regress. It begins with the birth of the complete placenta and lasts 6–8 weeks. It is characterized by:
- Involution processes.
- Wound-healing processes.
- Beginning of and continued lactation.
- Resumption of ovarian functions.

11.1 Process of involution

Definition. Return of maternal organs to their original position, size, shape and state. The final state does not, however, correspond to the original state from before the pregnancy in all anatomical and functional aspects.

Involution of the uterus, pelvic floor, abdominal wall, pelvic girdle, bladder, bowels, increased tone of the abdominal muscles, reabsorption of retained fluid. All organs of the female organism whose performance was affected by the pregnancy readjust once more to the nonpregnant state in the puerperium.

Causes. Once the placenta has been expelled, two changes are effected.

Uterine hormone supply is immediately almost completely shut off. The following are no longer supplied:
- Human chorionic gonadotropin (hCG).
- Human placental lactogen (hPL).
- Progesterones.
- Estrogens.

The **blood supply to the uterine musculature** is shut off to a large extent by the puerperal contractions.

Puerperal contractions. Three types: the tonic contraction (or retraction), spontaneous rhythmic contractions (afterpains), stimulus contractions (e.g., on breastfeeding).

Tonic contraction. In the first days after birth the uterus feels constantly quite hard or "tight". The tonic contraction of the uterine musculature begins in the hours after expulsion of the placenta and slowly decreases over the course of the next 4–5 days.

Spontaneous rhythmic contractions = afterpains occur in addition to the tonic contraction. They begin a few hours after delivery and stop on the second or third day postpartum. The intervals between them are initially short, and become increasingly longer. The primipara barely notices them. For multiparae, afterpains, which spread from the back towards the front, are usually associated with very unpleasant pains. Afterpains promote shortening of the muscle fibers.

Stimulus contractions = lactation contractions occur in particular when the baby is placed to the breast and sucks. The sucking stimulus on the nipple increases the amount of the contraction-stimulating oxytocin released from the posterior pituitary.

Consequences of the puerperal contractions
- Shutdown of a large part of the blood supply to the muscles of the uterus. This results in: contraction ischemia, which in turn brings about degeneration and autolysis of superfluous muscle fibers.
- Hemostasis of the uterine wound. Muscle contractions cause ligature and closure of the majority of the blood vessels because blood vessels and muscles cross over each other in the uterine wall.

- the so-called "living ligature". Complete closure of at least the large uteroplacental vessels occurs via thrombosis.
- Expulsion of the wound exudate = lochia.

Results. The reduction in weight and size of the uterus in the puerperium is mainly due to involution of its large muscle mass (Fig. 11.1).

Note. Weight of the uterus:
Directly after birth: approx. 1,000 g.
At the end of the puerperium (6–8 weeks postpartum): approx. 50–80 g!

11.1.1 Position and attitude of the uterus in the puerperium

Shortly after birth, the uterus is usually found severely anteflexed (Figs. 11.2 and 11.3). The heavy muscle mass of the uterine body has tipped forwards over the cervix. As a result of the looseness of the whole overstretched support system, the uterus is extremely mobile in the first days postpartum. For this reason, a uterus which was previously severely anteflexed, now smaller, can be briefly found to be retroverted or retroflexed a few days later.

11.1.2 Closure of the cervix

Closure of the cervix occurs extremely quickly:
- Day 2 p.p.: the cervix begins to reform.
- Day 3 p.p.: the cervix is almost completely formed and the cervical canal is largely contracted.
- Days 8–10 p.p.: internal os. Closed, or only wide enough to permit outflow of secre-

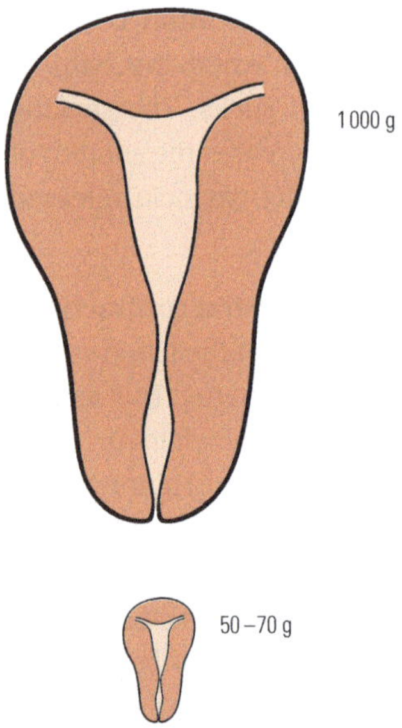

Fig. 11.1: Weight and size reduction of the uterus in the puerperium.

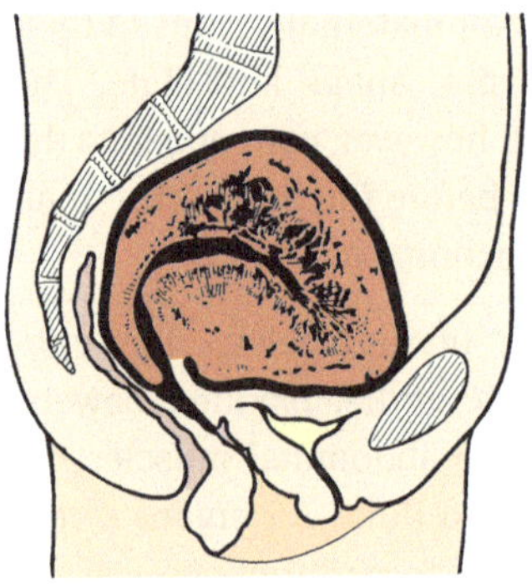

Fig. 11.2: Location of the puerperal uterus on day 5 p.p. (after Reist).

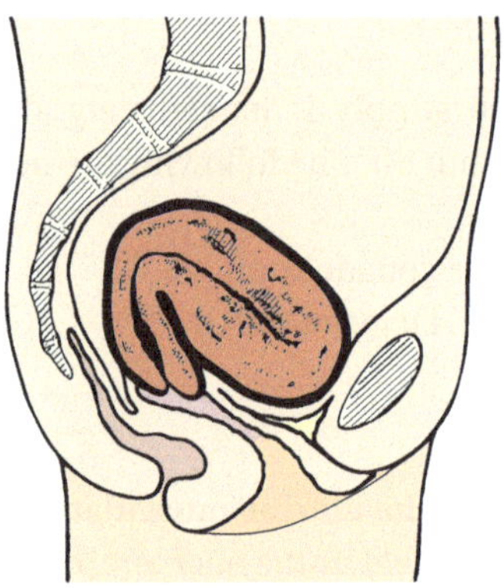

Fig. 11.3: Location of the puerperal uterus on day 12 p.p. (severely anteflexed; Reist).

tions. External os. At most 1 cm wide. It is no longer wide enough for a finger to pass through into the cervical canal.

After involution has been completed the cervix has a more conical form. The external os, which was dimpled before the first birth, becomes a transverse slit over 4–5 weeks.

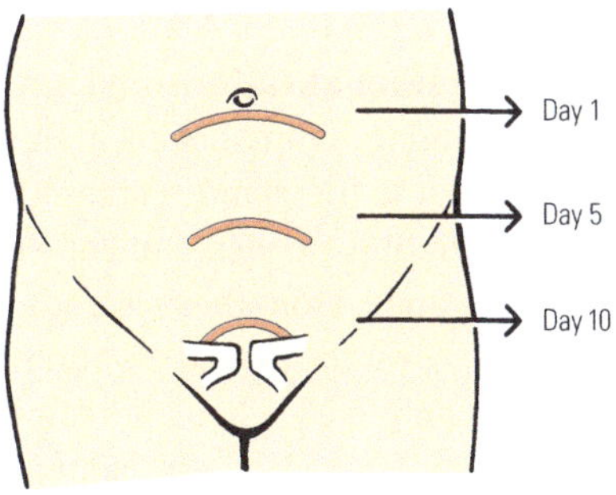

Fig. 11.4: Fundal height in the first puerperal days.

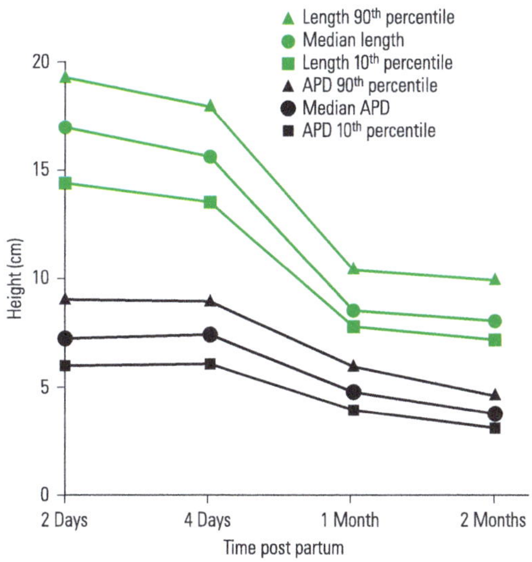

Fig. 11.5: Median values and 10th and 90th percentile of the sonographically measured uterine length, the anteroposterior diameter (APD) of the uterus during the puerperium (after Reles and colleagues, 1992).

11.1.3 Fundal height in the first days postpartum

- Directly after expulsion of the placenta: Approximately in the middle between navel and symphysis pubis.
- After 24 hours: At navel height or slightly lower (Fig. 11.4) .
  Causes. Lessening of the uterine contraction, increased pelvic floor tone in the first days p.p.
- In the next 10 days: Daily 1 finger-width lower.

Note.
On day 5 p.p.: approximately in the middle between navel and symphysis pubis.
On day 10 p.p.: approximately at the level of the symphysis pubis or 1–2 finger-widths higher.

After 2 weeks the uterus is no longer palpable from the abdomen. The change in size of the uterus can be followed with the help of ultrasound (Fig. 11.5).
The clinical value of this method of examination is most apparent in cases of impaired involution, not as a routinely applied method in the puerperium.

11.2 Wound-healing processes in the puerperium

Physiology. The wound surface of the uterus is caused by the detachment of the placenta and membranes, which were attached to the inner surface of the uterine cavity. This detachment occurs in the deep spongiosa layer, that is, close to the uterine muscle. After detachment the decidua of the whole inner uterine surface is exposed. The wound surface is only broken by the glands which have remained standing like islands in the stroma of the decidual spongiosa layer. Apart from these small epithelial islands the whole surface has been robbed of its protective epithelium.

In the first days after birth, the placental site is about the size of the palm of the hand. In contrast to its relatively smooth surroundings, its surface is rough, uneven and slightly lumpy. This is caused by tissue fragments which are still attached, blood vessel stumps and the remnants of the anchoring villi. Thrombi protrude button-like from some of the blood vessels. These ragged tissue remnants, which are much less profuse in the regions where the membranes have detached, are undernourished and become necrotic. The actual healing of the large surface wound begins when it has been cleansed. This cleansing is carried out by migrating granulocytes, lymphocytes and phagocytes. Large numbers are transported to the wound in the blood. They infiltrate below and above the necrotic tissue remains. The tissue debris is attacked by enzymes and for the most part liquefied (lochia). The remaining part becomes the foundation for the new endometrium.
The formed blood components also have another important job: in conjunction with masses of fibrin they create a **protective barrier** which extends far into the connective tissue septa of the uterus musculature. This protective barrier has an antibacterial effect. It seals off the whole wound area against attack by bacteria.
The second protective mechanism is the tonically contracted uterus. The wound area is reduced as a result, and closure of the blood vessels, which are the entry point for bacteria, is supported.

Note. Of the postpartum uterus for defense against bacteria: protective **two protective mechanisms** barrier and tonically contracted uterus.

Wound healing (epithelialization) and the regeneration of the endometrium begins in the epithelial islands, that is the gland remnants, which remained standing on detachment of placenta and membranes. From these islands, the epithelium grows over the exposed wound. Wound healing is completed when the complete stroma is again covered by epithelium. This is the case 4–6 weeks after birth.

11.2.1 Lochia

Definition. Secretion from the large wound in the uterine cavity. Description of lochia during the puerperium (see Tab. 11.1).

Tab. 11.1: Color of the lochia reflects the uterine wound.

Time	Color (consistency)	Term	Uterine wound
Day 1–3	Fresh blood	Lochia rubra	Hemostasis not yet complete
Second half of the first week	Brown/ brownish-red	Lochia fusca	Ligature of the blood vessels in the uterine wall increases, thrombi close the uteroplacental vessel openings. Decreased lochial flow, addition of serum, lymph and leukocytes
End of the second week	Dirty yellow (creamy)	Lochia flava	Expulsion of necrotic, usually liquefied cell materials of all types
End of the third week	Greyish-white (watery-serous)	Lochia alba	Increasing wound epithelialization, significantly less lochia
After approx. 4 weeks	Lochia cease		Wound healing concluded

Deviations are normal! More or less bloody lochia can be observed, particularly in healthy women, long after day 10 p.p. The odor is mild. Lochia contains bacteria from the vagina (streptococcus, staphylococcus, E. coli and other pyogenic bacteria). The bacteria multiply abundantly from day 2–3 p.p. in the lochia.

11.3 Lactation

Physiology. 5 phases:
- **Mammogenesis.** Development and growth of the mammary gland into a functioning organ.
- **Lactogenesis.** Preparation of the mammary gland for milk secretion.
- **Galactogenesis.** Triggering of milk secretion in the glandular cells.
- **Galactopoiesis.** Maintenance of milk production.
- **Galactokinesis.** Milk flow.

1. Mammogenesis. Development and growth of the mammary gland into a functioning organ, beginning at the onset of puberty. Growth of the mammary gland is controlled by the steroid hormones of the ovary, estrogen and progesterone. Estrogens bring about proliferation of the milk ducts and, together with progesterone, growth of the alveoli and the proliferation of the milk-producing alveolar epithelium.

2. Lactogenesis. Preparation of the mammary gland in pregnancy for its function of milk production. Further growth of the mammary gland and creation of new lobules increase breast volume. In addition, differentiation of the alveolar epithelial cells occurs. Parenchymal increase occurs as a result of the same steroid hormones, which are now produced in far greater amounts, first from the corpus luteum graviditatis, then from the placenta. The glandular cells differentiate as a result of the rapid increase in secretion of hPL (placenta) and prolactin (pituitary gland). Milk secretion is inhibited in pregnancy however, by the placental steroid hormones. Breast massage only allows expression of a few drops of colostrum (foremilk).

3. Galactogenesis. Milk production; triggering of milk secretion in the glandular cells after expulsion of the placenta. The production of the steroid hormones of pregnancy ceases immediately, as the ovaries slowly resume their duties. Milk secretion is triggered when the inhibitory effect of the high estrogen level on the secretory performance of the glandular epithelium is no longer present. This process is supported by the physiological sucking reflex. For this reason, early breastfeeding of the newborn promotes milk secretion. The effect of prolactin often first becomes apparent 3 days p.p., when milk flow begins (milk "comes in").

4. Galactopoiesis. Maintenance of lactation p.p., caused by endocrinal, mechanical and neural factors. The act of sucking on the nipple is of great importance, as it triggers a nerve reflex via the pituitary gland. This causes
- a) Continued production of prolactin in the anterior pituitary, which stimulates constant milk secretion from the glandular epithelium.
- b) Increased secretion of oxytocin from the posterior pituitary gland.

5. Galactokinesis. Ejection of the milk (letdown effect), triggered by oxytocin, which stimulates contraction of the myoepithelium of the alveolar wall and the narrower milk ducts; milk is ejected by muscle contraction. The uterine contractions it also triggers are a desired side effect of the increased release of oxytocin during breastfeeding.

Tab. 11.2: Comparison of the essential components of human and cow's milk (in g per 100 ml).

	Protein	Fat	Lactose	Minerals	Calories	Joule
Human milk						
Colostrum	1.8	3.0	6.5	0.35	65	165
Transition milk (days 4–14)	1.5	3.8	6.5	0.25	70	290
Mature milk	1.3	4.0	6.0	0.23	70	295
Cow's milk	3.5	4.0	4.5	0.7	70	290

Note. Breastfeeding promotes uterine involution! **Suckling and emptying of the breast** are most important for continued milk secretion.
If suckling does not occur and the breasts are not emptied the glands **atrophy** and **milk secretion ceases.**

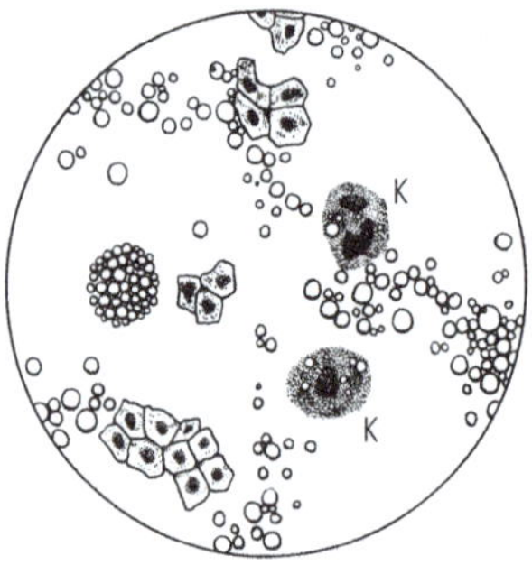

Fig. 11.6: Colostrum (microscope slide). C = colostrum corpuscles.

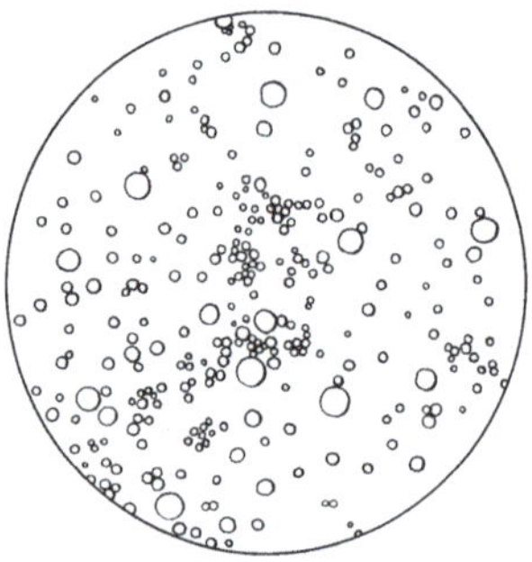

Fig. 11.7: Mature human milk showing fat droplets of different-sizes (microscope slide).

Components of human milk (Tab. 11.2).

Colostrum (Fig. 11.6) is secreted in the first days, transitory milk is produced from around day 4 to day 14 p.p., and from about day 15 p.p. approx. 700 ml per day of mature milk (Fig. 11.7) is produced.

11.4 Resumption of ovarian function

Secretion of the gonadotropins from the anterior pituitary gland is suppressed by the steroid hormones (estrogens and progesterone) in pregnancy, initially produced by the corpus luteum graviditatis of the ovary, and later by the placental steroid hormones. As a result, follicle maturation and ovulation do not occur in pregnancy. Initially only small amounts of steroid hormones are produced (relative steroid depletion) after expulsion of the placenta, as the ovaries do not immediately resume hormone production. The production of gonadotropins in the anterior pituitary is, however, no longer inhibited after removal of the placenta. Gonadotropins are once again produced, which leads to gradual resumption of ovarian function.

Note. When the **first cycle occurs after birth** is determined by the timepoint at which the relationship between the anterior pituitary interbrain system and the ovaries is taken up again.

Lactational amenorrhea. Amenorrhea during lactation. In most breastfeeding women the menstrual cycle resumes towards the end of the lactation period or on weaning.

Prolactin levels inhibit the hypothalamus-pituitary-ovarian feedback cycle. Prolactin levels are determined by the frequency of lactation. The more frequently the mother breastfeeds, the higher the levels of prolactin. Consequently: levels of LH, estradiol, FSH are low. Ovulation and menstruation do not resume until lactation frequency is reduced. A small number of women have a single bleed 6–8 weeks p.p., which interrupts the lactational amenorrhea. This bleed is often very like a menstrual period and is perceived as such by the women. It is, however, not a normal menstrual period.
In a small number of breastfeeding women, regular menstruation every 4 weeks resumes after lactational amenorrhea of 6–7 weeks.
The first period or periods after birth, regardless of when they occur, are usually not genuine menstrual periods. That is, not periods from a secretory transformed endometrium after ovulation and corpus luteum growth. These first periods, which the women consider to be menstrual periods, are almost always anovulatory periods; i.e., periods not preceded by ovulation. The first developing follicle/s do not completely mature, ovulation does not occur. The endometrium is correspondingly proliferated or overproliferated, not however secretory transformed. This mucosa bleeds when the serum estrogen concentration is no longer sufficient to maintain endometrial hyperplasia (relative estrogen deficiency). Hence the bleeding is caused by estrogen withdrawal (anovulatory bleeding).
When the first ovulation, and with it the first real menstrual period, occurs after a birth is individually very different and dependent on manifold factors, in particular on
- the length of lactation and
- the health of the woman.

In **nonlactating women** the first period occurs 5–6 weeks p.p. Large individual variations also apply here.

Breastfeeding and conception. Although the first period/s are usually anovulatory, and although breastfeeding women resume ovulation later than nonbreastfeeding women, an egg capable of being fertilized can still be produced during lactation. For this reason, breastfeeding is not a safe form of protection against another pregnancy.

11.5 Clinical picture of the puerperal period

Postnatal rounds. Questions:
- Quality of sleep? Disturbed by afterpains? Pain?
- Frontal headaches indicate lochial stasis, mid-abdominal pain endometritis and lateral lower abdominal pain adnexitis.
- Bladder voided? Flatus passed? Information about breastfeeding.

View chart. Pulse? Temperature? Fundal height and vaginal fluid loss must also be entered on the chart in the first days p.p.

Note. The main question in the puerperal period is whether the large uterine wound will heal normally or not.

11.5.1 The postpartum pulse

The pulse is a prognostically important indicator of possible problems. Normal postpartum heart rate is 60–80 bpm, extreme bradycardia is rare.

Practice tip. A rise in temperature coupled with a slow pulse is far less important than a rise in temperature with a rapid pulse!

11.5.2 Temperature postpartum

The normal axillary temperature is 36.5–37.0 °C. Temperatures from 37.1 to 38.0 °C p.p. are termed sub-febrile; over 38° is fever postpartum.
These classifications should be observed. Apart from the first and second days after birth, over 80 % of women have normal temperatures after birth.
Subfebrile temperatures may indicate endometritis (see p. 406). Women with sub-febrile temperatures after day 2 p.p. should be treated with uterotonics, e.g., 5 × oxytocin nasal spray/day, in particular if the lochia have a fetid odor and, as is often the case, uterine involution is delayed.

Practice tip. Women with sub-febrile temperatures after day 2 p.p. should be treated preventatively with uterotonics.

Temperatures of 38 °C and above are clear signs of abnormalities. Of course, puerperal fever (p. 405) is the first consideration, but not all fevers postpartum are due to puerperal fever.

Differential diagnosis of fever postpartum
Puerperal fever:
- Infected perineal wound, endometritis, endomyometritis.
- Salpingitis, pelveoperitonitis.
- Parametritis, puerperal septicemia.

Extragenital fever
- Urinary tract infection (UTI), pyelonephritis.
- Virus.
- Thrombophlebitis, leg/pelvic vein thrombosis, sinus thrombosis.
- Milk stasis, mastitis.
- Secondary healing of laparotomy wound.

Fever occurring in the first 2 days p.p. is often caused by extragenital infections, e.g., by cystitis, pyelonephritis, bronchitis, angina and others. Fever from day 3 or 4 usually has a genital origin.
Increases in temperature postpartum usually occur in the late afternoon or evening. It is important therefore, to measure temperature not only in the morning, but particularly between 5 and 6 pm.

11.5.3 Monitoring fundal height

Descent of the uterus from day to day postpartum (p. 393). There are, however, marked individual differences.

Factors to be considered on assessing fundal height:
- Size of baby! Twins? Hydramnios (overdistended uterus)?
- Prolonged labor (exhausted uterus!).
- Primi- or multipara?
- Cesarean? Involution is often markedly delayed; involution is also often delayed after other obstetric operations.
- Retained placenta or membranes? Endometritis?
- Retroflected uterus? Lochial stasis?
- Impaired lactation (lactation promotes involution!)

Most common reason for an unusually high fundus:
Full bladder! A full bladder lifts up the uterus (Figs. 11.8 and 11.9). Void bladder! Fundal height may only be assessed when the bladder is empty!
Impaired involution = delayed involution.

11.5.4 Monitoring lochia

Appearance and odor of the lochia (see p. 394) give an indication of the wound healing status. Pads are to be handled by doctors, midwives and nurses with gloves only. Used pads are disposed of directly in the rubbish bin.

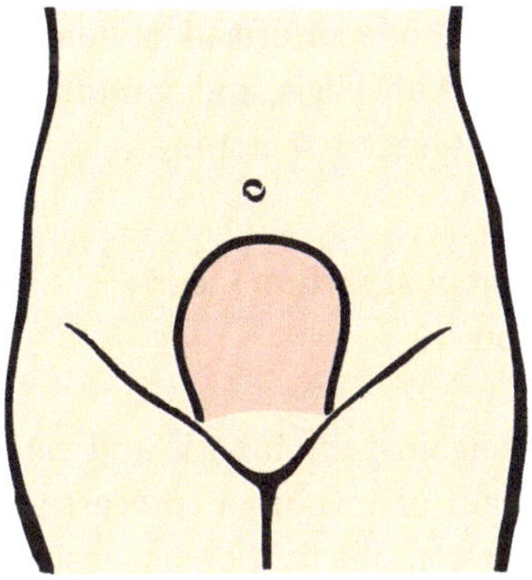

Fig. 11.8: Fundal height postpartum (day 2), bladder empty.

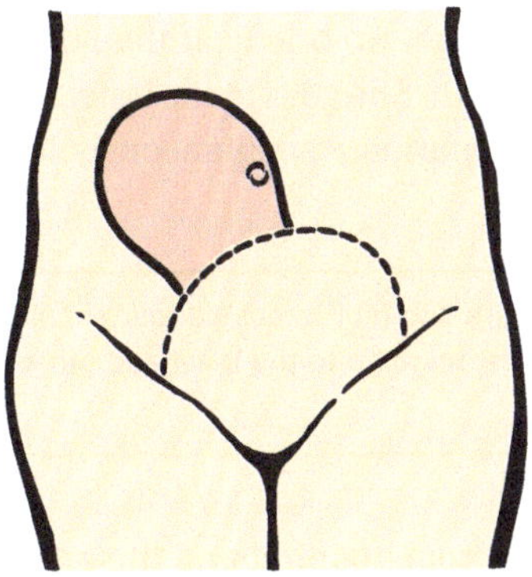

Fig. 11.9: Misleadingly high fundus postpartum due to full bladder.

11.5.5 Micturition in early puerperium

Early puerperium = first 10–14 days p.p.: women produce a lot of urine. Urinary "flooding" occurs in the first days after birth. The large volume of fluid which was retained in the tissues during pregnancy is now excreted via the kidneys.

Increased urine production in early puerperium = 2–4 l.

On the other hand, experience has shown us that voiding the bladder is often difficult in the first days postpartum. The woman should be allowed up to 6 h to empty her bladder for the first time after delivery. Micturition is not considered impaired (Ischuria puerperalis) unless it has not been possible to empty the bladder within 6h, at which point something must be undertaken.

Note. Care in the puerperal period: monitoring of regular voiding of the bladder!

Causes of impaired micturition postpartum. The main causes are lesions to urethra and bladder which occurred intrapartum as a result of these organs being crushed against the bony pelvic cavity on entry of the head into the pelvis. Mucosal tissue swells up (edema) in the bladder neck and blood is extravasated into the bladder wall.

Reflexive sphincter cramp. Occurs when urine comes into contact with perineal laceration or episiotomy wound.

Pregnancy and puerperal hypotonia. The tone of the bladder wall is still considerably reduced as a result of pregnancy.

Diagnosis. Measurement of residual urine, ultrasound estimation.

Incidence. Up to 10 %!

Complications. Retention of urine, cystitis.

Treatment. Support spontaneous micturition. Allow early ambulation after delivery.

If residual urine > 200ml, empty bladder with a single-use catheter. If problem persists (**impaired micturition**) the possibility of a UTI must be excluded and an in-dwelling catheter inserted. If micturition is impaired for longer than 3 days a suprapubic catheter and bladder training are indicated.
In cases of sphincter cramping: oxybutynin tablets (2.5–5mg) 3× daily.

11.5.6 Bowel movements

Constipation postpartum is seen as physiological to a certain degree.

Causes. The bowel tone is still reduced from the pregnancy, the intestines are "widened", abdominal wall and pelvic floor are relaxed, and the intestines are displaced now that the uterus is empty. Postpartum constipation is the continuation of pregnancy constipation.

The first bowel movement should occur at the latest on day 3 p.p. After that a bowel movement every second day is desirable.

Treatment

Laxatives postpartum. In order to get the bowels moving 1–2 tablespoons of paraffin can be given on the evening of day 2 p.p. If no success on day 3: enema

Drastic laxatives and purging salt solutions must not be used postpartum as they remove water and thus reduce milk secretion.
Once the bowels have reopened, they can usually be maintained with 1 tablespoon of paraffin or small enemas.

11.5.7 Postpartum exercises

Aim. Tightening of abdominal and pelvic floor musculature, cardiovascular training, prevention of prolapse problems and back pain. Careful exercising can be begun soon after delivery. To begin with, cardiovascular exercises are performed, and the level of physical difficulty is gradually increased.

There are different exercises:
- To stimulate circulation in the limbs.
- For breathing.
- For the pelvic floor muscles.
- For the abdominal muscles.
- For the back muscles.

These exercises can be performed regularly every morning on a daily basis, and continued after discharge for at least 3–4 months.

11.5.8 Ambulation postpartum – early ambulation

Aim. Prophylaxis against thrombosis and embolism, acceleration of involution processes; lochial stasis is rarer, micturition is easier, bowel, circulatory system and metabolism are stimulated. In addition, early mobilization promotes wellbeing, improves moods, and has no disadvantages.

The woman should get up briefly at the latest 6 hours after the birth. She goes to the toilet (in accompaniment) to urinate spontaneously for the first time.

Note. Women who are sub-febrile postpartum should only be allowed to get up to go to the toilet and otherwise have bed rest!

11.5.9 Discharge from hospital and the end of the clinical puerperium

Discharge examination
- Examination of the breasts (always done first!). Examination of the nipples (cracked?) and the whole breast (redness, swelling?), then palpation of the breast (pain, circumscribed pain in one location?).
- Fundal height (p. 393) via external examination.
- Assessment of vulva and perineum in those women with suturing after episiotomies and perineal lacerations.

Vaginal examination is not routinely performed before discharge, but on the 6 week postpartum checkup.

Counseling
- **Menstruation.** Breastfeeding women will not have their first menstrual period before week 6–8 p.p. (see p. 397). Any bleeding beforehand is not their period, but abnormal and a doctor should be informed immediately.
- **Breasts.** In particular, doctors must inform women to visit their doctor immediately if they have the slightest breast tenderness, swelling or (and) redness, especially if their temperature is raised (or even if not)! Home remedy attempts waste precious time.

Note. Puerperal mastitis (p. 416) is a very aggressive, tedious and dangerous illness if not immediately, correctly and actively dealt with!

- Any rise in temperature above 38 °C must be reported!
- Bathing should be avoided, showers only for the time being!
- Well-baby examination dates.
- Discussion about the baby and breastfeeding (see below).
- Intercourse from 2–3 weeks p.p.
- Family planning. Inform that breastfeeding is not a safe method of contraception! If desired, the woman can be informed about the different contraceptive possibilities in the puerperal period (condom, IUD, hormonal contraception, progestin-only pill, sterilization).

11.5.10 Breastfeeding

Note. Breast milk is the natural and therefore best nourishment for a newborn. Its composition of protein, fat, carbohydrates and salts cannot be matched even by the most expensive breast milk substitutes.

Advantages. Breastfed infants are far less susceptible to infection than formula-fed babies. For example the rates of bowel infections, dermatitis, rhinitis, chronic pulmonary infections and allergies are far lower in breastfed infants. They are more resistant to many illnesses than formula- fed infants.

In addition to these short-term advantages, studies have demonstrated formative effects and sparked debates as to whether breastfeeding has a protective effect against obesity, hyperlipidemia, hypertension, type 2 diabetes and atopic diseases. Some studies found that breastfeeding promoted neurocognitive development of the infants; others questioned the validity of these results.
In addition to nonspecific immune factors such as lysozyme or lactoferrin, the protective effects of breast milk are ascribed to the immunoglobulins it contains, in particular secretory IgA. Large amounts are secreted in colostrum and it prevents antigens and microorganisms from penetrating the bowel walls of the newborn by binding.
A prerequisite for breastfeeding is a willingness to do so by the mother, which is present in over 90 % of cases if widespread concerns and unwillingness are eliminated. Obstetricians, midwives and nurses can do much to promote willingness to breastfeed. The best opportunity for information about breastfeeding is during nursing.

Physiology of the act of suckling. The infant surrounds the nipple with the jaw and by airtight enclosure of the areola with the lips. By lowering the lower jaw, negative pressure is created in the infant's mouth cavity, through which the nipple is sucked into the mouth cavity. By lifting the tongue the nipple is compressed between tongue and palate. This process is supported by the let-down reflex caused by oxytocin.

Breastfeeding technique. Good instructions from nurse, midwife, lactation consultant, physician or experienced acquaintance are conditional for correct breastfeeding technique. Before each feed the nipple region and hands are thoroughly cleansed with water. Mother and baby should both be in a comfortable position (supine or supported sitting, otherwise back pain). In particular in the first few days, breastfeeding requires patience until the infant attaches to the whole nipple and sucks energetically. The baby must be able to breathe freely through the nose!

At every feed the baby is placed on each breast successively, whereby the first breast is alternated each feed. This breast is then emptied, whereas the other is often only partially emptied. This method ensures optimal milk production, which is not only stimulated by the emptying of the breast, but also by the frequency of stimulation brought on by the suckling of the infant. Attachment to only one breast per feed rarely leads to adequate milk production. The majority of the milk is received from the first breast. On the other breast it satisfies its sucking urge and stimulates milk production in the breasts.
The baby should not feed for too long! It should not be suck for longer than 5 minutes per breast in the first 1–3 days p.p. It receives 98 % of the milk volume in this time. It makes no sense to allow the baby to suckle for a further 10 min to receive the rest. The baby should not be allowed to fall asleep attached to the breast. Cracked nipples are definitely caused in this way.

Note. Prevention of cracked nipples = prevention of mastitis!

The duration of each feed can be lengthened to 10–15 minutes per breast later on in the period of lactation.

Nipple care. It is advisable to allow the breasts to air-dry in the puerperal period to prevent cracking.

If cracking occurs, treatment of the nipples with glucose powder after each feed is recommended.

Practice tip. Do not apply moist bandages to cracked nipples (causes maceration).

Avoid breathing on cracks – risk of mastitis! If the mother has a cold or flu she should at least wear a face mask while feeding and caring for her baby.
- If the cracks are deep and extremely painful, the baby is not breastfed on the injured breast and the milk is pumped at feeding time.

Some women find manual expression (Fig. 11.10) more pleasant and effective, as they control the amount of pressure on breast and nipple.

Note. If possible, the newborn should be breastfed for the first time in the delivery suite within the first hour after birth.

Breastfeeding according to the clock. Previously babies were fed 5 times a day at 4 h intervals. The first feed was early at 6am, then at

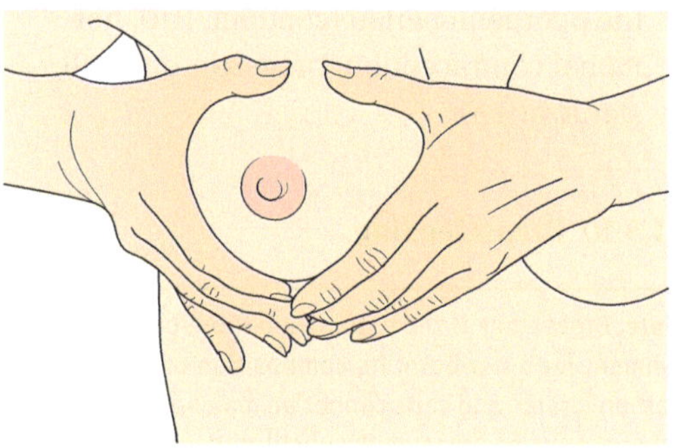

Fig. 11.10: Gentle breast massage with thumbs above and fingers below the breasts stimulates the let-down effect.

10 am, 2 pm, 6 pm, and then for the last time at 10 pm, with an 8 h break overnight. These 5 feedings per day and the feeding times were strictly adhered to. The number of feedings was often increased to 6 or 7 per day at 3 h intervals for babies which were underweight and poor feeders.

Demand feeding. Breastfeeding with no set feeding times; the rooming in system allows mothers and babies to observe, understand and get to know each other. This also means it is possible to fulfill the baby's basic requirements for contact with the mother and feeding at all times. After 4–6 weeks the baby spontaneously acquires a day-night rhythm involving about five meals per day and a break overnight. Introducing supplementary feedings too early disrupts development of this natural rhythm and leads eventually to reduced milk production.

Lactation duration. The mother should breastfeed her baby for at least 4–6 months.

Amount of milk drunk daily

Day 1: 50 g
Day 2: 100 g
Day 3: 100–150 g
Day 4: 150–210 g
Day 5: 200–280 g
Day 6: 250–350 g
Day 7: 300–420 g
Day 8: 350–490 g
Day 9: 400–560 g
Day 10: 450–630 g

Newborn's weight. Regular weight loss in the first 3–5 days, therefore known as physiological weight loss. Cause: fluid loss due to urination and defecation, in addition to breathing and evaporation. The weight loss should not exceed more than 10 % of the birth weight. Upwards growth curve from about day 5. The birth weight is regained between days 10 and 14.

In some cases drinking is difficult (breastfeeding difficulties) or impossible (breastfeeding obstructions).

Breastfeeding difficulties

Due to the mother. Flat or inverted nipples, cracks, mastitis, hypogalactia (unproductive breasts; insufficient milk production occasionally occurs as a constitutional defect, is far more commonly a result of reluctance to breastfeed or incorrect breastfeeding technique, however).

The existence of safe and effective remedies to increase milk production is questionable. In cases of milk stasis, oxytocin nasal spray is recommended: oxytocin nasal spray is applied 5 minutes before breastfeeding or pumping, in addition to the application of moist heat packs to the breasts 30 min beforehand.

Note. The best milk production stimulus is complete emptying of the breasts!

Breastfeeding difficulties due to flat or inverted nipples can be remedied with nipple shields (e.g., Dahlhausen Gentle Feed Nipple Shields).

Due to the baby. Ineffective sucking or drinking, head cold, congenital deformities (cleft lip and palate).

Breastfeeding obstructions (= **contraindications** to breastfeeding)

Due to the mother. Open tuberculosis infection (pathogen detectable in sputum) is an absolute contraindication to breastfeeding. Breastfeeding must be discontinued! Strict isolation and separation of mother and baby until no longer infectious (pathogen no longer detectable in sputum).

Further contraindications are HIV positive state and Hepatitis B (HBsAg positive), if the baby has not received hepatitis prophylaxis. Breastfeeding should be safe once the prophylaxis has been administered. Other conditions for which lactation is contraindicated today are: Hepatitis C (if PCR is positive), maternal phenylketonuria, galactosemia, drug addiction, breast cancer.

Due to the baby

Practice tip. Genuine breastfeeding obstructions are rare.

In particular for underweight babies, but also for other newborns, breast milk is important for the reasons listed above. Whether it is possible to maintain lactation by pumping and giving the baby the milk in a bottle or via another method (e.g., feeding tube) should always be checked.

Discontinuation of lactation

- Primary: suppression of lactation before it has been initiated.
- Secondary: discontinuation of lactation once it has been initiated.
- Physical measures. Cold compresses on the breasts, binding of the breasts, restriction of fluid intake, no soups, fruit; laxatives to promote purging bowel movements. Such physical measures are often not very effective. A diuretic can be administered in addition (e.g., furosemide), one 40 mg tablet once a day.
- Reduction of fluid intake, controversial measure. Although fluid restriction as a physical method for discontinuation of lactation is an old clinical measure, various authors have shown that fluid intake does not correlate with the volume of milk produced.
- Pharmacological measures. For the purposes of pharmacological suppression of lactation specific prolactin inhibitors are available today: Bromocriptine, Lisuride or Cabergolin.
- Dosage over 10–14 days for primary discontinuation:
  - Bromocriptin 2 × 5 mg daily.
  - Lisuride 2 × 0.2 mg daily.
  - Cabergolin 1 × 1 mg daily.
- Using these effective methods of lactation discontinuation, physical measures are no longer necessary.

Discontinuation of lactation can lead to painful congestion of the mammary glands. For relief of these symptoms the application of cold compresses – containing no further ingredients – is recommended.

Practice tip. Primary discontinuation of lactation should be practiced after late miscarriage (>12 weeks' gestation), as otherwise painful engorgement will occur in about 75 %.

References

ACOG educational bulletin No. 258: Breastfeeding: Maternal and infant aspects. Int J Obstet Gynccol 2001; 74:217

Kearney R, Cutner A: Postpartum voiding dysfunction. The Obstetrician & Gynaecologist. 2008; 10:71–74

Kramer MS: „Breast is best": The evidence. Early Hum Dev 2010; 86:729–32

Reynolds A: Breastfeeding and brain development. Ped Clin N Am 2001; 48:159

12 Pathological puerperium

12.1 Puerperal fever = childbed fever

Definition. Febrile disease process in the puerperal period caused by entry of pathogens into one of the birth wounds (placental site, injury to the lower uterine segment, the cervical canal, the vagina, the vulva. Vaginal and perineal lacerations, episiotomy wounds are large entry points for bacteria).

The question as to whether pyrexia (fever) in the puerperal period is puerperal fever or not does not in any way depend on the severity of the condition. The term puerperal fever must only be used when the fever is due to an infection of the **birth wounds**. All other disease processes as a result of infection of extragenital origin in the puerperal period, e.g., mastitis puerperalis, cystitis, pyelonephritis, as well as intercurrent diseases such as pneumonia, angina etc. are simply termed fever in the puerperal period and must not be termed puerperal fever.

Microbiology. Puerperal fever pathogens: aerobic bacteria such as E. coli, Proteus, Klebsiella, Pseudomonas, Groups A and B streptococcus. Anaerobic bacteria such as Bacteroides, Clostridium, Peptostreptococcus. Puerperal infections are almost always polymicrobial.

The particularly severe form of puerperal infection is usually caused by Group A streptococcus (GAS). These gram-positive bacteria line up in long chains, which explains the origin of the name. Lancefield distinguished 22 groups according to biological characteristics of the cell wall. Streptococcal bacteria partially produce exotoxins, which can have cell-damaging, cardiotoxic and lethal effects.

Path of infection

- **Exogenous infection:** foreign infection = infection with exogenous bacteria. This means the bacteria was introduced into the birth canal of the woman on vaginal examination or during a procedure in labor.
- **Endogenous infection:** infection with endogenous bacteria = infection with bacteria which are already present on the vulva, in the vagina or elsewhere on the woman's body, either as
- **Spontaneous infection:** spontaneous ascent of infection: the endogenous bacteria penetrate the upper, at first germ-free sections of the birth canal without contact by the laboring woman or new mother, or
- **Artificial endogenous infection:** the endogenous bacteria are spread on vaginal examination, manual exploration of the uterine cavity, obstetrical operation with instruments to the uterine cavity.

History

It is highly probable that childbed fever has existed for as long as children have been being born. Many of the oldest authors mention it (Hippocrates and Galen among others). It first appeared as a murderous plague on the introduction of birthing (or "lying-in") hospitals and the bedside instruction of students. The oldest reports on the occurrence of childbed fever as a serious endemic disease come from the Hôtel – Dieu in Paris, the oldest birthing hospital in the world.
The man who deserves eternal credit for the correct recognition of the nature of childbed fever and with that, the method of prevention, is Ignaz Philip Semmelweis (July 1, 1818–August 13, 1865). Semmelweis was the first to teach and prove that childbed fever, as it is now called, was transmitted by infection. He also already demanded that infected puerperal women be isolated. Washing the hands and instruments with chlorine as proposed by

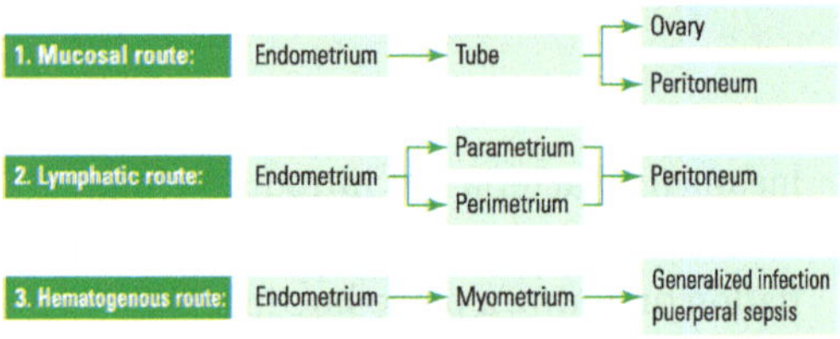

Fig. 12.1: Routes of puerperal infection.

Semmelweis resulted in a reduction of maternal mortality rates from 11.4 % to 1.27 %. He met with almost unanimous rejection from the authorities at the time (Scanzoni, von Siebold, Simpson, and others), to whom he wrote "open letters" in 1861. Main work: "Etiology, Concept and Prophylaxis of Childbed Fever" (1861).
Not until the bacteriological studies of Lister and Pasteur proved the correctness of Semmelweis' theory did it receive the worldwide recognition it deserved.

Clinical manifestation

Spread of puerperal infection

- **Local infection.** The infection is restricted to the birth wound and does not spread further = local puerperal infection.
- **Disseminated infection.** The infection is not restricted to one of the birth wounds. The bacteria migrate by different routes from the colonized wound, usually the placental implantation site, to other parts of the organism. Three routes are described for the progression of puerperal infection (Fig. 12.1).

12.1.1 Localized puerperal infections

Infected birth wound

Definition. Infection of a birth wound, e.g., a sutured perineal laceration: edematous swelling, redness of wound edges, opened sutures, wound dehiscence. The wound typically has a dirty, greenish-grey coating.

Infected wounds in these areas are seen relatively rarely these days; small abrasions and sutured perineal lacerations and episiotomy wounds tend to heal without reaction within a few days.

Symptoms. Edematous swelling of the vulva, considerable pain. If wound exudate is retained, elevated temperature and fever, unchanged pulse.

Treatment. Damp compresses with chamomile or rivanol solution to begin with. Sutures are to be removed if they are very tight. Wound exudate can begin to flow, discomfort is rapidly reduced. Chamomile sitzbaths several times a day. After wound cleansing with granulation promoting measures, await secondary healing. Secondary repair is recommended if perineal and vaginal wounds are large, dehiscent.

Endometritis puerperalis

Definition. Infection of the placental implantation site and endometrium. The upper muscle layers are also often affected. The endometritis puerperalis is then an endo**myo**metritis puerperalis.

Clinical manifestation. Subfebrile temperatures without feeling ill. Foul-smelling lochia. Impaired uterine involution (relatively large and soft, fundal height does not correspond to p.p. date). External palpation of the uterus often detects tenderness on the margins of the uterus–parametrial tenderness. Light bleeding.

Practice tip. Endometritis should always be assumed when a woman presents with subfebrile temperatures postpartum and she should be treated accordingly.

In this mild form of endometritis there is usually stasis of the vaginal discharge, often between days 4 to 7 p.p. = lochial stasis. The stasis is caused mechanically by clots blocking the internal os. A full bladder or rectum or retroflexed uterus causing a bend in the cervix must, however, also be considered as possible causes. Main characteristics: scanty and foul-smelling lochia or no lochia. The women complain of a typical frontal headache and generally not feeling well.

Note. Symptoms of endometritis puerperalis:
Subfebrile temperatures.
Foul-smelling lochia, lochial stasis frequently.
Impaired uterine involution (large, soft uterus).
Uterine tenderness on palpation, particularly laterally.
Often light bleeding.

Treatment. Uterotonics (e. g. oxytocin IM or nasal spray), possibly a spasmolytic to widen the cervical canal.

Women with endometritis must rest as much as possible.

Prognosis. Usually benign.

Practice tip. All localized childbed infections can be a stage on the way towards development of puerperal sepsis!

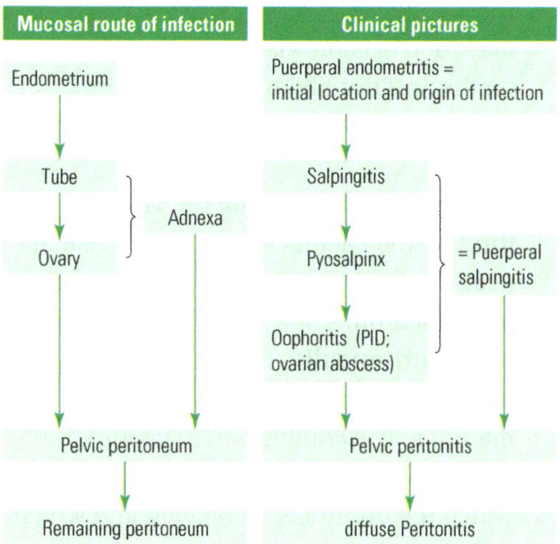

Fig. 12.2: Spread of infection via the mucosal route.

Dependent on:
- The virulence of the bacteria.
- The general resistance of the colonized organism. Long labors (> 18 h!), high blood loss, and operative procedures increase the risk of infection significantly, because they result in exhaustion and reduced resistance of the woman.
- The timepoint of the infection. If infectious bacteria from the woman's vagina ascend after ROM during a spontaneous delivery, it often takes about three days for the uterine cavity to be colonized with these bacteria.

12.1.2 Disseminated puerperal infection

Mucosal route = puerperal salpingitis

Definition. Infection of one or both tubes, arising from endometritis (Fig. 12.2).

Types
- **Endosalpingitis.** Mildest form. Inflammation of the tubal mucosa.
- If suppuration worsens, the mucosal epithelium is destroyed and adhesion of the folds occurs. If the inflammation spreads to the muscular and serosal layers of the tube it swells up and gradually becomes rigid.
- **Pyosalpinx puerperalis.** The fimbrial end usually adheres, and the exudate loaded with pathogenic bacteria cannot flow into the abdominal cavity.
- **Inflammation of the pelvic peritoneum = pelvic peritonitis.** In a severe infection with extremely virulent bacteria the purulent discharge containing pathogenic bacteria flows through the tube onto the peritoneum before the abdominal end of the tube is closed. This results in a localized peritonitis. Development of diffuse peritonitis is very rare in these circumstances. Pelvic peritonitis can however also occur when the pathogenic bacteria from a pyosalpinx

pass through the tubal wall, or a pyosalpinx ruptures.
- **Ovarian abscess.** In severe and prolonged processes the inflammation also (rarely) spreads to the ovary, which is usually broadly adhered to the tube. An ovarian abscess worsens the prognosis significantly: it can rupture, resulting in diffuse peritonitis.

Symptoms. Tearing and piercing pain, usually one-sided to begin with. Sudden temperature increase is common when the infection ascends into the tube. Severe pain in the lower abdomen in the acute stage; all abdominal contact is painful. Vaginal examination is often not possible as a result. Peritoneal symptoms are nausea and vomiting, reduced bowel peristalsis, retained wind, and bloated abdomen.

Prognosis. Must be made cautiously. It depends on whether only the tubes are affected, or pelvic peritonitis or diffuse peritonitis are also involved.

Treatment. Hospitalization. Immediate **pharmacological measures** (after bacteriological swab of cervix or uterine cavity): Ampicillin or Mezlocillin, 2 g IV 3× daily. See antimicrobial therapy p. 411 if puerperal sepsis is suspected.

Lymphatic route = myometritis → parametritis puerperalis

- **Myometritis puerperalis.** Circumscribed areas of myometrium with inflammatory edema and necrotic sections, development of smaller and larger abscesses in the muscle wall, puerperal uterine abscesses. Rarely a large, circumscribed section of uterus wall detaches and is expelled through the vaginally as a sequester. This process is called metritis dissecans.
- **Parametritis puerperalis. Phlegmonous** inflammation of the loose extraperitoneal connective tissue, originating from an infected section of uterine wall (lower uterine segment, cervical wall) or the upper vagina. The veins in the vicinity of the inflamed parametrial tissue become infected and thombosed. Women with cervical lacerations, pressure necrosis of the cervix or in the vaginal fornices are particularly susceptible to parametrial phlegmons.

Course of parametritis
- **Resorption.** The exudate is demarcated and reabsorbed = this is by far the most common outcome of parametritis. The possibility of resorption remains until colliquation occurs.
- **Colliquation = abscess development** with the possibility of perforation either into a hollow organ (usually the rectum, more rarely into the vagina, rarely into the bladder) or transcutaneously, usually above the inguinal ligament.
- **The exsudate (cellulitis) spreads** to the various connective tissue spaces:
  - **Upwards** to the lateral abdominal wall, whereby it appears as a doughy swelling slightly above the inguinal ligament.
  - **Anteriorly** to the bladder (bladder complaints!) or even prevesically into the retropubic space (cave of Retzius), where it may then become visible as a solid tumor on the anterior abdominal wall (rare).
  - **Posteriorly** to the rectum (tenesmus, diarrhea!).
  - **Downwards** (rare) along the Vasa iliaca through the Lacuna vasorum, where it appears on the inner thigh as phlegmonous inflammation.
  - **Retroperitoneally.** The phlegmonous inflammation can creep over the parametrial pelvic connective tissue into the loose retroperitoneal connective tissue in which the urethra is embedded and which stretches from the bladder to the kidneys (rare).

Symptoms. Rise in temperature, **pain radiates into one leg**.

Diagnosis. Vaginal examination. Pressure sensitive infiltrate in the parametrium.

Note. Characteristics of parametrial cellulitis:
Close to the pelvic wall.
Is not mobile, but completely fixed.
A characteristic wedge shape is usually found on palpation.

Treatment. To begin with, therapy as for puerperal salpingitis. If an abscess has formed, it must be widely incised in time, after which improvement is immediate. A typical location for threatened perforation of a parametrial abscess is the area above the inguinal ligament.

Hematogenous route = puerperal sepsis

Definition. Septic infection in connection with miscarriage or birth, caused by a septic source within the body. From here, pathogenic bacteria enter the bloodstream, either constantly or periodically over a short time, and to such an extent that the clinical consequences of this occurrence – not those of the local process at the source –eventually dominate the clinical picture. Synonym for severe or malignant childbed fever.

Sepsis is understood to be a systemic reaction of the organism to the infection with the following manifestations (systemic inflammatory response syndrome; SIRS. Two or more of the following symptoms must be present; American College of Chest Physicians, Society of Critical Care Medicine):

- Temperature > 38 °C or < 36 °C.
- Heart rate > 90 bpm.
- Respiratory rate > 20 breaths pm or $PaCO_2$ < 32 mmHg.
- WBC count > 12,000/mm^3 or < 4,000/mm$^{3.}$
- Proof of infection is required.

In **severe sepsis** multiple organ disfunction also occurs (hypoperfusion, hypotension, lactic acidosis, oliguria), in **septic shock** hypotension occurs despite volume replacement therapy (systolic BP < 90 mmHg).

Note. Pathophysiology of puerperal sepsis. The entry point, the primary site of sepsis, the secondary site of sepsis = the metastatic bacterial colonization.

In puerperal sepsis:
Entry point can be any birth wound. By far the most common entry point is the placental implantation site, here in particular endometritis with serious clinical picture and septic temperatures (septic endometritis). The occurrence of septic temperatures and the seriously ill appearance of the patient indicate that the bacteria have penetrated the protective wall.
Primary site of sepsis in the vicinity of the entry point of the bacteria, that is, in the area of the uterine wall. The primary site is usually a thrombophlebitis of one of the larger veins or a complete venous region in the drainage area of the uterus.

- Lower drainage area: innumerable uterine veins → internal iliac veins.
- Upper drainage area: innumerable veins → ovarian vein.

Thrombosis occurs in the inflamed veins. The bacteria invade the thrombi an infect them (septic thrombi) and spread through the peripheral uterine veins.
These inflamed veins with their infected thrombi represent the primary circulatory site = primary site of sepsis.
“Sepis” (septicemia) results when this primary site becomes connected to the bloodstream.
The bacteria, with or without miniscule particles of thrombus tissue, are continually or periodically dispersed into the bloodstream from the infected clots = bacterial embolism.

These emboli are the cause of the severe generalized infection (= puerperal sepsis).
Secondary sites of sepsis (= metastatic bacterial colonization) are most common.
- In the **lungs:** pulmonary abscesses and pulmonary gangrene, often with development of emphysema.
- On the **heart valves:** endocarditis ulcerosa (septica).

A bacterial source on the heart valve is found particularly in women with a history of rheumatic endocarditis. Because of its location in the bloodstream, this secondary sepsis site is extremely important. Great numbers of bacteria are found on the inflamed heart valve. From here, in addition to the primary site, large numbers of pathogenic bacteria constantly enter the bloodstream.

Practice tip. In around 20 % of cases a bacterial source is found on the endocardium = endocarditis septica.

Metastatic bacterial colonization of the following organs:
- **Internal organs.** Abscesses in kidneys, spleen, liver.
- **Joints.** Arthritides.
- **Musculature.** Myositides.
- **Bone marrow.** Osteomyelitis.
- **Eyes.** Panophthalmia of the retina and choroid (abscess development with destruction of the whole eye).
- **Skin.** Exanthema, petechial hemorrhages, skin abscesses.
- **Nervous system.** Brain (brain abscesses, purulent meningitis).

Due to the rapid course and the massive attack on many organs of the particularly severe form of sepsis caused by Group A Streptococcus, organ failure and death occur before secondary sites of sepsis can develop.

Clinical manifestation. High fever (over 39 °C):
- usually in the form of a remittent fever with 1–2 and more attacks of shivering over several weeks, or
- in the form of a more or less continuous fever (rare), possibly with only occasional shivering attacks.
- Uncharacteristic course of fever. Intermittent and remittent fever can become a continuous fever.

General appearance. The subjective feeling of wellbeing and the rosy appearance of the new mother, often also antimicrobial therapy, can mask the serious diagnosis.

Advanced sepsis. Looks unwell (facial appearance), rapid, weak pulse. At temperatures between 39 and 41 °C the pulse fluctuates between 130 and 160 bpm. The tongue becomes dry and cracked, breathing is rapid, in severe cases conspicuously restless. The cheeks are livid, the eyes have an unusual shine. Shortness of breath, pale and cyanotic. A strong feeling of illness accompanies every attack of shivering, the signal that bacteria have entered the bloodstream. In severe cases drowsiness and delirium alternate with euphoria, that is with elevated mood and subjective feeling of wellbeing. The euphoria must not mask the severity of the illness.

Hemogram
Depending on the severity of the case, an increasing leukocytosis of 20–30,000 leukocytes/cm^3 and a strong left shift, in addition to anemia with Hb levels below 9 g% are found. Leukopenia is sometimes observed in the early phase.

Prognosis. Even today, mortality rates are considerable. They fluctuate, depending on the pathogen, between 20 and 50 %. In these cases immune responses weaken rapidly and the woman dies within 2–3 days, during which the fever curve shows high spikes = fulminant sepsis.

Complications. Coagulation disorder. In some cases a falling platelet count can be an early symptom of the coagulation disorder caused by puerperal sepsis. This drop in platelet count is explained as follows: the endotoxin which is released, in particular by gram-negative bacteria, damages vascular endothelial cells. Platelets adhere to and are thus "consumed" at these sections of the blood vessel wall. In addition to the drop in platelets, some coagulation factors are present in plasma in increased concentration, which causes an increased tendency to coagulate (hypercoagulability). Moreover, the endotoxin triggers the release of tissue factor from monocytes. In this way, fibrin is precipitated and microthrombosis occurs in the capillary periphery, in particular in the kidneys and lungs (DIC; disseminated intravascular coagulation). When the consumption of coagulation factors exceeds the rate of synthesis as a result, a coagulation factor deficiency ensues, consumption coagulopathy. Thus, in addition to the septic process, severe bleeding complications occur.

Treatment. For this serious clinical picture interdisciplinary cooperation between obstetrician, intensive care physicians and microbiologists is necessary.

- **Intensive monitoring** with regular monitoring of temperature, heart and respiratory rates, blood pressure, urinary output and urimeter, bloodwork (hemogram, blood gases, electrolytes, creatinine, urea, fibrinogen, platelets, coagulation etc.).
- **Venous line**, preferably a central venous catheter (CVC), for measurement of central venous pressure (CVP).
- **Infusions.**
- Fresh frozen plasma, platelet concentrate in cases of thrombocytopenia .
- High corticosteroid doses.
- Albumin (human).
- Immunoglobulins, 0.5 ml/body weight i.v. weekly; IgM 5–10 ml i.m. every 3 days.
- In cases of hypotension and/or oliguria/anuria, Dopamine infusion, dosage about 200–350 µg/min depending on clinical success.
- In marked **respiratory insufficiency** (e.g., capillary $PO_2 < 60$ mmHg when breathing room air), intubation and artificial respiration with positive end-expiratory pressure (PEEP) of 4–10 cm H_2O.
- **Antimicrobial therapy.** Early initiation of antimicrobial therapy is the most effective weapon against puerperal sepsis.

Practice tip. The earlier antibiotics are administered on appearance of early symptoms (fever!), the more successful the treatment.

  - Before antimicrobials are administered, blood is taken for culturing and testing for sensitivity to the relevant antibiotics. A swab from the cervix or uterine cavity is also taken.
  - Until the results are available, immediate treatment as follows: Amoxicillin and Clavulanic acid, 3 × 2.2 g/day or Cefotiam, 3 × 2 g/day. The success of this antimicrobial therapy is monitored by regular temperature measurements and WBC hemogram. If the fever has not fallen by the third day of antimicrobial therapy, combination therapy with Metronidazole, which is effective against anaerobic bacteria, is recommended: 3 × 500 mg i.c.
  - If GAS has been detected, high-dose Penicillin G (up to 20 million units/day i. v.) is the remedy of choice.
- **Surgical treatment.** The conclusion that operative measures such as laparotomy and hysterectomy are indicated to remove the vascular bacterial source of the infection and the timing of these measures has changed over the last decades; even now, opinions are divided. This indecisiveness

while pursuing conservative management sometimes results in surgery being postponed for too long.

Note. Hysterectomy must be considered if the clinical picture is serious and the symptoms of shock have not improved after about 6 h of treatment.

The decision to perform a hysterectomy, particularly on a young woman who still wants children, is serious. There are no generally binding guidelines as to when the indication is warranted. It arises from the clinical picture, interdisciplinary advice, and the obstetrician's experience.

Puerperal (diffuse) peritonitis

Definition. Inflammation of the peritoneum in the puerperal period.

Symptoms. The most striking symptom of peritonitis is extreme pain involving the whole abdomen, sensitivity towards all touch and movement, pain in response to pressure and rebound pain. Eventually reflexive, involuntary abdominal guarding occurs, tension of the anterior and lateral abdominal muscles which can advance to a state of rigidity (movement of serosa is inhibited by the tension). Once the intestinal serosa has been infected and inflamed (usually beginning in the lower abdomen), the intestines are paralyzed (paralytic ileus; functional paralysis due to toxicity). This results in retention of stool and flatus, silent abdomen (bowel sounds are not even audible with a stethoscope).

Further: fermentation of the bowel contents trapped in the paralyzed bowel causes meteorism → abdominal distension, antiperistalsis of the unaffected intestines in the upper abdomen, belching, nausea, and vomiting.
Diarrhea and mild meteorism are often present in diffuse puerperal peritonitis to begin with.

General symptoms. Rapid, weak pulse, fever (often not high), subjective perception of extreme illness, cold sweaty forehead, cold pointy nose, anxiousness, extremely unwell appearance, tongue is dry, cracked, rough.

Treatment. Laparotomy without exception, as early as possible!

The procedure should be as minimal as possible. The abdominal cavity is suctioned and swabbed. Thorough irrigation with physiological saline solution. Antimicrobial solution in the abdominal cavity. Drainage, intravenous rehydration, monitoring of serum electrolytes, administration of potassium chloride to compensate the potassium deficiency. Stimulation of bowel motility. Suction of stomach contents.

12.2 Hemorrhage in the puerperal period

Causes
- Retained fragments of placenta or polyps and endometritis puerperalis cause two thirds of all puerperal hemorrhages.
- Functional causes are responsible for the remaining third.
- Hemorrhage due to birth trauma is rare in the puerperal period.

12.2.1 Retained placental tissue and placental polyp

Definition. A fragment of placental tissue which has remained in the uterus after incomplete detachment and expulsion. A placental polyp (Fig. 12.3) is retained placental tissue which has been encased by many layers of clotted blood.

Clinical manifestation. Bleeding ex utero. Cervix is not closed, but more or less wide open.

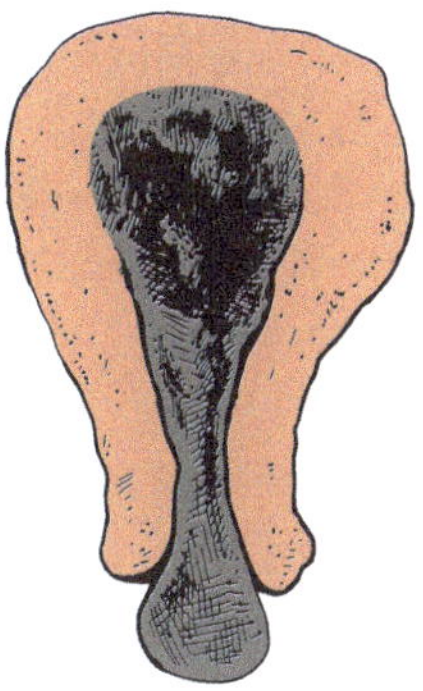

Fig. 12.3: Placental polyp = retained placental tissue, encased by layers of clotted blood.

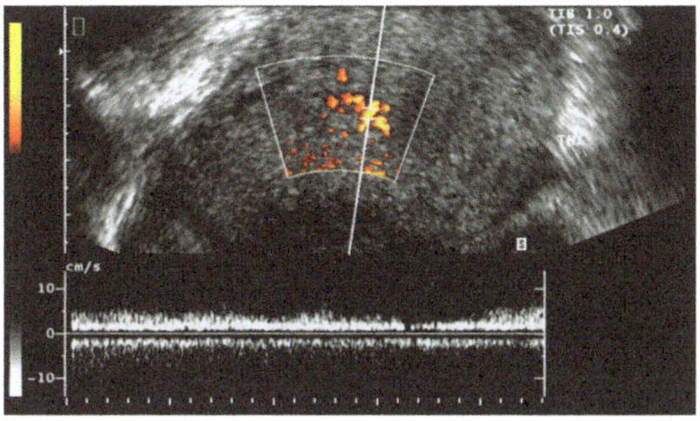

Fig. 12.4: Sonographic detection of retained placental tissue three weeks after birth; Doppler sonographic depiction of vascularization of the placental tissue.

Larger polyps trigger expulsive contractions. The lower pole is then expelled into the cervical canal, opening it. It is palpable and usually visible on speculum examination.

Ultrasonography (Fig. 12.4)

Hemorrhage in the puerperium after retention of placental tissue

- At the end of the first or in the course of the second week,
- Unexpected heavy bleeding, often life-threatening,
- Uterotonics only briefly bring about hemostasis if at all.

Heavy bleeding in the puerperal period is almost always due to retained placental tissue.

Complications. Infection of the placental tissue, the surrounding endometrium and the muscle layer below it (circumscribed endomyometritis). The thrombi of the blood vessels in the area are also infected.

Treatment. Removal of the placental tissue under antimicrobial protection.

Curettage of the puerperal uterus must be performed extremely slowly and very carefully, if possible under sonographic guidance, due to the significant danger of perforation.

Practice tip. All retained placental tissue causes endomyometritis. In no obstetrical condition is the uterus wall more susceptible to perforation than in endomyometritis.

It has also been reported that removal of the basal layer of the endometrium by curettage in the puerperium has resulted in Asherman's syndrome.
All retained placental tissue must be histologically examined, without exception. This is particularly important for differential diagnosis of trophoblastic tumor.
An alternative pharmacological treatment available today is misoprostol. An operative procedure, with all the associated risks, may thus be avoided, however monitoring is necessary.

Prophylaxis. Thorough examination of the placenta after birth.

12.2.2 Puerperal endometritis

The second most common cause of hemorrhage in the puerperium. Relatively harmless in comparison to retained placental tissue.

Hemorrhage type. Generally light bleeding, usually begins in the first day p.p., may persist for several days, can also cease for hours and days.

12.2.3 Functional hemorrhage in the puerperium

Bleeding in absence of retained placental tissue, puerperal endometritis and laceration. Usually as a result of the glandular hyperplasia which occurs in the course of the first anovulatory cycle in the puerperium (p. 396).

12.2.4 Bleeding from birth traumas in the puerperium

In rare cases lacerations are overlooked in labor or after birth when external or internal bleeding was not apparent for some reason. The main role is played by cervical lacerations which have been overlooked, silent rupture of the uterus, infra- or supralevatorial bleeding.

12.3 Injury to the symphysis pubis

Preliminary note. The connections of the pelvic girdle (Fig. 12.5), that is, the cartilage joining the symphysis pubis and the sacroiliac "joint" are a functional unit. In the pregravid phase of the cycle and particularly in pregnancy they loosen, primarily due to estrogens. They become more mobile = physiological pelvic relaxation. The gap between the pubic bones widens over the course of the pregnancy by up to 7–10 mm. Despite this physiological widening of the maternal pelvic girdle, lesions of these pelvic "joints", in particular the symphysis pubis occur not infrequently in pregnancy, but more often during labor. The lesions, known as pelvic girdle relaxation (Fig. 12.6), present a characteristic clinical picture once they have reached a certain degree.

Definition. Pain directly related to load-bearing in the region of the symphysis pubis, diastasis of the symphysis pubis, ranging from

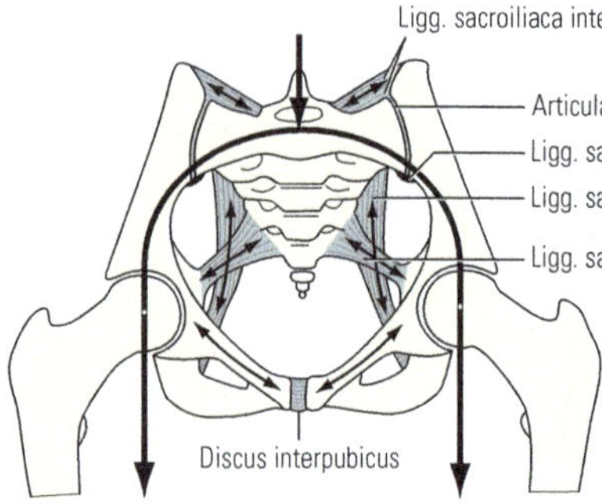

Fig. 12.5: The pelvis as a static construction. Frontal section at the level of the hip joints. Transferal of the trunk load onto the femur heads. Traction and pressure load on the symphysis pubis. Traction on the ligaments. Half-schematic.

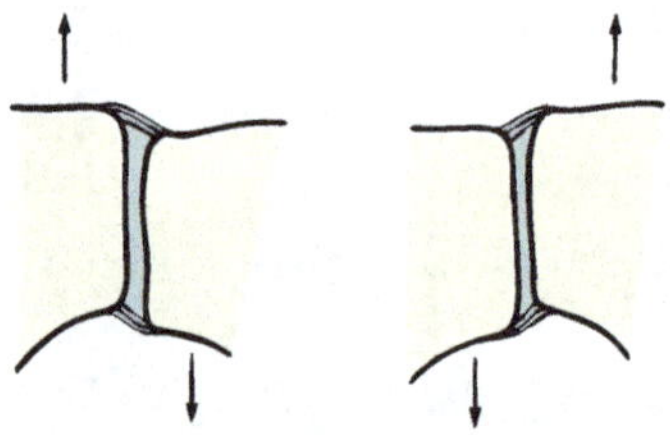

Fig. 12.6: Pelvic girdle relaxation. Misaligned pubic bones on transferal of weight from one leg to the other.

broadening of the gap to separation and dislocation of the pubic bones (Fig. 12.7).

Causes. Diastasis of the symphysis pubis is almost always the result of severe birth trauma (CPD, difficult forceps delivery). Severe birth traumas are rare today, and diastasis of the symphysis pubis correspondingly so. Today diastasis of the symphysis pubis is compared to the far more common injury of a lesser degree. Injury to the symphysis pubis, which can also be the result of trauma (overextension, small lacerations etc), almost always has a functional cause.

Interestingly, injury to the symphysis pubis as a result of birth trauma almost always occurs in spontaneous births. Only in 10 % of cases can symphysis pubis injury be attributed to cer-

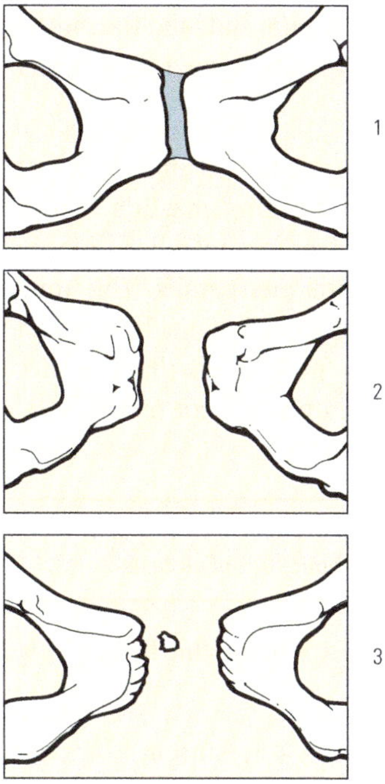

Fig. 12.7: Three cases presenting with relatively similar symphysis pubis symptoms. Postpartum x-rays: 1) injury to the symphysis pubis with a narrow gap between the pubic bones; 2) with a wide gap (diastasis of the symphysis pubis?); 3) very broad gap between the pubic bones, torn bone fragment? Obvious diastasis. In both 2 and 3 misalignment of the pubic bones is also visible, signifying pelvic girdle relaxation and dislocation.

tain labor difficulties. Therefore 90 % of cases have a functional cause. Functional symphysis pubis injury presents more or less the same clinical picture as traumatic injury.

Practice tip. Injury to the symphysis pubis can already occur in pregnancy, in labor or not until the puerperium.

Incidence. Incidence of 1 : 300 to 1 : 3,000 are given; rates of symphysis pubis injuries appear to have increased in the past years, in particular spontaneous injury.

Symptoms. The most common symptom is pain in the region of the symphysis pubis, which is usually commented on directly after birth or in the first days p.p. The pain increases on movement, on standing up, particularly on heavy lifting and carrying. It often radiates into the thigh and sacrum.

Practice tip. Lower abdominal pain of unknown origin which radiates into the thigh or sacrum indicates injury to the symphysis pubis.

When pressure is applied to the symphysis pubis pain is experienced at a certain spot. The same is usually valid for the sacroiliac joint. Patients often say they are unable to roll over in bed. In pronounced cases the legs are abducted and rotated outwards. In severe cases walking is difficult: waddling or complete inability to walk.

There is often swelling (hematoma?) in the region of the pubic symphysis. Vaginal examination: retrosymphysical hematoma as a cushion-like thickening behind the symphysis pubis. Often with temperature and fever. Sonographic examination (measurement of the gap) or x-ray (Fig. 12.6): widened symphysis pubis gap and dislocation of the pubic bones (step formation) are typical findings. However, a normal or even narrow gap does not contradict the diagnosis of injury to the symphysis pubis. Changes to gap width probably represent different stages of relaxation.

Practice tip. Injury to the symphysis pubis can already occur in the pregnancy with all characteristic symptoms.

Over half of the affected women complained about increased lower back pain, pelvic and pubic symphysis pain radiating into the thighs in the last weeks or months of pregnancy. They also complained of impaired ambulation (unsure footing, difficulties climbing stairs). The earliest symptoms (also in early pregnancy) are complaints of tiredness and aching limbs.

Prognosis. Generally good. Impaired ambulation is a complication which almost always resolves, even in severe cases.

Treatment. Physical rest, symptomatic (pain relief) treatment, strenuous activity should be avoided, sick leave. If complaints are severe, a firm belt with lateral supports e.g., after Kobes and Gölkel. Orthopedic follow-up.

12.4 Mastitis puerperalis

Definition. Inflammation of the breasts in the puerperium.

Incidence. Around 1% of all women postpartum.

Pathogen. In over 90% of cases, mastitis is caused by Staphylococcus aureus haemolyticus. In addition Streptococci, Proteus, and E. coli.

Transmission (Fig. 12.8). The main route of transmission is droplet transmission (nasopharynx) between hospital staff and the mother via the infant nasopharynx to the maternal nipple.

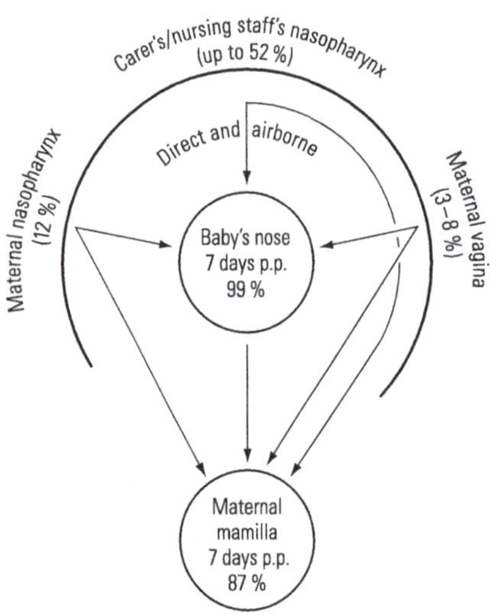

Fig. 12.8: Transmission of Staphylococcus aureus hemolyticus.

Mastitis is mainly transmitted during breastfeeding. It is "breastfeeding mastitis". Infection via the lochia (contact infection) plays a minor role in mastitis puerperalis. This route of infection was previously considered much more important. It is now known that hemolysing streptococci are only present in about 2% of lochial discharge.

Note. The maternal nipple is infected with staphylococci after breastfeeding in about 90 % of all cases.

Routes of infection within the breast (Fig. 12.9, 12.10).

In connective tissue (= interstitium): between the glands = interstitial mastitis or extracanalicular mastitis (Fig. 12.9).
Tiny tissue defects (cracks, abrasions, fissures) are a requirement for this route of infection. From these miniscule nipple defects the bacteria infiltrate via the lymph system deep into the connective tissue between the glands. A diffusely spreading (phlegmonous) inflammation results.
Interstitial mastitis, i.e., lymphogenous mastitis, is the most common form of Mastitis puerperalis.
If the lymphogenous inflammation is just under the skin of the nipple a subareolar abscess forms (Fig. 12.7).
If the phlegmon passes right through the breast tissue to the pectoral fascia:
- A sub- or retromammary abscess forms (Fig. 12.9).
- Intracanicular ascension occurs via open lactiferous ducts = glandular ducts (Fig. 12.10).

Each of the 15–20 glands = parenchyma of the breast has a special duct. Inflammation of the

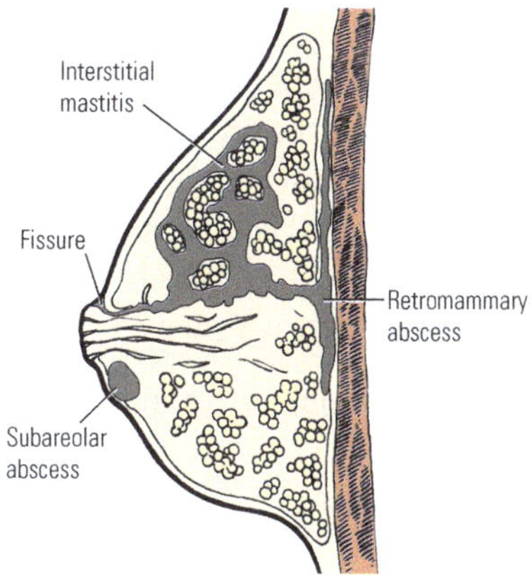

Fig. 12.9: Purulent interstitial mastitis (spread of infection in connective tissues, originating in fissures).

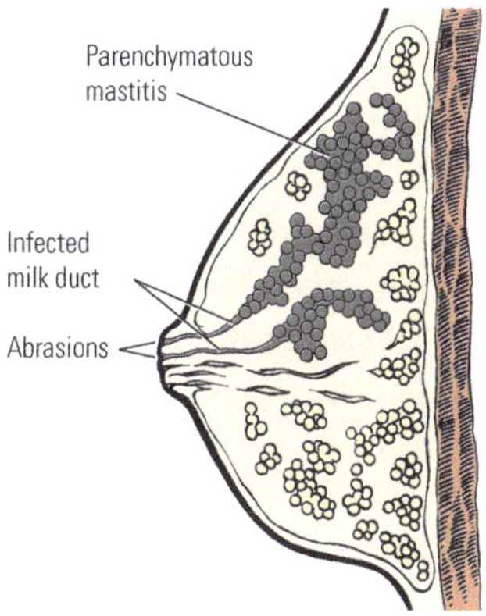

Fig. 12.10: Intracanalicular (parenchymatous) mastitis (spread of the infection from the open lactiferous ducts into the lobes).

ducts occurs first (= galactophoritis) and then inflammation of the milk glands, i.e., the parenchyma = parenchymatous mastitis.

As milk is an excellent breeding ground for germs, their growth is promoted if the breast is not sufficiently emptied (avoid milk stasis!).

Practice tip. Whether the route of infection was lymphogenous-interstitial or intracanalicular is practically irrelevant because as mastitis progresses one form merges into the other. Which of the forms is in the forefront is also unimportant for treatment.

Symptoms

- **Pain.** At a circumscribed location on one breast. In the beginning, however, the pain is usually only very mild.
- **Fever.** Usually begins after pain has begun; it is, however, not uncommon for fever to be the first symptom, and initially the only one.

Practice tip. Beginning mastitis is the first condition that should be considered if fever suddenly occurs or (more rarely) there is a slow rise in temperature at the end of the first week and over the course of the second week p.p., even if there are no apparent changes to the breast.

- **Redness.** Often only appears 12–14 hours after pain and rise in temperature occurred. One quadrant of a breast (most commonly the upper outer, next most common is the lower outer quadrant) is red and warmer than its surroundings. On palpation it is usually noticeably painful. The redness is often in connection with a **lymphangitis:** bluish-red lymph vessels cross over the reddened section to the swollen axillary lymph glands.
- **Abscess formation.** If mastitis is not detected in the early stages and immediately treated there is a risk of infiltration and abscess formation. Over the course of 2–3 days an infiltrate of 2–3 cm diameter forms which does not have clear edges. Palpation of the mass is extremely painful. The infiltrated area becomes liquefied over time (colliquation; can take days to several weeks) to a fluctuating abscess.

Treatment

Inhibition of lactation. In the early stage of mastitis, directly after appearance of the first symptoms, a low dose of a prolactin-inhibiting agent such as Bromocriptine or Lisuride is given, e.g., 1.25 mg once or twice, or one dose of

Cabergolin 0.5 mg. This pharmacological treatment reduces the volume of milk and should be supported by the resorptive treatment described below. The fever usually abates within 12–24 h. Further measures are usually not necessary. It is important to ensure that the breast is emptied during this period. This treatment plan allows lactation to be maintained, and in most cases it is possible to continue breastfeeding.

Antimicrobial treatment. If the clinical symptoms do not improve within 12–24 h after treatment to reduce lactation, 3–4 days of antimicrobial therapy is indicated. Penicillinase- resistant Penicillin derivatives are suitable, e.g., from the Oxacillin series.

Most experience has been made with Oxacillin. Dosage: 1 g 3 × daily = 3 g. Oral administration: 3 capsules → 0.25 g 4 × daily; i.v. injection 2 vials → 0.5 g 3 × daily. Because of its even better utilization, Dicloxycillin can be given in a lower dosage. Dosage: 0.5 g 4 × daily = 2 g. Oral administration: 2 capsules → 0.25 g twice a day (approx. 1 h before meals); i. v. injection 1 vial → 0.5 g 4× daily (dissolve as for Oxacillin).
Dosage can be increased if necessary, after observing and palpating to ensure that infiltration has not occurred.

Resorptive treatment with physical measures
Principle. Immobilization of the breast and cold applications.

Indication. Resorptive treatment is only of use in the early stages, if the breast inflammation has only just begun, or infiltration is very mild.

Method. The affected breast is firmly bound so that it is immobilized. Cold alcohol compresses or ice packs; voiding of the bowels, restricted fluid intake, no soups or fruit (98 % fluids!)

If, however, a patient presents with mastitis in which the infiltration has spread or colliquation has already begun, resorption of the site of inflammation can no longer be hoped for. Promotion of colliquation is to be actively and consistently pursued. It is most rapidly achieved by warm applications: moist warm compresses until the whole process has liquefied and marked fluctuation is noticeable all over.

Surgical treatment = aspiration or incision of the abscess.

Practice tip. Do not aspire or incise before the infiltrate has liquefied and fluctuates!

It is, however, equally wrong to **wait too long** with surgical treatment, as further tissue colliquation then results.

Aspiration. Once colliquation has occurred and the mass fluctuates, if the abscess is not too large it can be punctured under sonographic guidance with a cannula, suctioned, and irrigated. The cosmetic results are better than after incision and counterincision. In some cases the process may need to be repeated over the next few days.

Line of incision
Radial incision (Fig. 12.11). Simple incisions are always radial.

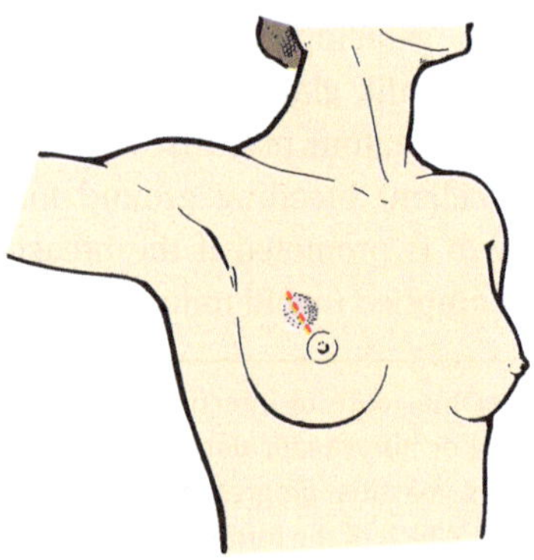

Fig. 12.11: Radial incision of an abscess due to mastitis.

Lactiferous ducts are damaged or severed on transverse incision (risk of degradation of parenchyma, formation of milk duct fistulae and milk cysts). The length of the incision is determined solely by the size of the abscess. A puncturing incision is only adequate in very small, superficial abscesses. Cosmetic aspects are to be considered. The incision should not extend into the nipple. As little healthy tissue as possible should be sacrificed.

Bardenheuer incision = lifting a flap of the breast (Fig. 12.12).

Technique. Depending on the size of the abscess, a 5–10 cm long arc incision is made on the lower margin of the breast directly in the fold. The wound is held open with dressing forceps, the finger is used to clear out the wound cavity and make it as smooth as possible. Abscesses in the upper quadrant are also easily reached. Rubber drainage tape is attached by suturing to the edge of the incision.

Bardenheuer's incision is suitable for:

- All extensive suppurations.
- All large, single abscesses in the lower outer and inner quadrant.
- Retromammary abscesses.

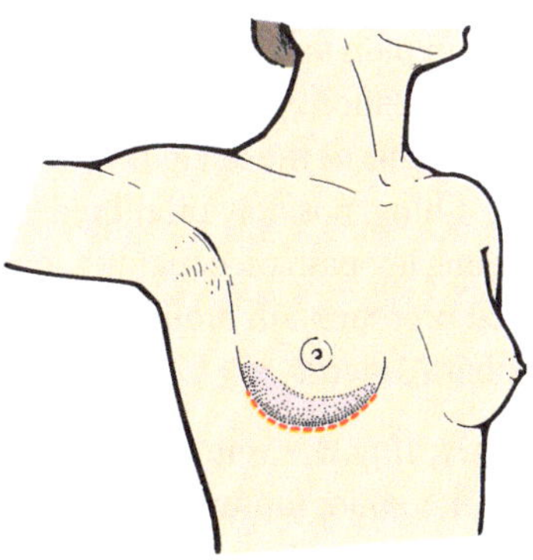

Fig. 12.12: Bardenheuer incision = lifting a flap of the breast.

Advantages. Excellent drainage, inconspicuous scar, no need for further incisions if the arc incision is correctly made.

If the abscess is large and at the deepest point of the cavity a counterincision should be made, and drainage tape applied. Tape/drain should not be removed until secretion has almost completely ceased.
Incision alone is not enough, however:
The wound must be evacuated. The finger is inserted into the cavity and thoroughly evacuates it. Remaining tissue bridges must be separated and the abscess cavity explored on all sides for soft sections of the wall. If another abscess is found, it is digitally opened and also evacuated. Counterincision and drainage tape through both abscesses!

Note. The **3 main mistakes** in treatment of breast abscesses due to mastitis:

1. The incision is made before colliquation has occurred.
2. The incisions for large abscesses are too small.
3. Counterincisions are not made when they are required.

Abscesses due to mastitis have a strong tendency to recur. If recurrence is to be avoided, these mistakes must not be made.

Discontinuation of lactation because of mastitis. Controversial. In mild cases breastfeeding should be maintained. If infiltration has occurred, breastfeeding should be discontinued. Absolute immobilization of the breast is now most important. If an abscess has formed breastfeeding is contraindicated as single cases of infant fatality due to colonized milk have been reported. Important rule: if lactation is discontinued due to mastitis, the infant must not drink from the healthy breast either. Discontinuation of lactation see p. 403.

Prophylaxis of puerperal mastitis. Goals:
- Prevention of abrasions and cracks, details see p. 402.
- Prevention of bacterial hospitalism (= colonization of hospitals with pathogenic bacteria).

Especially important is blockage of the staphylococci infection routes.

12.5 Pelvic vein thrombosis

Definition. Generally mild, i.e., noninflammatory, partial, or complete thrombotic obstructions of the internal iliac vein and its venous plexus and of the external iliac vein.

Consequences. Thrombi in the area of the internal iliac vein. Difficult to detect on clinical examination and therefore often the source of periodic pulmonary embolism (hypertension, Cor pulmonale in pregnancy, pulmonary embolism "out of nowhere" in the puerperium).

Thrombi in the external iliac vein rapidly result in thrombi development descending into the femoral vein, and are easily recognized due to the edema of the affected extremity and the typical pressure pain along the course of the main blood vessels of the leg. Both forms have a tendency to ascend to the inferior vena cava (IVC). The valves involved in the thrombosis are irreversibly damaged within days, so that conservatively "healed" iliac vein thrombi generally result in long-term complications ("postthrombotic syndrome; PTS).
PTS involves a many-layered clinical picture of chronic venous insufficiency, which presents differently in each case, depending on the course of organization of the thrombosis, its tendency to recur, and the efficiency of the collateral circulation. The symptoms range from edema, marks of congestion, secondary lymphatic edema with induration, secondary varicosity, trophic disorders (venous ulcers, Ulcera cruris).

Etiology and pathogenesis
- **Decreased venous flow velocity** from the legs occurs in normal early pregnancy and can achieve pathogenetic significance in late pregnancy as a result of the obstruction of venous flow by the large uterus and postpartum by bed rest.
- **Changes to the venous wall** are less likely to play a role in the etiology of pelvic vein thrombosis postpartum. Degenerative changes to the vein walls, which often extend to the venous plexus of the pelvis, do however play a role in varicosity in pregnancy.

Incidence. 1–2 %

Clinical manifestation
- Known history. History of thrombosis, adiposity, PIH, varicosity, operative delivery.
- General signs. Increasing pulse rate (Mahler's sign), often in the form of a "climbing pulse", elevated temperature (Michaelis sign), often only sub-febrile.
- Local signs. Asymmetrical pressure pain in the parametrium, fullness of the hemorrhoid veins, possibly hemorrhoid vein thrombosis, fullness of the collateral circulation (superficial epigastric vein), spontaneous groin pain and pain on pressure to the groin and along the course of the large blood vessels of the leg to the adductor canal. Shiny, possibly bright red skin. Spontaneous leg pain on coughing, on blowing a blood pressure cuff around the thigh (Loewenberg's sign).

Diagnostic imagery. If pelvic vein thrombosis is suspected, Doppler sonography is indicated to detect the thrombosis and if the diagnosis is confirmed to localize it, determine its extent and if possible to estimate its age.

Treatment. Treatment of pelvic vein thrombosis is by administration of high-dose Heparin: in the acute treatment phase bolus injection of 5,000 units Heparin IV, then 400 units/kg and 24 h adjustment after 1.5- to 2.5-fold lengthening of the partial thromboplastin time (PTT). Alternatively, low-molecular-weight Heparins are recommended, particularly in pregnancy, for example 3 × 5,000 units Dalteparin per day with the goal of antifactor Xa activity of > 0.2 units/ml. Immobilization with elevation and compression treatment of the affected leg can contribute to reducing the swelling and pain relief. These measures do not reduce the risk of embolism or improve the sequelae in terms of PTS.

Secondary prophylaxis with a lower dose of heparin or low molecular weight heparin is continued in the mobilized patient after the initial high-dose heparin treatment.
Coumarins are subsequently given; it must be considered, however, that Coumarins are contraindicated while breastfeeding. Treatment with oral anticoagulants can last for up to two years.
Monitoring for Coumarin treatment: prothrombin time (PT). Heparin antidote: Protaminsulfate 1 % or 5 % (against depot Heparin). Coumarin antidote: Vitamin K_1.

Deep vein thrombosis (DVT) of the leg/pelvis in pregnancy. Both pregnancy and puerperium predispose to thrombi, as in addition to the reduced velocity of venous bloodflow and increased varicosity in pregnancy, the concentration of the coagulation factors increases and that of the coagulation inhibitory factors and the fibrinolytic system decreases.

Incidence. Around 1 %. The risk of thrombosis is around 5 times higher for pregnant women than for nonpregnant women.

Risk factors. Women with a history of thrombosis have a higher risk, as do women with hereditary thrombophilias such as Factor V

Tab. 12.1: Thrombosis risk groups in pregnancy and the puerperium and management (after Bauersachs and colleagues, 2007); VTE = venous thromboembolism.

Low risk	Medium risk	High risk
– No prior VTE, but positive thrombophilia – No prior VTE, negative thrombophilia, but a number of risk factors present – No prior VTE, but presence of lupus/antiphospholipid antibodies – Prior (secondary) VTE, negative thrombophilia	– No prior VTE, but deficiency of Antithrombin I or II – Prior VTE with no trigger – Prior VTE in pregnancy or while taking ovulation inhibitors – Prior recurrent (secondary) VTE – More than 1 prior miscarriage with presence of lupus/antiphospholipid antibodies	– Pregnant woman on oral anticoagulants – Antithrombin deficiency with thrombi – Lupus/antiphospholipid antibodies with thrombi – Recurring VTE despite sufficient prophylaxis – Thrombosis/embolism in current pregnancy
Observation: – If additional risk factors are present heparinization as outlined for medium risk, continuing for 2 weeks p.p.	**Prophlaxis:** – Begin when risk has been established – Continue for 6 weeks p.p. – Dalteparin 50–100 IU/kg body weight per day	**Full anticoagulation:** – Begin when risk has been established, possibly pre-conception – Dalteparin 100–150 IU/kg body weight per day

Leiden mutation, Prothrombin Gene mutation, Protein-S, or Protein-C deficiency, Antithrombin deficiency, or acquired thrombophilias such as antiphospholipid syndrome (detection of antiphospholipid and lupus antibodies!)

Thrombosis prophylaxis. Rigorous prophylaxis in high-risk pregnant women and/or new mothers (e.g., extreme varicosis, abdominal operative delivery, adiposity, diabetes mellitus).

Measures:
- Early mobilization (see p. 400).
- Anatomically fitted gradient compression stockings (GCS; pressure lessens proximally).
- Pharmacological prophylaxis, today in the majority of cases with low-molecular-weight Heparins (see Tab. 12.1).

The following side effects must be considered if Heparin or low-molecular-weight Heparin is to be administered long-term: platelet levels are to be monitored twice a week from day 5 after beginning the prophylaxis because of the risk of thrombocytopenia (in around 3 % of cases; Heilmann and colleagues). These are rarer in low-molecular-weight heparins, as is the risk of severe hemorrhage, and of osteoporosis, which is described in 5–10 % of cases of long-term administration in pregnancy, also after low-dose heparinization.
Oral anticoagulants (Coumarin) should not be administered in pregnancy.
After delivery, post-operative prophylaxis is recommended until complete mobilization, if other risks exist continuation of the relevant prophylaxis is recommended for 6 weeks.

12.6 Postpartum thyroiditis

10 % of women develop thyroiditis postpartum, which is generally mild or clinically inapparent. Its course can have one or two phases with intermittent thyrotoxicosis. Symptomatic beta-blocker treatment is recommended in the periods of thyrotoxicosis, not antithyroid drugs! The cause lies in cytotoxic autoimmune reactions. The prognosis is good, complete healing can be expected within 3–12 months. However 5 % of women retain hyperthyroidism.

12.7 Psychiatric disorders

Mental upset and disorders after birth are widespread. Rapid mood swings between happiness and irritability, tearfulness (commonly known as **"baby blues"**) often occur on day 3–5 p.p. These mood swings last a few days and do not require specific treatment.

Post partem depression. Can occur days or weeks after birth. Depression may be of varying degrees from mild depression which does not require treatment, to severe delusional depression. Depressive symptoms which have been observed: concentration difficulties, sluggish thinking capacity, brooding, depersonalization, listlessness, disinterest, lack of motivation, depression, feelings of guilt and inadequacy, irritability, panic attacks, compulsive thoughts and impulses, sleeping difficulties, thoughts of suicide. Suicidal thoughts are to be taken seriously; the risk of suicide is considerable in severe postnatal depression.

Practice tip. If there is pronounced risk of suicide and compulsive behavior, for example wanting to do something to the baby, hospital admission is necessary. This should be to a psychiatric clinic with a mother-baby unit.

Puerperal psychosis. Puerperal psychoses, which demonstrate the whole spectrum of psychopathologies, must be clearly distinguished from "baby blues" and postnatal depression.

Incidence. 1–2 : 1,000 births.

Symptoms. Appear in the first weeks p.p. and affect primiparae in particular. Feelings of inadequacy and guilt, depression with compulsiveness, e.g., wanting to kill one's own baby, fear of loss of control, avoidance behavior, panic attacks, delusional convictions under the influence of ordering voices, optical or auditory hallucinations, euphoric or manic moods with flighty ideas, overstimulation, reduced sleep requirements, grandiose ideas.

Extremely high risk of recurrence after subsequent births.

Treatment. Hospitalization in a specialist mother-baby mental health unit.

Posttraumatic stress disorder. Occurs after experiencing a traumatic delivery. Reliving the birth with nightmares of the occurrence, sleep disorders, irritability. The stress disorder usually appears within six months of the event, does not last longer than one month. The best treatment lies in discussion to reconcile the woman's subjective experience with the procedures experienced. Psychotherapy and/or antidepressives may be indicated.

References

Branch DW, Silver RM, Blackwell JL, et al.: Outcome treated pregnancies in women with antiphospholipit syndrome: an update of the Utah experience. Obstet Gynecol 1992; 80:614

Centers of Disease: Toxic shock syndrome – United States 1970–1982. MMWR 1982; 31:201

Culligan P, Hill S, Heit M: Rupture of the symphysis pubis during vaginal delivery followed by two subsequent uneventful pregnancies. Obstet Gynecol 2002; 100:1114

Dixon JM: Repeated aspiration of breast abscesses in lactating women. Br Med J 1988; 297:1517

Gerhardt A, Scharf RE, Beckmann MW et al: Prothrombin and factor V mutations in women with a history of thrombosis during pregnancy and the puerperium. N Engl J Med 2000; 342:374

Gherman RB, Goodwin TM, Leung B, et al.: Incidencee, clinical characteristics, and timing of objectively diagnosed venous thromboembolism during pregnancy. Obstet Gynecol 1999; 94:730

Hackett SP, Stevens DL: Streptococcal toxic shock syndrome: synthesis of tumor necrosis factor and interleukin-1 by monocytes stimulated with pyrigenic exotoxin A and streptolysin O. J Inf Dis 1992; 165:879

Meaney JF, Weg JG, Chenevert TL, et al.: Diagnosis of pulmonary embolism with magnetic resonance angiography. N Eng J Med 1997; 33:1422

Scholefield JH, Duncan JL, Rogers K: Review of a hospital experience of breast abscesses. Br J Surg 1987; 74:469

Snow RE, Neubert AG: Peripartum pubic symphysis separation: A case series and review of the literature. Obstet Gynecol Surv 1997; 52:438

Stevens DL: Streptococcal toxic-shock-syndrome: spectrum of disease, pathogenesis, and new concepts in treatment. Emerg Inf Dis 1995; 1:69

Summers PR: Surgical aspects of peripartal infections. Clin Obstet Gynecol 1994; 37:324

Warkentin TE, Levine MN, Hirsch J, et al.: Heparin-induced thrombocytopenia in patients treated with low-molecular-weight heparin or unfractionated heparin N Engl J Med 1995; 332:332

Wolf JE, Rabinowitz LG: Streptococcal toxic shock-like syndrome 1995; 131:73

Zurawski B, Bardsley M, Beall B, et al.: Invasive group A streptococcal disease in metropolitan Atlanta: a population-based assessment. Clin Infect Dis 1998; 27:150

13 The newborn

M. Obladen

Important definitions
- Neonatal period: first 28 days of life.
- Gestational age: first day of the last menstrual period to birth; 280 days = 40 weeks.
- Liveborn: at least one vital sign present after birth: heartbeat, umbilical cord pulsation, respiration.
- Stillborn: vital signs absent (heartbeat, umbilical cord pulsation, respiration), birth weight > 500 g.
- Mature newborn: gestational age 259–293 days or 37–42 completed weeks.
- Preterm baby: gestational age < 259 days or < 37 completed weeks of pregnancy.

13.1 The healthy newborn

13.1.1 The baby and its parents

All mothers look forward to a healthy baby. Sex, weight, appearance and health of the baby are anticipated by the parents with excitement, often also with fear. The slightest deviation from what the mother perceives to be normal in a phase in which she is particularly vulnerable emotionally can be very distressing.

Note. A common criticism of hospital obstetrics is that the newborn is too often pathologized, and that unnecessary or contradictory information and advice is given by too many or inexperienced doctors and nursing staff.

Information. Parents must be informed by the doctor about diseases, defects, disabilities, and operations as early, honestly, and completely as possible and reasonable. It has proven valuable to conduct the first conversation with both parents, whereby ideally the consulting pediatrician and the obstetrician who knows the mother take part.

Neonatologist. Those looking after newborns in an obstetrical department must be informed about the advances of neonatology in recent years and the possibilities of intensive medicine, but must not upset or scare the mother with this knowledge. Extreme gentleness is necessary, particularly when parents are being informed about diseases, malformations, disabilities, operations, serious prognoses, or about a transfer. The baby belongs to its parents. They have the right to be proud of their baby. Those holding the conversation must always bear in mind the major changes which occur in a family as a result of the birth of a baby, and the emotional requirements of parents and baby.

The **obstetrician** must know the normal intra- and extrauterine development and most common newborn diseases until the end of the early neonatal period. Among the most important tasks for an obstetrician are recognizing dangers to and illnesses of newborns and coming to the right conclusions, requiring:
- Command of primary newborn resuscitation.
- Knowledge of pathogenesis and diagnosis of the most common dangers, diseases and defects.
- Immediate decision-making regarding transfers and transport of endangered and sick newborns.

13.1.2 Initial care

Definition. First procedures involving the baby directly post natum in the labor ward, dependent on maturity and condition of the newborn. Primary resuscitation (p. 439) is performed on vitally challenged babies. Our procedure:

- The umbilical cord is clamped and cut, the airways are freed.
- Status is evaluated (1 and 5 min Apgar scores).
- The baby is dried and kept warm.
- Contact between mother and baby.
- The baby is bathed.
- The baby is examined, and maturity evaluated.
- Eyes, vitamin K prophylaxis.
- Insertion of nasogastric tube (patency of esophagus).

Clamping and cutting the umbilical cord. Early (immediately) in children of diabetic mothers to reduce polycythemia (see p. 455), delayed (after pulsation of the cord has ceased, however not before 1 min p.p.) in preterm babies to reduce preterm anemia.

Freeing the airways. If mouth, nose, pharynx are blocked with mucus or blood. In order to avoid aspiration, first the mouth and pharynx, and then the nose are suctioned with a soft, not too thin catheter.

Practice tip. Suctioning of the nasal passages usually provokes a deep inspiration, which could lead to aspiration.

The baby is kept **warm** with a prewarmed cloth, in which it is completely wrapped. Placing a naked, wet newborn onto the mother's abdomen does not demonstrate empathy, but lack of knowledge about temperature regulation. It can cause significant hypothermia, in particular to newborns having difficulty adapting.
The **nasogastric tube** is used to exclude an esophageal and duodenal atresia (> 10ml secretion in the stomach).

Practice tip. The esophagus should not be probed in the first 10 min to avoid a dangerous vagal stimulus (bradycardia).

Dressing the baby can wait. It is unnecessary to clean the baby perfectly and remove the vernix.

13.1.3 Examination

Initial examination (within the first 24h post natum):

- Recognition of impaired respiratory or circulatory adaptation, congenital defects, birth trauma:
- Body measurements. Weight, length, occipitofrontal head circumference:
- Signs of maturity, condition and behavior, but not yet differentiated neurostatus:
- Skin. Color, hemorrhage, trauma:
- Cranial and mouth cavity. Trauma, asymmetry, facial paresis, cleft formation:
- Thorax. Breathing, heart sounds, sternal or subcostal recession:
- Abdomen. Tumors, umbilicus, genitals, femoral pulses:
- Skeleton. Extremities, spine, joints, clavicle fracture.

Well-baby examination, day 3–10.
An experienced pediatrician performs the examination, if possible in the presence of the mother. The notes are looked at beforehand: family history, age, social situation, maternal diseases and possibly treatments, course of earlier pregnancies, complications, diagnosis and treatment during this pregnancy, course of labor, Apgar score, resuscitation or other procedures performed on the baby. This examination focuses on:

- Skin. Color, turgor, pustules, icterus.
- Skull, mouth cavity. Head shape, oral thrush.
- Fontanelles. Size and consistency.

- Thoracic organs. Heart sounds, pulmonary ventilation, sternal recession.
- Newborn reflexes and muscle tone.
- Abdominal organs. Liver edge, spleen size, umbilicus, kidney size, tumors, testes descended.
- Skeleton. Hip placement, fold symmetry, spine.

Size of the anterior fontanelle (Fig. 13.1). 0.5–3 cm. Increase in diameter or bulging indicate an increase in intracranial pressure.

Newborn reflexes. Most important are: Moro reflex (Fig. 13.2), Galant reflex, traction response. Completeness and possible differences between the sides are vital for evaluation, not so much the response (almost always present).

- Moro reflex (present 0–5 months). Triggered by suddenly letting go of the head. Result: extension of the arms laterally, at right angles, fanning of the fingers, flexing of the arms, bringing them together in front of the chest.

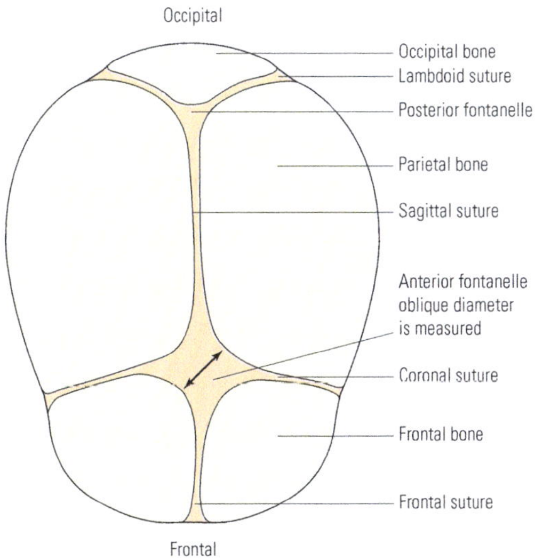

Fig. 13.1: The size of the fontanelle is measured diagonally.

Diagnosis. Detects cerebral asymmetries, arm plexus paresis.

- Galant reflex (present 0–5 months): Triggered by paravertebral stroking of the skin with wooden spatula. Result: homolateral contraction with simultaneous flexion of the trunk (towards the stimulated side). Diagnosis. Cerebral side differences, congenital scoliosis.

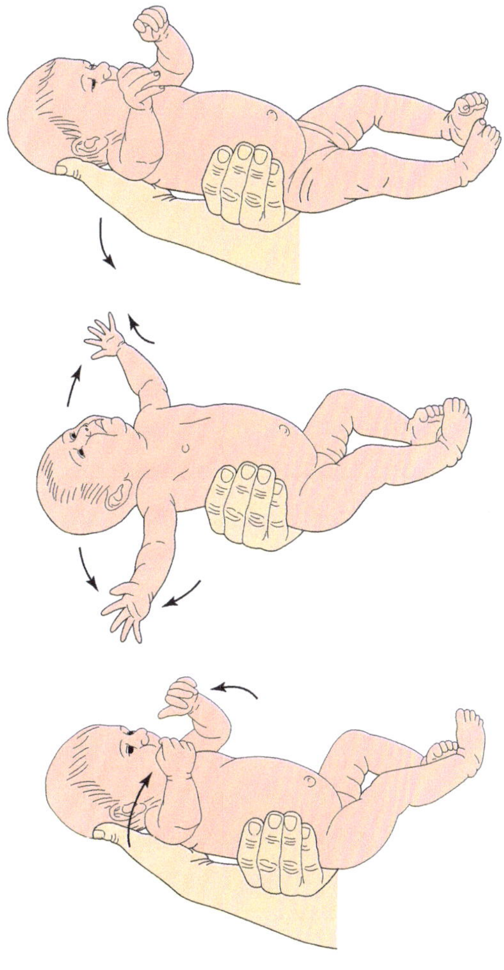

Fig. 13.2: Moro reflex. The head is briefly allowed to fall backwards, the baby responds with a complicated grasping reaction: sudden extension and abduction of the arms followed by flexion and adduction.

- Traction response (Fig. 13.3). Triggered by gently pulling on the hands. Result: light flexion from the elbows, when held in a sitting position the head can be held for 2–3 s. Diagnosis. Evaluation of muscle tone and head control

Practice tip. On examining the abdominal organs (Fig. 13.4), slightly elevating the legs helps to relax the abdominal muscles. At the same time it makes evaluation of the size of liver and spleen and localization of the kidneys easier.

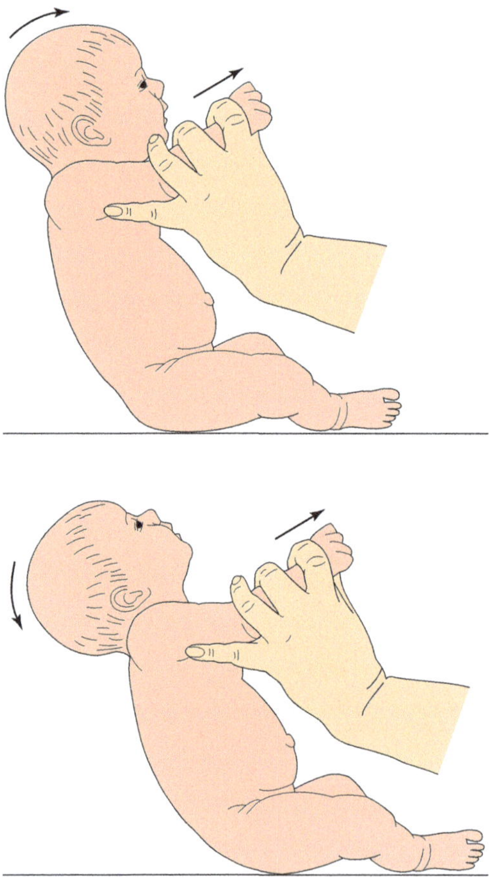

Fig. 13.3: Traction response and head control. Above: the mature, healthy newborn actively performs traction with the upper arm muscles and can hold the head for a few seconds. Below: reaction is absent in preterm newborns and those with hypotonic mobility disorder.

In a newborn, the margin of the liver can protrude below the ribs in the medioclavicular line by 2.5 cm.

13.1.4 Screening program

Note. Goal is the diagnosis of treatable congenital metabolic diseases before irreversible damage has occurred.

Blood is taken on day 3–4 after birth (often after discharge from the hospital) because an adequate intake of nourishment is necessary to trigger metabolic reactions.
If the baby is younger than 72 h on discharge the screening test is performed anyway, to be completed with a follow up test.

Note. Universal screening. Screening at hours of age is recommended for the following disorders (blood test of all newborns): Phenylketonuria (PKU), maple syrup urine disease (MSUD), galactosemia, hypothyreosis, adrenogenital syndrome (AGS), biotinidase deficiency (BIOT), errors of fatty acid metabolism (MCAD, LCAD, VLCAD), Carnitine palmitoyl transferase deficiency types I and II (CPT-I/-II), glutaric aciduria type I (GAT I), isovaleric acidemia (IVA). Effective treatment options and adequate tests are available for these "core disorders". The parents must consent to the screening.

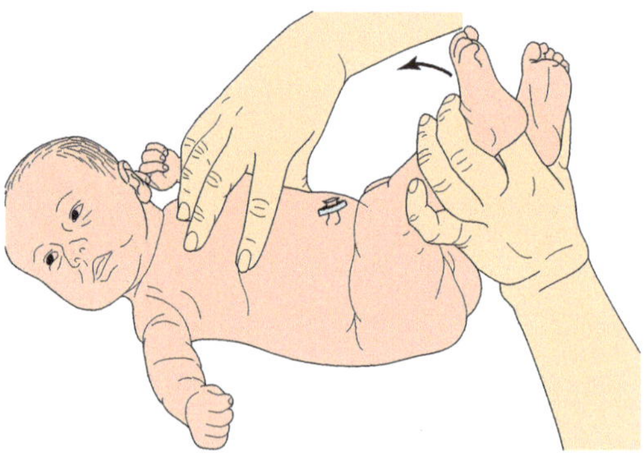

Fig. 13.4: Abdominal palpation: relaxation of the abdominal muscles by elevating the legs. The liver edge is palpated with the fingertip from caudal to cranial.

13.1.5 Other preventative measures

Credé prophylaxis. Preventative treatment against gonoblenorrhea by applying 1% silver nitrate solution (or Erythromycin, no Argentum catarrh) into the conjunctival sac.

Vitamin K deficiency prophylaxis. As breast milk does not contain vitamin K the body's depots are quickly depleted and factors II, VII, IX, and X reduced. Also, in cases of cholestasis, later sufficient vitamin K is not reabsorbed from food. There are two types of vitamin K deficiency hemorrhage:
- Early hemorrhage on day 3–7 after birth as Melaena (bloody stools), cephalhematoma, severe gastrointestinal and intracranial hemorrhages.
- Late hemorrhage, weeks 2–16 after birth, usually brain hemorrhage.

Method:
- High-risk newborns receive 1mg vitamin K s. c. after birth.
- Mature newborns receive 2 mg oral after birth, 2 mg on discharge from the hospital, and 2 mg at week 5.

Vitamin D. The daily application of 500 IU vitamin D in tablet form is recommended for prophylaxis of rickets in northern countries from day 5 to the first birthday. The tablet is to be dissolved and given in a spoonful of water, not placed in the baby's bottle.

Hearing test. An examination of the hearing ability is recommended and should take place in the first week of life, either using otoacoustic emissions (OAE) or brainstem audiometry.

Cardiac defect screening should be performed on day 2 or 3 after birth. Pulse oximetry on the foot, suspected cyanotic cardiac defect if $SO_2 < 95\,\%$, follow up with echocardiography.

Prophylaxis of sudden infant death syndrome (SIDS). Causes of SIDS are unknown. It is probable that different diseases are involved, e.g., conduction disorders (long QT syndrome) and brain stem damage (post asphyxial gliosis). SIDS is rarer in babies who are being or have been breastfed, from a nonsmoking environment, and who do not sleep lying on their belly. Information about these facts helps to make this catastrophe rarer.

13.2 Diet and care

13.2.1 Lactation, breastfeeding, medication in breast milk

Breastfeeding. Most newborns are fed naturally. Advantages of breastfeeding: breast milk is made for its purpose, sterile, warm, easy to obtain and administer, always available, cheap, particularly easily digested, and does not contain allergens. Breastfeeding promotes mother-baby bonding and protects the baby from infections.
Protection against infections is mainly due to secretory IgA, high levels of which are present in colostrum. It passes through the gastrointestinal tract of the baby and protects against enteropathogenic E. coli (EPEC) and intestinal viruses. In addition, protection against infections is promoted by nonspecific immune factors in breast milk (lysozyme, lactoferrin) and cellular components (macrophages, granulocytes, lymphocytes).
The easy digestibility of breast milk is due to:
- The fine coagulation due to the low casein content of milk protein.
- The high lipase content, which participates in intestinal lipolysis.
- The development of Bifidus flora, which prevents E. coli growth.

Lactation consultation should convey confidence and self-assurance; attachment should be practiced with an experienced nurse or midwife. The first feeding can take place shortly after birth, because the baby's sucking reflex is particularly strong at this time and the release of prolactin from the anterior pituitary is stimulated. The best stimulus for milk production is the emptying of the breasts.
The mammary glands do not reach full milk production levels until 7–10 days after birth, however. For the beginning, one breast should be emptied before the baby is moved to the other side.

Breastfeeding technique. The mother is instructed in breastfeeding technique in the labor ward (Fig. 13.5): the baby should be hungry, dry, dressed neither too warm nor too cold, and be held in a comfortable position for each feed. Half to two thirds of the meal is drunk in the first 5 min, after 15 min only very little is drunk. Longer feedings are exhausting for the mother, can cause cracked nipples, and "spoil" the baby.

As the mother can only be separated for brief periods while demand feeding, the resulting stress on some women should not be underestimated.

Breastfeeding volume. Daily weighing in the first week to determine whether enough milk is being produced. Weighing before and after each feeding to determine volume is pointless because the volume fluctuates and it puts the

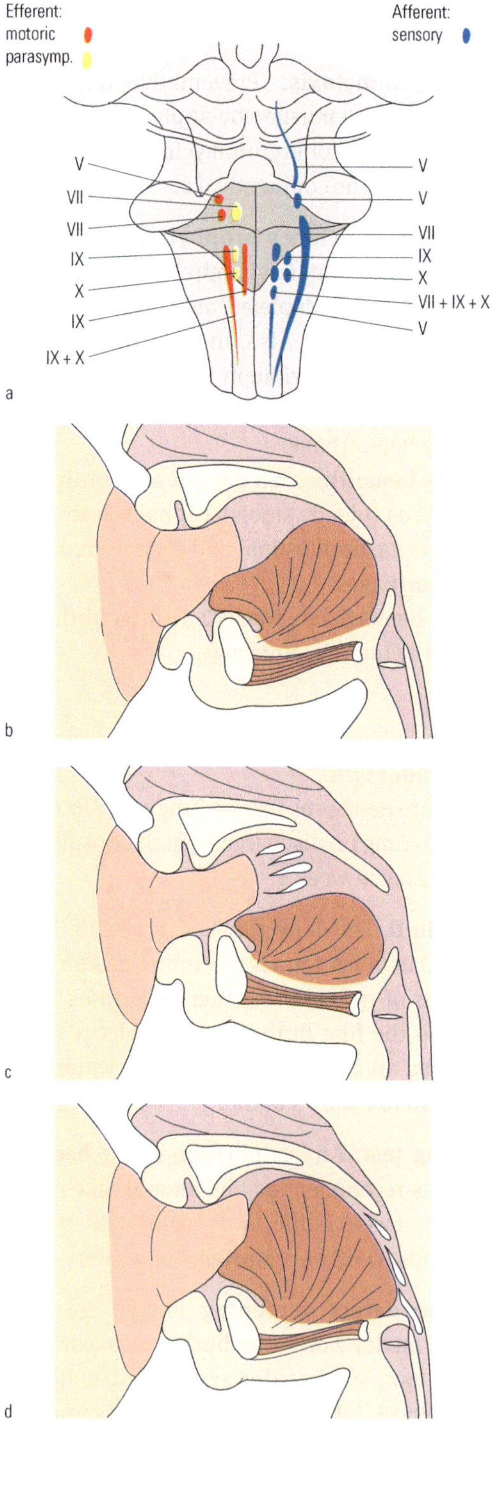

a
b
c
d

Fig. 13.5: The act of sucking. a) sucking and swallowing is controlled by the complicated interplay of a number of brain nerves. b) Areola (not mamilla) is encircled by the baby's mouth (suction pads). c) Pressing upper and lower jaw together forces the milk out of the milk ducts. d) The milk flows over the closed epiglottis into the esophagus. Although trachea (respiratory rate 50/min) and esophagus (swallowing frequency 30/min) cross, the baby doesn't choke.

Tab. 13.1: Components of infant formulae.

	Protein g/dl	Casein content %	Fat g/dl	Lactose g/dl	Other carbo-hydrates g/dl	Ca mg/dl	P mg/dl	Osmolarity mOsm/l	Calories pro 100 ml
Colostrum	2.7		1.9	5.3	–	31	14		54
Mature human milk	1.2	35	3.5	7.0	–	33	15	240	67
Initial formula	1.7	40	3.6	7.5	–	40	32	320	69
Formula for preterm babies	2.0	30	3.4	6.0	2.0	75	46	260	70
Cow's milk	3.3	82	3.5	4.8	–	125	95	380	66

mother under pressure. Weight loss of up to 10 % of the birth weight is normal in the first 10 days. Under no circumstances is cow's milk to be added.

Hypoglycemia is a danger for immature (< 37 weeks), LBW (< 2,500 g), postterm (> 41 weeks), or LGA (> 4,000 g) babies. Regular blood sugar testing is required and the feeding of 5 % dextrose or tea-dextrose solution.

Medication in breast milk. Most medications only pass over into the breast milk in low amounts and are harmless for the newborn. Some medications accumulate in breast milk and are toxic for the newborn. It may be necessary to restrict breastfeeding for a limited period in these cases. If in doubt, a neonatologist should be consulted before lactation is discontinued.

Note. The following medications/narcotics are **dangerous** for the breastfed baby: amphetamines, atropine, chloramphenicol, dicumarol, ergotamine, heroin, indomethacin, iodine, lithium, methadone, phenylbutazone, reserpine, scopolamine, sulfonamides, tetracyclines, thiouracil, cytostatics.

13.2.2 Dietary plan for artificial feeding

Artificial feeding only if breastfeeding is impossible! High quality commercial products which guarantee a reliable nutrient intake are available thanks to the scientifically based introduction of modified cow's milk which made the mechanization of infant formula possible. At the same time, artificial infant formula cannot replace the physiological, immunological and psychosocial benefits of breastfeeding. The baby should only be given artificial formula if breastfeeding is not possible.

Dietary plan (Tab. 13.1, Fig. 13.6). The first feed is given on day 2. The daily milk volume is cal-

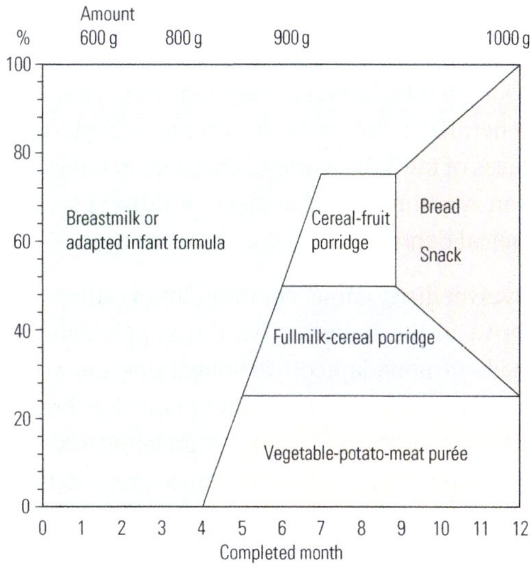

Fig. 13.6: Dietary plan in the first year of life.

culated, the amounts are calculated based on weight and increased.

Practice tip. The daily volume of milk usually reaches 1/6 of the body weight after 8 days.

An exclusive diet of breast milk or industrially produced infant formula is sufficient until the fifth month. From then on, stepwise introduction of vegetable and fruit juices, puréed vegetables with meat, and full milk cereal porridge (diet in first year; Fig. 13.6) to ensure that requirements for iron, vitamins, and roughage are being covered.

13.2.3 Dietary disorders

Exsiccosis, thirst fever. In cases of high weight loss and insufficient fluid intake in the first days of life, dehydration and fever as a result of thirst often occur, particularly in hypotrophic or postterm newborns. It can also develop if there is insufficient fluid intake (infusion) during phototherapy (see p. 456).

Failure to thrive. The most common dietary disorder is absent or insufficient weight gain.

Causes. Inadequate or excessive feeding with poor quality formula, maternal hypogalactia, generalized infection or serious organic diseases of the baby, chronic enteritis, malabsorption syndromes, and neglect, or rather psychological deprivation.

Overfeeding. More common than failure to thrive in the industrial world: supplementary feeds of nonadapted, carbohydrate- and calorie-rich formula in the assumption that breast milk is insufficient. Dietary counseling and the provision of a growth curve can be preventative.

Normal stool. The stool of a breastfed infant is thin, yellowish to orange in color, may contain clumps and often has a water ring.

Gastroenteritis. Acute diarrhea is rare in exclusively breastfed infants, can occur in septic generalized infections or as hospital epidemic (dyspepsia coli, rotavirus); often caused by candidiasis: whitish deposits in the mouth, scaly maculopapulous efflorescences in the perianal region. Sources of infection: inadequately sterilized pacifier or teat, vaginal candidiasis of the mother.

Vomiting. Causes:
- Meconium or bloody amniotic fluid which has been swallowed.
- Duodenal atresia or stenosis.
- Malrotation or intestinal obstruction.
- Sepsis.
- Hiatus hernia.
- Adrenogenital syndrome.
- Pyloric stenosis.

Distended abdomen. Causes:
- Postasphyxia syndrome, perforated bowel.
- Sepsis, peritonitis.
- Meconium ileus.
- Space-occupying mass, e.g., tumor, cyst, ascites, urinary tract obstruction.
- Occlusion ileus, e.g., atresia, stenosis, malrotation, tumor compression, meconium plug syndrome.
- Hirschsprung's disease (congenital aganglionic megacolon).
- Necrotizing enterocolitis (NEC; in preterm babies).

13.2.4 Care of the healthy newborn

The **carer's main tasks** are:
- Nursing and emotional support of the mother on learning how to look after her baby, breastfeeding and rooming in.
- Care and observation of the newborn with the goal of early recognition of anomalies and signs of disease.

Practice tip. The early diagnosis of sepsis is almost always attributable to an observant nurse!

The simpler basic care is, the easier it is for the mothers to learn. New, supposedly modern methods of care are continually suggested, often from a commercial interest and need to be tested before their introduction in order to avoid damaging the baby.

Passage of meconium. The passage of meconium usually occurs in the first hours of life. Meconium consists of bile, pancreas secretion, and desquamated epithelial cells, has a tough or sticky consistency, dark brown to brownish-green color. and is replaced on day 2 or 3 by transition stool.

Passage of urine. Can be expected immediately after birth, sometimes not until 24–36 h p.p.

Diaper change, cleaning is done before feeding. Removal of stool and cleansing of the bottom is done with tissue (cellulose) and oil. Girls are to be cleansed from front to back so that stool is not introduced into the vagina.
Washing is done under running water with a clean washcloth and mild, alkali-free wash lotion.
The first bath is not given until the umbilical cord rest has detached and the navel is completely dry, usually after day 12, before a feeding.
Vaseline without additives (medical or biological) is used as to cream the buttox.

Practice tip. Powder is unnecessary and dangerous in newborn care: talcum aspiration, umbilical granuloma.

- Single-use diapers are used which spread the legs, and which promotes development of the hip joint.
- The skin dries out once the vernix has disappeared and often peels in the first days p.p.
- Red skin, rash. A macular Erythema neonatorum often occurs temporarily. It can become an urticarial or vesicular exanthema in some babies (particularly in icterus and phototherapy).
- The umbilicus is cleaned with a sterile compress or cotton swab and alcohol (70 % or isopropyl). The cord clamp is not removed in the first 24 h. The cord stump should be kept clean and dry; plasters and bandages are unnecessary.
- The eyes are cleaned from outside to inside with running water. A harmless conjunctival catarrh often develops in the first few days of life as a result of the Credé prophylaxis with silver nitrate.
- Sterile swabs and water are best for cleaning the mouth.

13.3 Postnatal adaptation

13.3.1 Physiological adaptation

Note. Adjustments. The separation of the fetal organism from the maternal requires adjustments:
- Respiratory adjustment from placental to pulmonary gas exchange.
- Circulatory adjustment due to opening of the pulmonary circulation.
- Temperature adjustment to self-regulation.
- Dietary adjustment from parenteral to enteral.
- Metabolic adjustment: blood sugar, electrolytes, acid-base household.
- Bacterial colonization and confrontation with microorganisms and environmental toxins.

Respiratory adaptation

First breath. The fetus is born from apnea into a position of expiration. Cold, light, gravity, compression on passage through the birth canal, hypercapnia, acidosis, and hypoxia stimulate the first breath. The inflow of air creates surface tension, retraction force and negative interstitial pressure, lung fluid is reabsorbed, and after 2–3 breaths the residual volume is established. Beginning to breathe air triggers the transition from fetal to adult circulation.

Peculiarities of breathing in the first 24 hours of life (postnatal respiratory adaptation):
- Respiratory rate: 40–50/min.
- Regulation: Carotid body is immature = low pO_2 response.
  ain breathing stimulus at term is pCO_2.
- Morphology: Bronchial branching and alveoli growth 24–40 weeks.
  Capillarization from week 26.
- Surfactant: Lamellar bodies 24 weeks. Phosphatide glycerol 35 weeks.
  surface active film = alveolar stability
- Mechanism: Transpulmonary pressure 80 cm H_2.
  Airway resistance elevated.

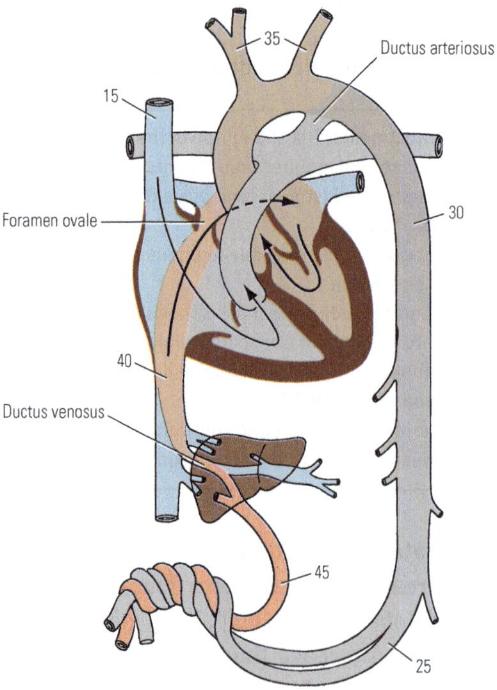

Fig. 13.7: Fetal circulation with partial oxygen pressure (mmHg) in varying vascular regions.

- Ventilation: Normal respiratory minute volume due to high respiratory rate and increased respiration.
- Diffusion: Interstitium 1–0.2 μm.
  Tendency to develop edema.
  Fluid content 40 ml = 60 % of lung weight.
- Perfusion: Foramen ovale closes within minutes, Ductus arteriosus within days.
  Right-left shunt drops from 90 to 20 %.
- Oxygen transport critical, as hematocrit 40–50 % (week 26–40).
  Left shift of the O_2 dissociation curve.

Circulatory adaptation

Pulmonary vascular resistance (PVR) is high before birth: < 1/10 of the cardiac output passes through the lungs, right-to-left shunt to 90 %. The circulatory system reverses at the onset of respiration: pulmonary vascular resistance sinks below the system resistance, the expanded lungs fill with blood which flows out via the pulmonary veins, increases the pressure in the left atrium and thus effects a functional closure of the foramen ovale (Fig. 13.7).
Closure of the ductus arteriosus (DA or ductus Botalli) does not usually occur for a few days due to increased partial oxygen pressure (see Fig. 13.7) and prostaglandin reduction.

Practice tip. Heart rate of a mature neonate: 120–160/min.

Persistent/patent ductus arteriousus (PDA)
Definition. Open ductus arteriosus (DA; fetal connection between the bifurcation of the pulmonal artery and the descending thoracic aorta, right-to-left shunt) with postnatal shunt reversal (left-to-right shunt).

The DA can remain open or reopen, particularly in preterm babies (< 32 weeks) as a result of hypoxia or increased prostaglandin production.

Note. The left-to-right shunt increases pulmonary perfusion, reduces cerebral perfusion and promotes chronic lung transformation.

Clinical presentation

- Varying heart sounds: systolic or continuous murmur.
- Precordial murmur.
- Bounding pulse.
- Respiratory worsening.
- Metabolic acidosis.
- Cardio-, hepatomegaly.

Persistent pulmonary hypertension of the newborn (PPHN)

Definition. Failure of transition of the fetal circulatory system with persistence of the right-to-left shunt as a result of pulmonary hypertension (= elevated blood pressure in the pulmonary circulation) due to PDA or open foramen ovale. Primary pulmonary hypertension is rare, secondary pulmonary hypertension results from spasm, closure or defective development of the pulmonary blood vessels (medial hypertrophy) or pulmonary hypoplasia.

Causes:

- Severe, prolonged hypoxia.
- Meconium aspiration syndrome (MAS; see p. 442).
- Surfactant deficiency (see p. 447).
- Polycythemia (in particular of receiver twin in TTTS).
- Fetal hydrops (see p. 457).
- Severe infections (early form of GBS sepsis, see p. 468).
- Pulmonary hypoplasia.
- Diaphragmatic hernia (see p. 460).

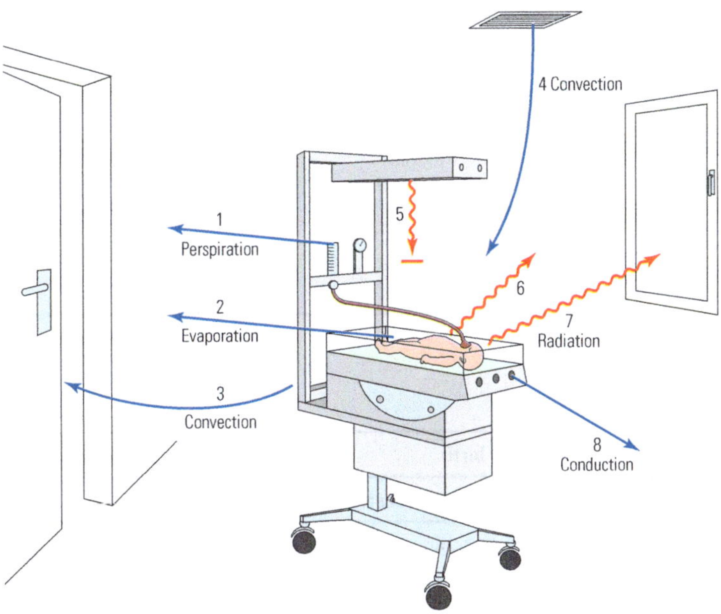

Fig. 13.8: Routes of heat loss and mistakes often leading to undercooling of the baby: 1) breathing gas/O_2 not warmed; 2) baby naked and wet; 3) draught through open door; 4) air conditioning with draught and cool room temperature; 5) radiant heater off; 6) tiled wall; 7) window too close; 8) mattress heater off, conductive mat (rubber).

Consequences. Various trigger mechanisms set a vicious circle in motion in the pulmonary circulation: hypoxemia and increased PVR are maintained.

Thermal adaptation

Postnatal drop in temperature (Fig. 13.8). In unfavorable circumstances the rectal temperature of a term baby drops by 1–2 °C and does not restabilize until 4–8 h postnatally. The danger of hypothermia is particularly high in cases of:
- Low birth weight.
- Pre- and postnatal hypoxia.
- Resuscitation without adequate equipment (e.g., heating device, warm towels).
- Birth in a cold delivery suite.
- Not drying the baby.
- Bathing too early after delivery.
- Maternal medication (e.g., opiates, diazepam, general anesthetic).
- Hypoglycemia.

Practice tip. Initial care takes place in a heated, draught-free room under a radiant infra-red heater.

In addition to postnatal adaptation the risk of cooling is present in:
- Preterm babies.
- Acute infection, particularly sepsis.
- Shock, cardiac insufficiency.
- Hypothyreosis.
- Transport of the baby.

Evaluation of adaptation

Apgar scoring system (Tab. 13.2). Postnatal adaptation and vitality of the term neonate is

Tab. 13.2: Apgar scoring system for evaluation of the neonate.

Apgar score Sign	0	1	2
Color	Blue or white	Acrocyanosis	Pink
Respiratory effort	Absent	Slow, irregular	Unimpaired
Heart rate	Absent	< 100	> 100
Muscle tone	Flaccid	Weak flexion	Active movement
Reflexes on suction	No response	Lowered	Crying

Tab. 13.3: Blood gas analysis: normal values in neonate.

	At birth		At 24 h
	Umbilical vein	**Umbilical artery**	**Arterial blood**
pH	7.32	7.24	7.37
pCO_2 (mmHg)	38	49	33
Standard bicarbonate (mmol/l)	20	19	20
Base excess (mmol/l)	−4	−7	−5
pO_2 (mmHg)	27	16	73

evaluated with the help of the Apgar score (appearance, pulse, grimace, activity, respiration), a scoring system to evaluate newborn condition.

The standardized evaluation is performed after 1, 5, and 10 min (stopwatch!). 7–10 points are normal; 4–6 points indicate a mild depression, < 4 a severely depressed neonate.
The 5 minute score has significant prognostic value: low scores correlate with later disability.

Evaluation of preterm neonates. The Apgar scoring system is of little use as respiratory effort, muscle tone, and reflex irritability are dependent on gestational age.

Practice tip. In our experience, rectal temperature before leaving delivery suite, blood pressure, and BGA of the LBW newborn provide more reliable information about the quality of the initial care and likelihood of survival than the Apgar scoring system.

Perinatal asphyxia. Acute failure of gas exchange in the organs pre- (Fig. 13.9) and postnatal (Fig. 13.10) with hypoxia, hypercapnia and metabolic acidosis.

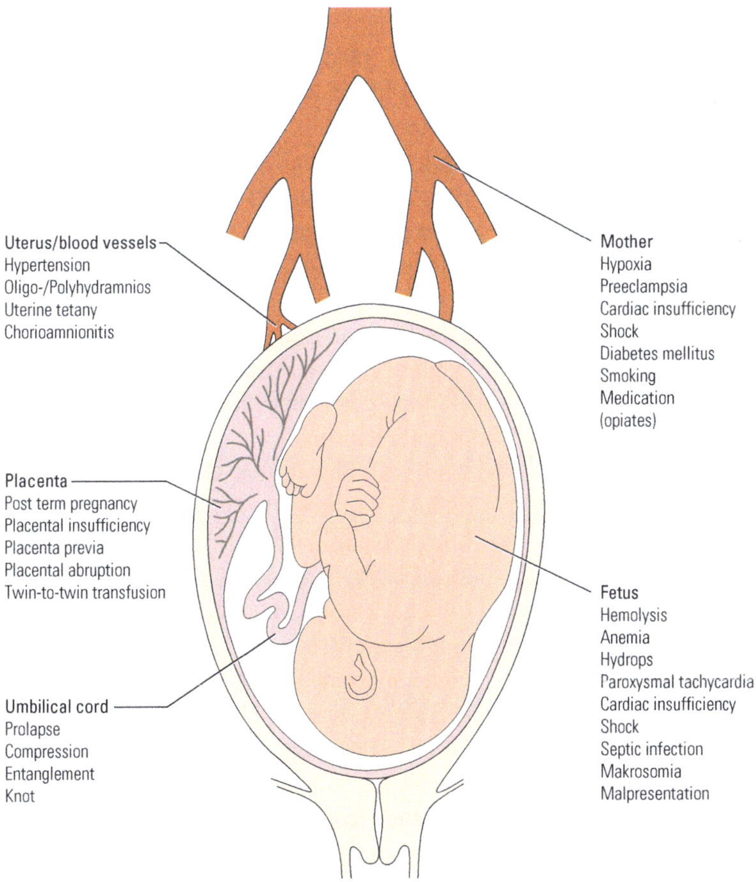

Fig. 13.9: Fetal blood supply and prenatal (circulatory) causes of asphyxia.

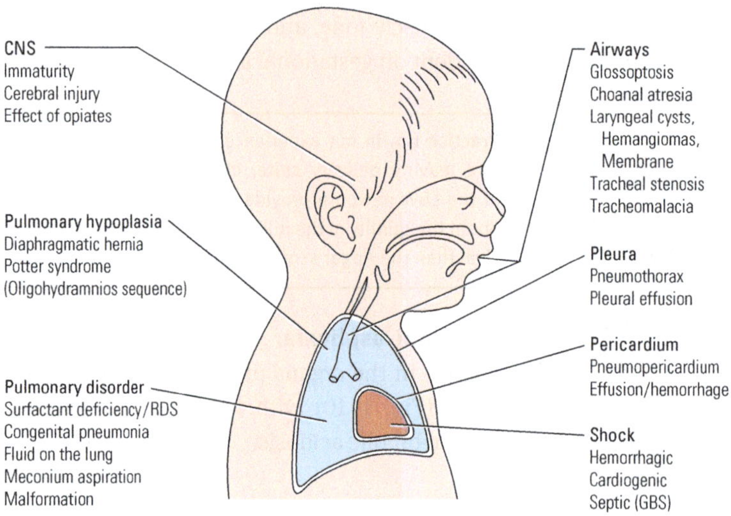

Fig. 13.10: Airways of the newborn and postnatal (respiratory) causes of asphyxia.

Hypoxemia. Reduced PaO_2. pO_2 of the fetal umbilical vein is 45, of the descending aorta 25 mmHg.

Hypoxia. Oxygen deficiency in the tissues, dependent on oxygen saturation, Hb concentration and perfusion; persistent hypoxia is associated with base deficit via increase in lactate.

Acidosis. Blood-gas analysis (BGA; Tab. 13.3) allows an objective evaluation of vitality.

Practice tip. Umbilical artery values of 7.20–7.38 are normal. A pH < 7.20 signifies mild acidosis, < 7.10 moderate, and below 7.0 severe acidosis. A pH of < 7.10 from the well-vascularized heel 15–30 min after birth signifies a severe acidosis.

Blood pressure. Measurement is possible in every labor ward. It enables recognition and treatment of blood flow centralization.

13.3.2 Pathological adaptation

Birth asphyxia

Hypoxia or ischemia and organ damage are threatened in cases of maternal hypotension, respiratory placental insufficiency, impaired umbilical blood flow, or insufficient newborn respiratory effort.

- Lungs. Meconium aspiration, PPHN with right-to-left shunt, RDS of the preterm baby, shock lung with secondary surfactant deficiency, pulmonary edema, pulmonary hemorrhage.
- CNS. Hypoxic-ischemic encephalopathy, cerebral edema, seizures. Increased risk of intra-/periventricular hemorrhage in preterm babies.
- Cardiovascular system. Cardiogenic shock, reduced contractility due to glycogen depletion, and papillary muscle necroses.
- Kidneys. Pre-/intrarenal kidney failure, tubular necrosis, renal vein thrombosis, inadequately increased secretion of antidiuretic hormone (ADH).
- GI tract. Mesenteric hypoperfusion, NEC, bowel perforation, liver necrosis.
- Metabolism. Lactate acidosis, hypocalcemia, hyponatremia, hyper- or hypoglycemia, impaired temperature regulation.
- Coagulation. DIC, hemorrhages.

The pattern of injury after asphyxia is dependent on extent and duration, whether ischemia or hypoxia is in the foreground and on maturity.

Resuscitation of term and preterm infants

Resuscitation means reviving; goal: maintenance of elemental vital functions and with that, cerebral and myocardial supplies of oxygen.

Success is determined by resuscitation team experience and preparation in the labor ward prior to birth. In cases of known risk factor/s (Figs. 13.9, 13.10), there is usually time before birth to summon a resuscitation team (a pediatrician with neonatal experience and a pediatric nurse with intensive care training) or to transfer the pregnant woman to the appropriate hospital.

Equipment (functioning must be checked daily):

- Resuscitation table with radiant heater and light source.
- Vacuum pump (suction 200 mbar), suction catheters sizes 6, 8.
- Blood pressure monitor with cuffs 1–4.
- Pulse oximeter, ECG monitor, BGA device.
- Warmed sterile towels.
- Oxygen source with flowmeter, humidifier and - line, conduction?
- Neonatal bag with PEEP valve and masks of various sizes, spare battery.
- Laryngoscope and Magill's forceps for infants.
- Neonatal endotracheal tubes 2.5, 3.0, 3.5 and connectors.
- Disposable suction device with fluid collector, size 8.
- Stopwatch.
- Disposable scalpel, cord clamps, pleural catheter size 8, suture, instruments for umbilical catheterization.

Medication

- Dextrose 5 % and 10 %.
- Sodium bicarbonate 8.4 %.
- Vitamin K_1 (phytomenadione) 1 mg.
- Adrenaline (epinephrine) 1 : 10,000.
- Possibly an emergency bag of 0 Rh positive blood (refrigerator).

Resuscitation of the mildly depressed preterm and term infant. Those with experience usually manage with little intervention (see below).

In preterm babies < 30 weeks, the filling of the lungs should be supported by brief mask ventilation (Fig. 13.11; auscultation), but we try to avoid primary intubation and ventilation. Only ventilation bags with a safety valve should be used because of the danger of pneumothorax as a result of excessive peak pressure. Nasotracheal intubation should only be performed if respiratory insufficiency persists for longer than 1 min or a long transport to the pediatric clinic is planned.

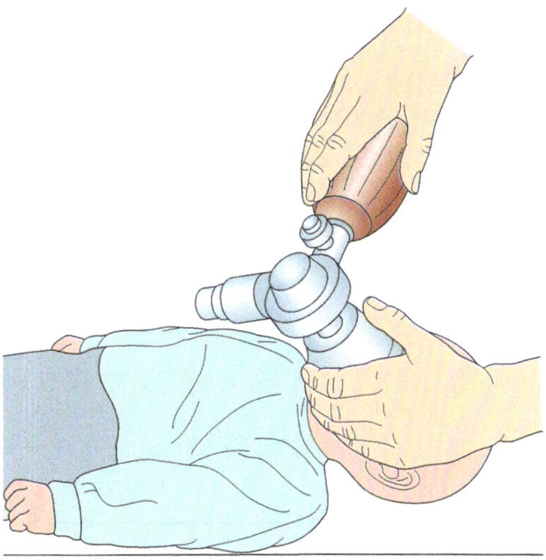

Fig. 13.11: Ventilation with mask and bag. The left hand presses the soft mask firmly over mouth and nose, the little finger pushes the lower jaw forwards (Esmarch's maneuver). Avoid pressure to the occiput!.

Resuscitation of the preterm baby and moderately depressed newborn (Apgar 4–6)
- Anticipate problems (EDD, exact history).
- Be present early.
- Remain calm and focused.
- Check equipment. Heater, towels, oxygen, bag and mask, stethoscope, vacuum pump, suction catheter, laryngoscope, Magill's forceps, tubes.
- Keep warm. Heater, drying, towels.
- Free airways. Suction pharynx and nose.
- Auscultation. Heart sounds on the left? Ventilation?
- Ventilation. Initially only with mask and bag.
- Vitamin K injection, 1mg s.c.

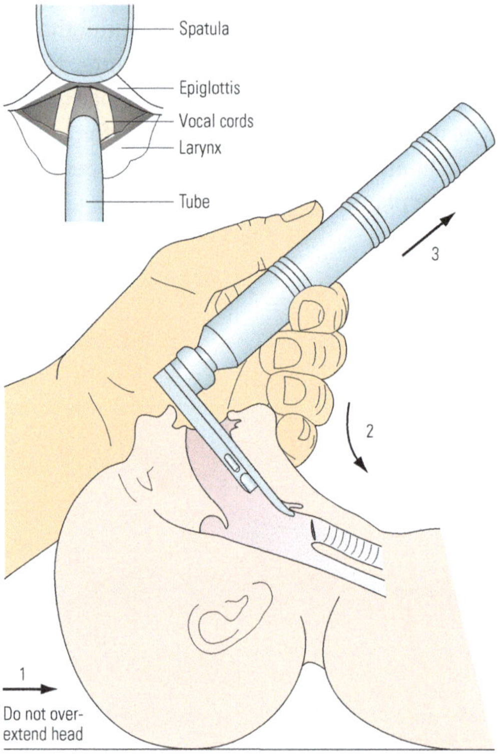

Fig. 13.12: Laryngoscope, positioning and insertion (1–3). Esmarch's maneuver and view in endotracheal intubation. The laryngoscope is held in the left hand, the epiglottis held with the spatula so that the laryngeal inlet is visible.

Further measures (if the baby does not recover)
- Endotracheal intubation (Fig. 13.12), nasotracheal tube 2.5–3.5 mm.
- Adrenaline 0.01–0.03 mg/kg endotracheal.
- Umbilical vein catheter in cases of shock (CVP).
- Volume replacement: serum replacement/ emergency blood.
- Buffering if metabolic acidosis persists.

Reanimation of the severely depressed newborn. Severe depression (Apgar 0–3) has become very rare with modern methods of labor monitoring. It occurs as secondary (terminal) apnea after prolonged hypoxia (e.g., cord prolapse) or in cases of severe hemorrhagic shock (e.g., hemorrhage from velamentous insertion). In addition to respiratory insufficiency, it is always accompanied by severe metabolic acidosis (umbilical artery pH < 7.0) and circulatory shock. In this situation the respiratory resuscitation described is not sufficient to stabilize the baby and further measures are necessary:

Placement of an umbilical vein catheter (once intubated and ventilation has begun), as in severe circulatory shock if peripheral veins are not accessible for cannulation.
Emergency blood transfusion. In hemorrhagic shock, lysine-free 0 Rh negative blood (as universal donor blood) can be transfused without cross-matching.
Catecholamines, cardiac massage, blind buffering: if cardiac effort is absent or bradycardia < 50/min 0.1–0.3 ml/kg adrenaline (epinephrine) 1 : 10,000 is administered via the endotracheal tube.

Resuscitation in severe depression (Apgar 0–3)
- Anticipate problems, e.g., cord prolapse, emergency cesarean section if bleeding ex utero occurs.
- Be present early.

- Remain calm and focused, check equipment, prepare umbilical vein catheterization and blood pressure monitoring, have emergency blood available, and warmed if necessary.
- Dry and keep the baby warm (additional heat source).
- Free airways (suction pharynx and nose).
- Immediate nasotracheal intubation.
- Oxygen ventilation is used less frequently. New studies show higher survival rates in resuscitation with air. Many newborns only have pre-ductal $SO_2 > 95\,\%$ after 10 min.
- Cardiac massage if heart rate < 50/min (Fig. 13.13)
- Endotracheal epinephrine: 0.01–0.03 mg/kg.
- Insert umbilical vein catheter (size 8) 8–10 cm deep (Fig. 13.14), measure central venous pressure (CVP).
- Intravenous (slow) $NaHCO_3$ 3 mmol/kg diluted 1 : 1 with 5 % glucose.
- Volume replacement (serum/emergency blood) till CVP positive.
- Vitamin K injection 1mg s.c.
- BGA and further treatment as required.

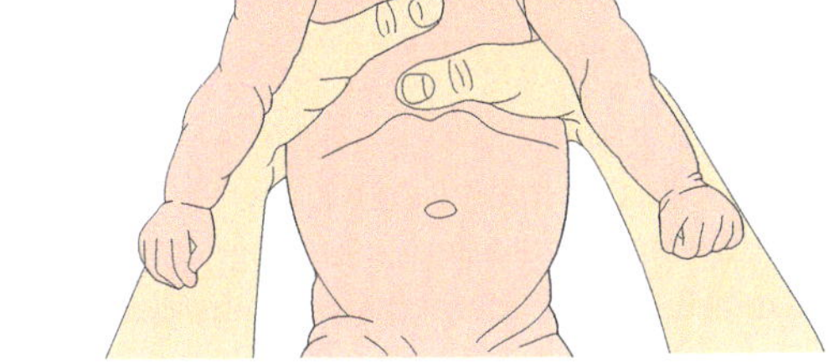

Fig. 13.13: External cardiac massage. After 4–5 compressions, one ventilation of 100 % O_2 is given.

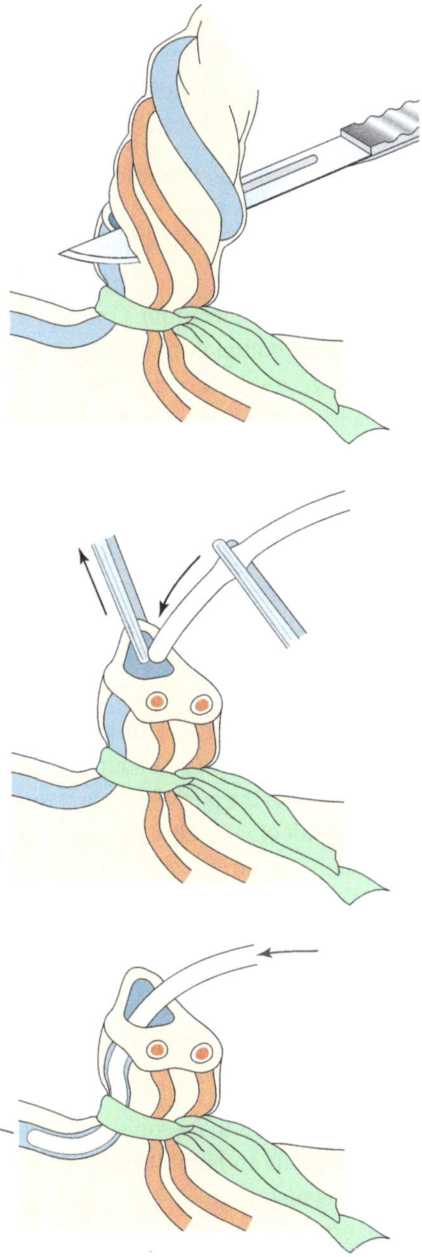

Fig. 13.14: Umbilical vein catheter. After cutting the cord the blood vessels become visible. The umbilical vein is the largest of the three vessels, is usually cranial, and is thin walled and not contracted. Catheterization is easier if the cord stump is pulled caudally with tweezers.

Meconium aspiration syndrome (MAS)

Definition. Respiratory insufficiency of the newborn (RDS, respiratory distress syndrome) as a result of meconium aspiration.

Pathogenesis. Cause is intrauterine hypoxia, often in hypotrophic term or postterm newborns, which results in mesenteric ischemia and hyperperistalsis of the intestines, inducing early passage of meconium. Consequences: aspiration of meconium intrauterine or directly postnatal with respiratory insufficiency due to bronchial obstruction. Impaired diffusion, atelectasis, emphysemous areas (gas overdistension), interstitial emphysema, hypoxia or chemical-toxic pneumonia with atelectasis and intrapulmonary shunts with hypoxia.

Practice tip. The passage of meconium-stained amniotic fluid is always an alarm signal.

To be expected in 10 % of all births. It is dangerous if it is thick green or pea soup-like and is aspirated deep into the airways on first inspiration or as a result of resuscitation.
Warning signs of intrauterine hypoxia with threatened MAS are:
- Heart rate decelerations.
- Absent variability.
- Prolonged, complicated labor.
- Passage of meconium-stained AF.

Clinical presentation
- The skin is covered in meconium at birth.
- Skin, fingernails and umbilical cord are stained greenish-yellow.
- Severe respiratory depression with gasping respiration, loud rattling noises
- Bradycardia, hypotension, shock symptoms.
- Tachypnea, dyspnea, intercostal retraction, expiratory moaning and cyanosis.

Complications. Pneumothorax and pneumomediastinum, persistent pulmonary hypertension (see p. 434), threat of bacterial superinfection!

Treatment
- Prompt expedition of delivery if fetal hypoxia persists!
- No primary mask ventilation if MAS is suspected!
- As much meconium as possible is to be removed from the upper airways after birth of the head and before the first in-breath. The efforts of obstetrician and neonatology team must be coordinated to this end.
- The baby should not be stimulated to breathe initially, but suctioned with a broad endotracheal catheter.

Hypoxic ischemic encephalopathy (HIE)

Definition. General term for central nervous system consequences of birth asphyxia.

Clinical manifestation. One third of mature newborns who experienced severe birth asphyxia develop hypoxic ischemic encephalopathy on day 1 after birth.

HIE is classified in three grades of clinical severity (Sarnat staging system):
- Grade I (mild). Irritability, nervousness, mild hypotonia, poor feeding.
- Grade II (moderate). Lethargy, seizures (beginning 12–24h), marked hypotonia, assisted feeding.
- Grade III (severe). Coma, prolonged seizures, severe hypotonia, spontaneous respiration often absent.

Grade I is usually rapidly reversible, grade III often leads to cerebral injury later, which–depending on the location–can range from mental retardation, hyperactivity syndrome, spastic tetraparesis and choreoarthrosis to epilepsy and intellectual impairment.

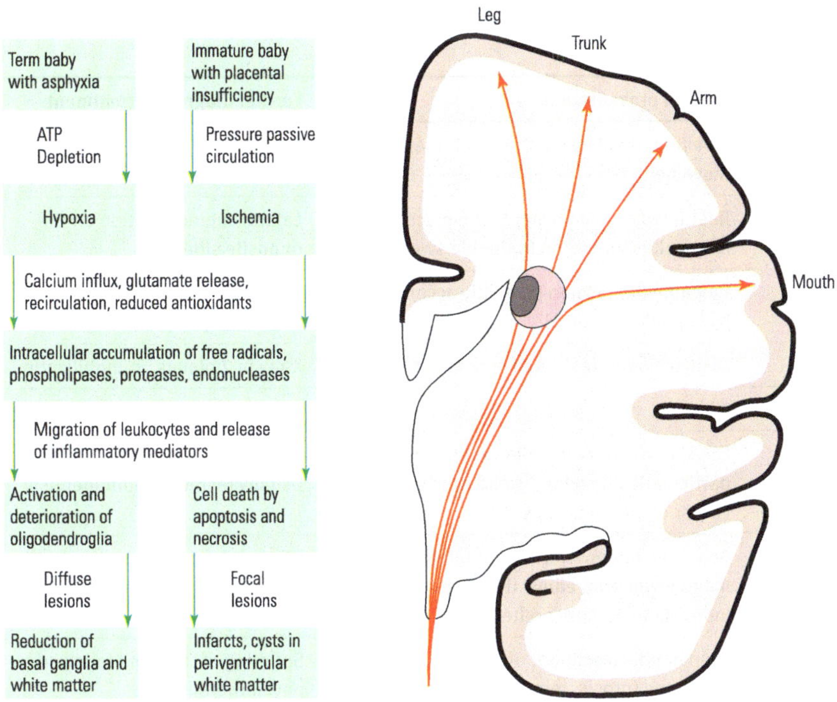

Fig. 13.15: Pathogenesis of hypoxic ischemic brain damage and typical localization of cystic periventricular leukomalacia.

Characteristic. (Cystic) periventricular leukomalacia (PVL) is a specific form in preterm infants as a result of reduced cerebral perfusion (ischemia) with periventricular necroses of white matter, sometimes with white matter lesions. Hypoxia plays a minor role here, inflammatory processes (chorioamnionitis) a large role.

The result is cerebral paresis, whereby spastic diplegia is more common than tetraplegia, as the neural pathways leading to the legs are closer to the ventricle and therefore already affected by smaller lesions (Fig. 13.15).

Pathophysiology. Hyperventilation (absent autoregulation) with ischemia, as cerebral perfusion is greatly restricted when pCO_2 is low; bacterial infection (PROM), in which toxic mediators are released.

Clinical presentation. Hypotension, hyperventilation.

Treatment

- Acute: adequate (not excessive) oxygenation, optimal ventilation and organ perfusion (caution: reperfusion injury) and maintenance of thermoneutral temperature (caution: fever).
- Neuroprotective treatment approach, e.g., systemic hypothermia over 3 days, is possible in specialized centers and can reduce the extent of brain damage.

13.4 Birth trauma

Table 13.4 lists the most common perinatal injuries.

Tab. 13.4: Common perinatal traumas with clinical presentation, diagnosis and treatment.

Type of trauma	Clinical presentation	Further diagnosis, treatment
Fracture	Swelling, displacement, hematoma, restricted movement	Immobilization
Clavicle fracture	Restricted arm movement if displaced. Step, later callus formation (palpable swelling)	Lateral supine position on the opposite side
Skull fracture	Palpable depression (possibly accompanied by cephalhematoma)	Exclude intracranial hemorrhage! Surgical repair of the depression
Fracture of long bones	Displacement, restricted movement	X-ray in 2 planes, immobilization
Nerve lesion		
Facial palsy	Facial asymmetry in unilateral paralysis, particularly on crying, eyelid does not close, corner of mouth droops	Regular moistening of the cornea. Usually resolves spontaneously
Brachial plexus paralysis: 1. Upper plexus paralysis (C5–C6) genetic Duchenne palsy	Adducted upper arm, inward rotation, pronated lower arm, elbow flexion not possible. Intact hand grasping reflex	DD: epiphyseal separation of the humerus, x-ray diagnosis. Physiotherapy to prevent contraction
2. Lower plexus paralysis (C7–T1) Klumpke palsy	Drop hand, claw hand, often also Horner's syndrome (ptosis, miosis, enophthalmos)	Splinting of the hand followed by physiotherapy
Spinal cord injury	Paralysis, depending on the height of the injury, paraplegia possible	Positioning; CT, MRI, surgery
Hemorrhage		
Sternocleidomastoid hematoma	Hematoma, firm mass, torticollis (crooked neck), restricted movement	Intensive physiotherapy
Caput succedaneum	Bloody-serous edema of skin and loose cell tissue of the leading part in labor → doughy edematous, bluish congested swelling, usually occipito-parietal, crossing sutures	No treatment required
Cephalhematoma	Hematoma between periosteum and bone, subperiosteal hematoma. Swelling does not cross the sutures	Spontaneous resolution in weeks to months. Resorption. Calcification possible
Intracranial hemorrhage		p. 446

Facial nerve paralysis

Usually caused by mechanical compression or edema, less commonly resulting from injury in forceps delivery.

Clinical manifestation. Only the healthy side of the mouth moves when the baby cries.

Treatment. None.

Prognosis. Good, usually resolves spontaneously.

Brachial plexus paralysis

Lesion of the brachial plexus (plexus cervicobrachialis), e.g., as a result of overstretching from breech presentation or shoulder dystocia.

Types: upper (genetic Duchenne palsy; segments C5–6), lower (Klumpke paralysis; segments C7–T1) brachial plexus paralysis.

Clinical presentation

- Adducted, medially rotated arm, pronation (Fig. 13.16).
- Parts of the Moro reflex are absent and indicate the height of the lesion.

Clavicule fracture

Fracture of the clavicle during birth.

Clinical presentation

- Swelling or irregular shape, crepitation on pressure, relief posture, sometimes cracking is audible or palpable.
- Asymmetric Moro reflex.
- Pain on passive movement of the arm.

Treatment. None.

Prognosis. Heals spontaneously, often not discovered until callus formation on day 7–10 on the x-ray image.

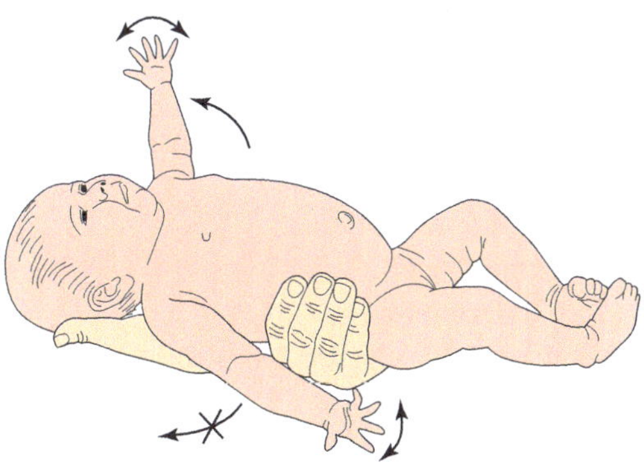

Fig. 13.16: Upper (Erb–Duchenne palsy) brachial plexus paralysis. The baby is depicted during the Moro reflex (see Fig. 13.2). The right arm cannot be raised and bent. The fanning of the fingers indicates functioning of the lower parts of the brachial plexus.

Humerus fracture

Occurs during arm extraction and is usually noticed immediately by the obstetrician.

Clinical presentation. Upper arm swelling, relief posture, occasionally bent.

Diagnosis is confirmed by x-ray.

Treatment. Immobilization of the arm (on the thorax) for three weeks.

Cephalhematoma

Hematoma between periosteum and skull bones, subperiosteal hematoma.

Cause. Torn blood vessels between periosteum and bone on passage of the head during birth due to friction between soft tissues and flat skull bones, usually after vacuum extraction or forceps delivery, occasionally occurs spontaneously.

Clinical presentation

- Markedly fluctuating, grape- to hen's egg-sized hemispheric swelling on the skull.
- Sutures are not crossed (as opposed to caput).
- Can occur bilaterally, over both parietal bones.

Treatment. Never puncture! Heals spontaneously within 3–6 weeks from the edge inwards. Large hematomas can be accompanied by anemia which requires treatment or by a severe resorption icterus.

Congestion hematomas

Cause. Umbilical cord wrapped tightly around the neck or presenting part.

Clinical presentation. Punctiform, partially confluent hemorrhages, also in the conjunctiva.

Treatment. None.

Prognosis. Spontaneous healing, usually harmless, occasionally reabsorption icterus.

Sternocleidomastoid hematoma
Torticollis, wryneck. Fixed lateral tilt to the head with a slight rotation to the opposite side.

Cause. Common after breech presentation.

Clinical presentation. A pea-sized thickening of the muscle is usually palpated on day 2 or 3, which becomes a cord-like fibrosis after a few days due to connective tissue organization of the birth hematoma.

Prognosis. Risk of scarring and contraction which leads to muscular shortening (torticollis).

Intracranial hemorrhage
Definition. Hemorrhage within the bony skull. The most common in premature babies are periventricular and intraventricular hemorrhages (PVH, IVH).

Four stages. 1) Subependymal hemorrhage. Common and harmless, no ventricular involvement. 2) Intraventricular hemorrhage: hemorrhage from the subependymal layer (germinal matrix) into the lateral ventricles. Spontaneous reabsorption usually occurs. Prognosis is also good here. 3) Ventricle tamponade: posthemorrhagic hydrocephalus can develop. 4) Intraparenchymal hemorrhage: more or less extensive sections of the brain and pathways are destroyed, so that permanent damage is to be expected.

13.5 The preterm baby

Definition. The gestational age of term newborns ranges from 37–41 weeks (259–293 days, calculated from the first day of the LMP). Preterm infants are babies born before completion of 37 weeks (gestational age < 259 days).

The following definitions apply regardless of gestational age:
- Low birth weight (LBW) infants. Birth weight < 2,500 g; 5–15 % of live births, however > 70 % of infant deaths in the neonatal period (1–28 days of life).
- Very low birth weight infants (VLBW). Birth weight < 1,500 g, 0.8–1.5 % of live births, however > 50 % of infant deaths in the neonatal period.
- Extremely low birth weight infants. Birth weight < 1,000 g; 0.4–0.6 % of live births, > 40 % of infant deaths in the neonatal period.

Incidence. 5–7 % of all neonates are preterm babies.

13.5.1 Gestational age

Signs of maturity. Assessment of maturity provides information about physical characteristics and functions and whether the baby is preterm (immature); made by quantitatively determining gestational age based on physical or neurological criteria using a scoring system with an accuracy of 2 weeks:
- Skin transparency.
- Ear cartilage (pinna; complete cartilage, shape of ear).
- Plantar surface creasing.
- Mammary gland diameter.
- Nipple differentiation.
- Fingernail length.
- Hair differentiation.
- Genitals (labia closure, testes descended).

13.5.2 Complications

Immaturity in preterm infants is accompanied by adaptational impairments, which must be taken into consideration on care and treatment:

- Thermoregulation: hypothermia, hypoxia, acidosis.
- Respiration: surfactant deficiency, RDS, asphyxia, apnea.
- Circulatory system: shock, right-to-left shunt, hypoxia, intracranial hemorrhage, necrotizing enterocolitis.
- Diet: catabolism, aspiration, subileus.
- Metabolism: hypoglycemia, hypocalcemia, hypoproteinemia, icterus, anemia.
- Excretion: edema, electrolyte imbalances.
- Immunity: pneumonia, sepsis, meningitis.

Note.
Preterm infants < 35 weeks should be transferred to special care wards (before manifestation of symptoms).
Preterm infants < 32 weeks: birth in perinatal center necessary.
Preterm infants < 30 weeks: initial care to be provided by neonatologist.

Initial care of the preterm infant

Phase 1. Preparation
- Telephone call: risk factors? CS: schedule.
- Prepare intensive care space: calibrate transoxode, incubator 35°, warm x-ray cassette.

Phase 2. Labor ward
- Warm resuscitation table, close doors, have warm towels ready.
- O_2 6–8l/min; suction: max up to 0.25 bar.
- Check ventilation bag and intubation instruments.

First minute
- Wrap the baby in a towel, suction pharynx and nose.
- Auscultate: heart sounds on the right?
- Mask ventilation to unfold the lungs, stethoscope: check ventilation.
- Bag-valve: 45 cm H_2O! Attach pulse oximeter.
- Do not unwrap towel!

Second to fifth minutes
- Either after a few minutes or before intubation: suction stomach (size 8 or 10) and measure contents.
- If mask ventilation does not result in stabilization or independent respiration: nasotracheal intubation.
- Blood sugar check, blood gases.
- Measure blood pressure: if systolic < 40 mmHg 5 % plasma 3 ml/kg slowly i.v., dextrose infusion 7.5–10 %.
- Viamin K 1mg s.c., cut the cord (long; swab!).
- Rectal temperature measurement, if necessary wrap in a new towel.
- Antibiotics if indicated; then bring forward blood sampling!
- Credé prophylaxis.

On arrival in the neonatal ward
- Baby is still in the original towel or incubator: measure temperature, blood gases, blood sugar, hematocrit, blood pressure.
- If necessary begin a ventilation protocol. Check incubator temperature.
- Weigh in towels under heat source.

13.5.3 Diseases of preterm babies

Reduced enzyme activity, bacterial colonization, inadequate immune defenses and the influx of oxygen radicals due to the premature transition from placental to pulmonary respiration all contribute to the pathogenesis of diseases of preterm babies. The incidence increases with decreasing gestational age. The most common diseases are subsequently discussed.

Surfactant deficiency (Respiratory Distress Syndrome; RDS)

Definition. Respiratory distress syndrome of the preterm baby due to surfactant deficiency, acute pulmonary disease within the first hours of life.

Pathogenesis. The main cause is the deficiency of pulmonary surface active system (surfactant), which is composed of phospholipids (lecithin, phosphatidylglycerol; PC) and proteins (hydrophilic surfactant protein A; SP-A, and hydrophobic surfactant proteins B and C; SP-B and C). The increased surface tension on the air-water interface causes an expiratory alveolar collapse after birth, atelectasis and right-to-left shunt. Hyaline membranes form due to plasma influx in the alveoli. Hypoxia, acidosis and right-to-left shunt create a vicious circle (Fig. 13.17).

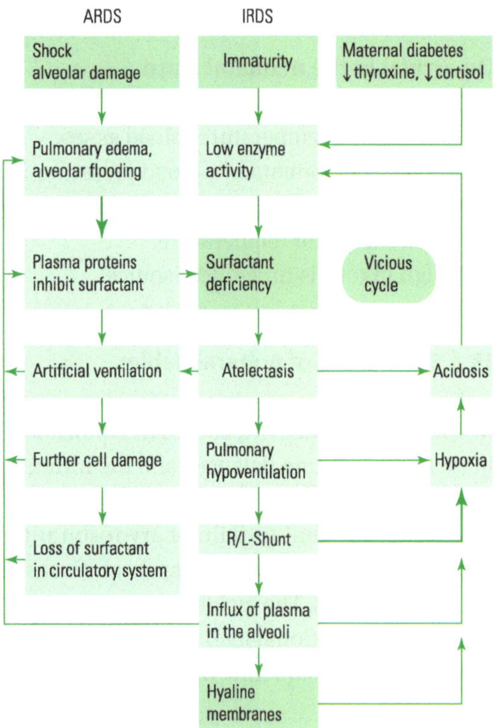

Fig. 13.17: Respiratory distress syndrome. Pathogenesis and factors which can influence its course. Left adult (ARDS), right immature (IRDS) pathogenic route, both of which occur in newborns (R/L shunt = right-to-left shunt).

Clinical presentation. Symptoms immediately after birth or within the first six hours of life.
- Tachypnea, dyspnea: sternal and intercostal retraction, nasal flaring, moaning on in- and expiration (grunting).
- Weakened respiratory sounds, greyish pallor and cyanosis.

Diagnosis
- Prenatal. Detection of surfactant metabolites in amniotic fluid (not routine): L/S ratio (lecithin/sphingomyelin) >2 : 1 indicates adequate pulmonary maturity.
- Postnatal. Clinical presentation, BGA and radiology. Chest x-ray (primary diagnosis): thick, finely granulated image (microatelectasis), if necessary air bronchogram.

Treatment. Warmth, application of surfactant, continuous positive airways pressure (CPAP).

Prevention. In cases of threatened preterm delivery induced pulmonary maturity by administration of glucocorticoids to the mother in order to stimulate fetal surfactant synthesis.

Persistent/patent ductus arteriosus (PDA)

Definition. In the term newborn the ductus arteriosus closes due to reduced prostaglandin E_2 production as a result of the postnatal increase in partial oxygen pressure. This mechanism can be impaired in preterm babies with RDS or other pulmonary diseases. The ductus remains patent or reopens whereby a left-to-right shunt is created, with pulmonary flooding, retrograde diastolic flow in the systemic circulation (reduced perfusion of mesenteric and cerebral blood vessels), cardiac insufficiency and pulmonary edema.

Complications. Chronic pulmonary disease, necrotizing enterocolitis, periventricular leukomalacia.

Bronchopulmonary dysplasia (BPD)

Definition. Chronic lung disease of the preterm infant with interstitial edema and fibrosis, atelectasis, hyperinflated basal lung sections and pulmonary hypertension (Cor pulmonale).

Pathogenesis. Two types:
- Classical form, caused by organ immaturity, barotrauma (ventilation) and oxygen toxicity (free radicals).
- "New" form, inflammatory mediators (interleukins) in primary pulmonary infection (e.g., ureaplasma, mycoplasma) play the main role here.

Clinical presentation
- Dyspnea (retraction, nasal flaring).
- Prolonged O_2 dependence, persistent hypercapnia, hypercrinia, recurrent bronchospasms.
- Right heart overload.
- Recurrent bronchopulmonary infections.

Diagnosis
- Clinical course (underlying pulmonary disease, duration of ventilation, persistent pulmonary insufficiency with severe obstruction).
- Chest x-ray. Hyperinflated areas next to atelectatic areas. Streaky marking, fibrotic thickening, cardiomegaly (particularly right cardiac enlargement).

Prevention. BPD has different, partly iatrogenic causes, the prevention, or rather avoidance, of which has priority. Gentle ventilation avoiding high peak pressures, early and strict withdrawal from the respirator (accepting the consequence of hypercapnia), avoidance or prevention of premature closure of a hemodynamically effective PDA.

Apnea of prematurity (AOP)

Definition. Brief (> 20 sec) and recurring episodes of stopped breathing. Complex disturbance of breathing regulation while sleeping.

Pathogenesis. Periodic breathing (Cheyne-Stokes) is physiological in premature babies < 35 weeks and due to the immaturity of the breathing center. pCO_2 is the main respiratory stimulus of the chemoreceptors. Premature babies donot often react to reduced oxygen tension with increased respiratory effort. Apneas > 20 s are often accompanied by bradycardia. It is possible to differentiate between central and obstructive apnea, but it has little practical consequence.

Apneas are more common and severe in preterm babies with intracranial hemorrhages, infection, anemia, PDA, gastroesophageal reflux (GER).

Retinopathy of prematurity (ROP)

Definition. Vasoproliferative retinopathy which causes scarring of the retina and blindness.

Synonyms: retrolental fibroplasia, retinopathia praematurorum.

Incidence. Indirectly proportionate to gestational age.

Pathogenesis. Immaturity (avascular retina) and the toxic effects of oxygen on the developing retinal blood vessels as a result of increased or disturbed expression of vascular endothelial growth factor (VEGF). Risk factors: multiples, hypercapnia, blood exchange transfusions, numerous transfusions.

Prevention
- Continuous transcutaneous paO_2 monitoring. Arterial control measurements.
- Timely examination of the ocular fundus by the ophthalmologist.

Intracranial hemorrhage

Incidence. Less common, as management of labor has become gentler, and postnatal transport is avoided.

Hypercapnia, and thus increased blood flow in the arterioles of the subependymal germinal matrix, result from dyspnea of premature babies. Ruptured vessels are then possible. Stages of intracranial hemorrhage: see p. 446.
Risk factors for intracranial hemorrhage of prematurity:
- Asphyxia.
- Birth trauma.
- Bicarbonate administration.
- Fluctuating blood pressure.
- Postnatal transport.
- Pneumothorax.

Necrotizing enterocolitis (NEC)

Definition. Hemorrhagic-necrotizing, ulcerating inflammation, usually multifocal, of the small and large intestines.

Pathogenesis. Causes are immaturity of the bowels, early enteral nutrition, mesenteric hypoperfusion from hypovolemia or PHA (retrograde diastolic flow), bacterial superinfection from gas producers. Regional accumulation and endemic occurrence show some characteristics of a nosocomial infection.

Prevention. Breastmilk has a partially protective function as opposed to formula for premature babies.

Anemia of prematurity

Definition. Absent erythropoiesis and rapid growth predispose all neonates to a certain degree of anemia (trimester reduction). This is more marked in premature babies.

Two types: early hemorrhagic anemia caused by early cord clamping and blood loss for diagnostic purposes in intensive care. Late hyporegenerative anemia caused by high pO_2, which inhibits erythropoietin production.

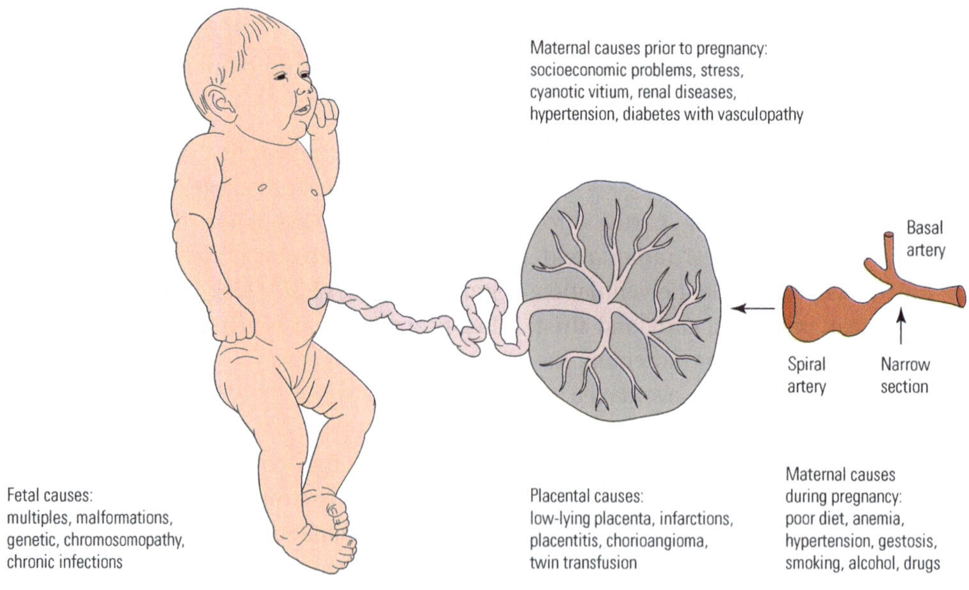

Fig. 13.18: Hypotrophic newborn. Causes of fetal growth restriction.

Practice tip. Delayed clamping of the umbilical cord limits the severity of the anemia.

13.6 Hypotrophic newborn

Definition. Newborns whose body weight is 10 % of intrauterine growth (SGA; Fig. 13.17).

Pathogenesis. Intrauterine growth is dependent on the genetic potential of the baby and influenced by (Fig. 13.18):
- Environmental factors (maternal health, diet, smoking).
- Hormones and growth factors, whereby in contrast to postnatal growth, fetal growth depends on insulin, less on thyroid and growth hormone.
- Size and condition of the placenta: thrombosis, diffuse fibrin deposits, edema, thickening of basal membrane and terminal villi.
- Classification of body measurements into population-specific percentiles at the time of birth allows assessment of fetal growth (see Fig. 13.19).
- Hypotrophic newborns have reduced umbilical artery glucose concentration at birth and more rapid postnatal drop in blood sugar.

Fetal growth restriction. Two main groups: In symmetrical restriction the fetus grows continuously but more slowly; head circumference and length are reduced in proportion to weight. Causes: chromosomal abnormalities, congeni-

Tab. 13.5: Damage to the newborn from maternal medication.

Medication	Neonatal risk
Alcohol	Microcephaly, developmental deficits
Anti-diabetics, oral anti-epileptics	Hypoglycemia, hemorrhages (atypical location)
Aminoglycoside (Streptomycin)	Ototoxicity
Anti-coagulants (Dicumarol)	CNS malformations
Diethylstilbostrol (DES)	Vaginal carcinoma
Cytostatics (Methotrexate, Aminopterin)	Malformations, anemia
Heroin, methadone	Withdrawal syndrome, hyperexcitability
Disinfectant containing iodine	Hypothyreosis
Morphine	Withdrawal syndrome, respiratory depression
Nicotine	Hypotrophy, microcephaly
Promethazine	Withdrawal syndrome, hyperexcitability
Reserpine	Obstruction of nasal mucosa
Sulfonamides	Hyperbilirubinemia, kern icterus
Tetracyclines	Tooth enamel discoloration
Thalidomide	Dysmelia
Thyrostatics	Goiter, hypothyreosis
Tocolytics	Hypocalcemia, hypoglycemia

tal malformations, some congenital metabolic disorders, viral infections.
In asymmetric restriction, fetal growth slows and can cease. Brain growth usually continues; liver, spleen, and body mass are more affected; head circumference is less affected than length; body weight is usually reduced.

Gestational age. As clinical determination of gestational age is not reliable, in particular in very immature preterm babies, and intrauterine growth is influenced by population and region, choice of the "correct" growth curve is not easy (Fig. 13.19).

Common problems of SGA newborns
- Continuation of the factors which caused the hypotrophy, e.g., vertical infection, exposure to cigarette smoke.
- Hypoglycemia (reduced glycogen reserves).
- Hyperviscosity/polycythemia (increased erythropoietin production).
- Hypothermia (reduced brown fat deposits).
- Dietary problems (intestinal hypomotility).
- After-effects of maternal medication (Tab. 13.5).

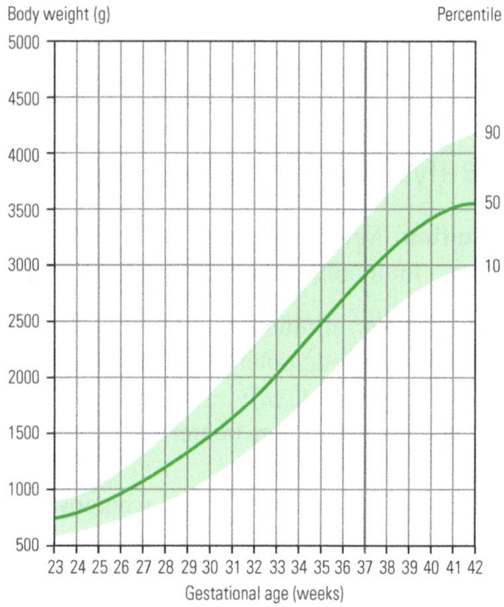

Fig. 13.19: Sheffield percentile curves for birth weight (both sexes) in relation to gestational age.

13.7 The infant of the diabetic mother (IDM)

13.7.1 Glucose metabolism and hypoglycemia

Note. Glucose is the most important substrate of oxidative brain metabolism and virtually the only form of fetal nourishment.

Supply ceases when the cord is clamped, blood sugar sinks to 50 mg/dl within 2 h; after 24–48 h a balance has been reached between glucose consumption and gluconeogenesis.
Glucose metabolism is susceptible in infants of diabetic mothers with increased insulin production and in those with a birth weight > 4,000 g (reduced glycogen reserve in premature babies, hypotrophic and postterm babies), in particular if no glucose is given in the first few days before milk production has begun.

Practice tip. Late hypoglycemia after the first two days of life occurs in congenital metabolic disorders: galactosemia, glycogen storage diseases.

Hypoglycemia of the newborn means blood sugar is < 35 mg/dl within the first 24 hours of life and < 45 mg/dl thereafter.

Clinical presentation
- Asymptomatic.
- Symptomatic. Neuromuscular hyperexcitability, trembling, tachypnea, seizures, hypotonia, apnea, pallor, cyanosis, coma, permanent brain damage.

Diagnosis
- Postnatal blood sugar monitoring at 2, 6, 12, and 24 hours of age.

Treatment

Early supplementary feeds with adapted formula or dextrose solution at 4 hours of age in:
- Hypotrophic newborns < 2,500 g.
- Postterm and dystrophic babies with reduced turgor.

Prevention. Early supplementation (see above) prevents hypoglycemia.

13.7.2 Fetopathia diabetica and complications

Definition. (Prenatal) developmental disorder in fetuses and neonates with macrosomia (hypertrophic or LGA newborn) and hyperinsulinism due to increased intrauterine blood sugar in gestational or maternal type I diabetes. Synonyms: diabetic embryo- or fetopathy.

Pathogenesis. Glucose crosses the placenta and brings about fetal and maternal hyperglycemia. The result is B-cell hyperplasia with hyperinsulinemia. As a fetal growth hormone, insulin stimulates lipogenesis and protein synthesis with organ enlargement, hypertrophy; birth weight > 90th percentile (Fig. 13.20). The chronic hypoxia stimulates erythropoietin production, resulting in polycythemia and hyperviscosity syndrome (hematocrit > 65 %), occasionally with vascular thrombosis.

Placental vasculopathy occurs in cases of severe maternal diabetes and the babies are born hypotrophic, or SGA.
Postnatally, the delayed regression of neonatal hyperinsulinism often causes hypoglycemia!

Complications

Before birth. Metabolic dangers:
- Malformations (heart, intestines, caudal regression).
- Delayed surfactant maturation.
- Placental insufficiency (primarily respiratory).
- Hyperviscosity (erythropoietin production).
- Depositing of glycogen in ventricular septum.
- Renal vein thrombosis (hyperviscosity).

At birth. Danger of asphyxia:
- Asphyxia (up to 10 % of hypertrophic neonates).
- Meconium aspiration.
- Persistent pulmonary hypertension.
- Clavicule or humerus fracture.
- Erb–Duchenne palsy.

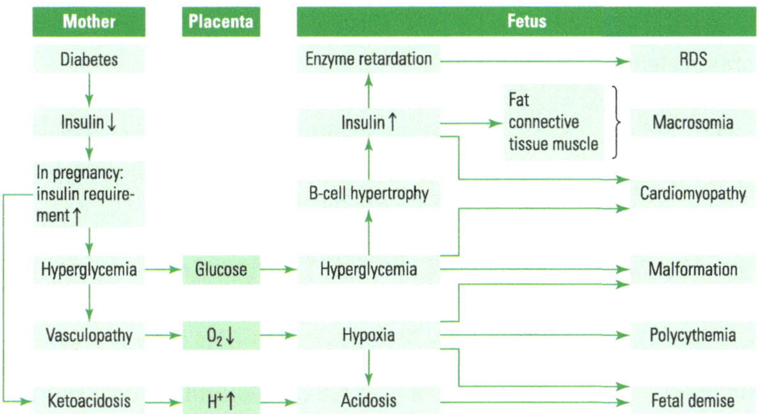

Fig. 13.20: Gestational diabetes. Effect on unborn baby.

After birth. Metabolic dangers:
- Hypoglycemia due to hyperinsulinism.
- Hypocalcemia (decreased production of parathyroid hormone).
- Hypomagnesemia (< 0.6 mmol/l).
- Hyperbilirubinemia (increased RBC breakdown).

Treatment. Glucose infusion (dextrose 10 % 5 ml/kg body weight/h).

Prevention. Strict control of gestational diabetes to ensure levels remain normoglycemic! Infants of diabetic mothers (IDM) and macrosomic newborns without diabetic history must be clinically and metabolically monitored.

13.8 Common newborn diseases

13.8.1 Respiratory disorders

Respiratory distress. The fetal lung is fully mature at 34 weeks; surfactant deficiency syndrome threatens those born earlier (respiratory distress syndrome; RDS, see p. 447) with dyspnea:
- Tachypnea > 60/min (maintenance of a normal respiratory minute volume despite high airway resistance).
- Sternal retraction (increased retraction strength of the lungs due to elevated surface tension and soft thorax skeleton).
- Expiratory moaning (improved gas exchange by delaying alveolar collapse).
- Nasal flaring (use of auxiliary breathing musculature).

Causes

Pulmonary
- RDS (see p. 447).
- Transitory tachypnea (wet lung).
- Aspiration syndrome (blood, meconium, see p. 442).
- Pneumonia (e.g., GBS, ureaplasmas).
- Persistent pulmonary hypertension (see p. 434).
- Pneumothorax and other extra-alveolar gas accumulations.
- Pulmonary hypoplasia (e.g., oligohydramnios sequence).
- Lobar emphysema and other lung malformations.

Extrapulmonary
- Post-asphyxia syndrome (see p. 438).
- Obstruction and malformation of the upper airways.
- Diaphragmatic hernia.
- High diaphragm due to other abdominal processes.
- Sepsis (see p. 468).
- Congenital cardiac malformations (see p. 463).

Wet lung

Definition. Increased fluid content of the alveoli, later the interstitium, with impaired or protracted reabsorption, e.g., due to too rapid birth, which overtaxes the pulmonary lymphatic system.

Note. Predisposed newborns are those born after cesarean, breech delivery, birth asphyxia, high maternal fluid intake.

Aspiration of amniotic fluid is not possible because AF is partially produced in the fetal lungs which are filled with fluid anyway.

Clinical presentation
- Tachypnea and nasal flaring directly after birth.
- Sternal retraction, occasionally also moaning or cyanosis, or requiring oxygen supplementation.
- The symptoms resolve within 24 h.

As it is difficult initially, to differentiate wet lung from RDS, congenital pneumonia or pneumothorax, all newborns with respiratory distress lasting longer than normal for direct postnatal adaptation should be transferred to the neonatal ward for clarification and treatment.

13.8.2 Anemia, polycythemia, hyperviscosity

Congenital anemia

Definition. Reduced hemoglobin (Hb) concentration and hematocrit (Hct) on the first or second day of life (Hb < 16.0 g/dl, Hct < 45 %) or third to fifth day (Hb < 14.5 g/dl, Hct < 40 %).

Classification according to pathogenesis.

Hypogenerative anemia. Inability to react to reduced erythrocytes with stimulation of erythropoiesis: anemia of prematurity, severe infections, hemodilution due to growth.

Main symptoms. Reduced reticulocytes, no erythroblasts in peripheral blood.

Hemolytic anemia. Rhesus, ABO-erythroblastosis, other blood group incompatibilities, erythrocyte enzyme defects, hemoglobinopathies (thalassemia).

Main symptoms. Increased reticulocytes and erythroblasts in peripheral blood.

Hemorrhagic anemia. Feto-maternal/-fetal transfusion, placenta previa, placental abruption, marginal sinus bleeding, skin, intracranial, intestinal bleeding (melena), diagnostic blood loss.

Clinical presentation/diagnosis/DD. Hypovolemia and shock are in the foreground in acute hemorrhage, Hb and Hct are normal to begin with.
- Main symptoms: tachycardia, elevated recapillarization time, hypertension.
- In unclear anemia HbF cells in maternal blood are counted and quantified if necessary to detect feto-maternal transfusion.

Treatment
- Transfusion! An O-Rhesus negative lysin-free CMV-negative unit of RBC is available in every maternity hospital: blood losses at birth can be considerable. The volume to be transfused is estimated, based on CVP (umbilical catheterization).
- In acute blood loss situations emergency transfusion (without cross-matching) is performed in the labor ward.

Practice tip. Obligatory for all other transfusions are: blood grouping, Coombs test, cross-matching.

Chronic blood loss can be significant, e.g., in feto-maternal or twin-twin transfusion.

Clinical presentation
- Pallor, despite apparent vitality.
- Apnea of prematurity.
- Tachycardia.
- Cardiac insufficiency (edema, hepatomegaly).
- Splenomegaly (extramedullary blood production).
- Fetla hydrops.
- Blood pressure is usually normal in chronic anemia.

Polycythemia

Definition. Venous Hct >55 % or Hb >22 g/dl. Synonyms: erythrocytosis, hyperviscosity syndrome.

Pathogenesis. Cause: placental insufficiency. Fetal hypoxia stimulates fetal production of erythropoietin, RBC production increases. Common in hypotrophic and postterm newborns; babies of smokers and diabetics.

Placental hypertransfusion. twin-twin, feto-maternal transfusion, delayed cord clamping,

placing the baby below the level of the placenta ("drainage" of placental blood).
Increased viscosity reduces blood flow velocity! Stasis in the terminal vascular bed, hypoperfusion, ischemia.

Types

Secondary polycythemia. The fetus produces too many erythrocytes because of chronic oxygen deficiency and increased erythropoietin production (smoker, post-term pregnancy, placental insufficiency, diabetic fetopathy). CVP and blood volume are normal.

Treatment. Hemodilution (concentrated blood is exchanged for plasma).

Hypertransfusion (plethora). Feto-maternal or twin-twin transfusion (receiver), delayed cord clamping or low placement of the baby before clamping the cord. CVP and blood volume are elevated.

Treatment. Phlebotomy (monitor BP!)

Dehydration. Reduction of birth weight by more than 10 % due to fluid deficiency, phototherapy or diarrhea. CVP and blood volume are reduced.

Treatment. Parenteral administration of fluids.

13.8.3 Hyperbilirubinemia, icterus, phototherapy

Physiological icterus. Increase of unconjugated serum bilirubin in 50 % of all breastfed newborns on day 2 or 3 (peaking on day 4 or 5) to 270 µmol/l = 16 mg/dl. Return to normal values by day 10.

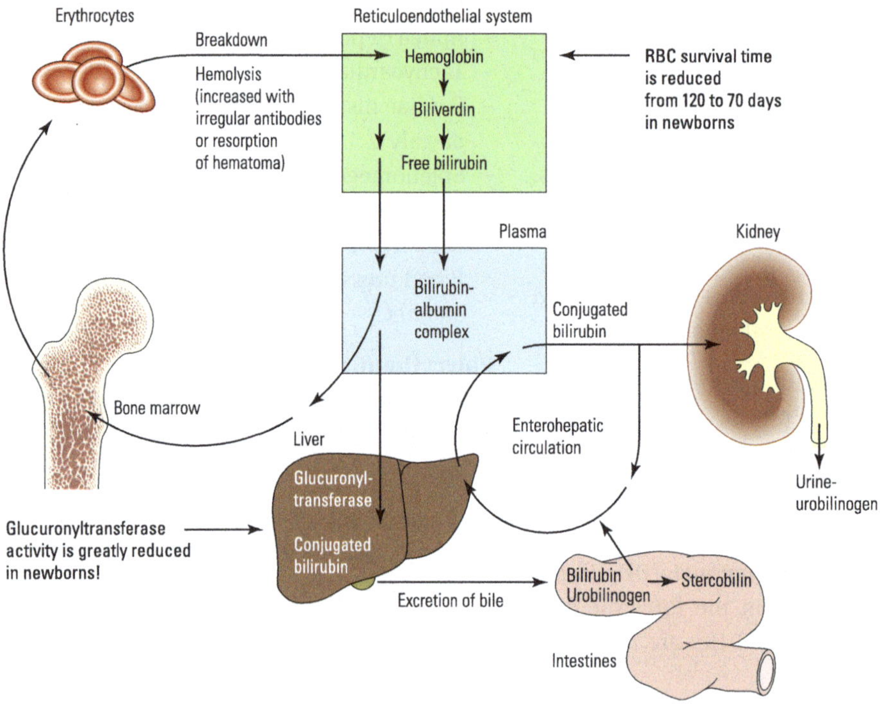

Fig. 13.21: Bilirubin metabolism and important causes of neonatal icterus.

Hyperbilirubinemia. Above 97 % of bilirubinemia for the reference population.

Physiology of bilirubin metabolism. Hb is broken down into unconjugated bilirubin in the monocyte-macrophage system. On release, it binds to albumin and is transported to the liver, where it is conjugated to water-soluble bilirubin via UDP-glucuronyltransferase.

Physiological characteristics of the newborn explain neonatal jaundice. Relatively high Hct/Hb and elevated bilirubin production. Shorter RBC survival time (Fig. 13.21; 70–90 days, adults 120 days). Immaturity of UDP-glucuronyltransferase. Enhanced enterohepatic circulation (intestinal glucuronidase activity and reabsorption) due to: delayed intestinal passage, colonization with intestinal flora still poor, breakdown of conjugated bilirubin into stercobilinogen, stercobilin.

Treatment

- Physiological icterus does not require treatment (early feeding, sufficient fluid intake).
- Pathological types require phototherapy (see below), in extreme cases exchange therapy. If therapy is indicated the critical levels are determined based on gestational age and birth weight.

Note. Phototherapy. Etiology must first be clarified, the extent and risks of elevated bilirubin must be checked and possible side effects monitored. It is the task of the obstetrics department to differentiate between physiological and pathological icterus types and to ensure timely transfer of sick newborns to the pediatric department for treatment.

Practice tip. The uncritical use of flow charts for treatment of hemolytic disease resulted in healthy newborns undergoing phototherapy unnecessarily in some places.

Principle. Blue light with an absorption maximum of 460 nm brings about the breakdown of

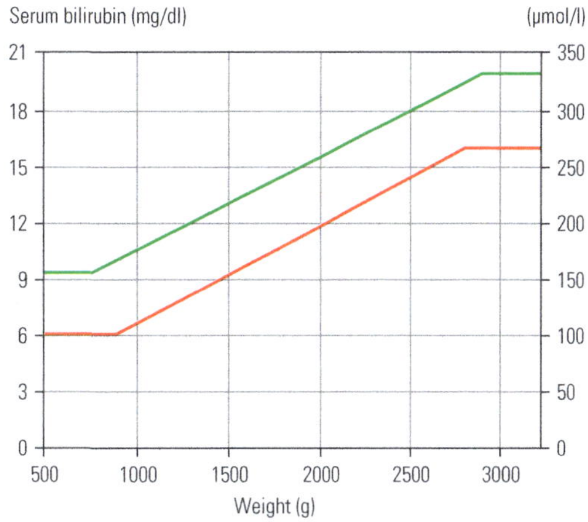

Fig. 13.22: Indication for phototherapy. Critical serum bilirubin levels for neonates without hemolysis. Green line without, red line with risk factors.

bilirubin in the skin, whereby photooxidation and photoisomerization create mono- and dipyrroles which are not toxic to the brain and can be excreted without glucuronization.

Indication (Fig. 13.22)

- Prophylactic phototherapy > 310 µmol/l (18 mg/dl).
- Illnesses involving jaundice listed (Tab. 13.6) must be ruled out. If this is not possible or if the baby is premature, it must be transferred to a pediatric hospital.

Side effects. Exanthemas, dehydration, thin stools and temperature regulation disorders.

Generally additional fluid must be administered parenterally during phototherapy to reduce the risk of dehydration and cholestasis (concentrated bile).
The eyes must be covered to avoid damaging the retina.

13.8.4 Hemolytic disease (HD)

Definition. Immune-mediated hemolytic disease due to blood group incompatibility (Rhe-

Tab. 13.6: Illnesses involving jaundice.

Diagnosis	Begin	Diagnostics
Reabsorption jaundice	Day 1–2	Hematoma, congestion hemorrhage
Hemolytic disease	Birth to day 4	Positive Coombs test, ↓ Hb
Congenital hemolytic anemia	From day 3	Spherocytosis, anemia
Drug-induced hemolysis	From day 3	History, anemia
Infections	Day 2–3	Conjugated bilirubin, hemogram, CRP, specific serology
Galactosemia	Day 2–3	Conjugated bilirubin, hypoglycemia
Biliary atresia	From day 7	Only unconjugated bilirubin

sus and ABO system) in newborns (synonyms: hemolytic disease of the newborn, HDN; erythroblastosis neonatorum) and fetuses (hemolytic disease of the fetus, HDF; erythroblastosis fetalis).

Rhesus incompatibility (Rhesus disease or erythroblastosis, hemolytic disease of the fetus). Blood group incompatibility in Rhesus system. Typical: mother Rh-negative, baby Rh-positive. Types:
- Anti-D antibody. Once common, rarer today after decades of immunological prophylaxis.
- Anti-C, anti-c, anti-E, anti-e antibodies however still just as common.

Diagnosis. To be made prenatally!
- Prenatal. Maternal blood group = Rh-negative: indirect Coombs test identifies irregular antibodies. Close sonographic monitoring (fetal hydrops?).
- Postnatal from cord blood. Baby's blood group and Rhesus factor → direct Coombs test (detection of irregular antibodies bound to erythrocytes). The direct Coombs test which shows antibodies bound to erythrocytes is positive. Usually negative in ABO incompatibility due to antigen immaturity!
- Bilirubin (↑ indirect bilirubin), hemogram (anemia → Hb < 12–15 g/dl, reticulocytosis).

Practice tip. Rh-negative women with irregular antibodies should be cared for in a perinatal center.

Treatment. Admission to neonatal unit if direct Coombs test is positive.

Prophylaxis. Anti-D immunoglobulin for Rh-negative women after birth of an Rh-positive baby, also after miscarriage, amniocentesis or unsuitable transfusions with Rh-positive blood. Prenatal anti-D immunological prophylaxis in week 28–29 of pregnant Rh-negative women.

ABO incompatibility (ABO HDN)

Pathogenesis. The mother usually has blood group O, the baby A or B. The regular iso-agglutinines (IgM) anti-A or anti-B are transformed to immune hemolysins (IgG), which cross the placenta and damage the fetus or newborn.

Practice tip. A negative Coombs test does not exclude sensitization in the ABO system.

Treatment. In the pediatric hospital!

Phototherapy, in ABO incompatibility often long-term, or infusion therapy to rebalance electrolytes.

13.8.5 Drug addiction, drug withdrawal

Definition. Addiction to addictive substances which act on the central nervous system (e.g., opiates such as heroin, codeine, methadone, cocaine, crack, barbiturates, benzodiazepines or amphetamines).

Drug use in pregnancy is increasing. In addition to the direct effects, the fetus is also at risk due to poor maternal diet, placental insufficiency and vertical infection (particularly hepatitis B, HIV).

Withdrawal after exposure to opiates. Newborns develop the following symptoms after birth:
- Trembling, irritability, myoclonia.
- Hyperactivity, muscular hypertension.
- Short sleep phases.
- Shrill screaming.
- Excessive sucking, feeding difficulties.
- Vomiting, diarrhea.
- Sneezing.
- Tachypnea.
- Sweating.

Prophylaxis. Special consultations for drug addicts in perinatal center. Cautious drug withdrawal with methadone can reduce neonatal withdrawal symptoms. The psychosocial situation must be taken into consideration when caring for mother and baby.

Tab. 13.7: Common causes of neonatal seizures

Causes	Mechanism of action
Days 1–3	
Perinatal hypoxia	Hypoxic ischemic encephalopathy
Difficult birth	Subdural hemorrhage
Infant diabetic mother	Hypoglycemia, hypocalcemia
Hypotrophic newborn	Hypoglycemia
Premature baby	Intraventricular hemorrhage, periventricular leukomalacia
Drug withdrawal	Maternal opiates
Days 4–14	
Infection	Meningitis, sepsis, toxoplasmosis
High phosphate intake	Hypocalcemia
Metabolic disorder	Galactosemia Nesidioblastosis Glycogen storage disease Hyperammonemia

13.8.6 Neonatal seizures

Pathogenesis. Causes: see Tab. 13.7

Clinical presentation
- Symptoms are uncommon (usually no generalized tonic-clonic seizures).
- Subtle eye movements, grimacing, focal automatism, yawning, sucking movements.
- Apnea.

Treatment. Transferal to neonatal unit if suspected!

13.9 Common congenital abnormalities

Definition. Developmental abnormalities of single or multiple organs or sections of the body due to a disruption of embryogenesis.

Incidence. 1–2 % of all newborns have abnormalities, 2–4 % exhibit malpositions as a result of the intrauterine situation, e.g., contractions due to anhydramnios.

Pathogenesis. A single cause can rarely be identified. A third of each are:
- Hereditary abnormalities (including new mutations).
- Multifactorial disorders of embryogenesis (including environmental factors).
- Unexplained.

Note. The type of injury (virus, hemorrhage, medication, radiation) is not important, but rather the timepoint (Fig. 13.23).

Practice tip. Honesty, empathy and experience are prerequisites for the dialogue with the parents. The baby must not be reduced to its abnormality in the discussion. It should always be shown to the parents. Negative terms such as deformity, defect healing, and high-risk baby should be avoided. A baby with a congenital abnormality is especially in need of acceptance and love from its parents.

13.9.1 Gastrointestinal tract

The most common malformations in the gastrointestinal tract are diaphragmatic hernia, omphalocele, gastroschisis, esophageal atresia, and intestinal atresia.

Diaphragmatic hernia

Definition. Diaphragmatic defect, usually unilateral (80 % left-sided), with displacement of abdominal organs into the chest cavity, crowding in the affected chest half, pulmonary hypoplasia.

Clinical presentation
- Acute, in some cases severe respiratory insufficiency. Dyspnea, cyanosis, asymmetric chest without breathing movements, breathing sounds not audible on auscultation (possibly bowel sounds in the thorax!); hypersonorous resonance.
- Heart displacement.
- Symptoms of shock.
- Concave abdomen.

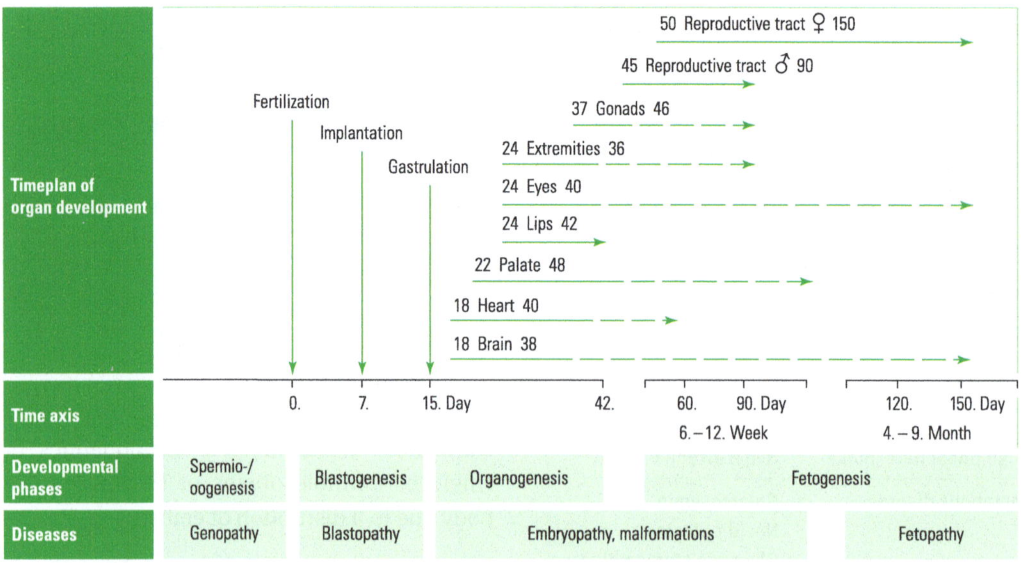

Fig. 13.23: Vulnerable phases for malformations of different organs. Determination in weeks or days.

Diagnosis
- Prenatal (sonography), perinatal care in specialized center.
- Postnatal. Chest x-ray in two planes.

Treatment
- Initial care. Primary intubation. Caution: no mask ventilation, danger of inflation of stomach, bowels in chest cavity.
- Nasogastric tube.
- Operative closure of the diaphragm once stabilized.

Prognosis. Dependent on the degree of pulmonary hypoplasia and accompanying malformations, which are present in 30 % of cases.

Omphalocele

Definition. Inhibitory malformation of the ventral abdominal wall with prolapse of abdominal organs in a hernia sac, made out of amnion, which did not return to the abdominal cavity. Synonym: umbilical hernia.

Clinical presentation
- Small and large intestines, parts of the liver, rarely also other abdominal organs are found in the hernia sac.
- Additional malformations are common (50 %), with an embryological explanation: cardiac defects, sternal cleft, Ectopia cordis, bladder exstrophy, vesicointestinal fissure, atresias; malpositioned bowel is obligatory.

Diagnosis
- Fetal sonography with diagnosis of sac contents on viewing!
- Chest x-ray (cardiac defects!), echocardiography.

Practice tip. 3 × S: suction, sack, side-positioning.

Treatment. Preoperative preparation is essential (12–24 (48) hours).
- Birth should be scheduled, if possible (cesarean?). In the foreground directly after birth are: shock, infection prophylaxis, cardiopulmonary adaptation, stabilization of acid-base and water and electrolyte household as well as disturbed temperature regulation.
- Nasogastric tube, lateral supine positioning to improve blood flow in the sac, minimize risk of infection and reduce fluid loss.
- Operative goal is to reposition the prolapsed abdominal organs and close the abdominal wall (and treat additional anomalies). Problems can arise in cases of large omphalocele due to the disproportion between abdominal cavity volume and abdominal organs!

Prognosis. Good, dependent on further anomalies.

Gastroschisis

Definition. Evisceration of abdominal organs (never the liver, however!) through a paraumbilical abdominal wall defect (usually on the right), whereby umbilical cord insertion is normal. Results from vascular insult on premature closure of the right vitelline artery.

Incidence. 1 in 10,000 newborns, 2/3 are premature.

Clinical presentation
- Small defect, no hernia sac.
- Prolapsed intestinal loops are strangulated, swollen, edematous, and can present as a compact bundle due to fibrous peritonitis or be torted and damaged as a result of chemical peritonitis.
- Further anomalies are rare.

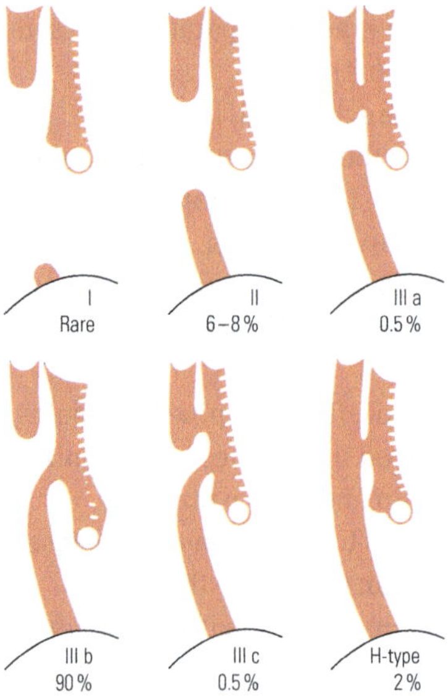

Fig. 13.24: Esophageal atresia. Classification and incidence acc. to Vogt (Types I, II, IIIa–c, H): I distal atresia without fistula (rare, 1 %); II atresia with distal lumen and no fistula; IIIa atresia with distal lumen and tracheo-esophageal fistula of the blind upper pouch; IIIb atresia with distal lumen and tracheo-esophageal fistula of the blind lower pouch = commonest type (> 90 %); IIIC atresia with distal lumen and tracheo-esophageal fistula of the upper and lower blind pouches; H-type: no atresia, trachea-esophageal fistula.

Diagnosis. Prenatal sonography.

Treatment. Initial care in the labor ward:
- Cover with sterile drapes, or place the baby up to its neck in a sterile plastic bag. The baby is kept warm, positioned on its side to avoid obstructing blood flow and a naso-gastric tube is inserted.
- Torsion is prevented; if strangulation occurs the opening is widened.
- Operation as soon as possible.

Prognosis
- In contrast to omphalocele, post-operative recovery is complicated, with long-lasting gastrointestinal atony, intensive care.
- Good results after successful post-operative treatment!

Esophageal atresia

Definition. Closure of the esophagus with or without tracheo-esophageal or broncho-esophageal fistula due to disturbed trachea-esophageal septation.

Incidence
- Commonest gastrointestinal tract malformation, 1 : 3 – 4,000.
- Combined with tracheo-esophageal fistula (TEF) in 80 % of cases.
- Often (1/3 of cases) associated with other malformations: Vitium cordis, gastrointestinal and urinary tract obstructions.
- 1/3 are premature babies, increased familial incidence.

Classification. After Vogt (Fig. 13.24); Type IIIB is most common (90 %).

Clinical presentation. Diagnosis is often made by the nurse!

Early symptoms:
- Hydramnios.
- Increased saliva, saliva is not swallowed.
- Collection of foamy secretion in nasopharynx.
- Coughing and sneezing.

Late symptoms: aspiration of food with choking, pneumonia.

Diagnosis
- Prenatal sonography (hydramnios and blind esophageal pouch).
- Postnatal. In the labor ward a tube cannot be passed through the esophagus (attempt is obligatory in all newborns after respiratory adaptation!).
- Chest x-ray depicts coiled feeding tube in the blind pouch. Stomach/bowels are filled with air in cases of distal fistula to the trachea.

Treatment. Operation. Neonatal intensive care!

- Immediate measures: tube is inserted into the blind pouch, continuous suction (or in brief intervals); possibly intubation, cardiorespiratory stabilization, operation (not an absolute emergency operation however).

Intestinal atresia

Definition. Occlusion (congenital obstruction) of intestinal lumen at various locations. Most common site is the duodenum.

Duodenal atresia

Pathogenesis. Multifactorial; extra- and intraintestinal causes: duodenal membranes, genuine atresias, annular pancreas, types of malrotation; common with Down syndrome.

Most commonly occurs distal to the papilla of Vater (vomiting therefore bilious).
Accompanying anomalies in 70 % (Trisomy 21, cardiac defect, malrotation).

Clinical presentation. Vomiting (usually bilious), symptoms of high small intestine ileus, prenatal hydramnios.

Diagnosis
- Hydramnios is an indication.
- Prenatal sonography.
- Postnatal stomach secretion volume > 10 ml.
- X-ray: double-bubble sign.

13.9.2 Congenital cardiac malformations

Note. Incidence. 1 in 100 live births. One in ten is a "critical" cardiac malformation, i.e., life-threatening in the neonatal period.

Signs

Screening for cardiac malformations see p. 429.
- Generalized cyanosis in transposition of the great arteries (TGA), pulmonary stenosis, anomalous pulmonary vein connection.
- Cardiac insufficiency, recognizable by grey skin tone, dyspnea, and liver enlargement, by hypoplastic left-heart syndrome, aortic isthmus stenosis.
- Systolic sounds in PDA, VSD, tetralogy of Fallot and other defects.

Diagnosis
- Pediatric cardiology examination, echocardiography!

13.9.3 Skeletal malformations

Note. The most common orthopedic and skeletal deformities are cleft lip and palate, premature closure of the cranial sutures (craniosynostosis), hip dysplasia, talipes, achondroplasia.

Malformations due to multifactorial inheritance with threshold effect, i.e., the malformation expresses itself when a number of genes or exogenous noxae come together.

Cleft lip and palate

Definition. Congenital vertical facial cleft (craniofacial dysplasia) of heterogeneous origin and in varying combinations; as isolated or complex cleft lip, and/or soft and/or hard palate. In 50 % of cases a unilateral cleft lip and palate is found.

Practice tip. Clefts do not generally cause respiratory distress, so that immediate transferal from the labor ward is not necessary. Parents who were poorly informed and whose baby was transferred immediately often urge speedy elimination of the cleft lip and palate.

Pathogenesis. Originates during late blastogenesis and early embryogenesis (weeks 3–8). Result of a singular or complex morphological disorder.

Incidence. 1 in 600–1,000 newborns. One symptom of other malformation syndromes, e.g., Trisomy 13.

Clinical presentation. Associated malformations?

Diagnosis. Clinical presentation!
- Prenatal. Fusion of upper jaw absent in sonogram.

Treatment. A silicon plate fitted within the first days of life closes the palate and makes normal sucking possible.
- Surgical closure of the lip after a number of months, the cleft palate much later (first operation from month 4, following operations up to the 6th year), as growth and arch of the palate are prerequisites for speech development.

Practice tip. Conditional for the rehabilitation program are multidisciplinary treatment and patience. Optimal long-term success can only be achieved through good cooperation between prenatal diagnosticians, obstetricians, neonatologists, oral surgeons, ENT physicians and speech therapists.

Prognosis. Good if disorders are isolated and with timely interdisciplinary treatment.

Craniosynostosis

Definition. Premature ossification of one or more cranial sutures with threatened deformation of the skull.

Types (overcompensated growth in the direction of the fused suture):
- Widening of the skull (brachycephaly) from fusion of the coronal sutures.
- Lengthening of the skull (dolichocephaly) from fusion of the sagittal suture.
- High-head syndrome (oxy- or turricephaly) from simultaneous fusion of coronal and sagittal sutures.
- Skull asymmetries from unilateral ossification of sutures (plagicephaly).
- Triangular skull (trigoncephaly) from premature fusion of the metopic suture: the forehead is narrow and has a triangular form, pointing towards the front.

Practice tip. Increased intracranial pressure is a danger in craniosynostosis, particularly if a number of sutures are affected.

Treatment. Multidisciplinary, assessment of functional and cosmetic risks and benefits.

Congenital hip dysplasia

Definition. Development disorder (flattening) of the acetabulum (hip joint socket) with threatened dislocation of the femoral head (hip joint subluxation or luxation; Fig. 13.25).

Incidence. 2–4 in 100 newborns, affects girls five times more often than boys.

Clinical presentation. The clinical examination, in particular Ortolani's test (hip clunk) is unreliable and can cause injuries. Inhibited abduction may also be completely absent or not occur till after luxation of the hip.

Diagnosis. Ultrasound examination at 4–6 weeks of age is advisable for all babies. Earlier tests are unreliable due to the immaturity of the joint, and should therefore only be performed on the basis of clinical suspicion (inhibited abduction, asymmetrical folds, breech presentation) or family history.

Treatment. Dysplasia. Early treatment with splint or harness (e.g., Pavlik) which flexes and abducts the hips. Goal: alignment of the femoral head centrally in the socket, avoidance of luxation and promotion of cartilage development and maturation of the socket by the movements allowed by the splint/harness.

Prognosis. The earlier the treatment, the more rapidly and uncomplicated good results can be achieved. Restitutio ad integrum (complete recovery) in mild to moderate dyplasias.

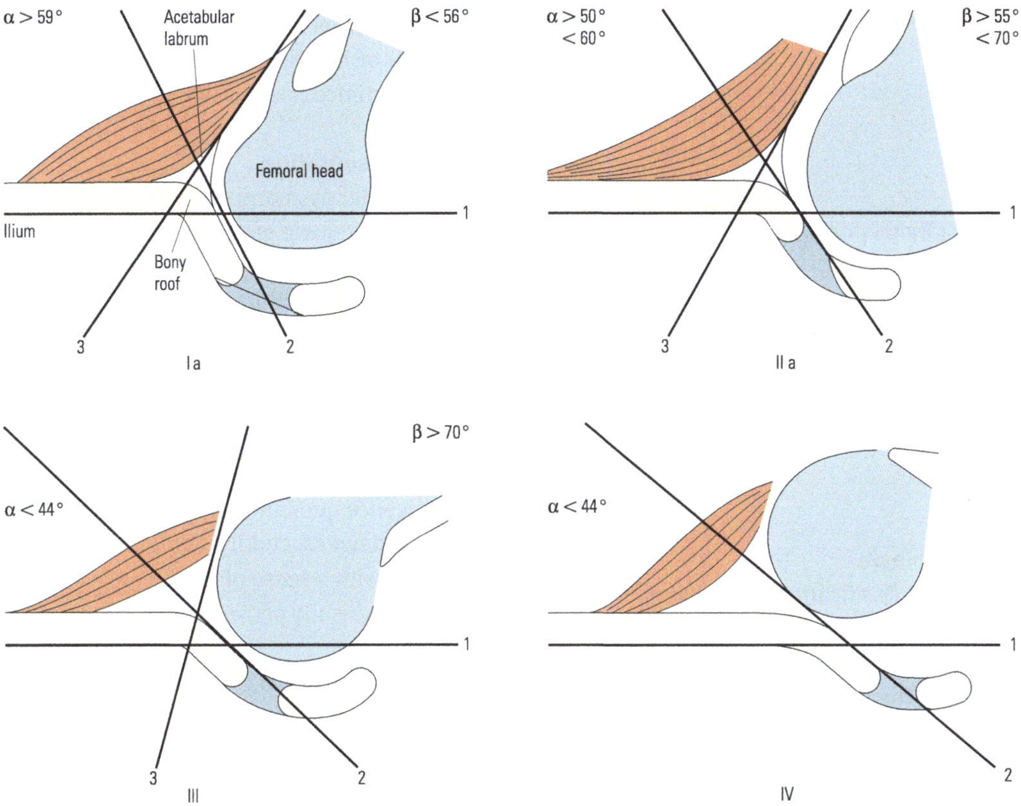

Fig. 13.25: Ultrasound classification of the hips according to the acetabular angle α and the angle of inclination β. 1) Baseline. 2) Acetabular roof line 3) Inclination line. Ia mature, normal hip, IIa immature hip with broadened, cartilaginous roof, III dysplastic (decentered) hip with shallow, bony roof, IV luxated hip with flat roof, β angle cannot be assessed.

Talipes equinovarus (TEV; club foot)

Definition. Malformation of the foot: inward rotation of the whole foot, adduction of the front part of the foot, in addition to supination and plantar flexion of the heel (Pes equinovarus), as the front part of the foot is flexed more than the heel.

Pathogenesis. Cause unknown, recessive inheritance with varying severity.

Clinical presentation (Fig. 13.26):
- Inward rotation and adduction of the front of the foot.
- Supination of the whole foot with subluxed talus.
- Varus malposition of the heel.
- Atrophy of calf musculature.

Differential diagnosis. Pigeon-toes and heel foot, harmless, result of enforced intrauterine position.

Complications. If untreated the infant walks on the lateral edge of the foot or even the back of the foot, which causes severe walking difficulties.

The club foot is always contracted, which means it can be neither actively nor passively corrected. Orthopedic correction of talipes (resetting and fixation with plaster or splinting)

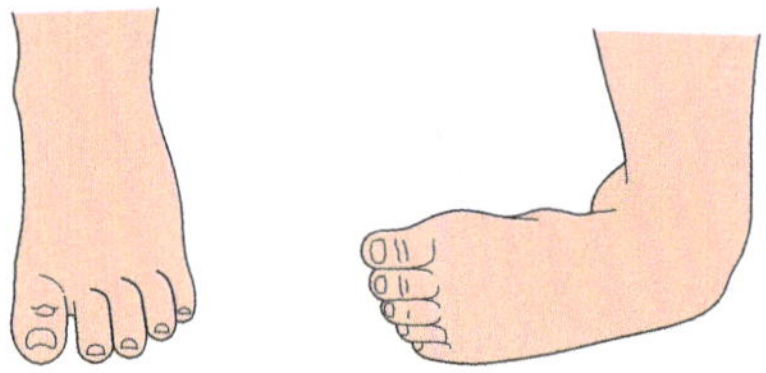

Fig. 13.26: Typical characteristics of talipes.

should begin in the first few days, as long as the tarsus is not ossified and the malformation is only fixation is only ligamentous and muscular. Early and rigorous orthopedic treatment enables normal walking and prevents operations later.

Achondroplasia

Definition. Ossification disorder of the long tubular bones and the pre-formed cartilaginous basis of the skull with disproportionate hyposomia (height 130 cm = dwarfism); caused by autosomal dominant genetic disorder or spontaneous mutation.

Clinical presentation
- Macrocephaly with saddle nose and prominent forehead.
- Short extremities, normal bone density.
- Marked lumbar lordosis.
- No mental retardation.

13.9.4 Down syndrome

Definition. Chromosomal abnormality, malformation, retardation syndrome with flat face, obliquely slanted eyes, small head, short neck, muscular hypotension, and excessive joint mobility. Synonym: Trisomy 21.

Incidence. Most common autosomal chromosome abnormality; prevalence: 1 in 700–1,000 live births.

Pathogenesis. Cause of free trisomy 21: 95 %. 47 chromosomes, of which 3 chromosome 21. Occurs during meiosis due to nonconjunction (meiosis I) or nondisjunction (meiosis II). Low risk of recurrence (1–2 %).

Clinical presentation
- Craniofacial dysmorphia. Rotund dwarfism (despite adequate growth hormone production); brachy- and microcephaly; Brushfield spots (thickening of the iris stroma), telecanthus (eyes abnormally far apart); broad bridge of the nose, low, small ears; open mouth with increased secretion of saliva and protruding, relatively large tongue.
- Intelligence quotient 25–50, individually varying degrees, cuddly, tender, some are musical with a sense of rhythm, to a certain extent physically active, friendly, generally cheerful.
- Muscular hypotonia, generalized connective tissue weakness, cutis laxa, low navel (often with hernia), single transverse palmar crease, foot deformity ("sandal gap": broad gap between first and second toe), clinodactyly, hip dysplasia. Underdeveloped jaw and teeth in addition to late fusion of the cranial sutures and the fontanelles without delayed development of the ossification centers.
- Congenital heart defects in 50 % (particularly endocardial cushion and septum defects: threatened pulmonary hypertension).
- Duodenal stenosis, Hirschsprung's disease (ileus!), anal atresia, rectal prolapse, tendency to constipation; primary hypothyreosis (25 %).
- Cryptorchidism is common (fibrous encasement of testes): masculine infertility, female patients are fertile with free trisomy: 50 % of their children are healthy, 50 % have trisomy 21.

Complications. High risk of leucosis (10–20 times more common!) From fourth decade on increasing dementia, among other things due to reduction of cholinergic neurotransmission enzymes (acetylcholinesterase, cholinacetyltransferase, catecholamines) and cerebral necroses.

Prognosis
- Average life expectancy reduced (see complications); with optimal support also over 50 years. Currently 80 % of patients reach 30 years of age; therefore medical and psychological–pedagogical care is of increasing importance.
- The type of cardiac defect determines life expectancy. Risk of leukemia is higher.
- With early, individually suitable and targeted support, the children are capable of learning to a limited extent and can be socially integrated!

13.9.5 Alcohol embryopathy, -fetopathy (fetal alcohol syndrome; FAS)

Definition. Disruption syndrome due to maternal alcohol abuse as well as in progressive or chronic phase of alcohol disease during pregnancy.

Incidence. Around 3 in 1,000 newborns!

Practice tip. Embryofetal alcohol syndrome is one of the most common congenital causes of mental disability!

Pathogenesis. Toxic effect of alcohol or its waste product acetaldehyde. Embryotoxic encephalopathy due to alcohol is in the foreground. Teratogenic mechanism is unclear; dose-effect correlation.

Clinical presentation. Dependent on the amount of alcohol consumed during the pregnancy.
- 50 g/day: stunted growth, reduced weight and head circumference (hypotrophy).
- 80–100 g/day: fetal growth restriction, muscular hypotonia and hyperactivity with dysmorphia:
- Laterally drooping eyelids, epicanthus, blepharophimosis, thin upper lip, missing philtrum, sunken bridge of nose, dysplasia of the pinna, microgenia, clinodactyly, abnormal hand creases.
- Malformations of genitals and joints, heart defects and cleft lip and palate are common.

Prognosis. Growth remains stunted, intelligence remains severely reduced.

Tab. 13.8: Immune status of the neonate.

	Natural (unspecific) immunity	Adaptive (specific) immunity
Humoral	Lysozyme: present in the fetus Complement: is not produced until week 22, chemotaxic activity and opsonisation are missing	IgA: not present at birth, exogenous supply (breastmilk) IgG: maternal origin (crosses the placenta; passive immunoprotection) IgM: only fetal immunoglobulin. 1–2 % of adult levels on birth
Cellular	Granulocytes: reduced reserves, chemotaxis absent, minimal moldability, phagocytosis normal, bactericidal effect normal Macrophages: extra- and intracellular destruction of pathogens functions	B-lymphocytes: production of antibodies does not begin until after birth T-lymphocytes: suppressor effect dominates, newborn does not yet have memory cells, reduced lymphokine production

13.10 Neonatal infections

13.10.1 Immune status of the neonate

Cellular and humoral immunity (Tab. 13.8) are present prenatally, with marked differences however. The phagocytic system is functional in the early embryonic phase. Peripheral lymphocytes are detectable from week 16; from week 20 T-lymphocytes in the thymus gland and immunoglobulins in the spleen.
Term newborns have high IgG antibody levels due to transplacental transmission. In contrast, concentrations of IgM and IgA are low because they cannot cross the placental barrier.

13.10.2 Sepsis and GBS infection

Sepsis. General infection due to spread of microorganisms (usually bacteria, rarely fungi) from the source of infection into the bloodstream (bacteremia, fungemia), most dangerous infection of term and premature newborns with high mortality. Synonym: septicemia. Early form in the first three days of life from intrauterine infection = fulminant course; late form after the third day of life = often nosocomial infection from intensive care!

Pathogenesis. Causes:
- *Early form.* Main cause is the inability of some GBS carriers to produce antibodies and pass these on to the fetus. Preferred location of the pathogen is maternal rectovaginal flora (β-hemolyzing group B streptococci, E. coli, Staph. aureus, listeria, Klebsiella, anaerobics).
- *Late form.* Pathogens are Enterococci, Haemophilus influenzae, Staph. epidermidis, Pseudomonaden, Klebsiella, Enterobacter, Serratia, anaerobics; fungi (Candida).

Route of infection. Ascending (chorioamnionitis in PROM >24h). Hematogenous (transplacental); via cutaneous or intestinal colonization; via ventilation tube, catheter.

Initiation of the inflammation by proinflammatory mediators (TNF, IL6) and activators of the complement and coagulation systems.
Chorioamnionitis due to GBS is a common cause of premature birth; therefore this infection must be expected in premature babies.

Clinical presentation. Always think of an infection if general condition worsens!

Practice tip. The experienced nurse notices the important early symptom: "I don't like the look of that baby, it looks poorly"!

In a preterm neonate the early form is similar to RDS or pneumonia; in a term newborn it is accompanied by sepsis, circulatory centralization and DIC.
The symptoms are uncharacteristic and take many forms:
- Variable temperatures (< 36° or > 37°).
- Apathy, hyperexcitability.
- Respiratory disorders (apnea, tachypnea).
- Apathetic feeding, failure to thrive, stomach contents, vomiting, bloated abdomen.
- Pallid grey skin tone, marbled skin, cold extremities, elevated recapillarization time.
- Icterus, hepatosplenomegaly.
- Petechiae, purpura, hemorrhaging tendencies.
- Metabolic acidosis.

Diagnosis. Infections!
- Swabs from placenta, membranes and ear; stomach contents immediately after birth. Hemogram. Leukocytosis (> 30,000/µl) or leukopenia (< 4,000/µl), left shift.

13.10.3 Other vertical infections

Pre-, perinatal infections. Innumerable pathogens are transmitted to the baby before or during the birth (usually initial maternal infection in pregnancy). Depending on the timepoint and severity they result in fetal death, embryopathies with malformations or fetopathies with generalized, localized or asymptomatic infection.

Note. The most common viral infections are: hepatitis B, genital herpes, HIV, rubella, cytomegaly. The most common bacterial infections are: GBS, listeriosis, syphilis. The most common zoonosis is toxoplasmosis.

Rubella

Symptoms. Cataract, glaucoma, deafness, myocarditis, cardiac defect, thrombocytopenia.
Procedures on delivery. Isolate baby, serology, IgM antibodies. No specific treatment possible.

Cytomegaly

Symptoms. 90 % asymptomatic. Low birth weight, hepatosplenomegaly, thrombocytopenia, icterus, microcephaly.
Procedures. Serology, detection of the virus. Consider Ganciclovir therapy.

Genital herpes

Symptoms. Herpes lesions on eyes, skin, mouth cavity, meningoencephalitis, generalized septic form.
Procedures. Cesarean section, isolate newborn. Consider Aciclovir therapy.

Hepatitis B

Symptoms. Initially usually asymptomatic. 10 % icterus at 3–5 months, often chronic hepatitis.
Procedures. HBsAg, HBeAg.

HIV

Symptoms. Initially asymptomatic. Possibly low birth weight, microcephaly; development of AIDS after months/years.
Procedures. Delivery by cesarean section, gloves during initial care and blood taking. Zidovudine prophylaxis. Do not breastfeed.

Syphilis

Symptoms. Maculopapular rash, desquamation, rhinitis, hepatosplenomegaly, periostitis, keratitis.
Procedures. IgM-FTA-Abs test. Hemogram, CRP. If suspected, penicillin therapy.

Tab. 13.9: Neonatal infection, clinical monitoring and laboratory diagnosis.

	Parameter	Reference value	Sensitivity	Problems
Clinical (every 2h)	Temperature	> 37.5, < 36.5 °C	< 50 %	
	Breathing	> 60/min	50 %	
	Pulse	> 160/min	< 50 %	
	Recap. time	> 2 s	> 50 %	
Laboratory	Leukocytes	> 30 < 4 × 1,000/µl	50 %	
	Neutrophil I:T ratio	> 0.2	60–90 %	elaborate
	IL-6	> 25 pg/ml	70–90 %	early
	CRP	> 1 mg/dl	40–60 %	late

Listeriosis

Symptoms. Early form with sepsis, shock, pneumonia. Late form with meningitis.
Procedures. Detection of pathogen (meconium). Treatment with Ampicillin.

Toxoplasmosis

Symptoms. Often asymptomatic. Low birth weight, chorioretinitis, seizures, hydrocephalus, hepatomegaly.
Procedures. Serology, specific IgM, liquor protein. Treatment with Pyrimethamine and Sulfadiazine.

Varicella

Symptoms. Fulminant disease possible, if mother contracts it 4 days before to 2 days after birth.
Procedures. Hyperimmunoglobulin, Aciclovir therapy.

Postnatal infections

Postnatal infections are among the most common neonatal illnesses. Predisposing factors are maternal illness in pregnancy or labor (particularly chorioamnionitis with intrapartum fever), operative delivery, PROM > 24 h, immaturity of the newborn, birth asphyxia, invasive treatment methods (e.g., venous catheter).
The most important pathogens are: GBS. Staphylococci, Pneumococci, E. coli, Klebsiella, Pseudomonas, Candida albicans.
Clinical picture. Pneumonia, sepsis, meningitis. Particularly at risk of infection are newborns with the following birth history:
- Fetal tachycardia.
- Maternal fever.
- PROM > 24 h.
- Duration of labor > 24 h.
- Meconium-stained or putrid fluid.

Clinical presentation, diagnosis see Tab. 13.9.

13.11 Level of Care and Regionalization

13.11.1 Prenatal transfer to a perinatal center

Laboring women are to be admitted/transferred to a perinatal center (i.e., those with a neonatal intensive care unit) under the following circumstances:
- Preterm birth < 28 completed weeks or 1,250 g.
- Triplets < 32 completed weeks and all higher order multiples.
- All prenatally diagnosed diseases for which emergency care directly after birth is necessary. This includes: maternal diseases which endanger the fetus (PKU, hypo-, hyperthyreosis, history of transplantation, autoimmune disease, HIV).
- Congenital abnormalities (e.g., critical cardiac defects, diaphragmatic hernia, myelomeningocele, gastroschisis).

Prenatal transfer of pregnant women to mid-level centers under the following circumstances:
- Preterm delivery from 28 to 31 completed weeks or 1,250–1,499 g.
- Twins from 28 to 32 completed weeks.
- Severe pregnancy-associated diseases (growth restriction < third percentile in preeclampsia and gestosis).
- Diabetic metabolic disorder requiring insulin with endangered fetus.

13.11.2 Neonatal consultation

Neonatology has its origins in obstetrics, and is today a part of pediatric medicine which concerns itself with disorders of postnatal adaptation and diseases of term and preterm neonates. Neonatologists are constantly present in perinatal centers. Other maternity hospitals should consult a neonatal on-call service as required.

Presence of a neonatologist in the labor ward is required in:
- Operative deliveries if the baby is endangered.
- Fetal-neonatal acidosis (pH < 7.10).
- Thick green (pea-soup) AF before birth.
- Maternal diabetes.
- Birth of an under- (< 2,500g) or overweight (> 4,000g) baby.
- Preterm birth < 36 weeks.
- Maternal fever, elevated CRP or other signs of infection.
- Fetal hemolytic disease, hydrops of all origins.
- Adaptation disorder (unusual breathing, blood sugar < 35mg/dL).
- Malformation.
- Infants of HBsAg –positive mother for immunization.

13.11.3 Indications for transfer to neonatal intensive care unit (NICU)

- Post-asphyxia syndrome (Apgar < 4, umbilical artery pH < 7.10, after primary resuscitation and intubation).
- Cardiorespiratory symptoms. Respiratory disorder, cyanosis, cardiac insufficiency, anemia, symptoms of shock.
- Birth weight < 2,000 g.
- Cerebral seizures, meningitis, apnea.
- Diabetic fetopathy, polycythemia, hemolytic disease.
- Severe malformations which must be treated immediately: diaphragmatic hernia, myelomeningocele, gastrointestinal atresia.
- Infection (see Tab. 13.9).
- Nutritional disorders: repeated vomiting, bloated abdomen.
- Hyperbilirubinemia, if clarification or treatment required.

The parents should be spoken to before transfer about their baby's disease, the necessity of transfer to a specialist hospital and visiting options.

13.11.4 Transfer to NICU not indicated

Conditions. The infant is in good condition postnatally, a pediatrician is available and diagnosis and monitoring are possible in the maternity hospital.
- Maternal illness or medication (e.g., steroids).
- After operative delivery (cesarean, forceps).
- Light birth asphyxia (Apgar 4–6, umbilical artery pH > 7.10), if the baby is stable at 10 min of age.
- Birth weight of 2,000–2,500 g, unless < 35 weeks.
- Meconium-stained fluid if no respiratory disorder present.
- Nonhemolytic icterus with a bilirubin level < 16 mg/dl (274 µmol/l) in an otherwise asymptomatic term newborn.
- Non-life-threatening malformation: hexadactyly, Down syndrome, cleft palate.
- Social problems (e.g., giving the baby up for adoption).

13.11.5 Postnatal transport

Postnatal transports involve risks: undercooling, intracranial hemorrhage, infection. If transport is unavoidable (transport was no longer possible antepartum because of advanced labor, severe APH, preeclampsia, fetal hypoxia) the hospitals must discuss the methods of birth and transport. In general, the baby is picked up with a mobile intensive care unit. Care and transport of the baby can only be adequately prepared for if qualified information has been provided or initial therapeutic measures suggested. During the transport skin color, respiration and motor function must be under continuous observation (switch on full lighting in the ambulance). Heart rate, temperature, oxygen saturation (pulse oximeter) in addition to O_2 concentration and inspirational pressure of the ventilator must be mechanically monitored and continuously displayed. The transport should be performed calmly and rapidly, without unnecessary stops and vibrations. If procedures need to be performed on the baby (e.g., suctioning) the vehicle should be stopped. Good cooperation with the regional ambulance services is essential for successful intensive care transport.

Advantages of maternal as opposed to neonatal transport:
- Increased survival rate of babies.
- Reduced incidence of intracranial hemorrhage.
- Reduced rate of permanent disability.
- Shorter hospital stays.
- Separation of mother and baby is avoided.
- Organization is simpler and faster.
- Lower costs (for transport and subsequently).

The chances for at-risk neonates are reduced by the postnatal transport. For this reason, women with high-risk fetuses belong in a hospital which has the resources (both equipment and staff-wise) to manage the birth and ensure adequate newborn care.

References

Avery GB, Fletcher MA, Macdonald MG: Neonatology. Pathophysiology and management of the newborn, 6th edn. Lippincott, Philadelphia 2005

Benirschke K, Kaufmann P, Baergen RN: Pathology of the human placenta. 5th edn. Springer, New York, Berlin, Heidelberg 2006

Briggs GG, Freeman RK, Yaffe SJ: Drugs in pregnancy and lactation. A reference guide to fetal and neonatal risk. 8th edn. Williams & Wilkins, Baltimore 2008

Garson A: The science and practice of pediatríc cardiology. 3rd edn. Williams & Wilkins, Baltimore 2005

Jones KL: Smith's recognizable patterns of human malformation, 6th edn. Saunders, Philadelphia 2005

Karotkin EH, Goldsmith JP: Assisted ventilation of the neonate, 4th edn. Saunders, Philadelphia 2003

MacDonald MG, Ramasethu J: Atlas of procedures in neonatology, 4th edn. Lippincott, Philadelphia 2007

Martin RJ, Fanaroff AA, Walsh MC: Neonatal-perinatal medicine. Diseases of the fetus and infant, 9th edn. Mosby, St. Louis 2010,

Milunski A, Milunski J: Genetic disorders and the fetus: Diagnosis, prevention and treatment. 6th edn. Wiley Blackwell, Oxford 2010

Munoz R, Morell V, da Cruz EM, Vetterly CG: Critical care of children with heart diseases. Springer, New York, Heidelberg 2009

Orkin SH, Nathan DG, Ginsburg D, Look AT: Nathan and Oski´s hematology of infancy and childhood. 7th edn. Saunders, Philadelphia 2009

Polin RA, Polin WW, Fox WW: Fetal and neonatal physiology. 4th edn. Saunders, Philadelphia 2011

Remington JS, Klein JA: Infectious diseases of the fetus and newborn infant, 6th edn. Saunders, Philadelphia 2006

Renníe J, Roberton NRC: Roberton´s textbook of neonatology, 4th edn. Churchill, Livingstone 2005

Royal College of Obstetricians and Gynecologists: Bacterial sepsis following pregnancy. Green-top Guideline No. 64b, April 2012

Scriver CR, Beaudet AL, Sly WS: The metabolic and molecular: basis of inherited disease. 8th edn. McGraw-Hill, New York 2001

Taeusch HW, Ballard RA, Gleason, CA, Avery ME: Diseases of the newbom, 8th edn. Saunders, Philadelphia 2005

The Cochrane Library of Systematic Reviews. www.cochrane.org/reviews, accessed 12.12.2010

Volpe JJ: Neurology of the newborn, 5th edn. Saunders, Philadelphia 2008

Yaffe SJ, Aranda JV: Neonatal and pediatric pharmacology: Therapeutic principles in practice. 4th edn. Lippincott Williams & Wilkins, Baltimore 2010

Index

Printed and bound by CPI Group (UK) Ltd, Croydon, CR0 4YY
22/03/2026
02075961-0001